ATLAS OF EQUINE ULTRASONOGRAPHY

DEDICATION

Jessica A. Kidd:

In memory of Professor Jack Fessler: my mentor from veterinary school to this day.

In appreciation and admiration of Professor Derek Knottenbelt: a true friend who provides boundless support and encouragement.

With love and thanks to my family, especially my husband Sam Millar: their ongoing support made the book a reality.

And finally, in memory of my father John Kidd: a true Renaissance man.

Kristina G. Lu:

To Carlin and Harper and to our endeavor to conquer life's challenges.

Michele L. Frazer:

To Oliver, Richard, Leah, and Gabrielle for their love and encouragement in this and all life's adventures.

To my mother, Betty, for her support through the years and, of course, for tolerating all my dogs.

To Lee for all those trips to Auburn.

ATLAS OF EQUINE ULTRASONOGRAPHY

Edited by

Jessica A. Kidd, BA, DVM, CertES(Orth), Diplomate
ECVS, MRCVS
Oxfordshire, UK

Kristina G. Lu, VMD, Diplomate ACT
Hagyard Equine Medical Institute, Lexington, KY, USA

Michele L. Frazer, DVM, Diplomate ACVIM, ACVECC
Hagyard Equine Medical Institute, Lexington, KY, USA

WILEY Blackwell

Library of Congress Cataloging-in-Publication Data
Atlas of equine ultrasonography / edited by Jessica Kidd, Kristina G. Lu, Michele L. Frazer.
      p. ; cm.
   Includes bibliographical references and index.
   ISBN 978-0-470-65813-0 (cloth)
   I. Kidd, Jessica, editor of compilation.   II. Lu, Kristina G., editor of compilation.   III. Frazer, Michele L., editor of compilation.
   [DNLM: 1. Horse Diseases–Atlases.   2. Ultrasonography–veterinary–Atlases.   SF 951]
   SF951
   636.1'089607543–dc23
                              2014000059

A catalogue record for this book is available from the British Library.

Wiley also publishes its books in a variety of electronic formats. Some content that appears in print may not be available in electronic books.

Cover image: Horse sketch: Reproduced with permission of Dr Jessica A. Kidd. Drawing by Serena Vignolini, www.serenavignolini.com. Ultrasound images from top to bottom courtesy of Stefania Bucca, Colin C. Schwarzwald, Fairfield T. Bain, Marcus Head and Roger K.W. Smith.
Cover design by Andrew Magee Design Ltd

Set in 10/12.5 pt Palatino LT Std by Toppan Best-set Premedia Limited
Printed and bound in Malaysia by Vivar Printing Sdn Bhd

3   2015

CONTENTS

Section 3b: Ultrasonography of the Abdominal Cavity

Section 3c: Ultrasonography of Small Structures

LIST OF CONTRIBUTORS

Debra Archer, BVMS, PhD, CertES(soft tissue),
    Diplomate ECVS, MRCVS
Professor of Equine Surgery
Philip Leverhulme Equine Hospital
University of Liverpool
Wirral, UK

Fairfield T. Bain, DVM, MBA, Diplomate: ACVIM,
    ACVP, ACVECC
Clinical Professor of Equine Internal Medicine
Department of Veterinary Clinical Sciences
College of Veterinary Medicine
Washington State University
Pullman, WA, USA

Sarah Boys Smith, MA, VetMB, CertES(Orth),
    Diplomate ECVS, MRCVS, RCVS Specialist in
    Equine Surgery
Senior Orthopaedic Clinician
Rossdales Equine Hospital and Diagnostic Centre
Newmarket, UK

Stefania Bucca, DVM
Associate Veterinarian
Qatar Racing and Equestrian Club
Doha, Qatar

Ann Carstens, BVSc, MS, MMedVet(large animal
    surgery), Diploma in Tertiary Education,
    MMedVet(diagnostic imaging), Diplomate ECVDI,
    PhD
Associate Professor Diagnostic Imaging
Faculty of Veterinary Science
University of Pretoria
Onderstepoort, South Africa

Eddy R.J. Cauvin, DVM, PhD, HDR, Diplomate
    ECVS, Associate member ECVDI
Partner
AZURVET Referral Veterinary Centre
Cagnes sur Mer, France

Michele L. Frazer, DVM, Diplomate ACVIM,
    ACVECC
Associate Veterinarian
Hagyard Equine Medical Institute
Lexington, KY, USA

Katherine S. Garrett, DVM, Diplomate ACVS
Director of Diagnostic Imaging
Rood and Riddle Equine Hospital
Lexington, KY, USA

Marcus Head, BVetMed, MRCVS
Senior Associate
Rossdales Equine Hospital and Diagnostic Centre
Newmarket, UK

Richard Holder, DVM
Senior Partner
Hagyard Equine Medical Institute
Lexington, KY, USA

Jessica A. Kidd, BA, DVM, CertES(Orth), Diplomate
    ECVS, MRCVS
RCVS and European Recognised Specialist in Equine
    Surgery
Surgeon
Oxfordshire, UK

Charles Love, DVM, Diplomate ACT
Associate Professor of Theriogenology
Texas A&M University College of Veterinary
    Medicine
College Station, TX, USA

Kristina Lu, VMD, Diplomate ACT
Theriogenologist
Hagyard Equine Medical Institute
Lexington, KY, USA

Massimo Magri, DVM
Practice Owner
Clinica Veterinaria Spirano
Spirano (BG), Italy

Peter R. Morresey, BVSc, MACVSc, Diplomate ACT,
    Diplomate ACVIM (Large Animal)
Internal Medicine Clinician
Rood and Riddle Equine Hospital
Lexington, KY, USA

Kimberly Palgrave, BS, BVM&S, GPCert(DI), MRCVS
Associate Veterinarian
Overland Animal Hospital
Denver, CO, USA

Caryn E. Plummer, DVM, Diplomate ACVO
Assistant Professor and Service Chief,
    Comparative Ophthalmology
Department of Small Animal Clinical Sciences
College of Veterinary Medicine
University of Florida
Gainesville, FL, USA

Malgorzata A. Pozor, DVM, PhD, Diplomate ACT
Clinical Assistant Professor
Department of Large Animal Clinical Sciences
College of Veterinary Medicine
University of Florida
Gainesville, FL, USA

Jonathan F. Pycock, BVetMed, PhD, DESM MRCVS,
    RCVS Specialist in Equine Reproduction
Clinical Director
Equine Reproductive Services
Ryton, UK

David J. Reese, DVM, Diplomate ACVR
Senior Lecturer, Diagnostic Imaging (Head of
    Section)
College of Veterinary Medicine
Murdoch University
Murdoch, WA, Australia

Barbara Riccio, DVM, PhD
Associate Veterinarian
Studio Veterinario Associato Cascina Gufa
Merlino (LO), Italy

Colin C. Schwarzwald, Dr. med. vet., PhD,
    Diplomate ACVIM & ECEIM
Director, Clinic for Equine Internal Medicine
Equine Department
University of Zurich
Zurich, Switzerland

Christine Schweizer, DVM, Diplomate ACT
Reproductive Specialist
Early Winter Equine PLLC
Lansing, NY, USA

Nathan Slovis, DVM, Diplomate ACVIM, CHT
Director, McGee Medical and Critical Care Center
Hagyard Equine Medical Institute
Lexington, KY, USA

Roger K.W. Smith, MA, VetMB, PhD, FHEA, DEO,
    Associate member ECVDI, Diplomate ECVS,
    MRCVS
Professor of Equine Orthopaedics
The Royal Veterinary College
North Mymms, Hatfield, UK

Walter Zent, DVM, Diplomate ACT (Hon)
Senior Partner
Hagyard Equine Medical Institute
Lexington, KY, USA

ABOUT THE COMPANION WEBSITE

This book is accompanied by a companion website:

www.wiley.com/go/kidd/equine-ultrasonography

The website includes:

- 54 videos referenced in the text.
- Videos 1–53 were compiled by Sarah Boys Smith and relate to Section 1 of the book, on musculoskeletal regions.
- Video 54 relates to chapter 17 of the book.
- A Powerpoint file showing recommended order of scanning for the stallion internal reproductive tract.

INTRODUCTION

Kimberly Palgrave[1] and Jessica A. Kidd[2]

[1]Overland Animal Hospital, Denver, CO, USA; [2]Oxfordshire, UK

Welcome to the first edition of the Atlas of Equine Ultrasonography.

The field of veterinary ultrasonography has blossomed in the last 30 years and the improvements in technology since its first use have been exponential. It is also now being used on structures and body systems that were not previously thought to be conducive to ultrasonography. Many vets in equine practice now have access to an ultrasound machine and, along with radiography, ultrasonography has become a mainstay of equine diagnostic imaging. It has the advantages of being non-invasive and complementary to radiography. The purpose of this book is to encourage further use of ultrasonography in clinical case management and expansion of the techniques utilized by vets in both general practice and at the referral level.

Ultrasonography is an excellent diagnostic tool which has many applications in veterinary practice. When considered in conjunction with relevant clinical information, such as patient history and physical examination findings, it can be an extremely useful aid in the clinical decision-making process. Developing the skills necessary to confidently acquire and interpret ultrasound images requires knowledge of normal equine anatomy and an understanding of the mechanisms displayed by individual body systems when reacting to various disease processes. We hope this book will help achieve this. A general appreciation of the physics of ultrasound is also necessary as this enables the ultrasonographer to optimize the diagnostic quality of ultrasound images obtained by appropriately altering their technique and machine settings. The aim of this introductory chapter is to provide an overview of ultrasound technology and the fundamental principles of image evaluation with a focus on the applications of ultrasound within equine practice.

HOW TO USE THIS BOOK

The book is divided into three main sections: musculoskeletal, reproduction, and internal medicine. Each section is then further subdivided into chapters by anatomical region. Within each chapter is information on scanning technique for that area, a review of the normal anatomy and discussion of some of the more common ultrasonographic abnormalities. This is then followed by images that demonstrate normal and abnormal findings. The end of each chapter lists Recommended Reading for more extensive references relating to the chapter topics.

PHYSICS OF ULTRASOUND

Ultrasound physics is a vast and theoretically complex subject; however, a thorough understanding of this topic is not required for performing and utilizing diagnostic ultrasonography effectively in the clinical environment. Therefore, this text will cover the aspects of ultrasound physics that directly relate to the interaction of ultrasound waves with tissue and how these interactions translate to the displayed image. Additional sources covering this subject matter in greater detail are listed at the end of this chapter under Recommended Reading.

Features of Ultrasound Waves

Ultrasound waves have features in common with audible sound waves although they are of a higher frequency than audible sound and cannot be heard by the human ear; hence the term *ultrasound*. They are both created through the vibration of an object resulting in movement of surrounding molecules.

Ultrasound waves are produced through the application of an electric current to piezoelectric crystals within the transducer (probe), causing the crystals to vibrate. This vibration is transmitted through the surrounding tissues in the form of sound waves. These waves interact with the tissues along their path of travel in various ways which may result in *attenuation* of the ultrasound beam.

Attenuation is defined as the progressive weakening in intensity of the ultrasound wave as it is transmitted through body tissues. Sound waves passing through tissues can either be *reflected*, *refracted*, *scattered* or *absorbed*. These are the primary causes of attenuation of the ultrasound wave and these phenomena are ultimately responsible for the formation of an ultrasound image.

Reflection and Acoustic Impedance

As ultrasound waves travel through the body, they come into contact with structures which reflect a proportion of the waves directly back towards the piezoelectric crystals, while the remainder of the waves continue to travel deeper into the tissues. The force of the returning waves or echoes results in vibration of the crystals and this vibration is then translated into an electrical signal, which is used to create the image displayed on the screen. Therefore, a unique feature of piezoelectric crystals is that they are capable of both emitting and receiving ultrasound waves.

It is important to realize that an ultrasound image is only produced when ultrasound waves are *reflected* back to the transducer. *Reflection* occurs when an ultrasound wave reaches an interface between two tissues as it is transmitted through the body and a portion of that wave is returned or "bounced back" to the probe while the remainder of the wave continues to travel deeper into the body. The strength of the returning wave and the length of time taken for that wave to travel through the tissues before returning to the probe is recognized and processed by the ultrasound machine in order to create the ultrasound image. These concepts will be later explored in the B-Mode and Echogenicity section.

The proportion of the emitted wave that is reflected back to the probe depends on the acoustic impedance of the interface between tissues and the angle at which the ultrasound wave strikes the interface. The acoustic impedance of a tissue is a product of the density of that tissue and the speed at which sounds waves travel through it. A dense tissue, such as bone, has a high acoustic impedance (7.8) compared to the relatively low acoustic impedance of air (0.0004), with soft tissues

Table I.1

Approximate acoustic impedance in commonly encountered tissues. (Source: Adapted from Curry, TS III *et al.*, 1990. Reproduced with permission of Lippincott Williams & Wilkins.)

Tissue	Acoustic impedance (in 10^6 Rayls)
Air	0.0004
Fat	1.38
Water (50°C)	1.54
Brain	1.58
Blood	1.61
Kidney	1.62
Liver	1.65
Muscle	1.70
Lens of eye	1.84
Bone (skull)	7.80

being in between (kidney – 1.62) (see Table I.1). However, it is the difference in acoustic impedance between tissue types that determines the reflective nature of a given tissue interface, not the acoustic impedance of a single tissue in isolation. For example, both a bone–soft tissue interface and an air–soft tissue interface have significant differences between the acoustic impedance values of the tissues at that interface, despite the fact that bone and air are at opposite ends of the acoustic impedance spectrum. Therefore, both bone–soft tissue and air–soft tissue interfaces are highly reflective, with the majority of the ultrasound waves being reflected back to the transducer in both scenarios. This also results in very little of the ultrasound wave remaining to penetrate into the deeper tissues beyond this highly reflective interface. By comparison, soft tissue–soft tissue interfaces (either between or within soft tissue structures) are less reflective due to the small differences between the acoustic impedances of these tissue types. Understanding this physical property of ultrasound wave propagation is essential to understanding how tissue variations translate into the ultrasound image appearance. This also justifies the need for appropriate patient preparation, including clipping of the haircoat where possible and application of ultrasound coupling gel to minimize the amount of air at the probe–skin interface. Differences in acoustic impedance also contribute to artifact formation, which will be discussed later in the chapter.

The angle at which the ultrasound beam strikes the tissues is also integral to the degree of *reflection* of the ultrasound wave. Only ultrasound waves striking an interface which is perpendicular to the direction in which the wave is travelling will result in reflection of the wave directly back to the probe. If the wave reaches the tissue interface at an angle, the waves will be reflected into adjacent tissues instead of back to the probe, resulting in a lack of direct information from that area of the body. Therefore, the true reflective nature of that particular tissue will not be accurately represented in the displayed ultrasound image. In practical terms, imaging a structure when the ultrasound beam is not directed perpendicular to the region of interest may result in a smaller proportion of the wave being reflected to the probe and the resulting ultrasound appearance of that structure may appear "patchy" or irregular, although this effect can be used to the ultrasonographer's advantage, by allowing the margins of structures to be more easily recognized, for example.

Refraction, Scatter, and Absorption

In addition to reflection, other types of interaction between the ultrasound beam and tissues include *refraction*, *scatter*, and *absorption*. If an ultrasound wave reaches an interface between tissues of different acoustic impedances at an angle other than perpendicular, the beam will change direction while continuing to travel deeper within the tissues before ultimately being reflected back to the probe. This phenomenon, known as *refraction*, is commonly observed in association with curved structures (e.g. endometrial cysts, embryonic vesicles) and will be covered in the section Ultrasound Artifacts.

The appearance of parenchymatous organs on ultrasound examination is primarily attributable to *scatter* of the ultrasound waves. Scatter occurs when the beam encounters small, irregular interfaces with minimal differences in acoustic impedance within an organ, as is present within the liver. The result of this interaction is the *scattering* of waves throughout the tissues in all directions instead of direct reflection back to the transducer. The strength of individual reflected echoes from these interfaces is relatively weak, compared to the strength of echoes being returned to the transducer from highly reflective interfaces, such as bone–soft tissue (e.g. interface between suspensory ligament–metacarpal III). However due to their abundant numbers, scattered waves contribute significantly to image formation of more homogeneous tissues, such as the spleen.

Absorption is the only interaction between the ultrasound beam and tissues which directly results in a reduction in the energy of the waves. This form of attenuation occurs when the mechanical energy of the ultrasound wave is converted to heat which is then contained in the tissues. The heat generated within

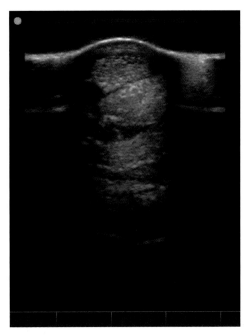

Figure I.1 B-mode, cross-sectional image of the soft tissue structures on the palmar aspect of the equine distal limb.

tissues from the use of diagnostic ultrasound is generally considered to be negligible.

B-Mode and Echogenicity

The production of an ultrasound image relies on information detailing the nature and location of structures within the region of interest being relayed effectively to the ultrasound machine. In real-time B-mode (*brightness* mode) imaging (Figure I.1), the strength of the signal received by the crystals within the probe correlates to the strength (amplitude) of ultrasound waves returning to the probe. These echoes are represented on the ultrasound screen by a series of dots on a black background. The brightness of each dot is determined by the strength of the returning echo that it represents. In practical terms, a strong returning echo will appear *brighter* (more white) while a weaker echo appears *darker* (grey or black).

The terminology used when describing the ultrasonographic appearance of various tissues is referred to as the *echogenicity* of that tissue. Structures which do not reflect ultrasound waves appear black on the ultrasound image and are termed anechoic. Fluid-filled structures, such as ovarian follicles and the vitreous chamber of the eye, are considered to be anechoic (Figure I.2).

The echogenicity of other tissues types must be considered in relation to one another. When comparing

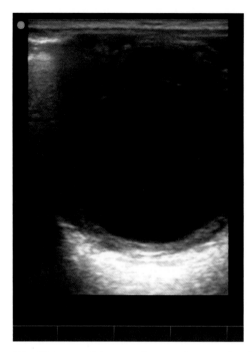

Figure I.2   Ultrasound image of an equine ovarian follicle containing anechoic fluid.

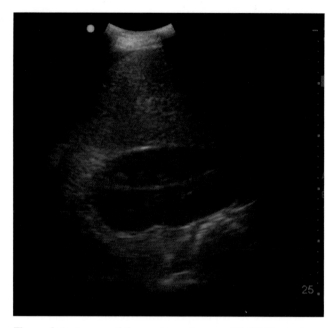

Figure I.3   Image of the equine spleen and left kidney demonstrating the mixed echogenic appearance of soft tissue structures; the spleen in this image is hyperechoic compared to the kidney.

two tissues in an ultrasound image, the darker structure is referred to as being more hypoechoic while the brighter structure is termed hyperechoic. Soft tissue structures within the body may exhibit varying echogenicities (Figure I.3), while the typical appearance of both a bone–soft tissue interface (e.g. region of the suspensory ligament and metacarpal III) and an air–soft tissue interface (e.g. parietal pleura and air-filled lung) is strongly hyperechoic (a bright-white line) (Figure I.4). If two tissues are represented by the same level of brightness in the ultrasound image, they are deemed to be isoechoic to one another.

The location (i.e. depth) of a reflective tissue interface is determined by the length of time taken for the ultrasound wave to be emitted by the crystals within the probe, travel through tissues to the reflective structure, and finally be transmitted back to the probe. An ultrasound wave which takes longer to be reflected back and received by the crystals within the probe will be represented on the ultrasound image as a dot located farther away from the transducer. This signifies a reflective structure positioned at a greater depth within the tissues.

M-Mode

M-mode imaging displays the movement of structures along a narrow, user-defined region of the ultrasound

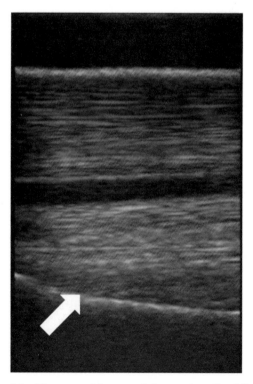

Figure I.4   Ultrasound image of the equine distal limb in the longitudinal plane demonstrating the appearance of the interface between the suspensory ligament and metacarpal III (bone–soft tissue interface) as a hyperechoic line (arrow).

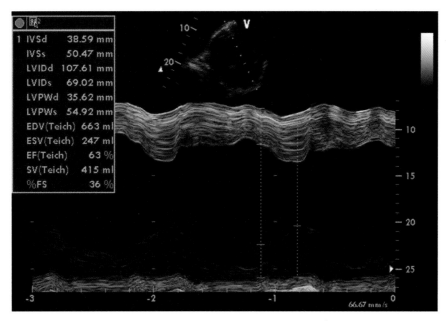

Figure I.5 M-mode image of the region of the equine mitral valve.

image in relation to time. A common example is cardiac ultrasonography. First, an optimal B-mode image is obtained and M-mode imaging is then selected. A linear cursor is displayed which originates from the midpoint of the transducer contact area and runs through the superficial structures into the deeper tissues. Depending on the type of ultrasound machine in use, the user will have a varying ability to position this cursor in the ideal location. M-mode imaging is activated and the movement of tissues along the cursor line is displayed as a function of time, with the horizontal axis representing time and the vertical axis representing tissue depth. As in B-mode imaging, the brightness of the displayed image correlates to the strength (amplitude) of returning echoes (Figure I.5). M-mode imaging enables the ultrasonographer to evaluate the relative movement of structures in a particular region of interest over time and perform relevant measurements/calculations relating to changes in dimensions of those structures. This imaging mode is particularly useful for cardiac applications, such as evaluating relative changes in chamber sizes throughout the cardiac cycle.

ULTRASOUND MACHINE

Console

The ultrasound machine setup includes the console and the transducer. Both are essential to the produc-

tion of a quality diagnostic ultrasound image. The console is responsible for activating the piezoelectric crystals within the transducer, functioning as the processing center for all information received by the crystals, providing the user with various controls necessary for optimizing the quality of the ultrasound image, and housing the screen which displays the final ultrasound image. Depending on the type of ultrasound machine being used, the console also provides the user with various image manipulation, storage, and file transfer options.

Transducer Frequency and Image Resolution

The primary function of the ultrasound transducer (probe) is to house the piezoelectric crystals which emit and receive ultrasound waves used in the production of a diagnostic image. The differences in transducer shape, size, and frequency options reflect the wide variety of ultrasound applications within equine practice and the requirement for specific probes which are most appropriate for particular uses (see Types of Transducer).

The ability to emit ultrasound waves of varying frequencies is a feature which will greatly enhance the versatility of an ultrasound probe. Frequency is defined as the number of times a wave repeats over a given time period (cycles per second). As previously described, ultrasound waves are similar to audible sound waves; however the frequency range of diagnostic ultrasound is much higher than that of audible sound. Diagnostic ultrasonography commonly utilizes frequencies in the range of 1–20 MHz compared to a range of 20–20 000 Hz for audible sound. The frequency of ultrasound waves passing through tissues has a significant impact on the quality of the ultrasound image produced. In particular, the resolution of a diagnostic image can be greatly enhanced through the use of an appropriate transducer frequency setting. This is largely due to the fact that as frequency increases, wavelength (the distance that a wave travels during a single cycle) decreases and the interaction of tissues with ultrasound waves of shorter wavelengths results in better ultrasound image resolution, although at the expense of depth of tissue penetration.

Image resolution can be defined as the ability of the ultrasound wave to distinguish between two separate structures within the tissues. In practical terms, resolution relates to the clarity of the ultrasound image displayed. *Axial resolution* concerns structures which are parallel to the direction of the beam (along the path of travel), while *lateral resolution* relates to structures which are oriented perpendicular to the direction of the beam (Figure I.6). Lateral resolution is primarily a function of ultrasound beam width while axial resolution is related to the ultrasound pulse length (wavelength multiplied by the number of cycles per pulse). Both axial and lateral resolutions are improved by the use of a higher-frequency ultrasound beam, however

increasing the frequency setting improves axial resolution to a greater degree.

When compared to lower-frequency waves travelling to the same depth within the tissues, higher-frequency ultrasound waves will interact with more structures along their path of travel. As ultrasound waves are physical pressure waves, they are attenuated by interactions with tissues and lose strength as a result of these interactions. In practical terms, ultrasound waves are stronger when they initially leave the transducer and arrive at superficial structures compared to when they have travelled deeper within the body tissues. Therefore, a balance must always be struck between image resolution and the ability of an ultrasound wave to penetrate to the required depth of tissue. In summary, a higher frequency setting will result in production of an image with better resolution but decreased ability to penetrate to the deeper structures. A lower frequency setting will enable the ultrasound wave to penetrate deeper into the tissues, however image resolution will be diminished.

Types of Transducer

There are two broad categories of ultrasound transducer – mechanical and electronic. Mechanical probes are characterized by the presence of single or multiple piezoelectric crystals mounted within the probe head. The crystal apparatus oscillates or rotates within the probe while the external housing of the transducer

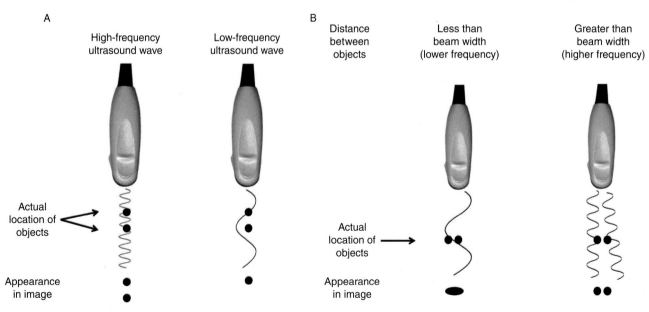

Figure I.6 Illustration of the relationship between frequency and image resolution: (A) axial resolution, (B) lateral resolution.

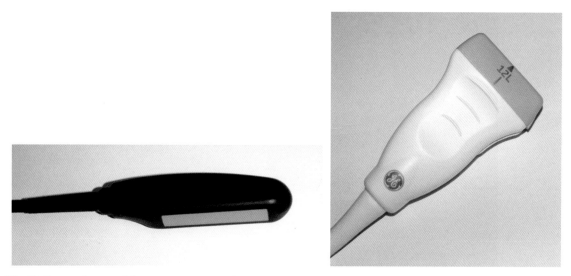

Figure I.7 Different forms of linear transducers for use in equine ultrasonography (rectal probe – left; musculoskeletal "tendon" probe – right).

remains stationary. Mechanical probes have been largely superseded by electronic (array) transducers, as these probes do not have moving parts that are liable to fatigue and wear over time.

Electronic transducers have several stationary crystal elements arranged within the probe head. These crystals are electronically stimulated to vibrate in particular sequences to create waves for specific types of ultrasound examinations. Several types of electronic transducers are manufactured, however the most common types found within equine practice are linear (rectal and musculoskeletal), convex, and phased-array.

Linear probes are most commonly used for evaluating the equine distal limb. They are also used for performing *per rectum* examination of the reproductive tract of the mare (Figure I.7). The crystal elements in linear probes are arranged along the scanning surface ("footprint") of the probe and these crystals are stimulated sequentially to emit ultrasound waves. This results in the formation of a rectangular ultrasound image. Linear probes usually emit ultrasound waves of higher frequency (7–13 MHz) and therefore provide images with enhanced resolution of superficial structures. However, they do not provide appropriate penetration for the evaluation of deeper structures.

Curvilinear transducers are similar to linear probes, however due to the crystal arrangement along a curved probe head, the resultant ultrasound image is sector ("pie")/wedge shaped. These probes are often referred to as convex or micro-convex, depending on the size and frequency range (typically 2–5 MHz for convex and 4–10 MHz for micro-convex) of the individual transducer (Figure I.8). Convex probes are primarily used for abdominal imaging and for scanning the sacroiliac and stifle regions in the horse. Micro-convex probes may be used in ocular ultrasonography.

Phased-array probes are designed almost exclusively for use in cardiac ultrasound applications with a typical frequency range of 1–5 MHz. The crystals are stimulated nearly simultaneously (<1 μsec intervals), resulting in the formation of a sector-shaped image which is updated more rapidly compared to those from curvilinear or linear probes. This is particularly useful when evaluating more rapidly moving structures, such as the myocardium. Phased-array probes generally have a smaller "footprint" which enables the ultrasonographer to access the intercostal space more readily when performing an echocardiographic examination (Figure I.9).

A *standoff* is frequently used when imaging superficial structures to minimize the appearance of reverberation artifacts in the region of interest (see Reverberation Artifacts). Commercially manufactured standoffs are available from various suppliers. These standoffs should be flexible to enable them to conform to the shape of the limb as well as the probe (generally manufactured for use with linear array transducers – either rectal or musculoskeletal configurations) (Figure I.10), have an acoustic impedance similar to that of soft tissue, be comfortable to use when scanning, and easy to clean.

Ultrasound Machine Controls and Image Optimization

The ability of the ultrasonographer to optimize the quality of the displayed ultrasound image relies on

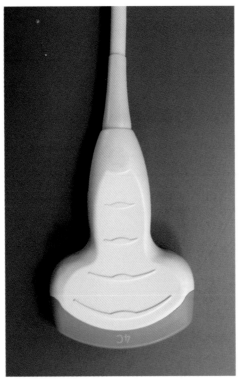
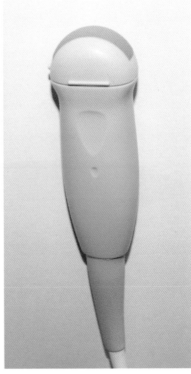

Figure I.8   Convex (left) and micro-convex (right) transducers.

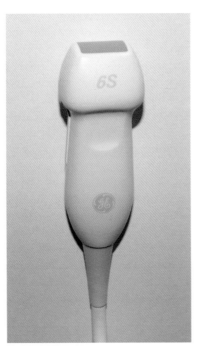

Figure I.9   Phased-array transducer.

several factors including adequate patient preparation and appropriate adjustment of the machine controls/ settings. The degree to which the ultrasonographer can alter the ultrasound wave characteristics and manipulate the image displayed is specific to each ultrasound manufacturer and model of machine. However, the fundamental controls used to optimize image quality are generally common to the vast majority of machines used throughout equine practice.

Machine Presets

Ultrasound machine presets enable the user to define a set of machine parameters which are generally suited to a specific type of ultrasound examination (e.g. abdominal, musculoskeletal, reproduction). Parameters that can be set within each preset include, but are not limited to, transducer frequency, gain, time gain compensation, and depth. The use of user-defined presets provides the ultrasonographer with an acceptable "starting point" for machine settings, so that only minor adjustments to the controls are required to optimize the appearance of the ultrasound image for individual patients.

Frequency

As previously stated, altering the frequency of the ultrasound waves produced by the transducer has a significant impact on image resolution. Therefore, choosing the correct frequency setting on a multi-frequency probe (mechanical or electronic) or selecting the most appropriate probe for a specific type of

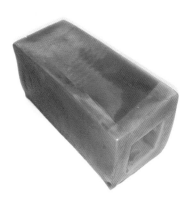
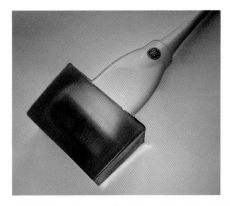

Figure I.10 Standoff for linear transducers: rectal (left) and musculoskeletal "tendon" (right).

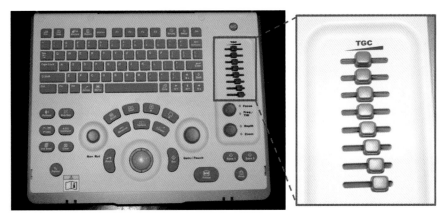

Figure I.11 Time–gain compensation control on an ultrasound console (red box).

examination (if single frequency probes are used) is essential for optimizing image quality. In general, it is recommended to use the highest frequency setting available to enhance image resolution, but which retains sufficient ability to penetrate to the required depth for the region of interest.

Gain

The purpose of the gain control is to increase or decrease the brightness of the image displayed through uniform, non-selective amplification or reduction of all echoes returning to the transducer. Altering the gain control has a more profound effect on the diagnostic quality of the image than simply adjusting the brightness of the console monitor. Increasing the overall gain setting will result in the strength of all returning waves being amplified. Although the appropriate level of image brightness is subjective and based on user preference, it is important that the gain control is not set too high as this will result in over-amplification of weaker echoes, and tissue contrast and resolution will

be compromised. Conversely, using a gain control setting that is too low may result in the loss of subtle tissue detail, as weaker echoes are not translated into the displayed image.

Time–Gain Compensation

Due to the physical properties of ultrasound waves, their interactions with tissues along the path of travel results in attenuation of those waves at increasing tissue depths. Stated another way, as sound waves travel through the tissues they lose strength and therefore echoes returning to the probe from greater depths will be weaker. If not compensated for, this results in an ultrasound image in which superficial structures nearer to the transducer appear brighter (*near-field*), whereas deeper structures farther from the probe (*far-field*) appear darker. The time–gain compensation (TGC) control enables the user to correct for this phenomenon by selectively amplifying returning echoes depending on their depth within the tissues, to create an image of uniform brightness (Figure I.11).

Depth

The region of interest should ideally occupy three-quarters of the displayed image. Altering the depth to the appropriate level for the structures being evaluated will also allow the user to make adjustments to the frequency settings to optimize image quality. For example, when imaging the equine distal limb, decreasing the depth such that the third metacarpal bone forms the far-field boundary of the image (approximately 4–6 cm depth depending on patient conformation) will enable a higher-frequency transducer setting to be used as increased penetration ability of the ultrasound waves is not required. This will optimize the quality of the ultrasound image displayed by enhancing image resolution.

Focus

As a conventional, unfocused ultrasound beam leaves the transducer and enters the tissues, it naturally begins to diverge/widen as it travels deeper within the tissues. This results in decreased resolution of structures in the far-field as beam width has a significant impact on lateral resolution. Focusing the ultrasound beam acts to narrow the beam width at a particular location along its length (the *focal zone*), resulting in improved resolution of the structures in the focused region (Figure I.12). Depending on machine capabilities, single or multiple focal zones can be selected and placed at specific intervals along the length of the ultrasound beam to correspond to the regions of interest within the ultrasound image. However, selecting multiple focal zones can result in

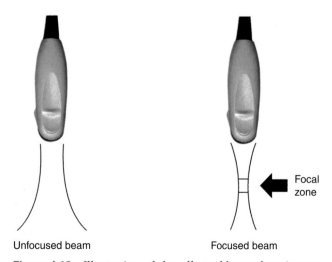

Unfocused beam   Focused beam

Figure I.12 Illustration of the effect of beam focusing on beam width.

a decrease in frame rate and may therefore limit the ability to effectively image rapidly moving structures (e.g. fetal heartbeat).

Frame Rate

The frame rate of an image is the number of ultrasound images displayed per second. Essentially, it is how quickly the image is updated. With respect to array transducers, a single ultrasound beam, which is created by stimulation of an individual crystal element within the probe, must be emitted, travel through the tissues, and be reflected back to the probe prior to the next crystal element in the sequence being activated. Therefore, echoes travelling deeper within the tissues will take longer to return to the probe and the sequential stimulation of the crystal elements within the probe is delayed. Therefore the frame rate decreases as the image depth increases and the length of the transducer surface or "footprint" increases. Higher frame rates are required to perform meaningful imaging studies of more rapidly moving structures, such as the heart.

Tissue Harmonic Imaging

Tissue harmonic imaging (THI) is an ultrasonographic technique utilizing the concept of harmonic frequencies to optimize both image resolution and penetration ability of the ultrasound beam. As described earlier in this chapter, conventional ultrasound imaging utilizes portions of the primary ultrasound beam which have been reflected back to the transducer to create the displayed image – the so-called *fundamental frequencies*. Throughout this process, additional waves are also being created which are returned to the probe alongside the fundamental frequency waves. These are referred to as *harmonic waves*. In conventional B-mode imaging, these harmonic waves are ignored and only the reflections from the primary beam are utilized for image formation.

By comparison, THI ignores the fundamental frequency waves so that only the harmonic waves are used to create the ultrasound image. Compared to the fundamental beam, harmonic waves are of a higher frequency but lower intensity. Intensity of the ultrasound wave is defined as the rate at which energy from the ultrasound wave is transferred to surrounding structures in a specific area. Therefore THI uses various signal-processing techniques to filter out echoes resulting from reflection of the primary ultrasound beam. In other words, THI emits a lower-frequency wave from the transducer but only "listens" to the higher-frequency waves returning to the probe to form the ultrasound image. The purpose of this is to provide the improved resolution and image quality achieved when higher-frequency ultrasound waves are used while overcoming the limitation of decreased penetration at increasing depth (attenuation) which is also associated with the use of higher wave frequencies. Benefits of THI include increased resolution, as the harmonic frequency beam is also narrower than the fundamental beam, and a decrease in some artifacts.

ULTRASOUND MACHINE AND TRANSDUCER SELECTION

There are various manufacturers and suppliers of ultrasound equipment for use in equine veterinary practice. The following are a few points which should be considered when acquiring new equipment, and personal requirements should be discussed with the supplier who can assist the user in selecting the most appropriate machine,

1. Who will be using the equipment? Is the machine in use for an equine-only or a mixed practice? What is the user experience level? Will the machine be used for ambulatory work (i.e. a portable machine is needed) or will the machine be used in a practice setting where portability may be less of a requirement?
2. What types of ultrasound examination are to be performed? Will they be predominantly musculoskeletal, or will they be reproductive, abdominal, cardiac/thoracic, or ophthalmic? This will determine the number and types of transducers required.
3. How many scans are to be performed on a weekly or monthly basis?
4. What is the available budget? This should include purchase of the equipment and any maintenance/ service fees.
5. What equipment features are required? Is a new machine necessary or is a refurbished machine suitable? Does the machine require color/Doppler capability? Is a human machine acceptable or is there need for veterinary specific software/presets and hardware? What image-storage capability is required (internal memory, storage to USB, printing of individual images, ability to network with practice management software/connect to PACS)?
6. What post-purchase support is provided by the manufacturer/supplier? This is extremely important for support after the initial purchase and should be taken into consideration – warranties, breakdown support/equipment repair, maintenance/ scheduled service costs, product training, clinical training, and provision of a loan machine while any servicing is performed.

PATIENT PREPARATION

Along with operator skill and the type of ultrasound equipment used for scanning, appropriate attention to patient preparation plays a key role in obtaining ultrasound images of diagnostic quality. Good preparation of the patient will greatly improve the images obtained. It is important that the patient be adequately restrained on a non-slip surface for the duration of the ultrasound examination, either by physical means (i.e. purpose-built stocks, assistant using a well fitting headcollar or bridle, use of restraint aids such as a twitch) and/or through the use of chemical restraint (i.e. sedation) if necessary (ensuring adherence to competition regulations regarding usage of pharmaceuticals). Horses should generally stand squarely to load the soft tissue structures evenly throughout the examination.

One of the most significant contributors to poor image quality is the presence of air between the transducer and the skin surface. The haircoat traps air which will degrade image quality and therefore, ideally, the regions of interest should be clipped with fine-bladed clippers prior to the application of coupling gel (Figure I.13). If the owner does not consent to clipping for esthetic reasons, in an animal with a light haircoat, water may be applied to the regions to be scanned. However, the owner should be made aware that the possible reduction in image quality may result in an inability to adequately visualize and diagnose more subtle lesions. Improved images may be obtained without fully clipping if the clippers are used in the direction of the haircoat ("down the leg") to remove the ends of the hair coat. This decreases the amount of air in the coat and is difficult to detect visually.

In an animal with a greasy or dirty haircoat, in addition to clipping, the area may be washed with a very dilute chlorhexidine scrub solution to remove excessive organic matter. Some users choose to apply surgical spirit to the region to be scanned, however if this practice is to be employed, caution should be taken to ensure that a sufficient amount of gel is used on the skin surface and that the probe is thoroughly cleaned following the ultrasound examination as surgical spirit may damage the transducer. Finally, ultrasound coupling gel should ideally be applied a few minutes prior to initiating the examination, as this will significantly improve the quality of images produced. It is useful to apply the gel in a proximal to distal direction to avoid the introduction of air bubbles.

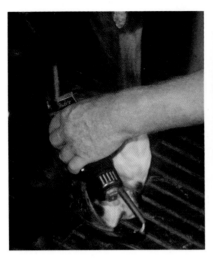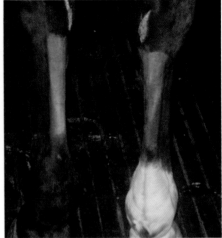

Figure I.13 Patient being prepared for an ultrasound examination of the proximal aspect of the distal hind limb. The haircoat has been removed from the caudal aspect of the distal limb in the regions of interest and extends a sufficient distance medially and laterally. (Source: BCF Technology Ltd. Reproduced with permission.)

Cobs and heavy breeds of horse present their own particular challenges for ultrasonography. A useful technique is to prepare them well in advance by clipping and cleaning the area thoroughly, applying copious amounts of ultrasound gel, wrapping the legs in plastic foodwrap/cellophane, and applying an external bandage to hold the gel and plastic wrap in place. This results in much better penetration of the gel into the skin and improves image quality significantly. These horses can also be difficult to scan due to the presence of skin folds, particularly in the palmar/plantar pastern region, and scanning with the leg in a non-weightbearing position may be of benefit.

ULTRASOUND ARTIFACTS

An *artifact* is defined as "something observed in a scientific investigation or experiment that is not naturally present but occurs as a result of the preparative or investigative procedure". In terms of ultrasonography, features of the ultrasound image which do not represent actual body tissues or misrepresent the relationship between tissues may be referred to as an artifact. The presence of these artifacts can significantly impede the user's ability to distinguish normal structures from pathological changes. However, understanding the causes of these artifacts enables the user to minimize them where possible, recognize and ignore the artifacts if they cannot be diminished, or even use them to their advantage by actively incorporating the artifact into the ultrasound examination.

Operator Error Artifacts

Artifacts in ultrasonography may be due to operator error or be directly related to the physics of ultrasonography. Common operator error artifacts include poor skin preparation/contact artifacts, which are created when the transducer cannot make uniform contact with the skin due to dirt, scabs, hair or other impediments. Air bubbles between the skin and the transducer also limit the ability of the ultrasound beam to effectively penetrate into the underlying tissues, resulting in artifact production. These artifacts are discussed in greater detail under Reverberation Artifact and Acoustic Shadowing Artifact.

Suboptimal gain, focal depth, or frequency settings will adversely affect image quality, as will scanning with the ultrasound beam being directed at an angle other than perpendicular to the tissue/region of interest (i.e. *off-incidence*). Optimal images are obtained when the ultrasound beam is directed 90° to the tissues being imaged, as this results in the most accurate representation of tissue location in the ultrasound image. If the ultrasound beam is not perpendicular to the tissues, a portion of the ultrasound beam will be reflected into surrounding tissues instead of back to the probe, resulting in fewer echoes returning to the transducer for image formation. For example, when imaging the distal limb in longitudinal section, the tendons will appear darker than normal (hypoechoic), although the borders will generally remain brighter (hyperechoic), which can give the misleading appearance of pathology. Being off-incidence even a few degrees can give rise to this artifact, although it can be utilized for diagnostic purposes as it can assist in the visualization and identification of structural margins.

If excessive pressure is applied to a region of the tissues containing either a discrete fluid-filled structure (e.g. ovarian follicle, embryonic vesicle, distended synovial structure) or "free" fluid (e.g. peritoneal effusion), the fluid may be displaced such that the true volume and location are distorted. This may result in the ultrasonographer being unable to detect small volumes of fluid or underestimating the total volume present. The application of excessive pressure can also cause soft tissue structures (e.g. tendons, vascular structures, anterior chamber of the globe) to be deformed, leading to inaccurate representation of margination and shape.

Other artifacts which are the direct result of the physics of ultrasonography are discussed in greater detail below.

Reverberation Artifact

Reverberation artifact is seen when imaging tissues with high acoustic impedance (highly reflective interfaces). There are three primary types of reverberation artifact which are classified based on the location and type of structures involved in the production of the artifact: a) transducer and reflective surface; b) reflective surfaces which are closely spaced together within the tissues such as a metallic object (*comet-tail* artifact); and c) fluid trapped within a collection of small gas bubbles (*ring-down* artifact).

Regardless of the structures involved, and therefore the individual classification of this artifact, reverberation is a result of the ultrasound beam encountering two highly reflective interfaces which are parallel to one another and subsequently being reflected back and forth between them. As this sequence takes place again and again, the ultrasound machine continues to receive echoes over regular intervals. As previously described, the ultrasound image is constructed by depicting the strength of the returning echo as the echogenicity (degree of brightness) and the length of time taken for the signal to be transmitted through the tissues and return to the probe as depth. These numerous echoes are therefore depicted as hyperechoic bands at regular intervals extending into the deeper field of the ultrasound image. However, the intensity of the returning echoes diminishes with each cycle of reflection between the interfaces due to the effect of attenuation, resulting in a decrease in the echogenicity of each band at increased depths on the image display.

For example, when scanning the equine distal limb, air trapped between the probe and the limb will act as a highly reflective interface. As the ultrasound wave leaves the probe and contacts air on the skin surface, the wave is reflected back towards the probe where it is registered and the skin surface is displayed as a hyperechoic line on the ultrasound image. However, some of the returning wave "bounces" off the surface of the probe and back towards the skin. This second wave encounters the highly reflective air–skin interface once more, returns to the probe, and a second hyperechoic line is represented on the image deep to the "true" image display. The process continues to repeat, resulting in a series of evenly spaced, hyperechoic lines appearing to extend into the deeper field of view which represents the number of times the wave has travelled from skin surface to probe and back (Figure I.14). Therefore, poor contact between the probe and the body will result in reverberation artifact and a loss of visualization of the soft tissue structures

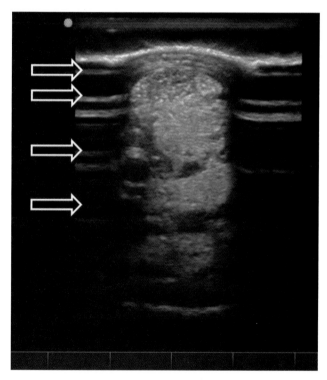

Figure I.14 Cross-sectional image of the equine distal limb with reverberation artifact (open arrows) on the lateral and medial aspects of the image resulting from lack of contact between the transducer and the limb in these regions (transducer within the standoff pad is wider than the surface of the leg in this scanning plane).

of the limb. To minimize this artifact, the patient should be appropriately prepared and additional ultrasound coupling gel should be used through the examination. However, it is important to recognize that this artifact will inevitably be seen at the medial and lateral margins of the ultrasound image when scanning the limb in the transverse plane. This is a result of the curved shape of the limb and the fact that the ultrasound probe will likely not be fully in contact with the patient when scanning in this orientation (variable with probe selection and patient conformation). This artifact is also routinely encountered when scanning the equine thorax and *per rectum* imaging of the reproductive tract, as both the aerated lung and gas within the colon/rectum are highly reflective interfaces just below the surface of the transducer (Figure I.15).

When the ultrasound wave encounters a metallic object (e.g. needle, surgical staple, orthopedic surgical implant) or calcification, a portion of the wave will become "trapped" inside the object where it reverberates back and forth within the object. With each reverberation, some of the wave "escapes" and returns to the probe where it is depicted on the image display as a hyperechoic line. Therefore, the collection of these returning waves has the appearance of a series of bright, white lines deep to the object. This is commonly referred to as *comet-tail* artifact.

Similarly, if an ultrasound wave strikes a pocket of fluid trapped within a collection of gas bubbles, such as in the gastrointestinal tract, the interface between the gas bubbles and the fluid is highly reflective. In this scenario, the ultrasound waves reverberate ("ring") inside the fluid, with a portion of the wave "escaping" with each reverberation and returning to the probe. These echoes are detected and displayed on the ultrasound image as either a continuous hyperechoic line or series of parallel hyperechoic bands extending deep to the collection of gas. This specific type of reverberation artifact is commonly referred to as *ring-down* artifact.

Reverberation artifacts in the near-field may also be a result of the ultrasound beam itself as waves released from the piezoelectric crystals in the transducer require a short distance to coalesce into an organized wave. This distance varies primarily with the frequency capability of the probe with higher frequency transducers producing less reverberation artifact in the near-field. If necessary, a *standoff* may be used to reduce the appearance of this artifact, particularly when evaluating superficial structures in the distal limb, such as the superficial digital flexor tendon.

Acoustic Enhancement Artifact

Acoustic enhancement artifact is created when the ultrasound waves pass through a tissue causing minimal attenuation, such as fluid, and appears as an artifactual brightness of tissues deep to that fluid-filled structure. As previously described, ultrasound waves are attenuated as they pass through the body, resulting in a loss of strength of echoes returning to the probe from deeper tissues. Without the appropriate usage of the time–gain compensation (TGC) controls, these tissues would therefore appear artifactually less echogenic (hypoechoic) than more superficial structures. Conversely, if the ultrasound beam is not attenuated by more superficial structures (e.g. because they are fluid filled), the waves reaching the deeper tissues will be relatively stronger than they should be at that given depth. Thus, the waves reflected back to the probe from these regions will also be stronger, resulting in an artifactual brightness (increased echogenicity or hyperechoic appearance) of tissues deep to the fluid-filled structure being displayed on the ultrasound image. This is referred to as *acoustic enhancement* and is commonly associated with ultrasonography of fluid-filled structures, such as tendinous "core" lesions, cystic lesions, ovarian follicles, early embryonic vesicles, and the eye, as ultrasound waves are not attenuated by fluid (Figure I.16). This can also be observed when imaging the distal limb

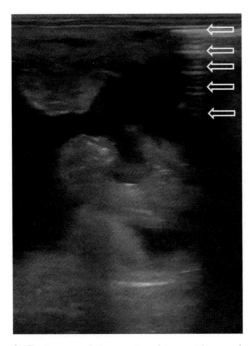

Figure I.15 Image of the equine fetus with reverberation artifact (arrows) resulting from the presence of gas within the rectum.

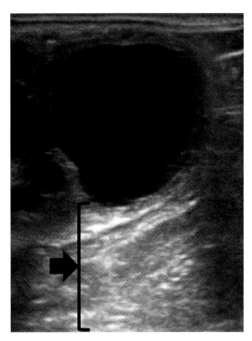

Figure I.16 Image of an equine ovary with acoustic enhancement artifact (arrow) deep to the anechoic ovulatory follicle.

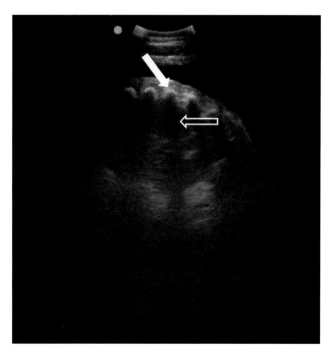

Figure I.17 Image of the equine fetus demonstrating acoustic shadowing artifact (open arrow) deep to the hyperechoic fetal rib (closed arrow).

as the metacarpal/tarsal vessels will not attenuate the ultrasound wave, thereby the underlying suspensory ligament will appear artifactually brighter (hyperechoic) when imaged through these vessels.

Acoustic enhancement may interfere with assessment of tissues deep to a fluid-filled structure as well as the deep margin/interface of the fluid and underlying soft tissue. The user may find it useful to decrease the degree of brightness in the far-field by adjusting the TGC controls for the areas deep to the fluid to minimize the appearance of this artifact. In other words, by decreasing the gain in the deeper field of view, the structures in the far-field (including the wall of the fluid-filled structure) may be evaluated more readily. It is important that the TGC is then reset for the remainder of the ultrasound examination.

Acoustic Shadowing Artifact

In contrast to acoustic enhancement, *acoustic shadowing artifact* results from the complete or near complete reflection of the ultrasound beam at a highly reflective interface.

As previously described, when an ultrasound wave reaches a highly reflective interface, such as mineral–soft tissue or gas–soft tissue, the vast majority of waves are reflected back to the probe resulting in a uniform, hyperechoic line being displayed for that correspond-

ing depth. Therefore the reflected ultrasound beam will not reach the structures deep to the highly reflective interface and that region will appear uniformly anechoic or hypoechoic as none/very few echoes are being received from that depth. This is termed *acoustic shadowing* and is observed deep to bony structures such as the metacarpals/metatarsals, ribs (Figure I.17), sesamoid bones of the fetlock joint (Figure I.18), and pelvis, as well as gaseous structures such as aerated lung and loops of intestine. It should be noted that acoustic shadowing and reverberation artifact may both be present when imaging these types of structures.

Edge Shadowing Artifact

Edge shadowing, also known as edge refraction, occurs deep to a curvilinear interface and is caused by the ultrasound wave striking such an interface at an angle. The interaction of an ultrasound beam with the lateral margins of a spherical/curved structure can result in the wave being redirected or "bent" away from the structure and into the deeper tissues with no ultrasound waves being transmitted directly below the edges of that structure. Therefore, no echoes are returned to the probe from these areas and an anechoic line or "cone" originating at both edges of the structure and extending into the deeper tissues is displayed

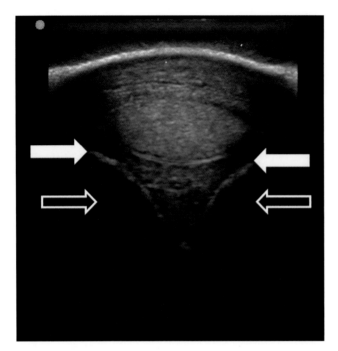

Figure I.18 Acoustic shadowing demonstrated in this cross-sectional image of the equine distal limb at the level of the sesamoid bones of the fetlock joint with anechoic regions (open arrows) deep to the hyperechoic cortex of the sesamoid bones (closed arrows).

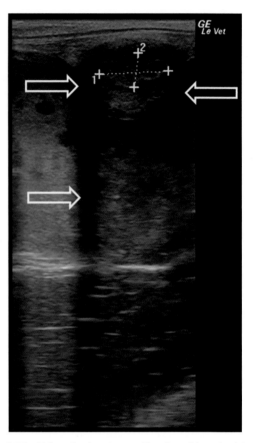

Figure I.19 Edge shadowing artifact is evident in this ultrasound image of the equine reproductive tract. (Source: BCF Technology Ltd. Reproduced with permission.)

(Figure I.19). This ultrasonographic appearance is known as the *edge shadowing artifact*. Uterine horns, ovarian follicles, ovaries, and the globe are all examples of structures causing edge shadowing artifact. It can also commonly be seen when imaging the suspensory branches from the palmar/plantar aspect of the limb.

Slice-Thickness Artifact

Slice thickness artifact is related to ultrasound beam width and is responsible for the artifactual appearance of soft tissue within a fluid-filled viscus ("pseudo-sludge"). The relationship between beam width and the distance between two points in the tissues has previously been described under the topic of image resolution. In addition to the negative effect on lateral resolution, a beam that is wider (thicker) than the distance between two defined points along its path ("slice") may also result in the production of an image artifact. This *slice-thickness artifact* is most appreciable when imaging near the periphery of a curved, fluid-filled structure. Depending on the cellularity of the fluid, these structures should appear on the ultrasound image as hypo-/anechoic with a more hyperechoic margin representing the wall. If the orientation of the

probe is such that the ultrasound wave is directed along the margin of a curved, fluid-filled structure and the beam is wide, tissue reflectors from the wall and surrounding tissues will be detected and reflect a portion of the wave, while the remainder of the wave passes through the fluid unimpeded. Thus, instead of the fluid appearing anechoic, the additional tissue reflectors will be represented as more hyperechoic material within this region of the ultrasound image, thereby giving the fluid an artificially flocculent appearance. For example, slice-thickness artifact may mimic the presence of reflective material within the vitreous chamber or particulate material within a preovulatory follicle (Figure I.20).

Distinguishing between fluid-containing tissue reflectors and slice-thickness artifact can be achieved by changing the position of the probe or altering the width of the beam. Moving the probe in relation to the anatomical region of interest will change the path of the ultrasound wave such that it will contact the fluid-filled structure at various angles. This will cause the artifact to disappear or be diminished at different orientations of the beam while true sediment or particu-

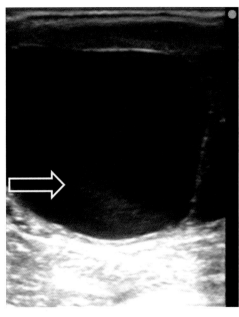

Figure I.20 Slice-thickness artifact (open arrow) is commonly observed when imaging curved, fluid-filled structures such as this preovulatory follicle.

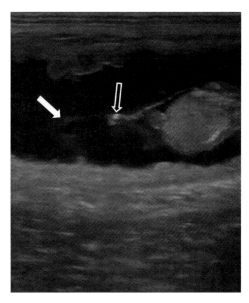

Figure I.21 Image of the equine fetus with the highly reflective bones of the distal limb causing reflection of side-lobes echoes and the inaccurate representation of the location of the limbs (closed arrow) adjacent to the actual location of the fetal limbs (open arrow).

late matter will have a more consistent ultrasonographic appearance. Narrowing of the beam also diminishes the presence of slice-thickness artifact and the user can accomplish this by focusing the beam in the region of the image where the artifact is observed. It may also be helpful to note the relationship of the fluid and the potential material within it. Artifactual sediment has a curved surface and true sediment/flocculent material generally has a flat surface and may be resuspended upon gentle agitation of the fluid-filled structure.

Side-Lobe Artifact

Side-lobe artifact occurs when accessory ultrasound waves contribute erroneous information regarding tissue location and echogenicity during image formation. The ultrasound beam emitted from the transducer is comprised of a primary beam, which is directed perpendicular to its point of origin on the probe and the tissues below it. However, there are also accessory beams (*side-lobes*) on either side of the primary beam which are weaker and do not travel perpendicularly to the underlying tissues. Due to their weak nature, interaction between these side-lobes and body tissues generally does not result in the production of echoes which will contribute to the displayed image. However, if a highly reflective interface is along the path of these accessory, non-perpendicular waves, the interaction may result in an echo of appreciable strength returning

to the probe. The location of this structure will be correctly represented by the primary beam, however it will also be represented as being located to the side of the actual structure. This *side-lobe artifact* will be less echogenic than the true structure appearance because it is originating from weaker echoes. This effect is most pronounced when a highly reflective structure is present within an anechoic region (e.g. the fetal skeleton within the fetal fluids) (Figure I.21).

Mirror-Image Artifact

Similar to reverberation artifact, a mirror-image artifact is caused by a disruption in the normal sequence of travel of an ultrasound wave as a result of an interaction with a highly reflective interface. A mirror-image artifact is characterized by a misrepresentation of a structure's location on both sides of the reflective interface. The "true" component of the image is created by the usual interaction of an ultrasound wave with a reflective structure within the tissues (echoes travelling from probe to tissue reflector and then directly back to the probe). The artifactual region of the image is produced by that portion of the beam which first contacts the highly reflective interface and is reflected into another area of the tissues instead of returning to the probe. The wave is then reflected back towards the interface and, upon reaching the interface for a second time, is finally returned to the probe. The ultrasound machine is only able to interpret the time taken for this portion of the beam to return to the transducer, not the diverted path of travel. As this travel time was prolonged by the additional reflections, the ultrasound machine translates this as the tissue reflector being farther away from the ultrasound probe (e.g. at a greater depth). Therefore, the final image construction combines the "true" image on the appropriate side of the highly reflective interface (more superficial) with the "mirror" image on the opposite side of that interface (deeper).

This is commonly appreciated in ultrasonography of the cranial abdomen in small animals at the highly reflective interface of the lung–diaphragm interface (gas–soft tissue interface) and may also be appreciated in equine patients at this same location. Mirror-image artifact may also be observed on ultrasonography of the equine reproductive tract (duplication of ovary or fetus is possible if a highly reflective loop of intestine or muscle is present). It is important to consider the possible presence of this artifact if additional, unexpected structures are visualized on the ultrasound image as these could otherwise be mistaken for pathology. Redirection of the transducer in different scanning angles/planes may diminish or completely eliminate this artifact, making it possible for the user to evaluate the actual region of interest more readily.

DOPPLER IMAGING

Doppler imaging enables the direction and velocity of blood flow within the patient to be determined and represented in an ultrasound image. The speed of ultrasound waves travelling in soft tissue is a known constant value. In addition, the frequency of the ultrasound wave being used is also known (dependent on the transducer frequency setting determined by the user). Using these two known values, the machine is able to calculate the movement of structures (e.g. red blood cells) relative to the ultrasound beam and display the speed and direction of this movement on the ultrasound image.

As the ultrasound wave strikes a moving object, the wave will be reflected and returned to the probe. The frequency of the wave will have been altered by the interaction with the moving object. An increase in the ultrasound wave frequency will occur if the object is moving towards the probe and is referred to as a *positive frequency shift*. Conversely, the wave frequency will decrease if the object is moving away from the probe and is recognized as a *negative frequency shift*. The difference between the frequency of the wave

transmitted from the probe and the frequency of the wave returning to the probe can be calculated and this difference in frequency is the *Doppler shift* (Figure I.22). Therefore, if an object, such as a red blood cell, is moving along the path of the ultrasound wave, the direction (away from or towards the probe) and the speed of the moving object can be determined by the ultrasound machine due to the change in the frequency of the returning ultrasound wave.

Doppler Modes

There are distinct Doppler modes which provide the user with additional information regarding tissue movement. More commonly available modes include spectral, color flow, and power Doppler.

Spectral Doppler

Spectral Doppler is useful for quantifying the velocity and direction of blood flow in relation to time. When the ultrasound machine is in spectral Doppler mode, the ultrasound probe receives the returning echo signal and the machine records the Doppler frequency shift in a graphical representation referred to as a *trace*. Each spectral waveform is thus representing the velocity of blood flow over time. This is depicted by a sharp line bounding the area of each waveform on the spectral trace, and is often referred to as the *envelope* (Figure I.23). Areas of the spectral trace above the baseline represent blood flow towards the probe (Figure I.23) while those areas below the baseline represent blood flow away from the probe (Figure I.24).

The two main types of spectral Doppler are pulsed wave (PW) Doppler and continuous wave (CW) Doppler.

Pulsed Wave Doppler In PW Doppler mode, the same crystal both sends and receives the ultrasound waves responsible for the Doppler display. While in B-mode, the region of interest is identified (e.g. blood vessel, valvular region) and the view is optimized for Doppler investigation. Most importantly, it is imperative that the ultrasound beam be parallel to the line of blood flow for the most accurate velocity readings to be obtained. PW Doppler mode is selected and an electronic "gate" is displayed which is then used to specify the sampling region (e.g. the region of the valve leaflets). Only echoes retuning from this region will be displayed. Thus, PW Doppler is very specific for identifying velocity of blood flow in a discrete location.

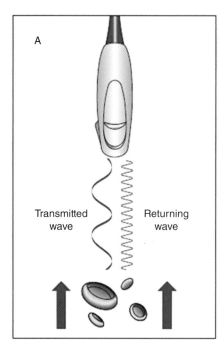
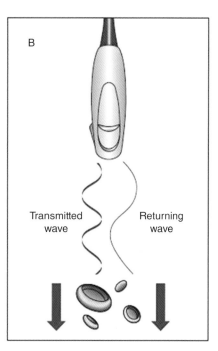

Figure I.22 Illustrations of Doppler shift: (A) positive Doppler shift when the flow of blood is towards the transducer and the returning wave is of a higher frequency than the transmitted wave; (B) negative Doppler shift when the flow of blood is away from the transducer and the returning wave is of a lower frequency than the transmitted wave. (Source: BCF Technology Ltd. Reproduced with permission.)

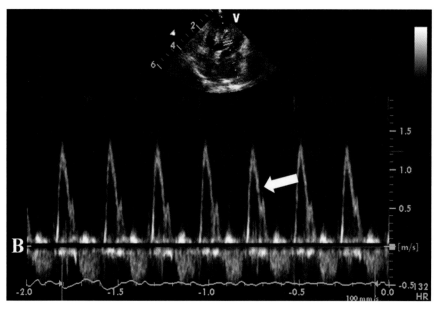

Figure I.23 Spectral Doppler trace with *envelopes* above the baseline (B) representing direction of bloodflow towards the probe (arrow).

In PW Doppler mode, the machine is also able to detect turbulence of flow, which is helpful when investigating possible valvular disease. Smooth (laminar) flow will be displayed with a *clean* envelope as the red blood cells are travelling at a near-uniform velocity (Figure I.25). Turbulent flow (where the red blood cells are travelling at various velocities due to an obstruction which results in abnormal blood flow) will result in spectral broadening (display of low, medium and high velocities) and possibly an increase in the peak

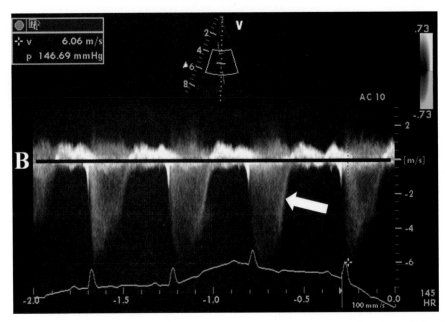

Figure I.24 Spectral Doppler trace with *envelopes* below the baseline (B) representing direction of bloodflow away from the probe (arrow).

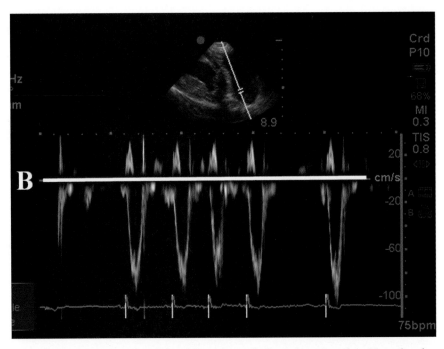

Figure I.25 Pulsed wave (PW) Doppler study of blood flow through the pulmonic valve. Note the *clean* envelope indicating laminar flow and display below the baseline (B), indicating primary direction of blood flow away from the transducer.

(highest) velocity. Therefore the envelope will not be clean as a wide range of velocities will be depicted.

The crystal sending the ultrasound wave must wait for the signal to return from the gated region before sending another wave. Therefore, if the red blood cells are travelling at a high velocity, they may overtake the returning ultrasound signal before it reaches the probe and the next ultrasound signal is emitted. Otherwise stated, the velocity of bloodflow is faster than the pulse repetition frequency. This results in aliasing, where the high-frequency portion of the signal is displayed on the wrong side of the baseline (*wrapped around*) resulting in the true measurement of this high-velocity flow being inaccurately represented on the spectral trace. Therefore PW Doppler is unreliable when measuring high-velocity blood flow.

Continuous Wave Doppler

In comparison to PW Doppler, CW Doppler is performed by two separate crystals housed within the transducer. One crystal continuously emits an ultrasound signal while the other crystal continuouly receives the ultrasound signal. Therefore there is constant sampling of Doppler frequency shift along the length of the ultrasound beam. As a result, CW Doppler is highly accurate for measuring Doppler shift (high sensitivity) and higher-velocity blood flow can be recorded compared to PW Doppler. However, as there are numerous velocities being recorded simultaneously, the envelope will not be *clean* (Figure I.26).

Color Flow Doppler

Color flow Doppler is a variation on PW Doppler where a gate is used to identify the sampling region of interest. Instead of the velocity and direction of flow being plotted against time on a spectral trace, the direction and relative velocity of blood flow are characterized and displayed through the use of color-coding (Figure I.27). The colors displayed are user defined, however convention dictates that the direc-

tion of flow in relation to the transducer should follow the acronym BART – blue away, red towards. Turbulent flow is indicated by a mosaic of color, with green usually indicating non-laminar flow. The relative velocity of flow may be indicated by the brightness of hue (i.e. higher velocity, brighter hue). Aliasing can occur with high velocities as this form of Doppler is a variation on PW Doppler.

Power Doppler

Power Doppler is a form of Doppler which analyzes the total strength of the returning echoes and ignores direction of flow. A color map of the Doppler frequency shift is created where the hue and brightness of the displayed color represent the power of the returning signal (superimposed on a B-mode image). When in Power Doppler mode, the machine is able to detect very low-velocity blood flow and may be useful for identifying blood flow within a suspected lesion.

SUMMARY/CONCLUSION

Ultrasonography is a versatile, powerful, and invaluable component of the equine veterinary diagnostic toolbox. In order to maximize the diagnostic quality of the information obtained during the ultrasound examination, a practical working knowledge of ultrasound physics is required. This will enable the clinician to

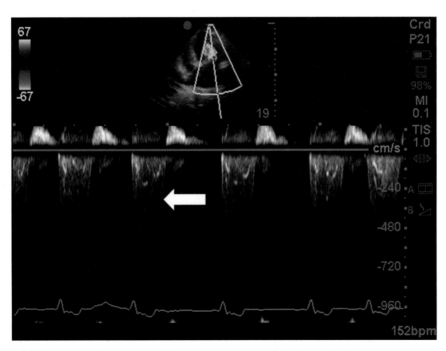

Figure I.26   Continuous wave (CW) Doppler trace exhibiting a *filled-in* envelope (arrow).

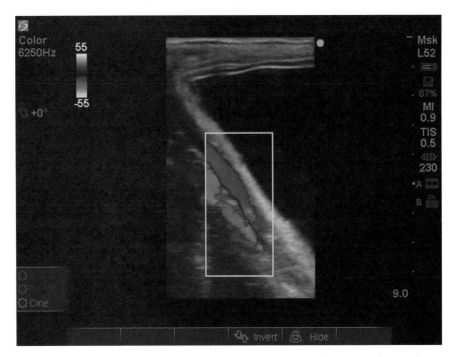

Figure I.27 Color flow Doppler image representing bloodflow in the region of the uteroplacental unit.

fully optimize the machine settings, understand and interpret the image displayed, and also avoid the potential pitfalls associated with the appearance of artifacts on the ultrasound image. Finally, and perhaps most importantly, this knowledge will also enable the ultrasonographer to perform the examination with greater skill and confidence.

RECOMMENDED READING

Choudhry, S., Gorman, B., Charboneau, J.W., *et al.* (2000) Comparison of tissue harmonic imaging with conventional US in abdominal disease. *Radiographics*, 20, 1127–1135.

Curry, T.S. III, Dowdey, J.E., & Murray, R.C. Jr. (1990) *Christensen's Physics of Diagnostic Radiology*, 4th edn. Lea & Febiger, Philadelphia.

Evans, D.H. & McDicken, W.N. (2000) *Doppler Ultrasound: Physics, Instrumentation, and Signal Processing*, 2nd edn. Wiley, New York.

Feldman, M.K., Katyal, S., & Blackwood, M.S. (2009) US artifacts. *Radiographics* 29, 1179–1189.

Ginther, O.J. (1995) *Ultrasonic Imaging and Animal Reproduction: Fundamentals, Book 1.* Equiservices Publishing, Cross Plains.

Goldstein, A. (1993) Overview of the physics of US. *Radiographics*, 13, 701–704.

Kremkau, F.W. (2002) *Diagnostic Ultrasound: Principles and Instruments*, 6th ed. W.B. Saunders Company, Philadelphia.

Kristoffersen, M., Öhberg, L., Johnston, C., & Alfredson, H. (2005) Neovascularisation in chronic tendon injuries detected with colour Doppler ultrasound in horse and man: implications for research and treatment. *Knee Surgery, Sports Traumatology, Arthroscopy*, 13, 505–508.

Merritt, C.R.B. (1991) Doppler US: The basics. *Radiographics*, 11, 109–119.

Matheson, J.S., O'Brien, R.T., & Delaney, F. (2003) Tissue harmonic ultrasound for imaging normal abdominal organs in dogs and cats. *Veterinary Radiology and Ultrasound*, 44(2), 205–208.

Penninck, D.G. (1995) Imaging artifacts in ultrasound. In: *Veterinary Diagnostic Ultrasound* (eds.T.G. Nyland & J.S. Mattoon). W.B. Saunders Company, Philadelphia.

Pozniak, M.A., Zagzebski, J.A., & Scanlan, K.A. (1992) Spectral and color Doppler artifacts. *Radiographics*, 12, 35–44.

Reubin, J.M. (1994) Spectral Doppler US. *Radiographics*, 14, 139–150.

Scanlan, K.A. (1991) Sonographic artifacts and their origins. *American Journal of Roentgenology*, 156, 1267–1272.

Shapiro, R.S., Wagreich, J., Parsons, R.B., Stancato-Pasik, A., Yeh, H.-C., & Lao, R. (1998) Tissue harmonic imaging sonography: evaluation of image quality compared with conventional sonography. *American Journal of Roentgenology*, 171, 1203–1206.

Tranquart, F., Grenier, N., Ader, V., & Pourcelot, L. (1999) Clinical use of ultrasound tissue harmonic imaging. *Ultrasound in medicine and biology*, 25(6), 889–894.

Zagzebski, J.A. (1996) *Essentials of Ultrasound Physics*. Mosby, Inc., St. Louis.

Ziskin, M.C. (1993) Fundamental physics of ultrasound and its propagation in tissue. *Radiographics*,13, 705–709.

SECTION 1

MUSCULOSKELETAL

CHAPTER ONE

ULTRASONOGRAPHY OF THE FOOT AND PASTERN

Ann Carstens[1] and Roger K.W. Smith[2]

[1]University of Pretoria, Onderstepoort, South Africa
[2]The Royal Veterinary College, North Mymms, Hatfield, UK

THE FOOT

Lameness associated with the foot is common and routinely evaluated using radiography. However, many causes of lameness are associated with soft tissue pathology where there are no or minimal radiographic changes. While magnetic resonance imaging (MRI) has become the imaging modality of choice for identifying such soft tissue causes, MRI is costly and not always available. Therefore, ultrasonography is a logical imaging modality to consider but its use is compromised by the presence of the hoof capsule, which precludes imaging through it. However, there are three ultrasonographic *windows* where images can be obtained of structures of the foot – proximal to the coronary band palmarly and dorsally, and transcuneally/transsolarly.

Ultrasonography Proximal to the Coronary Band

A number of structures within the foot extend proximal to the coronary band and so lend themselves to ultrasonographic examination.

Preparation

The hair should be clipped and cleaned as for other ultrasound examinations. Gel should be rubbed it the area and left for a few minutes to improve contact as this is often limiting.

Technique

For the palmar aspect of the foot a small footprint transducer (ideally a curvilinear probe) can be placed longitudinally between the bulbs of the heel, with the foot placed on a wooden wedge (as used for foot radiography – Figure 1.1) so as to have the fetlock partially flexed and the foot extended. This allows the assessment of the deep digital flexor tendon (DDFT), the palmar pouch of the distal interphalangeal (DIP) joint, the "T" ligament, and the navicular bursa down to the level of the proximal border of the navicular bone (Figure 1.2). However, the DDFT is off-incidence to the ultrasound beam and hence is hypoechoic, and the imaging window incorporates only the middle portion of the DDFT, making identification of DDFT tears, most commonly present in the lobes, difficult.

For the dorsal, medial, and lateral aspects, the transducer is positioned both transversely adjacent to the coronary band and longitudinally overlying the coronary band (Figure 1.3) and moved from the dorsal aspect to the dorsomedial and dorsolateral aspects where the dorsal joint capsule and collateral ligaments of the DIP joint (Figure 1.4) can be imaged immediately proximal to the coronary band. The collateral ligaments traverse the coronary band and so only the more proximal parts of the ligament are visible ultrasonographically. Care should be taken to ensure the transducer is on-incidence to the collateral ligament as it is easy to generate off-incidence artifacts in the ligaments that can resemble pathology (Figure 1.5). Further caudally lie the collateral cartilages, which are hypoechoic but can show areas of ossification (and therefore acoustic shadowing).

Ultrasonographic Abnormalities

Via the palmar window, only chronic DDFT pathology, where there is retained echogenicity and/or mineralization within the off-incidence hypoechoic DDFT, can

Atlas of Equine Ultrasonography, First Edition. Edited by Jessica A. Kidd, Kristina G. Lu, and Michele L. Frazer.
© 2014 John Wiley & Sons, Ltd. Published 2014 by John Wiley & Sons, Ltd.
Companion Website: www.wiley.com/go/kidd/equine-ultrasonography

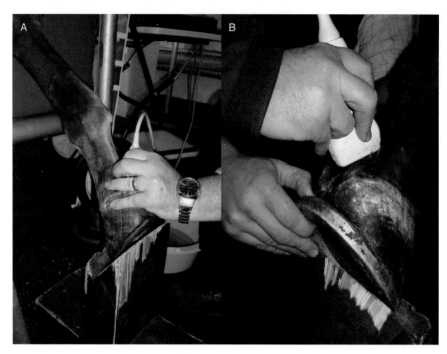

Figure 1.1   Positioning of either a curvilinear (A) or linear (B) transducer between the bulbs of the heels to image the palmar aspect of the foot.

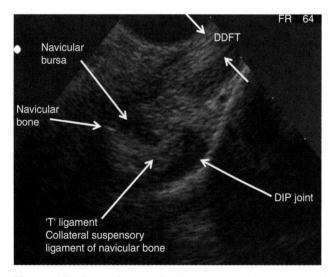

Figure 1.2   Normal sagittal ultrasonographic anatomy of the palmar foot. Proximal is to the right.

usually be visualized (Figure 1.6), limiting this view for comprehensive evaluation of the DDFT in this region of the foot. In some cases, DDFT pathology will extend sufficiently proximally to be visible in standard views within the distal pastern (see Pastern, later in this chapter).

Abnormalities of the distal interphalangeal joint can result in changes to the dorsal pouch which are visible ultrasonographically – both distension and synovial thickening (Figure 1.7) as well as osteophytosis in cases of osteoarthritis (Figure 1.8). Where ultrasonography of this region carries the most useful imaging is for collateral ligament desmitis, especially when there is palpable swelling in the region of the ligament (dorsomedially or dorsolaterally) at the level of the coronary band. Ultrasonographic abnormalities vary between enlargement and complete rupture (Figure 1.9).

Transsolar and Transcuneal Ultrasonography

The third phalanx (P3), distal sesamoid bone (navicular bone) (DSB), navicular bursa (NB), implantation of the deep digital flexor tendon (DDFT), distal sesamoid impar ligament (DSBIL), and other suprasolar structures can be evaluated ultrasonographically transcuneally (through the frog) and transsolarly (through the sole). A 7.5 MHz transducer, preferably curvilinear, should be used, although lower multi-frequency transducers such as a 3.5 MHz transducer used at 6 MHz can also give adequate images.

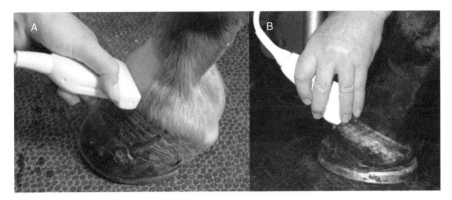

Figure 1.3 Linear transducer positioning to evaluate the dorsal and dorsolateral/dorsomedial aspects of the foot: (A) transverse, (B) longitudinal. Note the transducer spanning the coronary band in the longitudinal orientation.

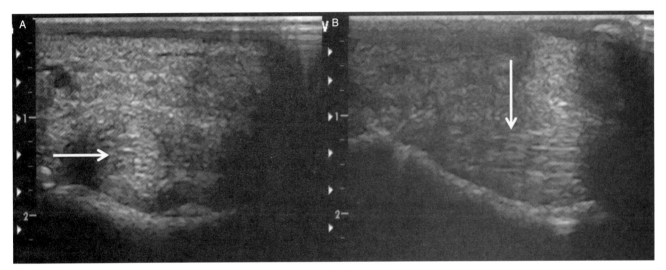

Figure 1.4 Normal ultrasonographic appearance of the distal interphalangeal joint collateral ligaments. (A) Transverse image – note the oval-shaped collateral ligament (arrow) lying in a depression in the underlying bony surface of the second phalanx. (B) Longitudinal image (proximal to the left) – the longitudinal striations of the ligament are visible (arrow). Note the acoustic shadowing over the hoof capsule.

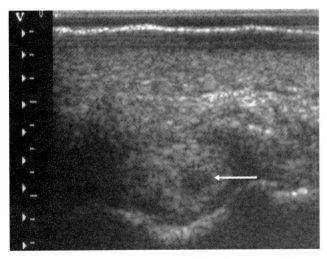

Figure 1.5 Hypoechoic region within the collateral ligament in a transverse image. There is no accompanying enlargement to the ligament and so such isolated hypoechoic areas should be interpreted with caution, as they can be generated artifactually by slight off-incidence orientations of the transducer.

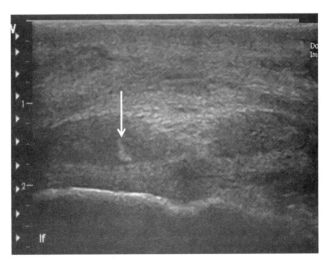

Figure 1.6 Retained echogenicity in an off-incidence transverse image of the distal deep digital flexor tendon consistent with chronic tendinopathy and/or mineralization.

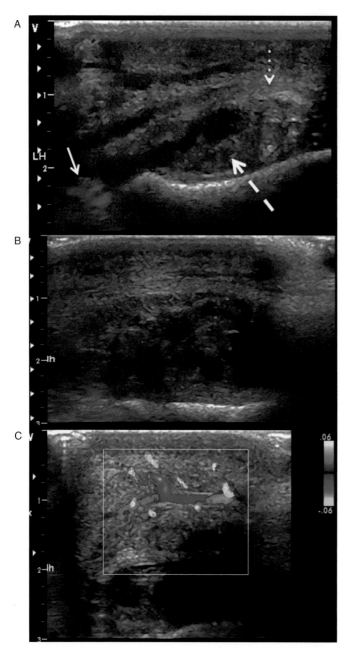

Figure 1.7 (A) Longitudinal image adjacent to the dorsal coronary band showing the extensor process of the distal phalanx (solid arrow), the digital extensor tendon (dotted arrow), and hypertrophied synovium (dashed arrow) together with a distended distal interphalangeal joint in a horse with distal interphalangeal joint sepsis (proximal to the right). (B) shows the corresponding transverse image and (C) the transverse image with Doppler imaging, showing the marked hyperemia of the joint capsule.

Preparation

Since the frog and sole are relatively impenetrable to ultrasound waves, and loose solar and frog keratin can trap air, it is important to prepare them to optimize the image. The sole and frog should be trimmed to get rid of loose scaly keratin and pared smooth. The foot should then be soaked in bandages/poultice for at least an hour in water. This may need to be prolonged to overnight soaking, if there is initially minimal softening of the sole or frog. Application of acoustic coupling gel (ACG) for 10–15 minutes prior to scanning also helps image visibility. Copious amounts of ACG that fill the collateral and central sulci of the frog also help to establish a clearer image with fewer artifacts and serve as a stand-off medium. A handler can hold the leg in a position so that the ultrasonographer can access the sole or the ultrasonographer may elect to hold the pastern between his/her knees with the sole facing upwards.

Scanning Procedure

For the navicular bone and associated structures (Figure 1.10), the area over the frog is scanned in both transverse and sagittal planes. The proximal aspect of the DSB is approximately at the middle of the frog and the insertion of the DDFT on P3 is just proximal to the apex of the frog (Figure 1.11). Using this technique, the hyperechoic collateral ligament of the DSB can be seen indistinctly on the proximal aspect of the DSB. The DSB flexor surface and distal aspect can be seen as a hyperechoic surface. Palmar/plantar to this is the hypoechoic DSB fibrocartilage, then the navicular bursa followed by the fibers of the DDFT, which, when followed distally, can be seen fanning out to implant on the *facies flexoria* of P3. Palmar/plantar and proximal to the DDFT and closely associated to it, is the very thin (hardly visible) distal digital annular ligament. From the distal aspect of the DSB the distal sesamoidean impar ligament (DSBIL) fibers can be seen extending distally to implant on P3 proximal to the *facies flexoria*. Between the DSBIL and the distal DSB is the hypo- to anechoic distal palmar recess of the distal interphalangeal joint (DIPJ). Between the DSBIL and the implantation of the DDFT is the distal recess of the navicular bursa, usually only a potential space. Between the DDFT and the sole is the inhomogeneously hyperechoic digital cushion (Figures 1.12, 1.13, 1.14, 1.15).

The entire solar surface of the distal two thirds of P3 can be evaluated if a small end-on footprint curvilinear transducer is used. Again the surface is evaluated both in the transverse and sagittal planes. The hyperechoic solar bone surface can be followed from centrally to its margin. A normal interruption can be seen at the tip of P3 if a crena is present. The overlying hypoechoic solar corium can be seen as well as the hyperechoic transitional line to the inhomogeneously hyperechoic keratinized epidermis of the sole (Figures 1.16, 1.17, 1.18, 1.19).

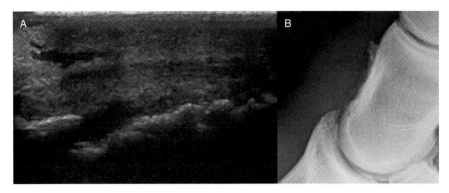

Figure 1.8 Distal interphalangeal joint osteoarthritis. Dorsal longitudinal ultrasonographic image (A – proximal to the right) showing irregular new bone on the dorsal surface of the second phalanx, as seen radiographically (B).

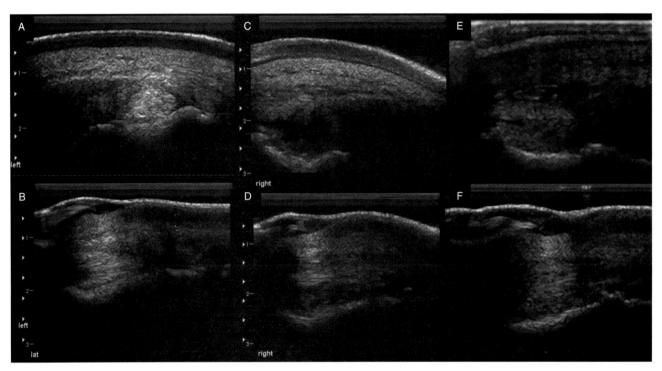

Figure 1.9 Ruptured collateral ligament of the distal interphalangeal joint. (A) and (B) show the transverse (A) and longitudinal (B) images of the normal contralateral medial collateral ligament. (C) and (D) show the corresponding ultrasonographic images of the ruptured ligament. Note the absence of any organized echogenic ligament tissue where the ligament should be. Images (E) and (F) show the "regeneration" of a new ligament after 2 months in a distal limb cast, indicating that these injuries, although seemingly severe, can heal satisfactorily when the joint is immobilized adequately.

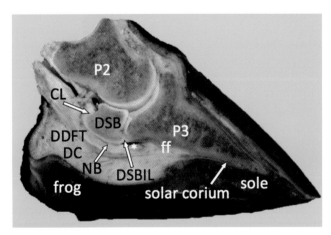

Figure 1.10 Anatomical structures in a sagittal section of the distal digit. CL: collateral ligament of the DSB; DC: digital cushion; DDFT: deep digital flexor tendon; DSB: distal sesamoid bone; ff: facies flexoria; NB: navicular bursa; P2: second phalanx; P3: third/distal phalanx; * distal recess of the NB.

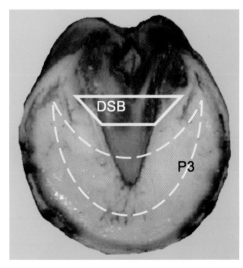

Figure 1.11 Diagrammatic illustration of the position of the DSB and P3 on a solar view of the foot. DSB: distal sesamoid bone; P3: third/distal phalanx.

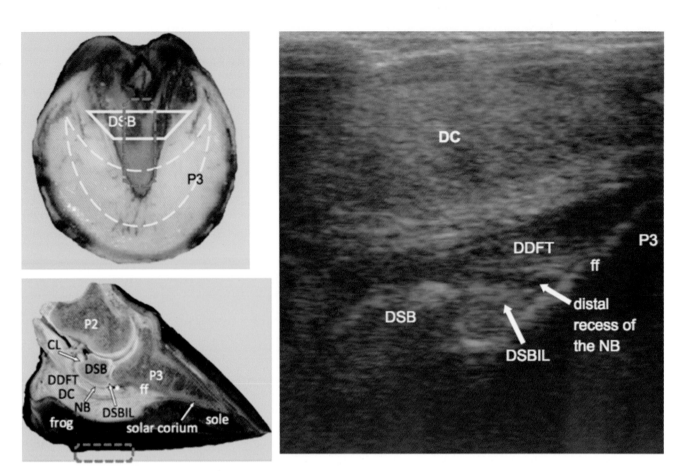

Figure 1.12 Sagittal transcuneal ultrasound image of the hyperechoic flexor cortical surface of the DSB and the solar surface of P3. DC: digital cushion; DDFT: deep digital flexor tendon; DSB: distal sesamoid bone; DSBIL: distal sesamoidean impar ligament; ff = facies flexoria = DDFT insertion on P3; NB: navicular bursa; P3: third/distal phalanx. Proximal is to the left and the solar surface is at the top of the image. The stippled red box in this, and all subsequent images in this chapter, indicates the probe position.

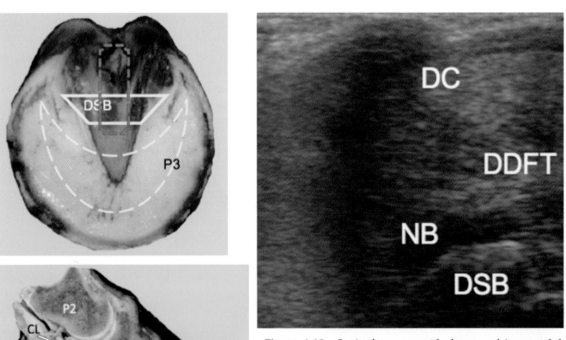

Figure 1.13 Sagittal transcuneal ultrasound image of the hyperechoic flexor cortical surface of the proximal DSB. Note the loss of image proximal to the DSB where transducer contact is poor and the DDFT is obliquely oriented to the angle of incidence of the ultrasound beam. DC: digital cushion; DDFT: deep digital flexor tendon; DSB: distal sesamoid bone; NB: navicular bursa. Proximal is to the left and the solar surface is at the top of the image.

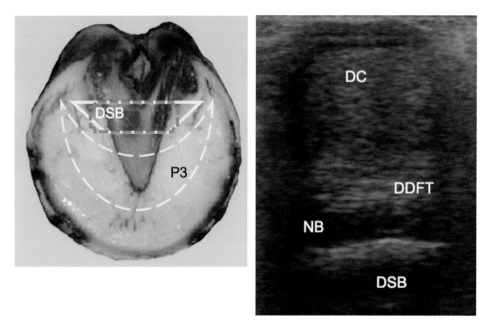

Figure 1.14 Transverse transcuneal ultrasound image of the hyperechoic flexor cortical surface mid DSB. DC: digital cushion; DDFT: deep digital flexor tendon; DSB: distal sesamoid bone; NB: navicular bursa. The solar surface is at the top of the image.

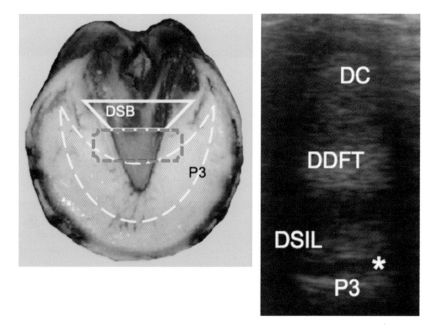

Figure 1.15 Transverse transcuneal ultrasound image of the DDFT and DSBIL immediately distal to the DSB. DC: digital cushion; DDFT: deep digital flexor tendon; DSB: distal sesamoid bone; P3: third/distal phalanx; *: palmar recess of the distal interphalangeal joint. The solar surface is at the top of the image.

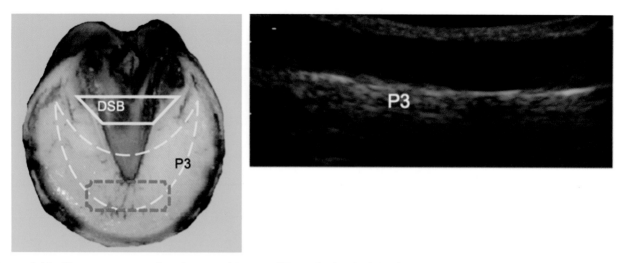

Figure 1.16   Transverse transsolar ultrasound image of P3 at the level of the frog apex. The solar corium is the hypoechoic structure above P3. DSB: distal sesamoid bone; P3: third/distal phalanx.

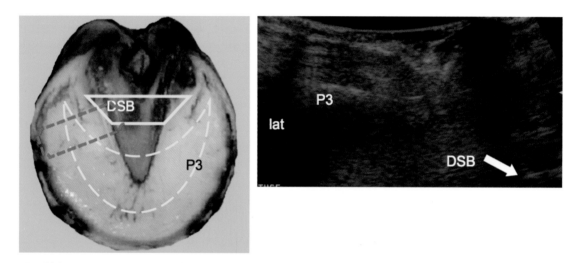

Figure 1.17   Oblique transverse transsolar/cuneal ultrasound image of the hyperechoic marginal solar surface lateral P3 with the DSB seen obliquely in the far field at the distal third of the frog. DSB: distal sesamoid bone; P3: third/distal phalanx. Laterodorsal is to the left.

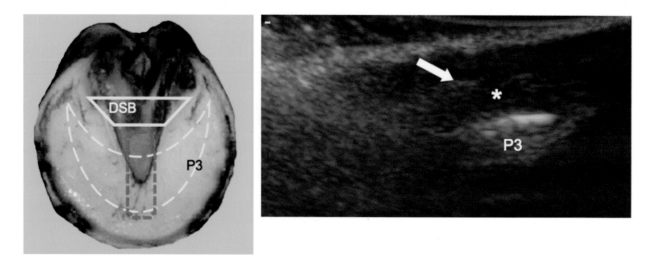

Figure 1.18   Sagittal transsolar ultrasound image of the hyperechoic solar tip of P3. Note the hypoechoic corium immediately solar to P3 (*) and the corium–solar keratinized epidermis interface (arrow). DSB: distal sesamoid bone; P3: third/distal phalanx. Proximal is to the left.

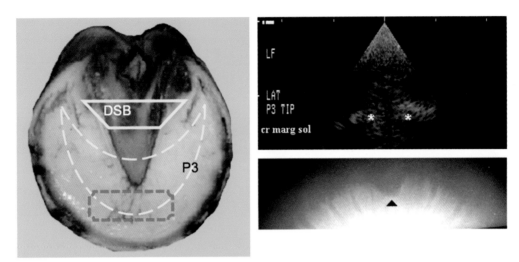

Figure 1.19 Transverse ultrasound image of the crena marginis solearis (crena) seen as a disruption of the hyperechoic margin of the tip of P3. Asterisks indicate the lateral and medial sides of the concavity. Sixty degree dorsopalmar oblique radiograph of the tip of the distal phalanx with a distinct crena marginis solearis (arrowhead); DSB: distal sesamoid bone; P3: third/distal phalanx. Lateral is to the left of the image. (Source: Ultrasound images – Olivier-Carstens, A. (2004) [1]. Reproduced with permission of John Wiley & Sons Ltd.)

Ultrasound-guided navicular bursocentesis can be quite easily performed by positioning the transducer in the sagittal plane over the DSB and placing the needle in the midline proximal to the bulbs of the heel and visualizing the tip of the needle when it reaches the proximal or flexor aspect of the DSB (Figure 1.20). Navicular bursa fluid can be aspirated or therapeutic or contrast agents can be deposited within the NB.

Ultrasonographic Abnormalities

Subsolar gas indicative of a solar abscess or penetrating foreign body will be seen as hyperechoic specks within the solar corium or at the corium–epidermis interface (Figure 1.21). Pedal osteitis changes (Figure 1.22) or marginal fractures of P3 (Figure 1.23) will be seen as an irregular P3 margin. In chronic laminitis (Figure 1.24), where capsular rotation of P3 or distal displacement of P3 relative to the hoof wall has taken place (sinking), the tip of P3 will be seen closer to the solar surface of P3 than normal (less than approximately 10.4 mm in the Thoroughbred). Abscessation or edema of the digital cushion will be seen as a change in its normal echogenicity.

Navicular bursitis with an effusion can be seen as an increase in fluid within the bursa and, depending on the nature of the fluid, will be more echoic if it is a modified transudate or exudate. Adhesions of the DDFT to the flexor surface of the DSB may be seen as increased echogenicity in this area and may be further evaluated dynamically while scanning by flexing and extending the tip of the foot while scanning in a longitudinal plane. If adhesions are present the normal gliding of the DDFT over the DSB will be impaired. Lesions of the DDFT can be seen as a thickening of the DDFT and, if acute or subacute (Figure 1.25), as a decreased echogenicity and loss of fiber alignment. A more chronic lesion will result in a more hyperechoic tendon. Rupture of the DDFT should be seen as an interruption of the normal fiber continuity, possibly with associated inhomogeneous echogenicities around and within it due to hemorrhage.

Doppler ultrasonography can indicate increased or decreased blood flow within the DDFT or DSBIL.

Fractures of the DSB and P3 can be seen as an interruption in the hyperechoic cortical line. Avulsion fractures of the DSB involving the DSBIL may result in a subluxation of the DSB and visualization of the underlying distal aspect of the second phalanx (P2). (Figures 1.26, 1.27). Distal sesamoid impar ligament rupture also result in proximal displacement of the DSB, allowing visualization of the distal condyle of P2 as well as fiber disruption of the DSBIL.

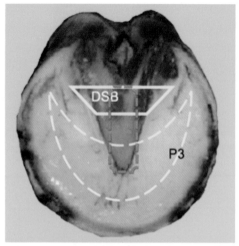

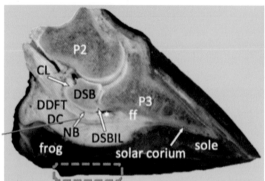

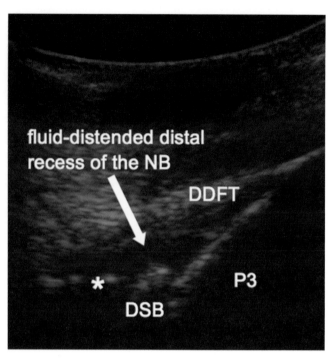

Figure 1.20   Ultrasound-guided injection of the navicular bursa. Sagittal image showing needle (red line) placement for NB arthrocentesis. Sagittal transcuneal ultrasound image showing the tip of the needle placement (*) to inject fluid into the NB. The distal recess of the bursa can be seen filled and distended with anechoic fluid depressing the DDFT solarly. Effusive navicular bursitis would appear similar with possible increase in echogenicity depending on nature of the fluid. DDFT: deep digital flexor tendon; DSB: distal sesamoid bone; NB: navicular bursa. Proximal is to the left.

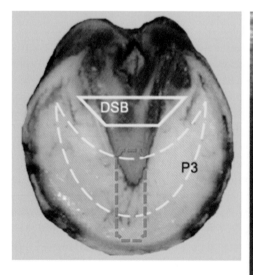

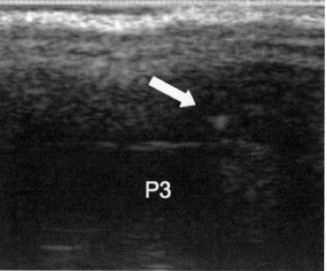

Figure 1.21   Subsolar abscess. Sagittal transsolar ultrasound image showing a focal hyperechoic area (arrow) immediately solar to the hyperechoic tip of P3, indicating subsolar gas. The adjacent dermis appears slightly thicker than normal and bulging slightly. P3: third/distal phalanx. Proximal is to the left.

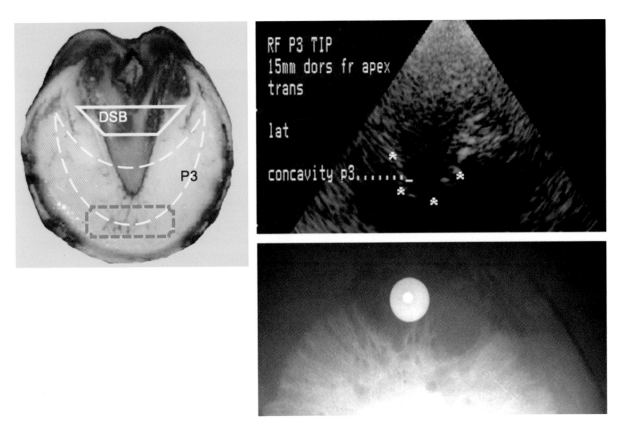

Figure 1.22 Septic pedal osteitis. Transverse ultrasound image of tip of P3; note the irregular hyperechoic areas (fragments – arrowheads) within the hypo- to anechoic fracture bed of the tip of P3. Dorsoproximal–palmarodistal radiograph of the tip of P3 of a clinical case of septic pedal osteitis. Note the irregularly marginated W-shaped radiolucent concavities of the tip of P3; metallic opacity drawing pin present. P3: third/distal phalanx. (Source: Ultrasound images – Olivier-Carstens, A. (2004) [1]. Reproduced with permission of John Wiley & Sons Ltd.)

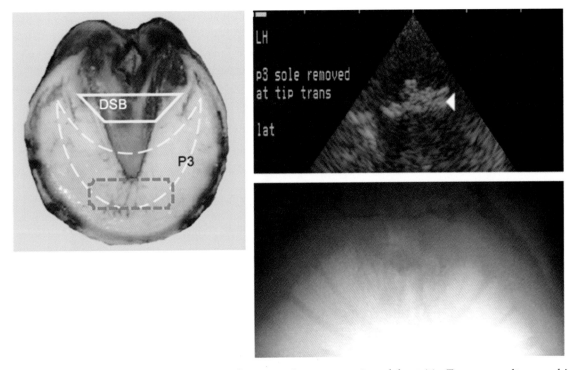

Figure 1.23 Pathological large marginal fracture of P3 secondary to a septic pedal osteitis. Transverse ultrasound image of tip of P3; note the irregular hyperechoic areas (fragments – arrowhead) within the hypo- to anechoic fracture bed of the tip of P3. Dorsoproximal–palmarodistal radiograph of tip of P3 of a clinical case with a pathological large marginal fracture of P3 secondary to chronic subsolar abscessation; note the irregular radiolucency at the tip of the distal phalanx and the bony opacities disassociated from the parent bone. The toe of the sole has been pared away. P3: third/distal phalanx. (Source: Ultrasound images – Olivier-Carstens, A. (2004) [1]. Reproduced with permission of John Wiley & Sons Ltd.)

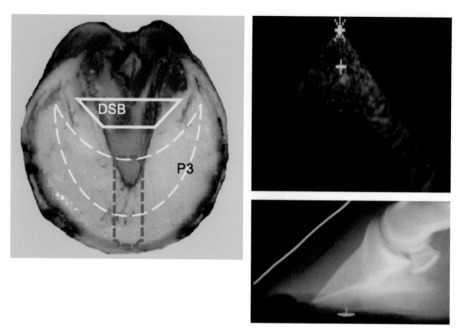

Figure 1.24 Chronic laminitis with capsular rotation of P3. Sagittal ultrasound transsolar image of distal tip of P3 (below cursor); the distance from the tip of the distal phalanx to the sole is 2.4 mm, indicating a marked decrease of the distance of the tip of P3 from the solar hoof surface. The normal distance in the Thoroughbred should not be less than 10.4 mm. Latero-medial radiograph of P3, showing marked capsular rotation of P3; metallic linear marker indicates dorsum of hoof wall of the same case; the magnification corrected distance between the tip of the distal phalanx and the solar margin is 3 mm; metallic drawing pin indicates frog apex. P3: third/distal phalanx. (Source: Ultrasound images – Olivier-Carstens, A. (2004) [1]. Reproduced with permission of John Wiley & Sons Ltd.)

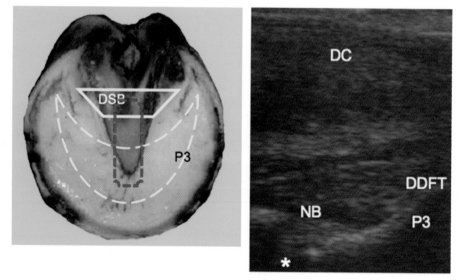

Figure 1.25 Implantational deep digital flexor tendinopathy. Sagittal transcuneal ultrasound image showing a thickening and bulging of the most distal aspect of the DDFT with decreased echogenicity and a decrease in the distinct fiber alignment as seen normally. There also appears to be an increase in the fluid within the distal recesses of the NB and DIPJ (*). DDFT: deep digital flexor tendon; DIPJ: distal interphalangeal joint; NB: navicular bursa; P3: third/distal phalanx. Proximal is to the left.

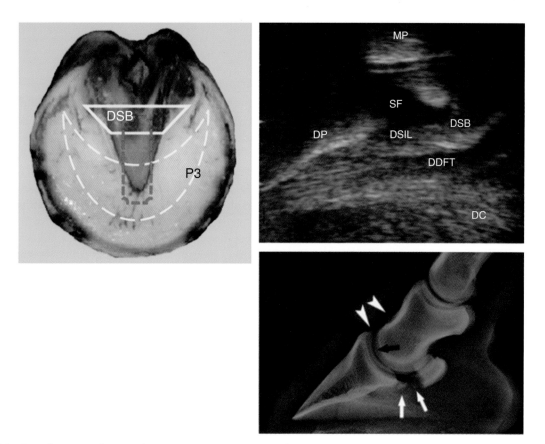

Figure 1.26 Distal sesamoid impar ligament rupture. Sagittal ultrasound image; note the hypoechogenic appearance of the DSBIL with fiber disruption, proximal displacement of the DSB, and a large pocket of synovial fluid (SF). The proximal displacement of the DSB allows visualization of the distal condyle of the second/middle phalanx (MP). The DDFT looks slightly less echogenic than normal but it is within the normal range of size. The architecture and variation in imaging representation is related to the orientation of the probe. LM radiograph of the right hind digit. Note several avulsion fracture fragments (white arrows) and the proximal displacement of the navicular bone as well as the dorsal periarticular remodeling of the DIPJ (arrowhead). The joint space is enlarged dorsally (black arrow) compared with the plantar aspect consistent with DIPJ instability. DC: digital cushion; DDFT: deep digital flexor tendon; DIPJ: distal interphalangeal joint; DP: third/distal phalanx; DSB: distal sesamoid bone; DSBIL: distal sesamoidean impar ligament; NB: navicular bursa. Proximal is to the right and the solar surface is to the bottom of the image. (Source: Ultrasound images – Heitzmann, A.G. & Denoix, J.-M. (2007) [2]. Reproduced with permission of John Wiley & Sons Ltd.)

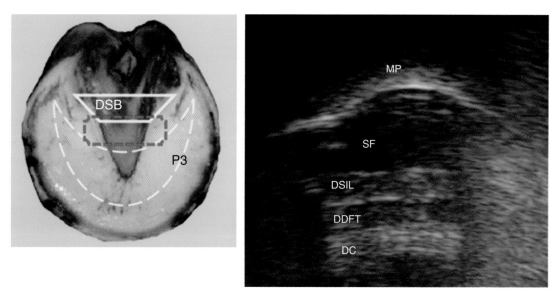

Figure 1.27 The same case as in Figure 1.26. Transverse ultrasound image; proximal displacement of the DSB allows visualization of the distal condyle of the second/middle phalanx (MP) and of a large pocket of synovial fluid (SF). Note the hypoechogenic appearance of the DSBIL. The solar surface is to the bottom of the image. DC: digital cushion; DDFT: deep digital flexor tendon; DSIL/DSBIL: distal sesamoidean impar ligament. (Source: Ultrasound image – Heitzmann, A.G. & Denoix, J.-M. (2007) [2]. Reproduced with permission of John Wiley & Sons Ltd.)

THE PASTERN

The pastern is an area that, with a little practice, can be evaluated very satisfactorily using the ultrasound machines and probes available in general practice. The use of ultrasonography to investigate lesions in this region of the distal limb is particularly applicable as many injuries to the soft tissue structures on the palmar aspect of the limb result in non-specific subcutaneous fibrosis which prevents accurate digital palpation of the area. Certainly, with the advent of ultrasonography, it has become apparent that many cases previously diagnosed as distal sesamoidean ligament desmitis were probably tendinitis of the superficial digital flexor tendon branches or digital sheath abnormalities.

Ultrasonography is particularly useful for "superimposing" the soft tissue components onto the information obtained from radiographs. The fetlock and pastern regions are particularly complex in the arrangement of its soft tissue attachments and the tendons running over the palmar/plantar aspect. Many primarily soft tissue abnormalities will also have bony lesions in this region of the limb and vice versa. Therefore the combination of ultrasonographic and radiographic techniques is frequently indicated. The most diagnostic information is usually obtained by performing a radiological appraisal *first*, followed by ultrasonography.

A variety of transducers can be used to examine these areas. Both sector and linear probes are applicable – the linear probe offers superior longitudinal images, while the small curvilinear probe can scan further distally in the pastern region by placing it between the bulbs of the heels.

Preparation and Scanning Technique

The skin is prepared as for other areas and the transducer applied using couplant gel and a standoff pad. The latter is usually used, as many of the structures being assessed are superficial. However, appreciable subcutaneous edema or fibrosis, common in this region, will provide a "natural" standoff and a separate standoff pad will therefore not be needed.

The ultrasound examination is normally performed with the limb fully weightbearing and the horse standing square. Exceptions to this include placement of the limb further caudally to hyperextend the DIP joint to allow scanning further distally in the pastern region and placement of the foot on a block to improve access and maneuverability of a large transducer.

Because many injuries to this region involve the digital sheath, an ultrasonographic examination of this area should stretch from the proximal limit of the digital sheath (mid-metacarpal) to the bulbs of the heels.

The palmar/plantar pastern region is also divided into a number of levels (1–3) or zones (P1a–c; P2a–b). The distal two zones correspond to the more distal position that can be frequently achieved with a sector probe between the bulbs of the heels, although one of those levels can be obtained with a linear probe if the limb is placed caudally so as to hyperextend the DIP joint. A single longitudinal level is usually achievable with a linear transducer (although a rectal probe may require reversing so that the lead is positioned proximally and does not contact the heels, compromising the required probe orientation).

Because a number of structures pass obliquely across the first phalanx (oblique distal sesamoidean ligaments proximally; SDFT branches distally), oblique 45° views should be used to perform a complete examination. Hence the skin should be clipped to the medial and lateral limits of the pastern when preparing the limb.

A full examination should therefore include transverse and longitudinal images obtained from both the palmar/plantar and oblique probe positions. The contralateral limb should, as usual, be scanned as well, both for comparative purposes but also as many soft tissue injuries in this region can be bilateral.

Line drawings of the normal anatomy are shown in Figure 1.28.

In addition to the digital flexor tendons within the digital sheath (see Chapter 2), both the oblique (ODSL) and straight (SDSL) distal sesamoidean ligaments (DSLs) can be identified ultrasonographically. The straight distal sesamoidean ligament (SDSL) is the most echogenic structure within the pastern region. The ODSLs require oblique views to image them adequately. The short and cruciate DSLs cannot be distinguished but can sometimes be identified adjacent to the joint capsule in oblique views of the palmar/plantar aspect of the fetlock joint.

Beware of the insertion of the SDSL onto the middle scutum on the palmar/plantar aspect of the PIP joint. This area will frequently have a hypoechoic "core" or "sandwich" in the transverse views (P3 only) and a hypoechoic "wedge" with its apex directly proximally in the longitudinal view (Figure 1.29). The hypoechoic region does not usually extend further proximally than the distal limit of insertion of the ODSL. These are normal anatomic variations and should not be mistaken for pathology.

Both proximal and distal digital annular ligaments exist within the pastern; they cannot be easily

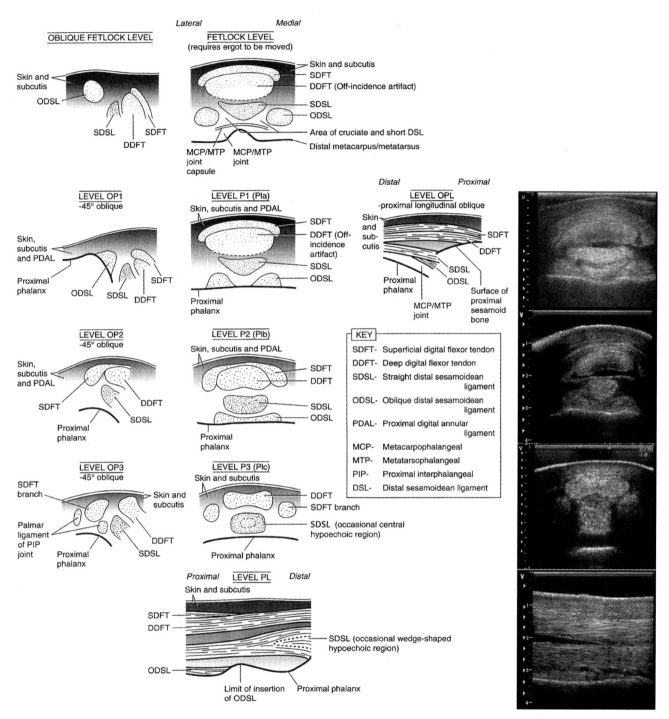

Figure 1.28 Diagrammatic representation of ultrasonographic anatomy of the pastern region. (Source: Smith, R.K.W. & Webbon, P.M. (1997) [3]. Reproduced with permission of Elsevier.)

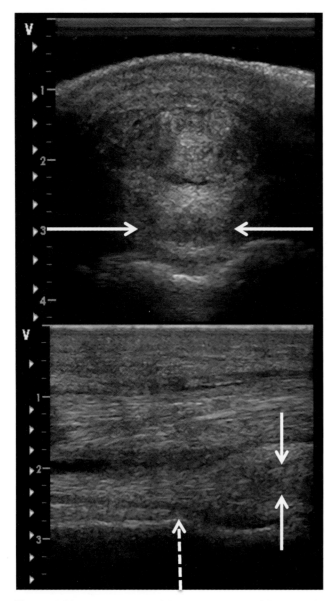

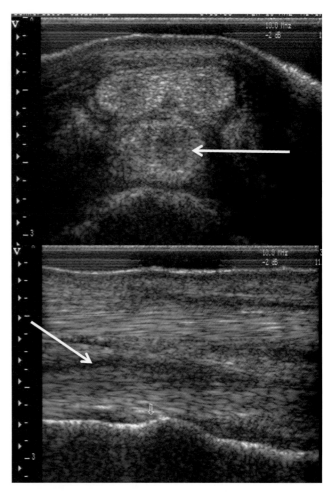

Figure 1.30 Straight distal sesamoidean ligament desmitis. Note the hypoechoic area seen in both transverse and longitudinal images extending further proximally than the limit of insertion of the oblique distal sesamoidean ligaments (open arrow).

Figure 1.29 Appearance of the insertion site of the straight distal sesamoidean ligament (SDSL) via the middle scutum onto the proximal aspect of the middle phalanx. Note the normal hypoechoic area with the distal SDSL/middle scutum (arrows) which should not be mistaken for SDSL desmitis. This hypoechoic area should not extend further than the limit of insertion of the oblique distal sesamoidean ligaments indicated by at bony prominence on the palmar/plantar aspect of the proximal phalanx (dashed arrow).

Ultrasonographic Abnormalities

Most soft tissue injuries to the pastern region are associated with the digital sheath so Chapter 2, relating to this structure, should be consulted in conjunction with this section.

Distal Sesamoidean Ligament Abnormalities

Injury to these ligaments is relatively rare but injuries to either the single straight distal sesamoidean ligament (SDSL) or the one of the paired oblique distal sesamoidean ligaments (ODSL) can be identified ultrasonographically. The changes identified ultrasonographically are similar to those seen in other strains involving tendons and ligaments (enlargement, alterations in echogenicity, shape, and loss of the normal striated pattern) (Figure 1.30). Enlargement of

visualized in the normal horse (they are usually less than 1 mm in thickness) but can be seen when enlarged. The proximal digital annular ligament can be identified proximal to the distal outpouching of the digital sheath, especially medially and laterally where they are more discrete structures grossly.

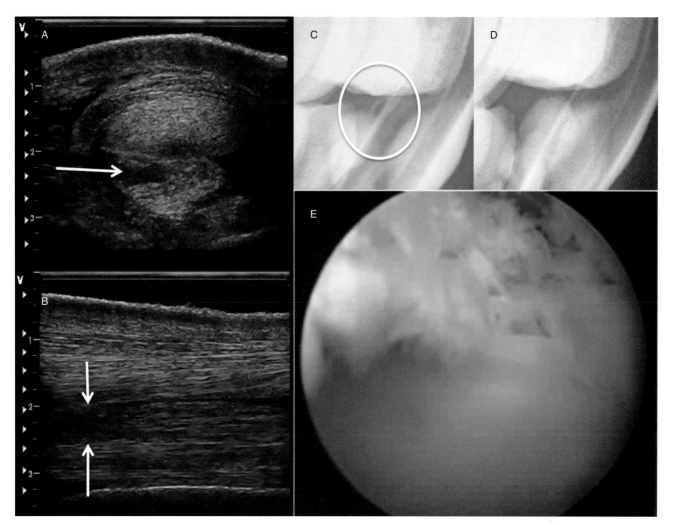

Figure 1.31 (A) and (B) are transverse and longitudinal ultrasound images showing an anechoic asymmetrical lesion in the proximal straight distal sesamoidean ligament (arrows). Its anechoic appearance in this location strongly suggests communication with the adjacent digital sheath, which was demonstrated in this case with contrast tenograms (C circled; contralateral limb for comparison, D) and tenoscopically where torn collagen fibers are seen prolapsed from the ligament (E).

the SDSL is manifested by occlusion of the space between the palmar/plantar surface of the first phalanx/ODSL and the SDSL, and between the DDFT and the SDSL. Once again subcutaneous fibrosis is a common concurrent finding. Many SDSL injuries can tear into the adjacent digital sheath resulting in digital sheath distension and can benefit from tenoscopic debridement (Figure 1.31). Radiography can be helpful in these cases to assess any subluxation of the PIP joint, which can result from damage to the DSLs (or the branches of the superficial digital flexor tendon). Severe disruption of the DSLs can result in proximal displacement of the proximal sesamoid bones (cf. severe SL disruption giving distal displacement). Avulsion fractures can also be present and these will also

be identifiable ultrasonographically where they can be linked to specific structures.

ODSL injury can be difficult to identify ultrasonographically, especially if the injury is restricted to its proximal limits; this requires oblique ultrasonographic views that are difficult to obtain devoid of artifacts. Injuries to these structures have been a relatively common diagnosis on magnetic resonance imaging (MRI), although care must be taken to avoid misinterpretation due to the magic angle artifact associated with the obliquity of these ligaments. Convincing changes on ultrasound include enlargement and heterogeneity, together with overlying subcutaneous fibrosis and enthesophytosis at the base of the proximal sesamoid bones (Figure 1.32).

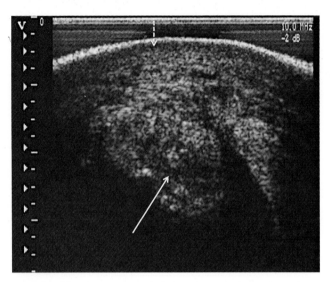

Figure 1.32 Transverse ultrasound image from the palmarolateral aspect of the proximal pastern region showing desmitis of the oblique distal sesamoidean ligament (arrow). This injury is invariably accompanied by subcutaneous fibrosis over the affected ligament (dashed arrow).

Enthesophytosis associated with the insertion of the ODSL onto the palmar/plantar aspect of the proximal phalanx is characterized as an irregularity to the bone surface. Although this is most commonly identified at this site, it is rarely a cause of lameness.

Digital Annular Ligaments

They are poorly visible ultrasonographically and rarely a cause of lameness, but they have been implicated in constriction syndromes similar to the palmar/plantar digital annular ligament (PAL). In these situations, they appear as thickened structures in the subcutaneous space and can be traced to their attachments to the palmar/plantar aspect of the proximal phalanx. Like the PAL, the identification of such thickening does not confirm constriction, which ideally relies on tenoscopic confirmation. These ligaments may also enlarge secondarily to many soft tissue conditions of the pastern region.

A small number of cases have been seen where horses have been presented with acute lameness referable to the proximal pastern region. Both radiography and ultrasonography have shown the presence of avulsion fractures at the origin of the proximal digital annular ligament. As with many avulsion fractures, the ligaments themselves have been largely normal in appearance.

Proximal Interphalangeal Joint Abnormalities

Synovial effusion can be identified ultrasonographically during ultrasonographic evaluation of the distal pastern as an anechoic region deep to the straight distal sesamoidean ligament.

With degenerative joint disease of the PIP joint, osteophytes and enthesophytes can be visualized ultrasonographically around the periphery of a joint by a roughened bone surface echo. Osteophytes can be imaged on the palmar surface at the limits of the anechoic synovial cavity when scanning longitudinally over the pastern.

PIP joint disease can be related to ligamentous damage either of the collateral ligaments or the palmar ligaments (Figure 1.33). Acute injury to these ligaments can be identified by enlargement and hypoechogenicity of the ligaments and occasionally avulsions. More chronic pathology is manifest by osteoarthritis and enthesophytosis, which are best identified ultrasonographically when the transducer is oriented longitudinally and moved over the lateral and medial aspect of the PIP joint.

The articular cartilage of the PIP joint is very thin which makes accurate identification of cartilage lesions difficult. Osteochondrotic lesions are usually identifiable by their bony changes (visible radiographically) rather than the articular cartilage changes *per se*. Ultrasound can be useful to differentiate some of the bony fragments on the palmar/plantar aspect of the fetlock joint, some of which are considered to be osteochondrotic in origin, while others are fractures or ossification within the DSLs.

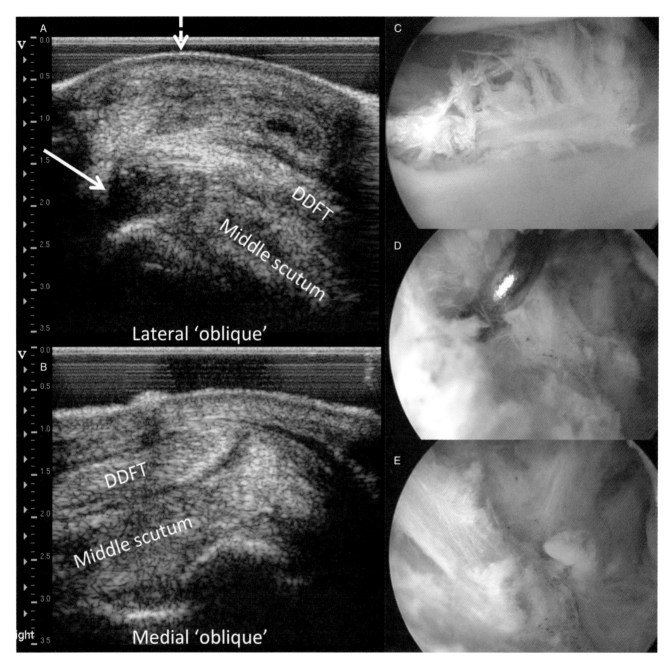

Figure 1.33 Desmitis of the palmar ligaments of the proximal interphalangeal (PIP) joint. Transverse ultrasound images obtained obliquely over the distal pastern region at the level of the proximal interphalangeal joint from the palmarolateral (A) and palmaromedial (B) aspects. The dashed arrow shows the subcutaneous fibrosis and the solid arrow the hypoechogenic palmar ligaments of the PIP joint. This disruption extended into the palmar pouch of the PIP joint, seen arthroscopically (C). An arthroscopic probe could be inserted into the damaged ligament (D). Image E shows the arthroscopic appearance of the ligament after debridement.

RECOMMENDED READING

Busoni, V. & Denoiz, J.-M. (2001) Ultrasonography of the podotrochlear apparatus in the horse using a transcuneal approach: technique and reference images. *Veterinary Radiology & Ultrasound*, 42, 534–540.

Dik, K.J., Boroffka, S., & Stolk, P. (1994) Ultrasonographic assessment of the proximal digital annular ligament in the equine forelimb. *Equine Veterinary Journal*, 26, 59–64.

Dyson, S.J. (1992) Ultrasonographic examination of the pastern. *Equine Veterinary Education*, 4, 254–256.

Heitzmann, A.G. & Denoix, J.-M. (2007) Rupture of the distal sesamoidean impar ligament with proximal displacement of the distal sesamoid bone in a steeplechaser. First published in *Equine Veterinary Education*, 19, 117–120.

Kristoffersen, M. & Thoefner, M.B. (2003) Ultrasonography of the navicular region in horses. *Equine Veterinary Education*, 15, 150–157.

Olivier-Carstens, A. (2004) Ultrasonography of the solar aspect of the distal phalanx in the horse. *Veterinary Radiology & Ultrasound*, 45, 449–457.

Sage, A.M. & Turner, T.A. (2002) Ultrasonography of the soft tissue structures of the equine foot. *Equine Veterinary Education*, 14, 78–283.

Sage, A.M. & Turner, T.A. (2000) Ultrasonography in the horse with palmar foot pain: 13 cases. *Proceedings of the American Association of Equine Practitioners*, 46, 380–381.

Smith, M. & Smith, R. (2008) Diagnostic ultrasound of the limb joints, muscle and bone in horses. *In Practice*, 30, 152–159.

REFERENCES

[1] Olivier-Carstens, A. (2004) Ultrasonography of the solar aspect of the distal phalanx in the horse. *Veterinary Radiology and Ultrasound*, 45, 449–457.

[2] Heitzmann, A.G. & Denoix, J.-M. (2007) Rupture of the distal sesamoidean impar ligament with proximal displacement of the distal sesamoid bone in a steeplechaser. *Equine Veterinary Education*, 19, 117–120.

[3] Smith, R.K.W. & Webbon, P.M. (1997) Soft tissue injuries of the pastern. In: *Current Therapy in Equine Medicine 4; Section 1: The Musculoskeletal System* (ed. S. Dyson). WB Saunders, Philadelphia, 61–69.

CHAPTER TWO

ULTRASONOGRAPHY OF THE FETLOCK

Eddy R.J. Cauvin[1] and Roger K.W. Smith[2]

[1]AZURVET Referral Veterinary Centre, Cagnes sur Mer, France
[2]The Royal Veterinary College, North Mymms, Hatfield, UK

THE FETLOCK JOINT

Preparation and Scanning Technique

High-frequency (7.5–16 MHz) linear array transducers provide optimal information in this area, although a micro-convex probe may be useful to image the distal aspect of the proximal sesamoid bones. A standoff pad may be used to improve probe-to-skin contact and structure alignment. However, with copious amounts of coupling gel, placing the probe directly on the skin provides finer control of the pressure exerted on the skin and underlying structures. Excessive pressure may cause pain, alter the shape of structures examined, and displace an effusion, which may thus be overlooked.

Images obtained in a *longitudinal (parasagittal) plane*, i.e. in a direction perpendicular to the joint space, are easier to interpret, although both longitudinal and transverse planes should be used in combination (Figure 2.1). The joint is examined with the horse weightbearing. Examination starts on the dorsal aspect, then both abaxial aspects are assessed, including the collateral ligaments, abaxial aspect of the sesamoid bones, and the palmar/plantar joint pouch. The intersesamoidean ligament is assessed from a palmar approach through the flexor tendons and proximal scutum (fibrocartilage covering the palmar aspect of the sesamoid bones). The limb is eventually picked up and flexed to evaluate the distal metacarpal/metatarsal joint surfaces.

Ultrasonographic Anatomy of the Normal Fetlock Joint

The ultrasonographic anatomy of the fetlock has been described by Denoix (see Recommended Reading at the end of the chapter). The fetlock is grossly similar in the thoracic and pelvic limbs. "Metacarpus" and "palmar" will therefore be used for both "metatarsus" and "metacarpus", and both "palmar" and "plantar" in the following text.

The structures at the dorsal aspect of the joint are schematically reviewed in Figure 2.2. The distal metacarpus forms a smooth, cylindrical surface, horizontally oriented and separated into two condyles (lateral and medial) by the sagittal ridge. The latter is perfectly round and smooth in longitudinal section and triangular in cross-section (Figure 2.3). The cartilage is anechogenic and regular in thickness. It is thickest over the sagittal ridge (usually 1–1.2 mm) and thinner over the condyles, typically less than 0.7 mm. The mineralized part of the cartilage and underlying subchondral bone cannot be differentiated; they form a smooth, hyperechogenic interface, producing shadowing and reverberation.

Proximal to the condyles and sagittal ridge, the cartilage is interrupted and there is often a small step between the edge of the cartilage and bare bone proximal to it. In this location, bone is actually covered by synovium up to the proximal insertion of the joint capsule. This area may be variable in shape, slightly irregular or concave (Figure 2.4).

The dorsoproximal edge of the proximal phalanx (P1) is rounded and smooth and its proximal articular surface is not visible (Figure 2.3). The dorsomedial and dorsolateral eminences of P1 are slightly convex, the medial one being slightly more prominent. In normal joints, the capsule and synovium are tightly applied against the bone surfaces. With severe effusion, the capsule may be displaced away from the bone surfaces.

The joint capsule on the dorsal aspect of the joint is thick, fibrous (isoechogenic to the extensor tendons),

Atlas of Equine Ultrasonography, First Edition. Edited by Jessica A. Kidd, Kristina G. Lu, and Michele L. Frazer.
© 2014 John Wiley & Sons, Ltd. Published 2014 by John Wiley & Sons, Ltd.
Companion Website: www.wiley.com/go/kidd/equine-ultrasonography

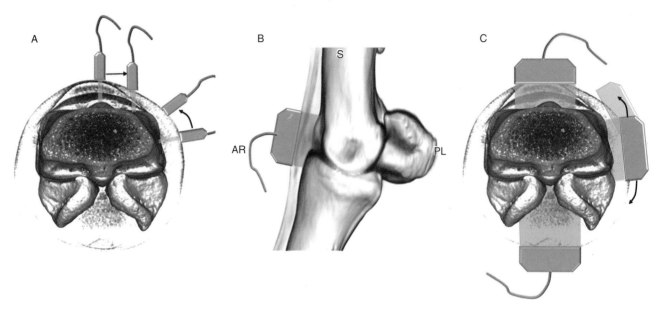

Figure 2.1 Schematic views showing the position of the transducer to examine the four quadrants of the fetlock. Each time the probe is rotated 90° to obtain both longitudinal (A and B) and transverse plane (C) images. In between, oblique positions are often necessary to better visualize the various structures. The examination starts on the dorsal aspect, in a sagittal plane (A and B), bringing the sagittal ridge into view. The probe is then slid sideways into a parasagittal plane (A) to image the medial and lateral condyles. The same examination is performed in transverse planes (C). The abaxial aspects are imaged longitudinally in a frontal plane (A), although 20–30° clockwise and anticlockwise rotation is necessary to align the beam with the ligament branches. In between, oblique positions may be useful to assess all the surfaces. Finally the palmar aspect is imaged in both transverse and longitudinal planes (C).

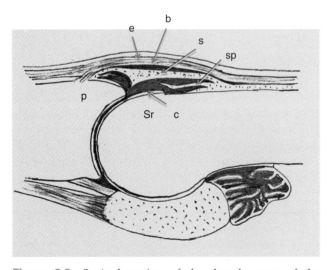

Figure 2.2 Sagittal section of the dorsal aspect of the fetlock. The schematic shows the organization of the soft tissue components. The smooth sagittal ridge (sr) is lined by hyaline cartilage (c); the proximal dorsal aspect of P1 (p), capsule lined with synovial membrane (s), and common (or long) digital extensor tendon (e) are highlighted by the synovial cavities (in black). Note the synovial reflection in the proximal aspect of joint (sp). The subtendinous bursa (b) is not visible in normal horses, little or no fluid is usually visible in the normal joint space.

and elastic (Figures 2.2 and 2.3). It inserts proximally on the metacarpus 3–4 cm proximal to the edge of the condyles and distally on the dorsoproximal aspect of P1, approximately 2 cm distal to the proximal edge. There the capsule adheres to the common/long digital extensor tendon. The lateral digital extensor tendon blends broadly into the fibrous capsule.

Dorsally the synovial membrane forms a transverse ridge, triangular in longitudinal section, which fills the space between the metacarpal condyles and P1. Proximally, the membrane reflects back to form a thin, flat, and transversely oriented fold or pad, normally not visible unless there is marked thickening and/or effusion. No fluid is normally visible.

The thin (2–4 mm) common (or long) digital extensor tendon (CDET) is separated from the joint capsule by a small subtendinous bursa. The latter is virtual and rarely visible in normal horses (Figure 2.3).

Abaxially (laterally and medially), the medial (MCL) and lateral (LCL) collateral ligaments are mere focal thickening of the joint capsule (Figure 2.5). Their borders are therefore difficult to differentiate from the rest of the fibrous capsule in cross-sections. In longitudinal (frontal) planes, parallel striation similar to that of tendons is clearly identified. Each ligament is made

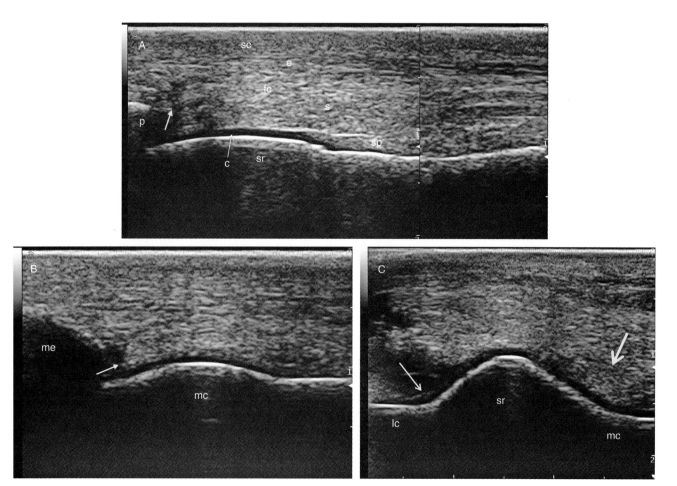

Figure 2.3 (A) Sagittal ultrasound scan over the sagittal ridge, showing the smooth sagittal ridge (sr) with overlying hyaline cartilage (c), the proximal dorsal aspect of P1 (p), synovial membrane (s), and common (or long) digital extensor tendon (e). Note the synovial pad reflection in the proximal aspect of joint (sp). The subtendinous bursa (b) is not visible in normal horses, little or no fluid is usually visible in the joint space. fc: fibrous capsule; sc: subcutaneous tissue. Note the hypoechogenic area within the synovial membrane proximal to P1 (arrow). This is an artifact due to the use of a linear array transducer. (B) A parasagittal image obtained medial to the sagittal ridge shows the round medial metacarpal condyle (mc) and dorsomedial proximal eminence of P1 (me). The cartilage is thinner than on the sagittal ridge. The triangular, dorsal space between the joint surfaces (arrow) is filled by synovial membrane which forms a pointy transverse ridge. (C) Transverse image over the dorsal aspect of the fetlock. The sagittal ridge (sr) and condyles (lateral [lc] and medial [mc]) are smooth and even. The cartilage is clearly visible except over the sides of the sagittal ridge where it is off-incidence. The synovial membrane fills the space on either side of the ridge (thick arrow). A small amount of fluid may be seen on the side of the sagittal ridge, a thin interface is seen between the anechogenic cartilage and the fluid (thin arrow).

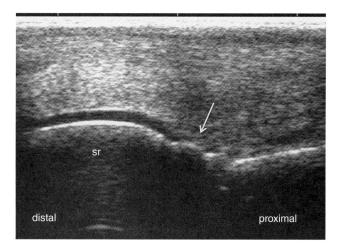

Figure 2.4 Sagittal view of the dorsoproximal aspect of the sagittal ridge, showing a common variation in the normal bony contour, proximal to the sagittal ridge (SR) the cartilage thins out gradually at its edge. The bone surface proximal to it is lined by synovial membrane (arrow). The bone there may be irregular. Although this may be associated with joint disease, it is often encountered in clinically normal horses.

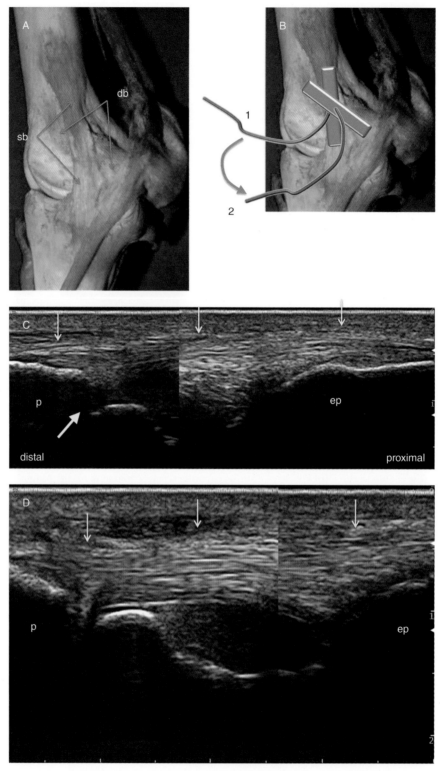

Figure 2.5   (A) Dissected specimen showing the structure of the collateral ligaments (db: deep branch; sb: superficial branch). (B) Positioning of the transducer, along the axis of the metacarpus to image the sb (1) and after an approximate 30° rotation to image the db (2). (C) Ultrasonographic image obtained in a frontal plane (probe aligned with the metacarpus) showing the superficial branch of the collateral ligament (thin arrows) extending from proximal to the epicondyle (ep) to the abaxial aspect of P1 (p). The joint space is indicated by the thick arrow. (D) Rotation of the probe will bring the deep branch into view (yellow arrows). Its extends from the underside of the epicondyle to the proximal edge of P1.

out of two separated branches: a long, superficial part and a shorter, deep part. The superficial branch extends from the metacarpal epicondyle down to the abaxial border of P1, 2 cm distal to the joint space. The deep branch originates dorsodistal to the epicondyle, crosses in a distopalmar direction under the superficial branch and inserts on the edge of P1, close to the joint space. The collateral ligaments are therefore X-shaped and each branch must be examined separately. The transversely oriented collateral ligaments of the proximal sesamoid bones blend into the deep branches of the collateral ligament.

The palmar aspect of the joint is largely hidden by the proximal sesamoid bones (Figure 2.6). The sagittal ridge of the distal metacarpus is visible from the palmar aspect of the limb between them, through the transversely oriented intersesamoidean ligament and hypoechogenic proximal scutum.

The palmar recess of the fetlock joint is a large synovial pouch located between the metacarpus, the apex of the sesamoid bones, the branches of the suspensory ligament, and the distal extremity ("button") of the splint bones (second and fourth metacarpal bones). In normal horses, it is mostly filled by synovial folds and

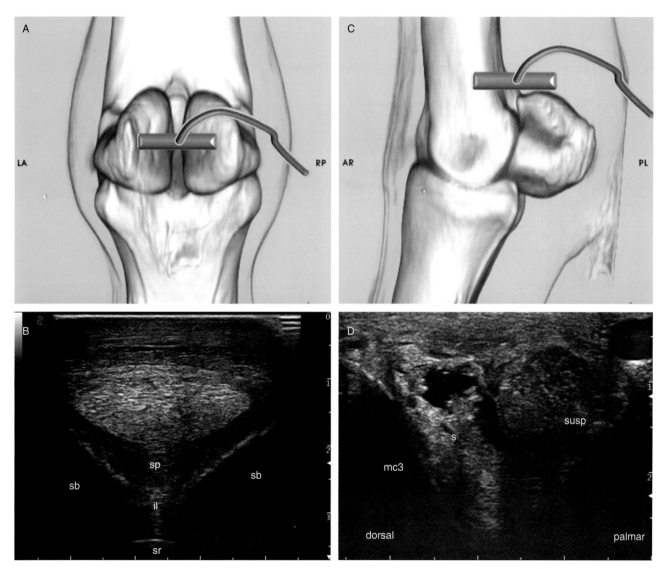

Figure 2.6 Imaging of the palmar aspect. (A) Position of the transducer. (B) Ultrasonographic image with the transducer as in (A). The scutum proximale (sp) forms a thick fibrocartilage, which encloses the sesamoid bones (sb). The intersesamoidean ligament (il) should be homogeneous and regular with a transverse fiber pattern. Only a small width of the sagittal ridge (sr) is visible between the two sesamoid bones. (C) The palmar recess of the metacarpophalangeal joint is imaged through a palmaroabaxial approach. (D) The palmar recess is located in a triangle between the metacarpus (mc3), proximal sesamoid bone, and branch of the suspensory ligament (susp). It is filled with synovial villi (s) with little fluid normally visible.

contains little fluid. It can however fill up with a moderate amount of fluid in clinically normal horses.

ULTRASONOGRAPHIC ABNORMALITIES OF THE FETLOCK

Synovitis/Arthritis

Synovitis refers to inflammation of the synovial lining of the joint. It is a feature of most joint diseases but may occur as a primary entity, particularly in sports and race horses. It should not be mistaken for a non-inflammatory joint effusion ("cold effusion") where abnormal amounts of anechogenic fluid are present without any thickening of the synovium.

Acute synovitis is characterized by mild to severe thickening of the synovial layer of the capsule (this layer is not normally visible) because of edema, vascular hyperemia, and distension of the synovial pouches by joint fluid (Figure 2.7). The inflammation is most obvious dorsoproximally. The dorsal fold ("synovial pad") is displaced away from the articular surface, and becomes hypoechogenic, mildly thickened, and clubbed (Figure 2.8). The palmar pouch contains large synovial villi that rapidly become hypertrophied and fill up the pouch within a matter of days. These form dense, amorphous, and highly vascularized masses.

The fluid is normally anechogenic. In early, acute stages, mildly echogenic, "cellular" and grainy fluid may be present (Figure 2.9). This is typical of hemarthrosis, although this appearance is very similar to that of septic exudate. Bleeding probably occurs through trauma and tearing of the capsule and synovium. The fluid rapidly becomes anechogenic unless recurrent bleeding or sepsis is present, although fibrin clots and pannus may remain adhering to cartilage for several days to weeks (Figure 2.10).

Chronic synovitis may develop as a complication of nearly any fetlock joint pathology that has been left untreated for too long or has not responded to treatment. The echogenicity of the synovial membrane increases, mostly because of a cellular infiltrate and secondary fibroplasia. It becomes more homogeneous and isoechogenic relative to the fibrous capsule. Fibrosis and retraction lead to rounding of the synovial pads and ridges (Figure 2.11).

Assessment of the synovial fold on the dorsal aspect of the joint is usually used as a reference point to confirm chronic inflammatory changes. There currently is a lack of quantitative data regarding what tissue thickness should be regarded as abnormal. Denoix suggests that thickening of the dorsoproximal

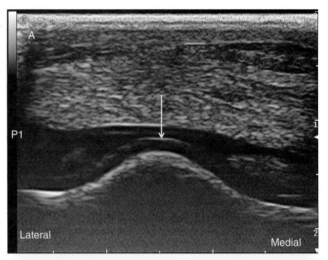

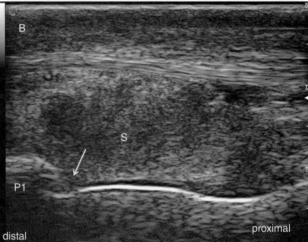

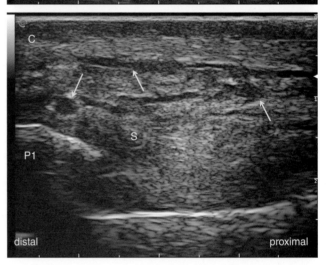

Figure 2.7   Acute synovitis. (A) Dorsal aspect, transverse plane: the dorsal pouch is filled with anechogenic fluid displacing the capsule and extensor tendon dorsally. The cartilage interface is visible (arrows). (B) Dorsal aspect, sagittal plane: the synovial membrane (s) is hypoechogenic, the transverse synovial ridge remains sharp and triangular (arrow). (C) Dorsomedial aspect, parasagittal plane: in severe cases, very enlarged capsular vessels are seen (arrows), edema causes the synovium to appear heterogeneous (s).

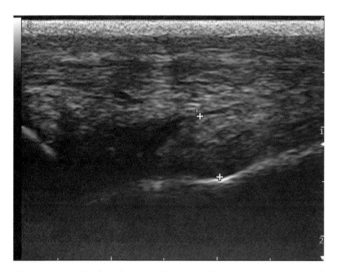

Figure 2.8 Within hours of injury, the proximal synovial pad thickens up and takes on a clubbed appearance (calipers), though remaining hypoechogenic (dorsomedial aspect, parasagittal plane).

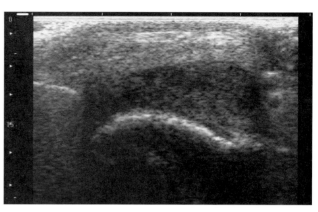

Figure 2.9 Hemarthrosis (dorsomedial aspect, parasagittal plane, distal to the left). The joint fluid is abnormally echogenic and grainy. This may be indistinguishable ultrasonographically from purulent septic fluid.

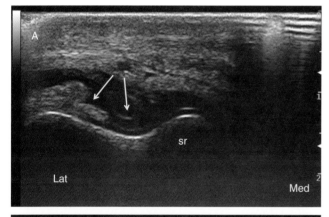

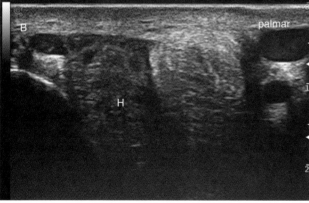

Figure 2.10 In the subacute stage, blood is removed but fibrin pannus or strands (arrows) may be visible (A: dorsal aspect transverse oblique plane), and an organizing hematoma (H) may become visible in the redundant palmar pouch (B: palmar lateral aspect, transverse plane).

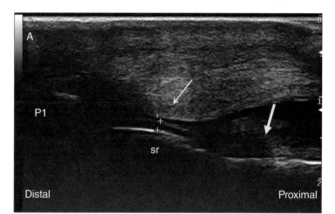

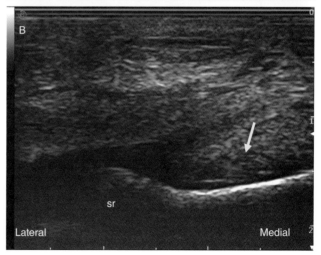

Figure 2.11 In chronic synovitis, the synovial membrane becomes more echogenic and rounded (thin arrow). Note the cartilage interface (calipers) and thickened proximal synovial reflection (thick arrow) (A: dorsal aspect, sagittal plane). The dorsoproximal synovial pad becomes clubbed, forming a dense, mass-like structure most prominent abaxially (arrow) (B: dorsal aspect, transverse plane).

synovial fold over 2 mm in thickness is a sign of inflammation while other authors use a cut-off thickness of 4 mm. (See Recommended Reading for further information.)

In the palmar pouch, hypertrophic villi may be clubbed or rounded or form localized, dense masses, which can eventually undergo fibrocartilaginous metaplasia or even become mineralized (thus producing hyperechoic acoustic shadowing artifacts).

Synovial hypertrophy and hyperplasia can form space-occupying lesions (Figure 2.12). Initially referred to as villonodular synovitis, they are most frequently recognized in the dorsal proximal pouch, where a pressure-induced, smooth, and rounded defect is often observed on the dorsodistal aspect of the metacarpus on radiographs as on ultrasound images. Similar hyperplastic masses are also common in the palmar pouch. This condition is purely inflammatory in horses

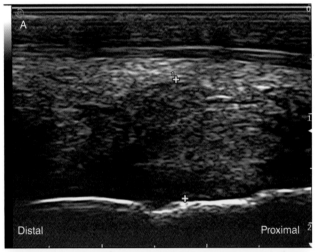

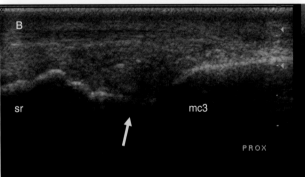

Figure 2.12 Chronic hypertrophic synovitis can produce firm synovial masses (between calipers) filling the joint recesses and displacing the extensor tendons (A: dorsal aspect, sagittal plane). These are space occupying and can eventually cause pressure remodeling of the underlying bone (arrow) (B: dorsal aspect, sagittal plane). mc3: third metacarpal bone; sr: sagittal ridge.

and should therefore be referred to as *chronic hypertrophic synovitis*. In-between stages, spanning from mild proliferation to very large mass formation, are encountered.

Enthesophytes, characterized by an irregular capsule-to-bone interface and the presence of hyperechogenic spurs at the capsule insertions, often occur at the collateral ligament insertions and at the capsule and extensor tendon attachments on the dorsoproximal aspect of P1.

Traumatic Cartilage/Subchondral Bone Injury

Traumatic arthritis of the fetlock can include bone contusion and various degrees of bone surface damage (subchondral bone or cartilage injuries, fragmentation etc.). Although radiography, using specific oblique views, can show the presence of fragmentation or defects, radiographs are often non-diagnostic. Scintigraphy and magnetic resonance imaging (MRI) are the most sensitive techniques to confirm such lesions. Ultrasonography will often confirm the presence of subchondral bone defects or cartilage erosions (Figure 2.13). Lesions located on the palmar part of the metacarpal condyles are hidden from view by the sesamoid bones. Large lesions may, however, be identified with the joint fully flexed. Proximal P1 subchondral injuries are not amenable to ultrasonographic diagnosis. Further investigations may be indicated if there is ultrasonographic evidence of severe synovitis without specific lesions identified on either radiography or ultrasonography.

Osteoarthritis (OA)

Fetlock OA is extremely common. Radiographic signs are often subtle and occur late in the disease process, at a stage where cartilage damage has become irreversible. Ultrasonography provides much earlier signs of joint disease and permits identification of very subtle lesions or new bone production.

Typically the earliest signs of OA include mild to severe synovitis and subtle cartilage changes, with focal or diffuse irregularity and discrete hyperechogenic foci. Thinning is most obvious on the sagittal ridge (although care should be taken not to misinterpret the incidental irregularity frequently seen at the dorsoproximal end of this ridge). Erosions may be visible on the distal aspect of the metacarpal condyles (Figure 2.14). In severe cases, there may be barely any visible cartilage left, the capsule coming into contact with the subchondral bone. Focal defects may result

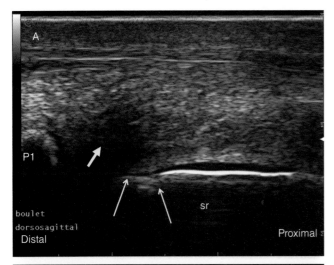

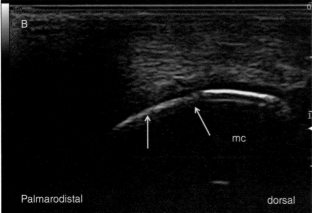

Figure 2.13 Trauma or concussion to the joint surface can cause focal destruction of the cartilage and erosion or chipping of the underlying subchondral bone. (A) A focal defect is seen on the sagittal ridge (thin arrows), with loss of cartilage and direct contact between the synovium and subchondral bone (dorsal aspect, sagittal plane). Subacute synovitis is present with synovial edema and effusion (thicker arrow). (B) Parasagittal view over the distal aspect of the metacarpus (lateral condyle) with the fetlock fully flexed, showing focal loss of cartilage and an irregular defect in the subchondral bone (arrows). mc: medial condyle; P1: proximal phalanx; sr: sagittal ridge.

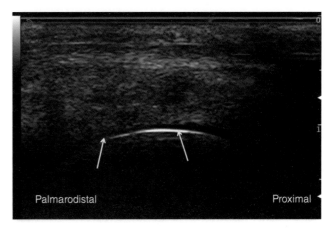

Figure 2.14 Flexed parasagittal view over the dorsomedial aspect. The subchondral bone is smooth and even but there is diffuse thinning of the cartilage (arrows), which appears slightly hyperechogenic.

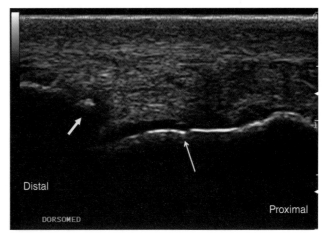

Figure 2.15 There is small chip fragment at the dorsomedial proximal border of the proximal phalanx (thick arrow). A discrete defect is noted in the cartilage and subchondral bone on the medial condyle, at the area of contact of the fragment during hyperextension ("kissing lesion", thin arrow). The rest of the cartilage is slightly irregular.

from contact ("kissing") lesions induced by osteochondral fragments (Figure 2.15). High-frequency probes (12–18 MHz) may be required to provide details of cartilage integrity.

Osteophytes are bony proliferations at the ends of the subchondral bone plate, where the synovial membrane replaces cartilage. True osteophytes form irregular to spiky, hyperechogenic interfaces that protrude into the joint (Figure 2.16). They are typically in alignment with the joint surface. They are most commonly encountered at the dorsoproximal border of P1, along the proximo-abaxial edges of P1 and the disto-abaxial edges of the metacarpal condyles, along the dorsoproximal margin of the cartilage-covered condyles and at the apex of the sesamoid bones. There may also be marked irregularity of the proximal extremity of the sagittal ridge.

Enthesophytes are bony new bone productions within the insertion of capsules, ligaments, or tendons. They may secondary to chronic inflammation, OA, primary capsulitis, or collateral desmitis. They are encountered within the dorso-abaxial insertion of the

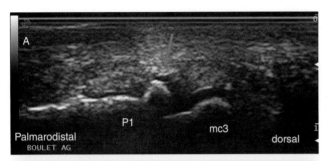

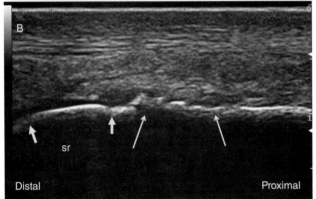

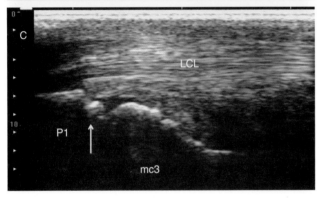

Figure 2.16 Various locations and appearances of osteophytes (A) Spur-like exostosis at the dorso-abaxial proximal border of P1, with remodeling of P1 and of the proximal edge of the metacarpal condyle. (B) Irregular new bone at the dorsoproximal aspect of the sagittal ridge (thin arrows), with focal erosions and areas of hyperechogenicity in the sagittal ridge cartilage (thick arrows). (C) Lateral abaxial articular edge of P1 (arrow), underneath the insertion of the collateral ligament (LCL). mc3: third metacarpus; sr: sagittal ridge.

capsule, and at the collateral ligament attachments on P1 and the metacarpus.

Chronic hypertrophic synovial hyperplasia is usually present in OA, although repeat intra-articular medication with steroid drugs may prevent chronic inflammatory changes, especially in young racehorses, making the diagnosis more difficult to confirm on ultrasound examination.

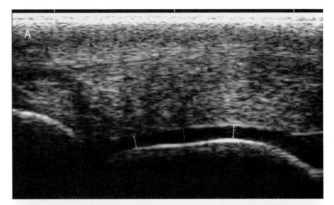

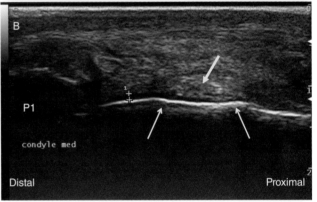

Figure 2.17 (A) Osteochondrosis lesion of the sagittal ridge, with an abnormally flat to slightly concave shape of the subchondral bone and focal thickening of the overlying cartilage (calipers). The latter is regular and anechogenic, there is no sign of dissection. This is usually an incidental finding. (B) More severe OC lesion on the dorsal aspect of the medial condyle, immediately medial to the sagittal ridge. The subchondral bone is irregular and concave, the cartilage is irregular and heterogeneous (arrows). Thickened synovium adheres to the lesion. Note the chronic synovitis.

Osteochondrosis and Cyst-Like Lesions

Subtle erosions or defects in the subchondral bone outline are more readily identified ultrasonographically than radiographically. The extent of the lesion in both longitudinal and transverse planes can be accurately established. Associated soft tissue inflammatory changes, cartilage thinning, and adhesions can also be detected. Depending on the stage of the lesion, it may be difficult to differentiate osteochondrosis from osseous cyst-like lesions, subchondral bone trauma, and erosions secondary to OA.

Osteochondrosis (OC) is common in the fetlock. The most common site is the dorsal aspect of the sagittal ridge where it can span from mild, usually clinically silent flattening of the ridge, to various degrees of subchondral bone defects (Figure 2.17). Lesions may also occur immediately lateral and/or medial to the

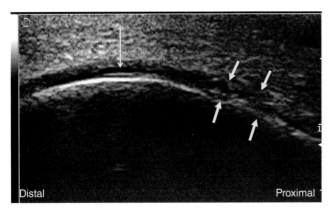

Figure 2.18 Osteochondrosis of the dorsal sagittal ridge. The subchondral bone is irregular proximally with thickened, echogenic, and heterogeneous cartilage (between large arrows). A linear interface (thin arrow) is noted between the deep portion of the cartilage and a shallow subchondral bone defect, characteristic of cartilage dissection (OCD). The cartilage flap is thinned and heterogeneous.

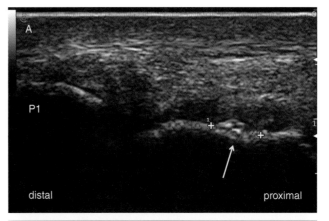

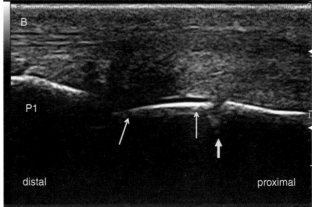

Figure 2.19 (A) Dorsal aspect of the medial condyle, parasagittal plane: mineralization of abnormal cartilage is evidenced by hyperechogenic foci within the thickness of the cartilage (arrow). The synovial membrane adheres to the defect (calipers). (B) Large OCD lesions on the dorsal aspect of the sagittal ridge can give rise to large, smooth mineralized fragments sitting in place (thin arrows). What looks like subchondral bone is actually a partially calcified cartilage fragment. The defect (thick arrow) indicates the real thickness of the cartilage (sagittal plane). The cartilage proximal to the lesion is abnormally thin.

sagittal ridge dorsoproximally. The thickness and echogenicity of the cartilage are both increased in OC, although thinning of the cartilage will eventually occur as a result of fragmentation and fibrillation of the damaged cartilage, and secondary OA. Cartilage dissection (osteochondrosis dissecans or OCD) may be identified by the formation of an interface between the cartilage and bone defect in some cases (Figure 2.18). Hyperechogenic areas of mineralization may be seen within affected cartilage and loose cartilage or osteochondral fragments ("joint mice") may be identified within the joint space (Figure 2.19).

Osseous cyst-like lesions are rare in the fetlock and may occur either in the proximal P1, in which case they are not visible ultrasonographically, or in the distal metacarpal condyle. They appear as localized defects on the subchondral bone surface with associated defects or abnormalities of the overlying cartilage, which becomes thickened, echogenic, and irregular. They may be indistinguishable from subchondral bone injuries.

Osteochondral Fragments

Hyperechogenic fragments are most frequently encountered on the dorsal aspect of the metacarpophalangeal joint. It can be difficult to differentiate between fractures, osteochondrosis, and ectopic bone or mineralization on radiographs. Ultrasonography has been shown to be more sensitive and specific than radiography to identify and localize osteochondral fragments in the dorsal fetlock region. Furthermore, it

can provide useful information regarding the clinical significance of such fragments, including secondary synovitis, OA, or associated cartilage injuries.

Chip fractures occur most commonly at the dorso-medio-proximal eminence of P1 (Figure 2.20), occasionally the lateral eminence. They form hyperechoic, convex interfaces that cast an acoustic shadow, separated from the bone by a hypoechogenic gap. The fragment typically retains the dimensions and shape of the normal eminence with a sharp interruption of the bone interface at the fracture site. There is usually marked soft tissue thickening dorsal to the fracture.

The fragments may be loose within the joint space, moving freely when the joint is manipulated or if pressure is exerted on the capsule with the probe

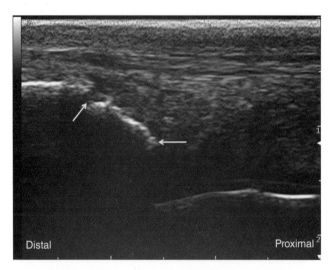

Figure 2.20 Dorsomedial parasagittal image showing a large fragment broken off the dorsomedial eminence of P1 (arrows). There is marked capsule thickening and anechogenic effusion.

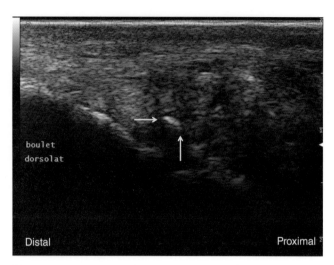

Figure 2.22 Small P1 fragment embedded in the thickened synovial membrane which completely surrounds the hyperechogenic interface (arrows). These fragments may be difficult to see arthroscopically.

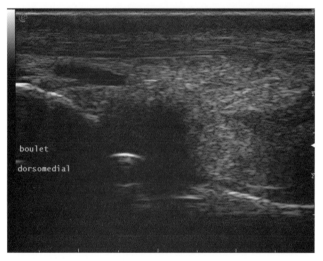

Figure 2.21 Bone fragment (arrows) moving freely within the fluid-distended joint space (dorsomedial aspect, parasagittal plane).

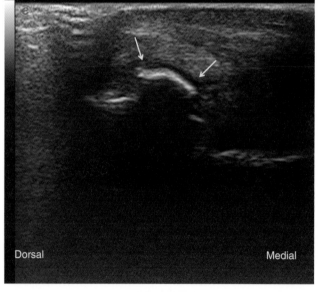

Figure 2.23 Large osteochondral fragment in the synovial membrane, on the dorsomedioproximal aspect of the fetlock (transverse plane). There is a thin, anechogenic layer around the fragment (arrows). This, together with the abnormally large size of the fragment, are suggestive of chondromatosis or continued cartilage growth.

(Figure 2.21). Most fragments are, however, attached to some extent to the capsule or synovium. The extent of soft tissue attachment should be evaluated. These fragments may be embedded within the synovial membrane or capsule (Figure 2.22), which may have important repercussions on the decision for or against surgery and the favored technique for its removal.

Partially mineralized fragments may arise as a result of cartilaginous metaplasia of unclear origin within the synovial membrane (*osteochondromatosis*). Contrary to fracture fragments, they are usually very smooth and rounded, sometimes with a hypoechoic, superficial layer (Figure 2.23). They can be very large, with no corresponding defect being identified on radiographs. They are usually located within the synovium, especially in the dorsal synovial pad. They may be an incidental finding with no associated inflammatory

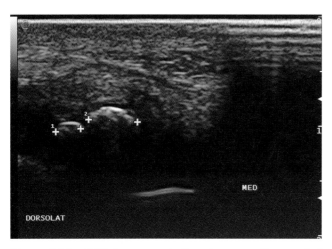

Figure 2.24   OCD fragments (calipers) are usually rounded and smooth and often attached to synovial membrane (transverse plane, dorsolateral aspect).

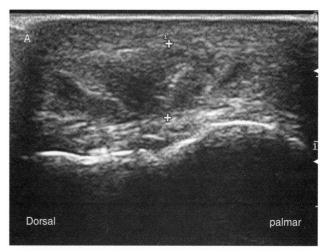

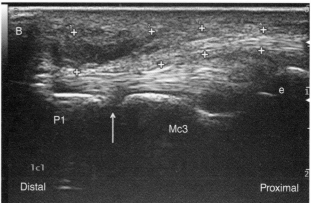

changes, unless there is mechanical interference with the joint. Looking for secondary joint injury, particularly synovitis and cartilage erosions (kissing lesions), helps with establishing the prognosis and with making a decision for or against surgery.

Developmental osteochondral fragments commonly arise at the dorsoproximal aspect of P1. These are often suspected to be a form of osteochondrosis, although there is controversy regarding their pathogenesis. These may be difficult to differentiate from chip fractures (Figure 2.24), unless located within the original defect in the subchondral bone (see Figure 2.19). No associated fracture bed is identified in P1, although a smooth underlying defect may be present. They may be hypoechogenic but most commonly become partially or fully mineralized. Loose osteochondral fragments may be free within the joint cavity. Most commonly, however, they are attached to the capsule by fibrous adhesions or are completely surrounded by synovial membrane. They are often an incidental finding with no other associated sign of joint disease.

Collateral Ligament Desmopathy

Injured collateral ligaments present with features similar to those of injured tendons. Although there may be focal, hypoechoic areas ("core lesions"), the most common ultrasonographic changes include increase in size, diffuse decrease of echogenicity, loss of fiber pattern, and edema (hypoechoic halo) around the ligament (Figure 2.25). These changes may affect one or both branches of the affected ligament. The injuries can be subtle or discrete (Figure 2.26) so the

Figure 2.25   Severe collateral ligament injury in a horse (A, transverse plane; B, frontal plane): there is marked disruption in the fiber pattern with a large, hypoechogenic area in the superficial branch of the lateral collateral ligament (calipers). The branch is enlarged with loss of contours. e: epicondyle of the third metacarpal bone (mc3); P1: proximal phalanx. The arrow indicates the joint space.

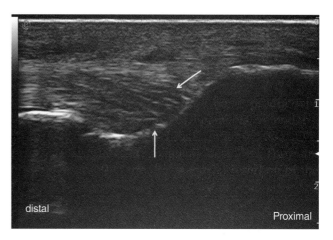

Figure 2.26   More discrete lesion affecting the metatarsal origin of the deep branch (arrows).

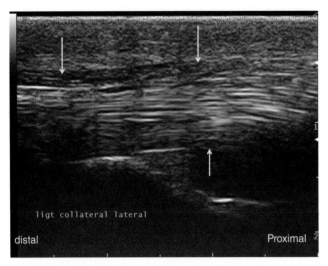

Figure 2.27 Diffuse injury with minimal fiber loss but with marked periligamentous swelling creating a hypoechogenic halo (arrows).

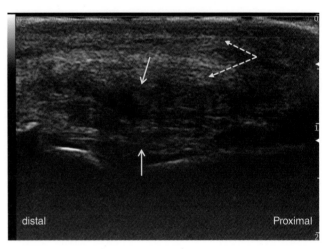

Figure 2.28 Complete rupture of a collateral ligament leads to severe enlargement and loss of the normal striation. The amorphous, hypoechogenic pattern (yellow arrows) is due to hemorrhage; there is marked periligamentous swelling (dotted arrows).

ligaments should be compared with the contralateral limb. In less severe sprains, there is diffuse decrease of echogenicity of the ligament without obvious fiber disruption (Figure 2.27). Periligamentous swelling often forms a hypoechogenic halo around the ligament. There is currently no published data regarding normal thickness for these ligaments.

Rupture may be partial (desmitis) or complete, with both deep and superficial branches being damaged in the majority of cases, although occasionally only one branch is affected. The lateral collateral ligament (LCL) was more frequently injured than the medial one (MCL) in Tenney and Whitcomb's review of 2008. In their study, rupture of both LCL and MCL was not observed but the contralateral ligament usually showed some thickening and heterogeneity (desmitis).

Complete rupture is evidenced by complete loss of fiber alignment and outline of the ligament. Often, the proximal and distal portions of the ligament are still visible, separated by mottled or honeycomb material, representing hematoma and necrosis (Figure 2.28). No longer under tension and crimped, the retracted ends appear hypoechoic and enlarged, with a faint linear fiber pattern. Avulsed pieces of bone may occasionally be seen.

Joint instability may be confirmed by imaging both separation of the ligament stumps and joint space widening while manipulating the joint.

Fibrous tissue gradually replaces the granulation tissue, with associated increase in echogenicity. Ligaments heal via scar tissue formation and rarely recover

a normal linear pattern. However, unlike for flexor tendons, a less than optimal linear pattern is often functional for ligaments. Healing normally takes several months in optimal conditions (stability) and ultrasonography is by far the most accurate way to assess the progress of healing and determine if and when the horse may resume exercise.

As for tendon injuries, chronic desmitis can lead to chronic thickening, poor fiber orientation, and ectopic mineralization (Figure 2.29). Enthesophytes are seen as hyperechoic artifacts near the insertion of the ligaments, or irregular bone-to-ligament transition (Figure 2.30). These are noticed much earlier than on radiographs and they tend to be more irregular and prominent than those secondary to chronic capsulitis.

Desmitis of the Intersesamoidean Ligament (Palmar Metacarpophalangeal Ligament)

This condition is rare but causes severe lameness. Ultrasonography from a palmar approach shows ligament thickening, marked bone–ligament interface irregularity, loss of the normal transverse linear pattern, and hypoechogenic areas within the ligament (Figure 2.31). The space between the two proximal sesamoid bones (PSBs) may be slightly widened. Avulsed fragments are occasionally seen.

Insertional injuries are associated with osteitis of the axial aspect of the sesamoid bones. There may be radiographic evidence of erosion or irregular lucency on

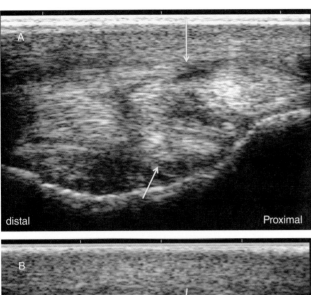

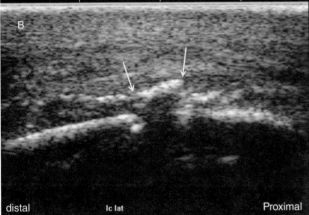

Figure 2.29 (A) Chronic desmitis, as for tendinitis, leads to a poorly organized, hyperechogenic, and thickened ligament (arrows). (B) Ectopic calcifications (arrows) create discrete, hyperechogenic interfaces casting acoustic shadows within the thickness of the ligament scar (transverse view).

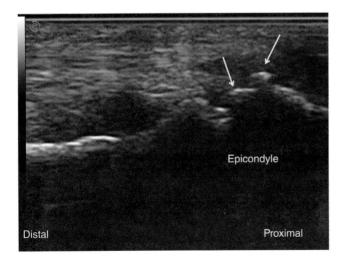

Figure 2.30 Enthesophytes are bone production spikes at the insertion of the ligament branches (arrows).

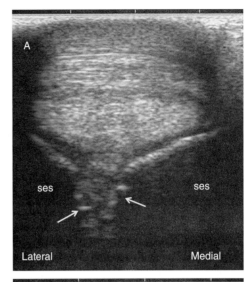

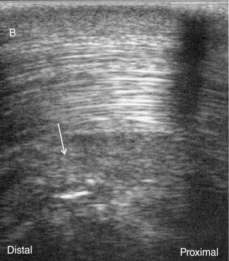

Figure 2.31 Transverse (A) and sagittal (B) ultrasonographs from the palmar aspect of the limb showing severe intersesamoidean ligament desmopathy (arrows), with loss of the striated transverse pattern, decreased echogenicity, and marked irregularity of the bony insertions on the axial surface of the sesamoid bones (ses).

the axial borders of the proximal sesamoid bones, which should be differentiated from osteomyelitis, usually secondary to septic tenosynovitis.

Proximal Sesamoid Bone (PSB) Fractures

The PSBs are parts of the metacarpophalangeal joint, as they are entirely located within the palmar joint capsule. Fractures are readily identified on radiographs but careful ultrasonographic evaluation is often useful to assess the amount of joint damage, rule out or confirm the involvement of the suspensory ligament

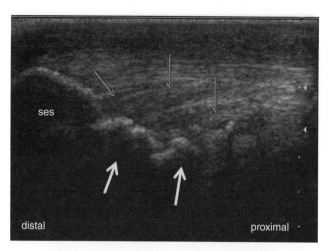

Figure 2.32 Longitudinal image over the abaxial aspect of the proximal sesamoid bone (ses): apical sesamoid bone fracture with several bone fragments tightly attached to the suspensory ligament branch (thick arrows). There is a focal, hypoechogenic lesion in the ligament insertion (thin arrows).

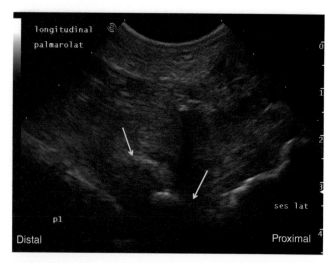

Figure 2.33 Type II plantar P1 fragments (arrows) located dorso-abaxially to the deep distal sesamoidean ligament. This image is obtained in a longitudinal oblique plane from the plantaro-abaxial aspect of the fetlock, distal to the sesamoid bone (ses slat), with a curved array (micro-convex) probe angled slightly proximad.

branches, and clarify the configuration of the fracture. Bony fragments may be loosely attached to the capsule (Figure 2.32) or may have large capsule or suspensory ligament attachments. Such details may be helpful for preoperative planning. Furthermore, associated joint surface damage and associated suspensory ligament branch injury have major repercussions on the postoperative prognosis.

Palmar/Plantar P1 Fragments

Type I (axial) palmar or plantar P1 fragments develop within the capsule between the base of the sesamoid bones and the proximopalmar articular border of the proximal phalanx. They are difficult to visualize ultrasonographically. The more abaxially located type II (*Birkeland*) fragments are commonly very large but rarely cause lameness. Their etiology is uncertain, although there is evidence that they may be fractures occurring at an early age, and they are often discovered incidentally on survey radiographs. They are extracapsular, usually located deep to the origin of the oblique distal sesamoidean ligaments and lateral to the deep distal sesamoidean ligaments without an obvious link to these structures (Figure 2.33). Ultrasonography may be useful when there is suspected pain associated with them, in order to evaluate the location of the fragment(s) in relation to the collateral ligaments, distal sesamoidean ligaments (DSL), and joint capsule.

Articular Long Bone Fractures

These injuries present as linear defects on the bone interface and ultrasound may be useful to establish the three-dimensional (3-D) configuration of a fracture and most importantly to provide information regarding associated cartilage damage, the presence of combined ligament or capsule injury, and potential fragmentation. It is also useful pre- or postoperatively to control adequate reduction of the articular fracture component.

Periarticular Injuries

Tendons, tendon sheaths, and bursae may be affected alone or in combination with joint disease. Ultrasonography is particularly useful to differentiate periarticular swelling (whether due to wounds, tenosynovitis, acquired bursae, abscesses etc.) from joint diseases. Extensor tendinitis is common and is nearly always traumatic in origin (Figure 2.34). Complete rupture may be ascertained, especially in the case of deep wounds. Abscesses, hematomata, and foreign body granulomas are common in the fetlock region. There may also be acquired subcutaneous bursae, either septic or not, that develop over the dorsal aspect of the fetlock. Bursitis of the subtendinous extensor bursa is rare but may be occasionally recognized between the joint capsule and the extensor tendon (Figure 2.35).

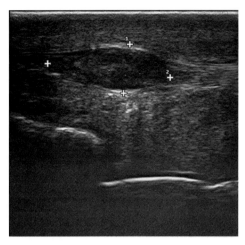

Figure 2.34 Focal extensor tendinitis (long digital extensor tendon) with focal rupture of the tendon (calipers) over the dorsal aspect of the fetlock (sagittal image).

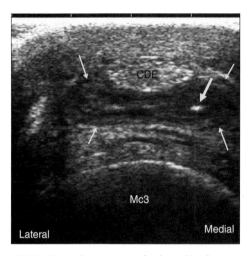

Figure 2.35 Dorsal aspect of the distal metacarpus (Mc3) at the dorsoproximal extent of the fetlock, transverse image: septic extensor bursitis due to a penetrating thorn (thick arrow). Note the thickened subtendinous bursa (thin arrows) containing echogenic, heterogeneous material. CDE: common digital extensor tendon.

Septic Arthritis

Articular contamination and infectious synovitis may be confirmed on ultrasound examination. Wounds and sinus tracts may be traced back to the joint (Figure 2.36). Occasionally, small, strongly hyperechogenic gas bubbles casting comet tail artifacts may be seen in the proximal recesses of the joint.

Initially, especially in foals, the joint fluid remains anechoic, but synovial membrane inflammation and edema are tremendous. As time goes on, the synovial membrane thickens and becomes more echogenic. The joint fluid rapidly becomes heterogeneous and echo-

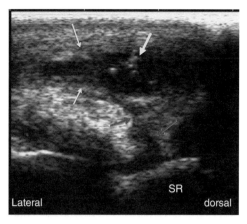

Figure 2.36 Dorsolateral aspect of the fetlock, oblique transverse plane: a hypoechogenic cavity is present in the subcutaneous tissue (thin, yellow arrows), containing small gas bubbles (thick arrow). A fistulous tract runs into the joint through the joint capsule (red arrows). SR: sagittal ridge.

genic, because of fibrin deposits and highly cellular, purulent exudate. When pressing with the probe on the joint pouch, the dense material can be seen to "float" in the fluid. It may be difficult in early cases to differentiate blood from exudate. In such cases, sample collection and cytological examination are warranted. Cartilage erosions and subchondral bone defects (osteomyelitis and osteitis) appear at a more advanced stage of infection.

Foreign bodies (thorns, needles, wires etc.) may be found in the soft tissues, in or around the extensor tendons, within the joint capsule, or even in the joint space. These may cause septic inflammation or may be an incidental finding.

THE DIGITAL FLEXOR TENDON SHEATH

As discussed in Chapter 1 in the context of ultrasonography of the pastern region, ultrasonography is particularly useful for "superimposing" the soft tissue components onto the information obtained from radiographs. The fetlock and pastern regions are particularly complex in the arrangement of their soft tissue attachments and the tendons running over the palmar/plantar aspect. Many primarily soft tissue abnormalities will also have bony lesions in this region of the limb and vice versa. Therefore the combination of ultrasonographic and radiographic techniques is frequently indicated. The most diagnostic information is usually obtained by performing a radiological appraisal *first*, followed by ultrasonography.

As the digital flexor tendon sheath (DFTS) is a major component of the palmar/plantar pastern and extends from the distal quarter of the metacarpal/metatarsal region to the foot, a full ultrasonographic examination should extend over this entire region.

A variety of transducers can be used to examine these areas. Both sector and linear probes are applicable – the linear probe offers superior longitudinal images, while the small footprint curvilinear probe can scan further distally in the pastern region by placing it between the bulbs of the heels (see Chapter 1). The skin is prepared as for other areas and the probe applied using couplant gel and a standoff pad. The latter is usually used, as many of the structures being assessed are superficial. However, appreciable subcutaneous edema or fibrosis, common in this region, will provide a "natural" standoff and a separate standoff pad will not always be needed.

Normal Ultrasonographic Anatomy of the Digital Sheath

In the distal metacarpal and metacarpophalangeal joint regions, the deep digital flexor tendon (DDFT) is considerably larger than the SDFT, which has become a thin structure superficial to the DDFT. In the hind limb, the dorsal surface of the DDFT usually has a well

circumscribed hypoechoic region within it in the proximal limit of the digital sheath (Figure 2.37). This is a normal finding and should not be confused with pathology.

The proximal pouch of the digital sheath contains synovial plicae, which join the DDFT to the digital sheath wall both medially and laterally (Figure 2.38). The lateral synovial plica is usually more substantial

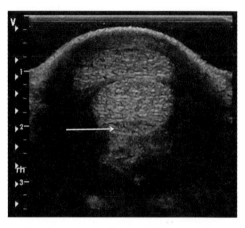

Figure 2.37 Transverse ultrasound image (lateral to the left) from the distal metatarsal region showing the normal dorsal hypoechoic region in the deep digital flexor tendon (arrow) at the proximal limit of the digital sheath. This should not be confused with pathology.

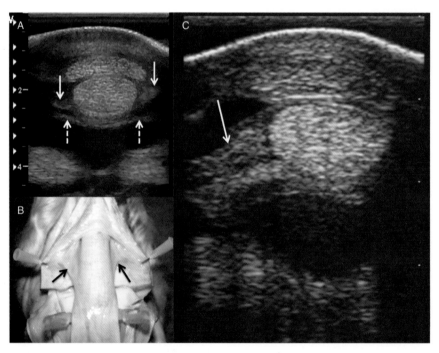

Figure 2.38 Synovial plica of the proximal digital sheath. (A) Transverse ultrasound image from a distended proximal digital sheath showing the medial and lateral plica attaching to the borders of the deep digital flexor tendon (arrows). (B) Gross dissection of the proximal digital sheath showing the plica (black arrows). (C) Thickened plica in a chronically distended sheath with hypertrophied synovium.

and extends further distally than the medial one. Furthermore, the lateral part of the proximal pouch of the digital sheath is more distendable and these factors result in the lateral plica being the most frequently identified. Although not normally visible in the non-distended sheath, they are easily identified with the improved contrast associated with sheath distension. The plicae should not be confused with adhesions, but they are useful structures with which to assess the status of the synovial membrane (i.e. if hypertrophied, etc.) (Figure 2.38).

Immediately proximal to the fetlock joint, there is a loop of the superficial digital flexor tendon which surrounds the deep digital flexor tendon, known as the manica flexoria. Its free distal edge is very thin and enters the fetlock canal when the fetlock joint is extended. Attached to its proximal border is a layer of synovium that is attached to the proximal limit of the digital sheath, thereby dividing the proximal digital sheath into two separate cavities dorsal to the flexor tendons (see Figure 2.38A). The manica flexoria can often be more easily evaluated using longitudinal views in the midline where it can be seen tightly opposed to the dorsal surface of the deep digital flexor tendon with its free end level with the proximal limit of the sagittal ridge (Figure 2.39).

Identification of the palmar/plantar annular ligament of the fetlock (PAL) in normal horses is difficult because of its size (1–2 mm in thickness). However, moving the probe medially or laterally away from the midline (where the annular ligament is joined to the superficial digital flexor tendon by the vinculum) will improve definition of the ligament by the relatively hypoechogenic synovial lining (+/− synovial fluid) between it and the SDFT. If it still cannot be identified with confidence, the probe should be moved further medially or laterally to visualize its attachment to the palmar/plantar border of the proximal sesamoid bones. Further confirmation can be provided by a longitudinally oriented scan (Figure 2.40).

Some authors prefer to assess the PAL by measuring the distance between the palmar/plantar surface of the SDFT and the skin surface, although this distance will include the skin, subcutaneous tissues, PAL, and synovial membrane, all of which can be affected to a variable degree in the condition of annular ligament syndrome. A normal measurement of 3.6 ± 0.7 mm for the ligament alone has been quoted, hence, anything over 5 mm should be considered significant, although this can be considerably larger in normal cob-like horses.

The intersesamoidean ligament is situated between the proximal sesamoid bones although, at the proximal

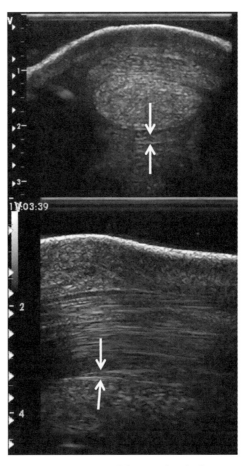

Figure 2.39 Transverse and longitudinal ultrasonographs from the distal metacarpal region showing the manica flexoria (arrows). Note the tapering of the manica flexoria in its normal position terminating distally at the level of the apex of the proximal sesamoid bone.

limit of the intersesamoidean ligament, the surface of the proximal sesamoid bones will *not* be visible on the same transverse image. Longitudinal images are frequently more useful to evaluate this structure adequately. The axial margin of the proximal sesamoid bones can be irregular in normal horses.

The ergot can result in a "blind" region at the base of the proximal sesamoid bones. To avoid missing localized pathology, the ergot can be moved medially/laterally or proximally/distally to minimize this "blind spot".

Immediately distal to the proximal sesamoid bones, the DDFT will frequently contain a central hypoechoic region, which is a normal finding and represents an off-incidence artifact resulting from the change in angle of the DDFT as it passes over the palmar/plantar aspect of the fetlock and its fibrocartilage-like phenotype in this region. Thus different orientations of the

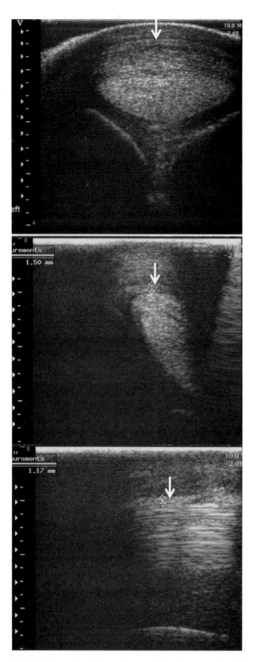

Figure 2.40 Imaging the palmar/plantar annular ligament (PAL). This can be achieved from the midline (top image), in an oblique image, where the attachment of the PAL to the respective proximal sesamoid bone can assist in its identification (middle image), and longitudinally, where the PAL has a stippled pattern in contrast to the adjacent striated pattern of the tendons and often has an "upturned" proximal edge (bottom image).

probe are frequently necessary for comprehensive evaluation of the DDFT in this region.

The distal manica of the SDFT is usually visible deep to the DDFT in the mid-pastern region. The distal palmar/plantar pouch of the digital sheath can be sometimes identified superficial to the DDFT as a thin anechoic region. Its size will vary depending on the amount of fluid within the sheath and frequently it is obliterated by the pressure applied with the probe. In the distal pastern region, synovial plicae are present between the dorsal surface of the DDFT and the dorsal wall of the digital sheath and, again, these should not be confused with adhesions. In the distal digital sheath, the SDFT divides into two branches which lie in the wall of the digital sheath and distally lie dorsal to the bilobed DDFT (see Figure 1.28).

ULTRASONOGRAPHIC ABNORMALITIES

Digital Sheath Abnormalities

Tenosynovitis of the digital sheath can be either non-septic or septic. Septic tenosynovitis is common because it is an area frequently subjected to trauma. Because of the close proximity of the digital sheath to the skin, puncture wounds, even though they may appear innocuous, are often associated with digital sheath penetration and underlying soft tissue trauma, which will frequently lead to septic tenosynovitis. Therefore such wounds should always be imaged ultrasonographically. Large skin defects result in poor contact with the transducer, so that ultrasonography is less applicable in these wounds. Digital exploration and visualization of the damaged structures frequently then offers sufficient information. However, as penetrating injuries can lacerate tendons when the metacarpophalangeal joint is hyperextended, the tendon laceration is frequently at a site different from the wound. Therefore, ultrasonographic evaluation of the area above and below the wound is useful to identify such lacerations.

Sepsis of the digital sheath will produce ultrasonographic signs of marked considerable effusion within the sheath, which can range from anechoic to hypoechoic dependent on the fibrin and cellular content of the fluid. The subcutaneous tissues and synovial membrane will be markedly thickened and edematous (hypoechogenic) and, depending on the duration of the sepsis, adhesions may be seen. The DDFT epitenon becomes thickened, giving rise to a hypoechoic halo around the tendon (Figure 2.41). The original trauma can also damage the tendons and ligaments in the area so the entire length of the digital sheath should be carefully evaluated (Figure 2.42). These changes should be taken as strongly suggestive of digital sheath sepsis although they are not pathognomonic; synovial fluid analysis is still needed to establish a positive diagnosis.

Foreign material can be introduced following traumatic injuries. Ultrasound is very sensitive at detecting

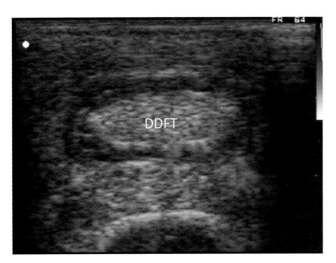

Figure 2.41 Characteristics of an infected digital sheath. The marked inflammation causes a hypoechogenic halo around the tendons (here demonstrated around the deep digital flexor tendon in the mid-pastern region).

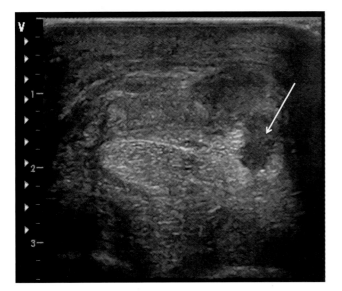

Figure 2.42 Percutaneous trauma to the deep digital flexor tendon in the distal pastern region. Because of the close proximity of the digital sheath and the DDFT to the palmar/plantar aspect of the pastern, injuries to this area are common and ultrasound is invaluable in identifying the nature of the damage to the tendons, especially when the pastern is swollen. This image is of a transverse ultrasonograph from the distal pastern region showing a defect in the medial border of the DDFT (arrow) associated with a barbed wire injury. This had been missed on a previous ultrasound examination because the scan had not been continued sufficiently distally. Note also the marked synovial and subcutaneous thickening and the presence of a hypoechoic region adjacent to the tendon defect, which raises the suspicion of a developing abscess. This was confirmed during surgery.

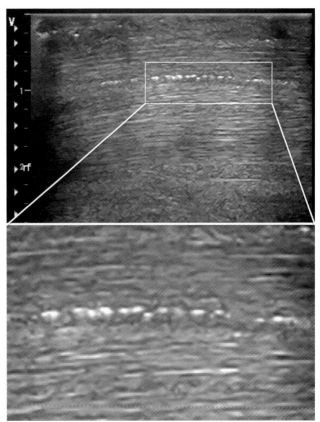

Figure 2.43 Percutaneous laceration in the distal metacarpal region showing a collection of air bubbles between the digital flexor tendons in this longitudinal ultrasound image. Note the presence of scattered hyperechoic foci with small central reverberation artifacts highly suggestive of gas/air and therefore confirming violation of the digital sheath.

foreign bodies, which are all hyperechogenic and cause variable amounts of acoustic shadowing. Radiolucent foreign bodies such as vegetation (including wood) are easily detectable with ultrasonography. Some metal foreign bodies can produce a reverberation artifact depending on their shape and size. Air/gas can be present as a result of aspiration through an open wound (Figure 2.43) where it can be a useful indicator of synovial penetration, it can be iatrogenically introduced (e.g. following nerve blocking), or, least likely, it can be produced by gas-forming bacteria. Air will tend to be present as bubbles, which often collect at the more proximal limits of the viscus/cavity. The shape of the bubbles is responsible for the characteristic ultrasonographic appearance of air – a combination of acoustic shadowing and reverberation artifact.

Non-septic tenosynovitis will produce an effusion that is usually anechoic and is most easily identified especially lateral and medial to the digital flexor tendons in the proximal pouch and/or palmar/plantar to the DDFT in the mid-pastern region often matching the location of the pathology. It need not be associated with lameness where it can be considered an incidental finding. Its presence will often improve the definition of the flexor tendons within the sheath and the digital sheath wall. Such improved definition can also be provided by scanning the area after injection of, for example, local anesthetic into the sheath. Care has to be taken, however, to avoid introducing air at the same time, as this will compromise the image because of the shadowing caused by the air.

Synovial hypertrophy is another common finding. The best assessment of the synovial membrane is made in the proximal pouch region, from either the lateral and medial synovial plicae, or the synovial layer that attaches to the proximal margin of the manica flexoria and extends proximally to divide the sheath into two cavities on the dorsal side of the flexor tendons (see Figure 2.38). This synovial hypertrophy and/or accumulation of fibrinocellular conglomerate can be responsible for synovial "masses" within the sheath (Figure 2.44).

Adhesions are associated with chronic tenosynovitis but accurate identification of adhesions can be challenging to the ultrasonographer. Caution is advised in the interpretation of indistinct borders of the flexor tendons being a sign of adhesions. This change more often reflects the degree of contrast supplied by the synovial fluid and membrane rather than adhesions *per se*. Adhesions can, however, be diagnosed with confidence if

extra echogenic material can be identified within anechoic synovial fluid. Adhesions can be associated with a focal hypoechogenicity on the surface of the tendon to which they are attached, which may be the cause or the consequence of the adhesion (Figure 2.45).

Calcification can occur in the wall of chronically damaged digital sheaths. It will produce a bright hyperechoic reflection with acoustic shadowing deep to it.

Digital sheath abnormalities are often secondary to other soft tissue pathology – either the flexor tendons lying within the sheath or immediately adjacent structures such as the palmar annular ligament (see next section). There is some evidence to suggest that tendon lesions can occur secondary to chronic inflammatory tenosynovitis.

Palmar/Plantar Annular Ligament Syndrome

Annular ligament syndrome (ALS) is characterized by relative constriction of the digital flexor tendons within the PAL. It can be either primary, when it is thought to result from primary desmitis of the PAL following direct or indirect (repeated over-extension of the fetlock joint) trauma, or secondary to other pathology, such as tendinitis, digital sheath tenosynovitis, and septic tenosynovitis.

Changes seen ultrasonographically include variable amounts of thickening of the synovial membrane, PAL

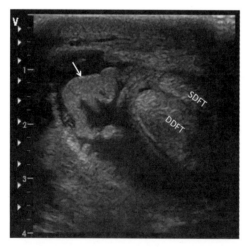

Figure 2.44 Oblique transverse ultrasound image from the palmarolateral aspect of the distal metacarpal region of a horse with marked inflammation of the digital sheath associated with tendon and sheath wall tear. Note the accumulation of fibrinocellular conglomerate within the cavity of the digital sheath.

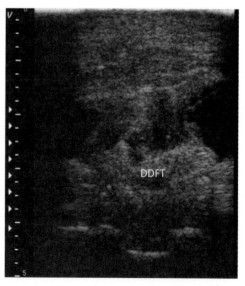

Figure 2.45 Blunt trauma to the deep digital flexor tendon (DDFT) in the distal pastern region showing marked distension of the distal digital sheath but also an adhesion between the damaged DDFT and the palmar sheath wall.

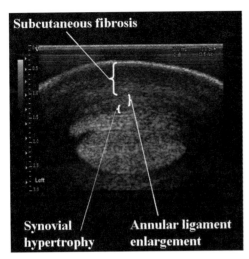

Subcutaneous fibrosis

Synovial hypertrophy

Annular ligament enlargement

Figure 2.46 Transverse ultrasonography of the palmar/plantar fetlock region in a case of annular ligament syndrome. Thickening of the palmar/plantar annular ligament (PAL) is usually accompanied by variable amounts of synovial hypertrophy and subcutaneous fibrosis. True constriction is difficult to establish ultrasonographically which requires either contrast tenography or tenoscopy for a more confident diagnosis.

(which can be hypoechoic if active desmitis is present), and subcutaneous tissues (Figure 2.46). It remains to be seen if prognosis or treatment is altered by the preponderance of each component. Digital sheath tenosynovitis will also be present and if the annular ligament syndrome is secondary, the primary pathology may also be identifiable. ALS has been classified into a number of types based on the characteristics of the soft tissues adjacent to the PAL as well as the PAL itself. Many chronic cases of ALS also have enthesophytosis at the insertion of the PAL which can be identified both radiographically and ultrasonographically (as a roughening to the palmar/plantar border of the proximal sesamoid bones, seen best with the probe positioned longitudinally over the palmar/plantar border).

The treatment for true constriction by the PAL is surgical transection of the PAL. However, it is often not clear if true constriction is present. Treatment is probably more appropriately directed at the primary cause (if identified), although there have been no definitive studies to compare outcomes of different intrathecal pathologies treated with or without PAL transection; current data suggest transection is not associated with improved prognosis when primary pathology is present. Consequently, the authors believe that PAL transection should only be considered after evaluation of the digital sheath tenoscopically, when passage of

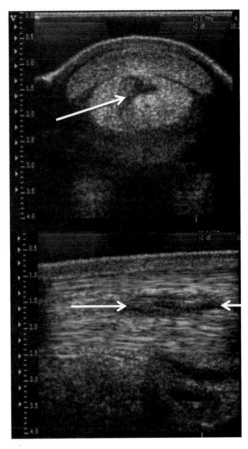

Figure 2.47 Deep digital flexor tendinopathy. Midsubstance tendinopathy of the deep digital flexor tendon (DDFT) can affect the DDFT in any part of the digital sheath (or distally within the foot) but is rare proximal to the digital sheath. These are transverse and longitudinal images from a case of deep digital flexor tendinopathy present in the proximal digital sheath (arrows). The location of the lesion can usually be identified clinically by a painful response to digital palpation and distension of the digital sheath, proportionately greater in the region of the lesion.

the arthroscope through the fetlock canal can give information on the degree of constriction and primary pathology can be identified.

Deep Digital Flexor Tendon Abnormalities

Strain Injuries

Strain injuries of the DDFT can occur anywhere within the digital sheath but are often centered at the fetlock. The lesions vary widely in appearance from a considerably enlarged tendon containing multiple hypoechoic foci to more focal hypoechoic/anechoic lesions (Figure 2.47). Very anechoic lesions may represent communication of the lesion with the cavity of the digital sheath.

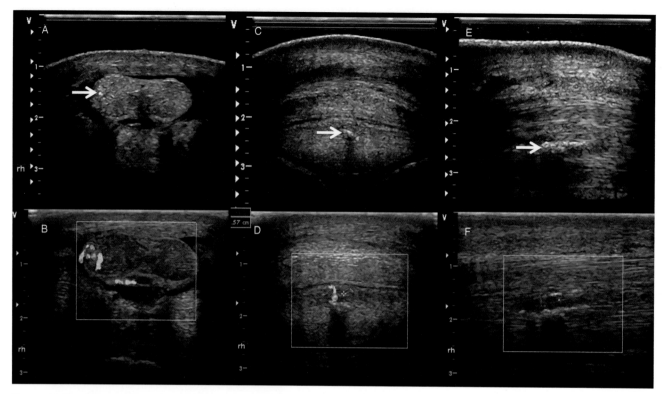

Figure 2.48 Chronic deep digital flexor tendinopathy characterized by mineralization of the tendon. (A) A transverse ultrasonograph from the distal pastern region where pin-point mineralization is difficult to identify (arrows). This can be improved by tilting the transducer (off-incidence artifact) or by the use of Doppler imaging for those cases with an active signal (B). Transverse (C) and longitudinal (E) images show mineralization in the deep digital flexor tendon at the level of the proximal sesamoid bones. While this lesion is very evident ultrasonographically, mineralization is not always clinically significant, although the concurrent presence of a Doppler signal ((D) and (F)) suggests greater significance.

As with any intra-sheath tendinitis, there will frequently be an accompanying tenosynovitis, which tends to be more severe if the lesion communicates with the digital sheath. Lameness is often severe and unremitting.

Mineralization/ossification is a frequent consequence of chronic injury in this tendon. This will show up as a brightly hyperechoic reflection which will cause a variable amount of acoustic shadowing, depending on its size and degree of mineralization/calcification (Figure 2.48). Not all mineralizations are significant but those associated with lameness often have a positive Doppler signal (Figure 2.48).

Tears

Damage to the surface of the deep digital flexor tendon can occur as a variant of over-extension injury to the tendon. These most frequently occur on the abaxial borders of the deep digital flexor tendon in the region of the metacarpophalangeal joint (i.e. usually in the fore limb), presumably due to excessive forces during over-extension which compress the tendon and cause a pressure-induced rupture. Due to their intrasynovial location and being bathed in synovial fluid, healing does not occur and these lesions will persist, relatively unaltered for long periods of time, being responsible for persistent digital sheath tenosynovitis and lameness. The larger of these tears are visible ultrasonographically as an irregular tendon border or defect in the proximal digital sheath (Figure 2.49). However, many are difficult to identify and require high-quality machines and experienced operators. Even then many lesions are focal and centered at the level of the ergot, which is a "blind spot" on ultrasound scanning, and are best seen immediately distal to the proximal sesamoid bone using oblique views (Figure 2.50). Hence a negative finding on ultrasound does not rule out the presence of a tear. Contrast tenography (undertaken at the same time as diagnostic analgesia) can demonstrate the presence of a tear immediately distal to the proximal sesamoid bones in the standing horse as a

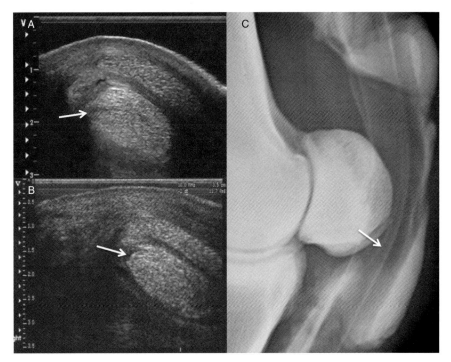

Figure 2.49 Marginal deep digital flexor tendon (DDFT) tears. (A) An oblique transverse image from the distal metacarpal region showing a deep longitudinal tear in the lateral margin of the DDFT (arrows). Deep tears are readily visible ultrasonographically. Less deep tears can be more difficult to identify ultrasonographically because the tension in the tendon under weightbearing load tends to close the defect. Greater sensitivity in detection can be provided by using non-weightbearing views proximal to the fetlock, oblique imaging (B), or contrast tenography where the tears are visible distal to the proximal sesamoid bones in the weightbearing limb (C – arrowed). This area should also be evaluated ultrasonographically to identify tears in the weightbearing limb – see Figure 2.50.

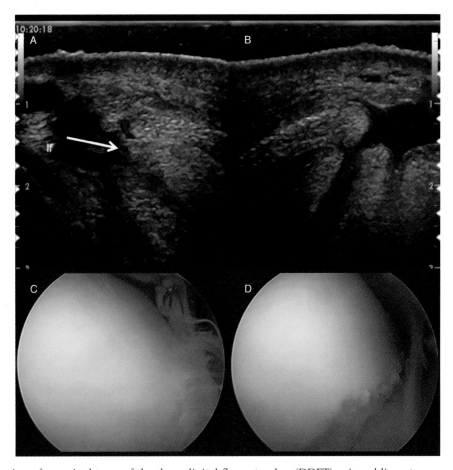

Figure 2.50 Detection of marginal tears of the deep digital flexor tendon (DDFT) using oblique transverse images immediately distal to the proximal sesamoid bones. (A) shows the "lateral" oblique with the transducer centered over the palmarolateral aspect of the proximal pastern where irregularity of the lateral margin of the DDFT is evident in contrast to the medial border (B). The corresponding tenoscopic images (lateral to the right) are shown before (C) and after (D) debridement.

line of contrast overlying the space-filling lucency of the DDFT in a lateromedial view (Figure 2.49). However, tenoscopy is still the gold standard for evaluation of these tears and is recommended to identify occult tears. It should certainly be considered in those cases of tenosynovitis that have failed to respond or recurred after intrathecal medication.

Treatment consists of tenoscopic debridement, although the prognosis remains poor. Open closure is not advised, as this has also been associated with a poor prognosis.

Penetrating Injuries

Penetrating injuries to the DDFT are most common in the pastern, are very common and can have potentially disastrous consequences if the extent of the soft tissue pathology is not recognized early. The ultrasonographic abnormalities range from very subtle palmar/plantar defects to penetrations extending from the palmar/plantar surface dorsally (see Figure 2.42). The digital sheath may not necessarily develop sepsis as a consequence of either the penetrating body entering the DDFT without significantly contaminating the sheath, or blunt trauma damaging the DDFT without actually entering the sheath. Consequently, superficial wounds in the pastern region should be evaluated ultrasonographically, especially if the lameness is severe or persists. DDFT lesions may not always be visible ultrasonographically immediately after bruising, so follow-up examinations are recommended if lameness and/or digital sheath effusion persists.

Adhesions can subsequently develop attaching to the tendon defects. The affected tendon can become septic. In such cases the ultrasonographic characteristics are a rapidly destructive (hypoechoic/anechoic lesions) condition with minimal tendon enlargement. Alternatively, appreciable tendon defects within the digital sheath may not show healing in the long term, with anechoic defects persisting.

Superficial Digital Flexor Tendon Abnormalities

Strain Injuries

The fetlock region of the SDFT is usually spared injury in equine superficial digital flexor tendinitis. However, severe cases of tendinitis, or, more commonly, re-injury, can result in tendinitis of the branches of the SDFT or that portion of the SDFT immediately proximal to the branches within the pastern region. Hence if SDFT tendinitis is identified ultrasonographically within the pastern region, the mid-metacarpal region should also be examined.

To image the branches satisfactorily, the probe needs to be moved to the medial and lateral aspects of the limb (45° oblique) where the branches appear as comma-shaped structures which enlarge as their insertion point is approached. The ultrasonographic changes include enlargement, heterogeneous echogenicity, and subcutaneous fibrosis (Figure 2.51). Estimation of size is made by comparing with the other branch of the same limb and with the branches on the contralateral limb, which has to be made at the same level on the limb.

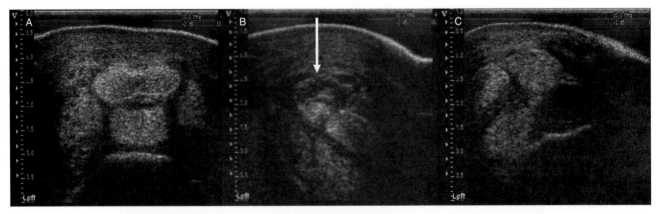

Figure 2.51 Tendinoapthy of the lateral branch of the superficial digital flexor tendon (SDFT) in the pastern region. Because of the oblique angle of the branches, the lesion is not readily visible in midline transverse images (A – lateral to the left) although asymmetrical subcutaneous fibrosis is evident. Full visualization requires movement of the transducer to the palmarolateral aspect of the pastern (B) where the branch can be seen as hypoechoic (arrow) and covered with subcutaneous fibrosis in contrast to a normal medial branch (C).

Manica Flexoria Tears

Most commonly in the hind limb, partial or complete tearing of the attachments of the manica flexoria (the loop of tendon that surrounds the deep digital flexor tendon) to the medial and lateral borders of the superficial digital flexor tendon results in secondary tenosynovitis and lameness. This injury is difficult to identify ultrasonographically. If the manica flexoria is absent this suggests severe disruption. Tilting the transducer to the plantaromedial and plantarolateral aspects of the limb can sometimes also demonstrate a disruption in the attachment of the manica to the tendon. However, in more subtle cases, instability of the manica can be identified using a longitudinally oriented transducer in the midline at the level of the apices of the proximal sesamoid bones in the weight-bearing or non-weight-bearing limb (Figure 2.52) or

else by the use of contrast tenography which can be undertaken at the same time as diagnostic analgesia and where the manica is outlined very effectively by contrast (Figure 2.53). However, as for deep digital flexor tendon tears, a negative ultrasonographic examination does not rule out this as a cause of digital sheath tenosynovitis associated with lameness, and tenoscopy represents the gold standard for diagnosis. The best therapeutic approach consists of complete removal of the manica flexoria tenoscopically.

Intersesamoidean Ligament Abnormalities

Injuries to this structure are probably more common than have been previously recognized. These include small avulsion fractures from the axial borders of the

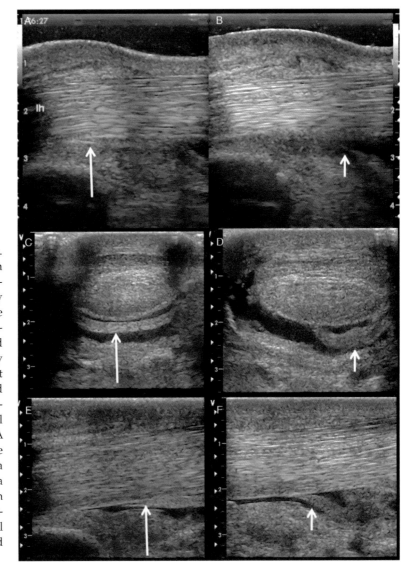

Figure 2.52 Tearing of the manica flexoria. Images A, C, and E are normal, for comparison with abnormal images B, D, and F. A more specific diagnosis can be achieved preoperatively using a midline longitudinal image from the distal metatarsal (metacarpal) region where displacement of the torn manica can be identified as a thickened, proximally displaced and wavy manica which is indicative of tearing (B – short arrow). This is compared to the straight and tapering normal manica which terminates distally at the level of the apex of the proximal sesamoid bone, as in the contralateral limb (A – long arrow). Non-weight-bearing transverse (C,D) and longitudinal (E,F) scans produce a degree of displacement of a normal manica flexoria thereby improving its identification (C,E). Taking this normal degree of displacement into consideration, this can also be useful to identify more proximal displacement and thickening associated with tearing (D,F).

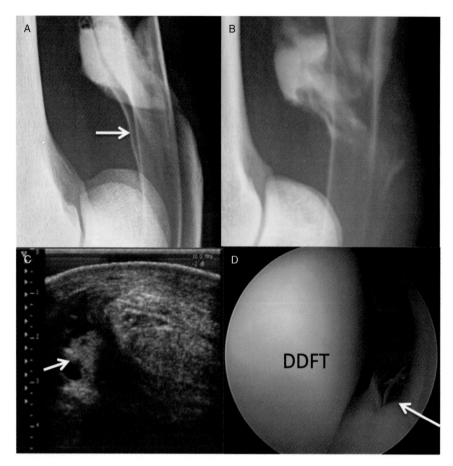

Figure 2.53 Tearing of the manica flexoria. (A,B) Contrast tenography where the contrast agent is introduced at the same time as diagnostic analgesia. A normal manica position is represented by parallel contrast columns tapering together at the level of the apex of the proximal sesamoid bones (A – arrow) in contrast to an absence of the columns in a fully displaced manica flexoria (B). (C) Oblique transverse image from the distal metatarsal region showing echogenic material lateral to the digital flexor tendons. This is a non-specific sign of digital sheath pathology. (D) The tenoscopic appearance of the torn margin of the superficial digital flexor tendon (arrows) in a case of a torn manica flexoria.

proximal sesamoid bone (often more easily identified ultrasonographically than radiographically because of the superimposition of the axial border on the distal metacarpus in most projections), and abscessation (localized hypoechogenicity) within the ligament (associated with septic osteitis of the axial border of the proximal sesamoid bones, first described by Wisner *et al.* 1991). Arthroscopy and tensocopy can also be used to evaluate the surfaces of the intersesamoidean ligament.

RECOMMENDED READING

Barclay, W.P., Foerner, J.J., & Phillips, T.N. (1987) Lameness attributable to osteochondral fragmentation of the plantar aspect of the proximal phalanx in horses. *Journal of the American Veterinary Medical Association*, 191, 855–857.

Dabareiner, R.M., White, N.A., & Sullins, K.E. (1996) Metacarpophalangeal joint synovial pad fibrotic proliferation in 63 horses. *Veterinary Surgery*, 25, 199–206.

Denoix, J.M., Jacot, S., Bousseau, B., & Perrot, P. (1996) Ultrasonographic anatomy of the dorsal and abaxial aspects of the equine fetlock. *Equine Veterinary Journal*, 28, 54–62.

Denoix, J.M. (2000) *The Equine Distal Limb: Atlas of Clinical Anatomy and Comparative Imaging.* Iowa State University Press: Iowa.

Dik, K.J., Dyson, S.J., & Vail, T.B. (1995) Aseptic tenosynovitis of digital flexor tendon sheath, fetlock, and pastern annular ligament constriction. *Veterinary Clinics of North America: Equine Practice*, 11, 151–162.

Redding, W.R. (1993) Evaluation of the equine digital flexor tendon sheath using diagnostic ultrasound and contrast radiography. *Veterinary Radiology and Ultrasound*, 34, 42–48.

Steyn, P.F., Schmidt, D., Watkins, J., & Hoffman, J. (1989) The sonographic diagnosis of chronic proliferative synovitis in the metacarpophalangeal joints of a horse. *Veterinary Radiology*, 30, 125–127.

Tenney, W.A. & Whitcomb, M.B. (2008) Rupture of collateral ligaments in metacarpophalangeal and metatarsophalangeal joints in horses: 17 cases (1999–2005). *Journal of the American Veterinary Medical Association*, 233, 456–462.

Vanderperren, K., Martens, A.M., Declercq, J., Duchateau, L., & Saunders, J.H. (2009) Comparison of ultrasonography versus radiography for the diagnosis of dorsal fragmentation of the metacarpophalangeal or metatarsophalangeal joint in horses. *Journal of the American Veterinary Medical Association*, 235, 70–75.

Weaver, J.C.B., Stover, S.M., & O'Brien, T.R. (1992) Radiographic anatomy of the soft tissue attachments in the equine metacarpophalangeal and proximal phalangeal region. *Equine Veterinary Journal*, 24, 310–315.

CHAPTER THREE

ULTRASONOGRAPHY OF THE METACARPUS AND METATARSUS

Roger K.W. Smith[1] and Eddy R.J. Cauvin[2]

[1]The Royal Veterinary College, North Mymms, Hatfield, UK
[2]Centre d'Imagerie, Cagnes sur Mer, France

PREPARATION AND SCANNING TECHNIQUE

It is important that the animal be examined fully weightbearing, so that tendinous structures are under tension, but it is still useful to examine the non-weightbearing limb, to assess the motion of each tendon in relation to the others and for Doppler evaluation. Careful preparation of the skin is paramount, including fine clipping, cleansing with scrub and alcohol, and liberal application of coupling gel. The area to be clipped depends on the structure being imaged but for complete evaluation of all the palmar soft tissue structures in the metacarpal/metatarsal region, the skin should be clipped from the palmar carpal region, immediately distal to the accessory carpal bone, to distal to the ergot of the fetlock and over the whole palmar aspect of the metacarpus from the palmaromedial to the palmarolateral aspect of the third metacarpal bone. As regards the hind limb, clipping should involve the metatarsal region up to the chestnut. It is possible in some thin-haired horses to perform ultrasonography without clipping, but the image quality will always be impaired and an acceptable image may not be obtained in all cases.

High-frequency (7.5–16 MHz) linear array transducers are preferred. A micro-convex transducer may be useful to image the proximal aspect of the suspensory ligament in some horses. A standoff pad is recommended to improve probe-to-skin contact and permit imaging of the whole width of the tendons in one picture. However, some operators prefer to scan the limb without the use of a pad, particularly with high-frequency transducers. In this case it is important to image the limb from both palmar and palmaro-abaxial approaches to obtain a comprehensive assessment of the palmar limb structures.

Images should be obtained in both transverse and longitudinal orientations in sagittal and, when appropriate, frontal planes. For reference purposes, several systems have been described to determine the level of the section on the limb. None of these has gained general acceptance. The most widely used system consists of dividing the metacarpal region into three equal tiers from the carpometacarpal joint to the proximal extent of the fetlock palmar annular ligament, termed I to III from proximal to distal. The metatarsal region is divided into four zones (I–IV), with zone I extending from the tuber calcis to the tarsometatarsal joint. Each of these zones is further divided into two halves, named a and b. The palmar fetlock area (at the level of the palmar fetlock annular ligament) is usually referred to as IIIc area in the fore limb, and IVc in the hind limb. It may be simplified further by dividing the distance from the level of the carpometacarpal joint to the distal sesamoid bones into seven regions (1–7) in the fore limb, and nine in the hind limb. This system has the advantage of not depending upon the animal's size but is based on specific anatomic features (Figure 3.1). One alternative is to measure the distance from the distal palpable border of the accessory carpal bone or from the tuber calcis to the ultrasonographic section examined. Although this only allows comparisons in the same individual, it may be useful for follow-up.

Typically the examination is performed from proximal to distal, first in transverse and then in longitudinal planes, followed by any appropriate oblique views. The authors start by examining the superficially

Atlas of Equine Ultrasonography, First Edition. Edited by Jessica A. Kidd, Kristina G. Lu, and Michele L. Frazer.
© 2014 John Wiley & Sons, Ltd. Published 2014 by John Wiley & Sons, Ltd.
Companion Website: www.wiley.com/go/kidd/equine-ultrasonography

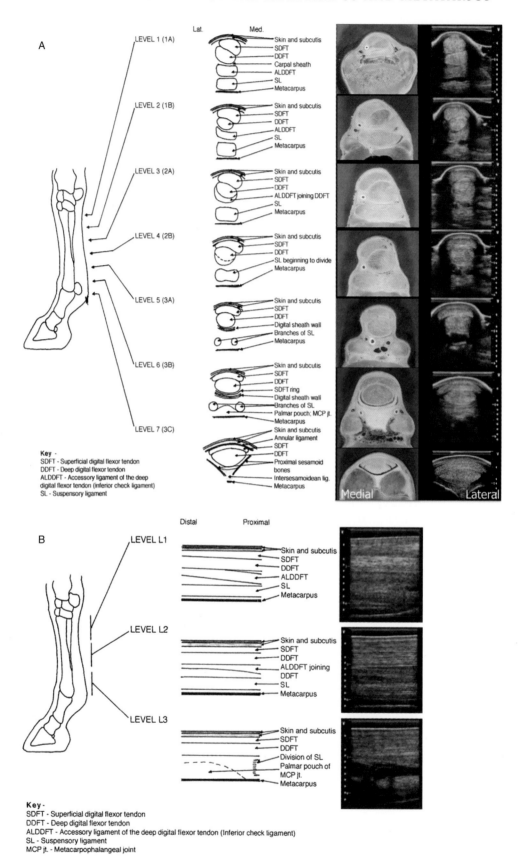

Figure 3.1 Normal ultrasonographic anatomy of the palmar aspect of the metacarpus. (A) Transverse ultrasonographic images are presented on the right side with comparative anatomy sections in the center and diagramatic representation of the location of the transverse images on the left side for the seven standard levels (labeled 1 (Ia) to 7 (IIIc)). (B) Longitudinal midline sagittal images in the three thirds of the palmar metacarpus. (Source: David R. Hodgson, Catherine McGowan and Kenneth McKeever (2013) *The Athletic Horse*, Second Edition. Reproduced with permission of Elsevier.)

located flexor tendons in both planes, then the deeper structures by altering the settings on the machine, and then finally the branches of the suspensory ligament. Off-incidence views are routinely obtained by tilting the transducer by about 10 degrees as an assessment of tissue organisation post injury. The limb may eventually be picked up and flexed to evaluate relative motion of the tendons and for Doppler imaging of pathology.

ULTRASONOGRAPHIC ANATOMY

The anatomy of the equine "tendon" region has been reviewed in numerous texts (see Recommended Reading at the end of the chapter). The anatomy in this region is fairly simple, although with improving imaging, subtle anatomic details may be evaluated.

General Appearance of Tendons and Ligaments (Figure 3.2)

In normal tendon, the striation imaged in sagittal or frontal plane scans does not correspond to fiber fascicles as such but rather to discrete interfaces between groups of fascicles. Nevertheless an even, regular striation aligned with the long axis of the tendon and that extends over the width of the image closely follows the

underlying microstructure, and has been used recently to provide objective assessment of structure, so-called *ultrasound tissue characterization* (van Schie *et al.*, 2003). The use of higher-frequency probes (>12 MHz) permits finer assessment of intraparenchymal structure. Tendon is highly vascularized but the endotenon (loose connective tissue separating the collagenous fascicles) and associated vessels are usually of a caliber well below the resolution of diagnostic ultrasound (0.1–0.5 mm). Endotenon and the size of fiber bundles do participate in the heterogeneity of tendon parenchyma and account in part for the differences in appearance between different tendons.

Thoracic Limb

There are four tendons running over the palmar aspect of the metacarpus (Figure 3.1), respectively from palmar (superficial) to dorsal (deep) they are the superficial digital flexor tendon (SDFT), deep digital flexor tendon (DDFT), accessory ligament of the DDF muscle (ALDDF), and tendon of the third interosseous muscle, more commonly referred to as the suspensory ligament (SL). These will be reviewed in turn.

Superficial Digital Flexor Tendon The SDFT arises from the SDF muscle in the distal antebrachial area, 2–6 cm proximal to the accessory carpal bone. The musculotendinous junction is short but progressive, extending from the distal quarter of the caudal

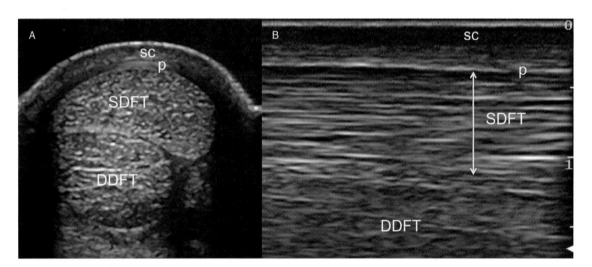

Figure 3.2 Ultrasonographic appearance of tendons and ligaments. (A) In transverse sectional images, the tendon parenchyma typically appears as a "granular" substance with densely packed echogenic dots. The subcutaneous tissue (sc) is hypoechogenic, the paratenon and overlying fascia form a hyperechogenic interface (p). (B) The tendon parenchyma (SDFT) presents in the long axis (sagittal scans) as series of coarse, transversely oriented hyperechogenic interfaces. These do not represent fibers as such, but rather discrete interfaces between fiber packets. They are separated by anechogenic spaces that represent endotenon (loose, vascularized connective tissue) but also non-resolvable (visible) fibers located before the next visible interface. DDFT: deep digital flexor tendon; SDFT: superficial digital flexor tendon.

antebrachium to the proximal edge of the accessory carpal bone (ACB). Hypoechogenic muscle strands extend more distally in young horses, often well into the carpal canal. The accessory ("radial check" or "superior check") ligament of the SDFT (ALSDFT) lies dorsomedial to the SDFT. This thick ligamentous structure derives from an atrophied SDFT radial head and runs obliquely from the caudomedial aspect of the radius at the level of the chestnut to join the SDFT proximal to the ACB.

Within the carpal region, the SDFT is oval to circular in cross-section. In the proximal metacarpal region, it becomes oval in cross-section and is located palmaromedial to the DDFT. Its dorsal aspect becomes concave as it runs distally, giving it an asymmetric crescentic shape with a thicker medial border and a tapered lateral margin in zone II. It is located at the palmar aspect of the limb in this region. It becomes gradually thinner dorsopalmarly in the distal metacarpus and fetlock regions, with its dorsal surface tightly molded around the palmar contour of the DDFT. In zone IIIb (distal part of the metacarpus) it forms a thin membranous ring around the deep digital flexor tendon called the manica flexoria, which arises from the sharp lateral and medial edges of the SDFT. The SDFT eventually divides into two branches in the proximal pastern area, distal to the ergot, each branch blending into the middle scutum (fibrocartilaginous palmar capsule of the proximal interphalangeal joint) before inserting on P2. The SDFT is a very dense, echogenic tendon, although it is normally less echogenic than the DDFT and ALDDFT. Using high-frequency ultrasound transducers (14 MHz and over), fiber fascicles can be differentiated within the parenchyma. In longitudinal sections the tendon has a regular, continuous striated pattern, and the striation is similar to that of the DDFT.

Deep Digital Flexor Tendon   The DDFT also originates in the distal antebrachium from the reunion of three muscular heads (humeral, ulnar, accessory or radial), and its musculotendinous junction occurs at the same level as that of the SDFT. The muscle heads, along with that of the SDFT, are indistinguishable ultrasonographically. The DDF tendon is initially dorsolateral to the SDFT in the carpal region, where it runs over the medial surface of the ACB. It lies dorsal to the superficial digital flexor tendon in the middle and distal thirds of the metacarpus. It is oval in shape throughout its path. In the pastern area, it becomes bilobed, with a "ski goggle" appearance on ultrasonographs. It becomes flatter in the foot over the palmar aspect of the navicular bone before inserting on the palmarodistal surface of the distal phalanx.

Accessory Ligament of the Deep Digital Flexor Tendon   The ALDDFT ("inferior check ligament") originates on the palmar aspect of the carpus as a distal continuation of the palmar carpal ligament. It joins the deep digital flexor tendon at the mid-metacarpal region (zone II). The junction is very gradual from Ia to IIb. As the fibers of the ALDDFT are oblique, this creates a *hypoechogenic, off-incidence artifact* within the dorsal aspect of the DDFT in this area (see level 4 or zone 2b in Figure 3.1). The ALDDFT is rectangular in cross-section in zone I (levels 1 and 2), then becomes crescent shaped in zone II (levels 3 and 4), curving mostly around the lateral aspect of the DDFT. The carpal flexor tendon sheath forms a hypoechoic space between the deep digital flexor tendon and the ALDDFT down to their junction, and it occasionally contains some anechogenic fluid.

Suspensory Ligament   The SL is formed by the atrophied interosseous III muscle and its tendon. It is anatomically divided into three portions: the proximal origin (3–5 cm long), the body (main portion down to the bifurcation), and the two branches (lateral and medial). The origin and body of the suspensory ligament are examined from the palmar aspect of the limb, whereas the branches should be examined in turn from the lateral and medial aspects. Some muscle fibers remain in young horses, giving the ligament a mottled, hypoechoic appearance. These decrease with age. Most studies have showed that the SL in normal horses is always bilaterally symmetrical at any level. The SL originates from the proximal palmar cortex of the third metacarpal bone. It blends into the joint capsule of the carpometacarpal joint and palmar carpal ligament. The origin and body of the SL are rectangular in cross-section, although the origin is divided into two distinct lobes separated by hypoechogenic tissue. These two lobes are molded on slightly concave surfaces on the palmar aspect of the third metacarpal bone, separated by a variably prominent bony ridge. The body of the SL has a coarser, less echogenic appearance than the tendons. The SL divides in the distal third into two branches (medial and lateral). Each inserts over the abaxial surface of the ipsilateral proximal sesamoid bone. The medial branch is slightly larger than the lateral, but both are initially oval and then become "tear-drop'" in shape more distally. The striated pattern is regular over the whole length of the SL, although it is not uncommon in adults and older horses to have a thinner or less marked striation at the origin and proximal body.

The SL branches are continued distodorsally by the extensor branches which course dorsally and join distally in the pastern onto the common digital extensor tendon. The sesamoid bones are an integral part of the suspensory apparatus, as are their distal ligaments (see Chapter 1); these should therefore ideally be examined along with the SL, as combined injuries can occur.

Extensor Tendons In the metacarpal area, the extensor tendons are easily identified over the dorsal aspect of the third metacarpal bone (MC3). They have a less echogenic, coarser appearance than flexor tendons. They are very thin and flat in cross-section. The common digital extensor tendon (CDET) is dorsolateral proximally and dorsal in the distal half of the metacarpus. The lateral digital extensor tendon (LDET) is much smaller, round in cross-section, and situated laterally in the proximal metacarpus. It runs obliquely to follow the lateral edge of the CDET in the distal third, where it becomes flatter and blends into the fetlock joint capsule.

Other structures of interest include the surface of MC3, which is round and smooth, and the overlying periosteum which is clearly visible as an echogenic, 2–3 mm thick, homogeneous layer over the hyperechogenic bone interface. The splint bones (MC2 and MC4) can also be assessed; they are smooth and regular in long-axis scans and sharply rounded in cross-section. The interosseous ligament between the splint bones and the third metacarpal bone forms an echogenic space between the bone interfaces, and it may become mineralized in older horses.

All tendons, except in sheathed areas, are surrounded by a thin connective tissue layer (the paratenon). This is less echogenic than the tendon parenchyma and contains numerous small vessels that are not visible in normal tendons. The carpal and digital flexor tendon sheaths are described in other sections of this text.

The neurovascular bundles are well identified in this part of the limb (Figure 3.3). In the proximal and mid-metacarpal area, the medial palmar artery and nerve are identified close to the skin surface on the dorsomedial aspect of the DDFT, while their lateral counterpart is more deeply located. The corresponding veins are large and located in the connective tissue space dorsal to the ALDDFT/DDFT and palmar to the SL; the lateral vein is more axially located. In the distal third of the metacarpus, the bundle becomes more superficial and follows the abaxial borders of the DDFT before running over the abaxial aspect of the proximal sesamoid bones palmar to the SL branch insertions.

The nerves have a coarse striated pattern on long-axis scans, and the veins are anechogenic with thin, deformable walls, although echogenic whorls of

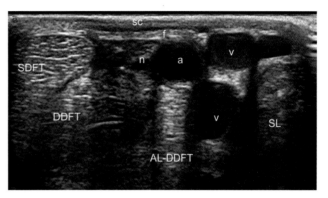

Figure 3.3 Transverse ultrasonograph from the mid-metacarpal region using a palmaromedial approach. Neurovascular structures are identified: the medial common palmar nerve (n) has coarse, grainy appearance; the associated artery (a) is round in section with a thick wall, the veins (v) are easily compressed due to thin walls. Note the thick superficial fascia (f). AL-DDFT: accessory ligament of the deep digital flexor tendon; DDFT: deep digital flexor tendon; sc: subcutaneous tissue; SDFT: superficial digital flexor tendon.

moving blood cells may be identified in the veins and larger arteries. Venous valves are usually visible and can be seen to open and close. The arteries are of much smaller caliber and have thicker walls. They are always round in cross-section. The arterial flow is fairly regular with indistinct systolic surges in Doppler studies.

Pelvic Limb Differences

The overall arrangement is similar to that of the thoracic limb. It is virtually the same in the distal two thirds of the metatarsus. Proximally, the SDFT is slightly flatter than in the fore limb, and is located plantarolateral to the DDFT as it runs over the plantar aspect of the tuber calcis of the fibular tarsal bone (*calcaneus*) and overlying long plantar ligament. This tendon has a poorly developed or no muscular body in the hind limb. The DDFT is formed by the fusion of two tendons: the lateral digital flexor tendon (LDFT) is the main part, running medial to the tuber calcis over the sustentaculum tali and then plantar to the distal tarsal bones; the medial digital flexor tendon (MDFT) is a small, cylindrical tendon that runs over the medial aspect of the tarsus, in a groove within the medial collateral ligament, before joining onto the medial border of the LDFT in the proximal quarter of the metatarsus to form the DDFT *sensu stricto*.

Contrary to what has long been described in many anatomy textbooks, there is an ALDDFT in the hind limb also. It is often rather thin but varies between individuals from an aponeurotic membrane to a fully developed ligament, similar to that encountered in the thoracic limb. It arises from the short plantar ligament of the tarsus.

Finally, the SL in the hind limb has a large lateral head that fills the concave space over the medial aspect of the 4th metatarsal bone. It is more triangular to oval shaped than in the fore limb. The intercapital ridge on the plantar proximal metatarsus is rather less marked than in the fore limb. A strong deep fascia is sometimes identified plantar to the SL, running between the heads of the two splint bones. In the proximal part of the metatarsus, it may be difficult to image the SL from a plantar approach, because of the prominent and axially concave head of the fourth metatarsus (lateral splint bone). It may therefore be useful to use a plantaromedial approach. In some horses, the use of a microconvex array transducer can be very useful to image the origin of the ligament as the pie-shaped beam easily encompasses the whole cross-section of the SL from a plantaromedial to plantar entry point.

Quantitative Assessment of Flexor Tendon and SL Size

Reference measurements are difficult to establish because of a greater than two-fold variation in tendon size between normal individuals and depending on breed or type of horses. A review by Reef (see Recommended Reading) yields cross-sectional areas (CSA) of 0.8–1.2 cm^2 in Thoroughbreds in the United States, while a larger range (0.72–1.93 cm^2) has been reported as being normal for Thoroughbreds in Great Britain, with 7.7–13.9 cm^2 in zone 4 (IIb) in National hunt horses. Tendon CSA varies with breed and size, and is smaller in Arabian-type horses (0.6–0.8 cm^2) and in ponies. Smith and co-workers (1994) did not find a significant difference between Thoroughbreds and heavier horses. The cross-sectional area varies with the anatomic level; it is smallest in the mid-metacarpal area and largest in the fetlock region. It may vary somewhat with age and training. The lateromedial dimension varies between 1 and 3 cm, depending on the location. The dorsopalmar thickness has been reported to be 0.7–0.8 cm proximally, decreasing to approximately 0.4 cm distally although these are less sensitive measurements.

Dimensions for the SL have also been reviewed by Reef (1998). For racing Thoroughbreds and Standardbreds in the United States, the cross-sectional area ranges from 1.0–1.5 cm^2, most horses having a cross-sectional area of 1.0–1.2 cm^2 in the body part. It is slightly larger in the pelvic limb (1.2–1.75 cm^2). The branches measure 0.6–0.8 cm^2 proximally to 1–1.2 cm^2 distally. Measuring the dorsopalmar/plantar thickness

of the ligament is probably of greater clinical interest than for the SDFT, especially in the origin and proximal body area, as it is difficult to image the entire SL in one image necessary for CSA measurement. It is normally less than 1 cm in average sized horses (0.8–0.9 cm in Thoroughbreds). The branches are less than 1 cm thick in a dorsopalmar direction.

ULTRASONOGRAPHIC ABNORMALITIES

Tendinopathy/Desmopathy

General Ultrasonographic Changes

Tendinitis/desmitis refers to spontaneous loss of structural integrity of the fibrous parenchyma of tendons and ligaments respectively. The complex pathogenesis of this condition has been reviewed elsewhere (Smith, 2010) and will not be reviewed here. As inflammation is not always a major pathophysiological component of the condition, *tendinopathy/desmopathy* is more appropriate. However, the terms *tendinitis/desmitis* remain more widely used.

Ultrasonography allows us to detect variations in gross anatomy (size and shape of the tendon or ligament) but also in the overall structure of the parenchyma (refer to the Ultrasonographic Anatomy section). Acute damage is associated with an increase in size, and a reduction in echogenicity with loss of the normal striated pattern, often affecting the central area of the tendon. Immediately after the injury, the lesion fills up with blood and debris, which are variably echogenic (hypo- to hyperechogenic) and heterogeneous. The lesion in the first few days may be subtle or even missed, as matrix debris and clots may have similar echogenicity to that of the normal parenchyma (Figure 3.4). The acute lesion is usually poorly defined and heterogeneous but long-axis images will confirm loss of fiber alignment (Figure 3.5).

Edema leads to increased water content and decreased echogenicity in the surrounding tendon, paratenon, and subcutaneous tissues (Figure 3.5). The tendon may be swollen, although this is variable initially, but one should detect peritendinous and subcutaneous tissue thickening. Comparison with the contralateral limb (which may not be completely normal with many overstrain injuries) may help confirm increased size. After a few days, organized hematoma and early, immature granulation tissue fill the lesion. They are hypoechogenic and provide the typical, discrete appearance of many tendinitis lesions (Figure 3.6).

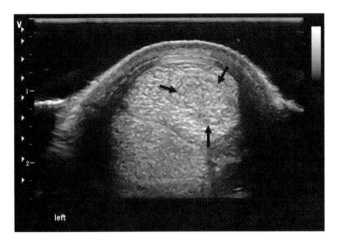

Figure 3.4 Transverse ultrasound scan image at level 1 showing a poorly defined area within the SDFT that is grossly isoechogenic to the remaining parenchyma but with altered echotexture. More subtle lesions are easily missed at this early, acute stage.

The lesion may increase in size for several days after injury, because of repeat bleeding and local release of degrading enzymes by invading inflammatory cells. It may become more evident after several days. In fact, to establish a baseline severity scan, all lesions are best examined ultrasonographically at 7–10 days after injury: this is usually the stage when the lesion is largest and most obvious. If any doubt persists, the animals should remain box-rested and be re-evaluated 2 weeks later.

SDF Tendinopathy

A common manifestation of acute SDFT injury is a discrete hypoechoic lesion visible in the central region of the tendon (hence the usual term, "core lesion"; Figure 3.6). It is most commonly located in the mid-metacarpal region. Lesions can also occur more

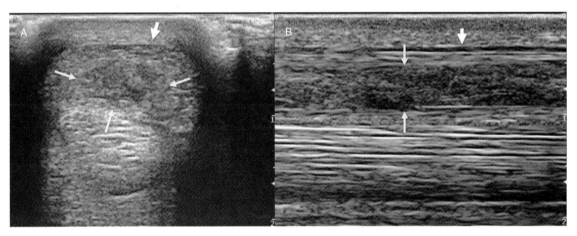

Figure 3.5 Transverse (A) and sagittal (B) ultrasound scan images showing a poorly defined, heterogeneous and slightly hypoechogenic area in the transverse plane within the SDF tendon (yellow arrows). The sagittal plane image shows severe fiber disruption and decreased echogenicity. Note the increased cross-sectional area of the SDFT and peripheral swelling of the paratenon (white arrow).

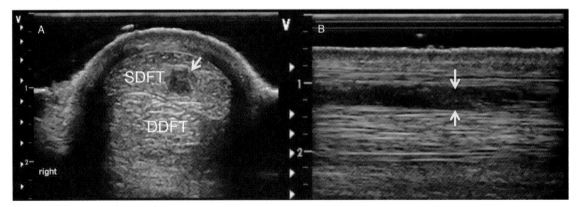

Figure 3.6 Transverse (A) and sagittal (B) ultrasound scan images of the palmar mid-metacarpal region (level 3). A well defined, hypoechogenic "core" lesion is present in the central part of the tendon. This appearance is related to early granulation tissue which appears homogeneously hypoechogenic. DDFT: deep digital flexor tendon; SDFT: superficial digital flexor tendon.

eccentrically within the tendon (Figure 3.7). Lesions occurring at the periphery of the tendon are often associated with extension of the hematoma into the paratenon or even peritendinous tissues. These may be traumatic in origin (see Local Trauma). Such lesions often alter the shape of the tendon. There is also an increase in tendon cross-sectional area, which is highly variable between lesions. The size of the lesion relative to the cross-sectional area of the tendon, and also its proximodistal length, should be ascertained to aid in prognostication (see Semi-Objective Assessment of Severity) and for future reference.

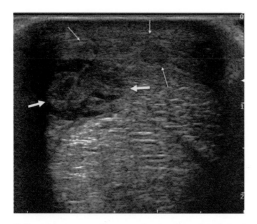

Figure 3.7 Transverse image obtained at level 4, showing an acute, hypoechogenic lesion with a honeycomb pattern, typical of organized hematoma. It distorts the lateral aspect of the SDFT (thick arrows). The paratenon is markedly thickened (thin arrows) around the lesion, extending around the SDFT.

Diffuse lesions are more challenging to visualize: the tendon becomes enlarged, hypoechogenic, and very heterogeneous (Figure 3.8). Sagittal ultrasound scans confirm diffuse loss of striation.

Tendon enlargement can be measured objectively by measuring the cross-sectional area (CSA) of the tendon on transverse images. Injured tendons have a CSA greater than normal (see Quantitative Assessment of Flexor Tendon and SL Size). A greater than 20% difference between limbs is considered significant, although this may not be the case if both limbs are affected or may be due to previous injury.

In very subtle cases, often the only finding can be enlargement and/or change in shape of the tendon. This can be accompanied by peritendinous edema, which is not specific for tendinitis and can also result from local trauma (Figure 3.9). Providing there is no evidence of tendon injury and the edema disappears, work can be resumed after a short period of rest. If edema persists, however, the presence of tendinitis should be suspected and repeat examinations are warranted.

There is some controversy as to the ability to detect subclinical or preclinical lesions with ultrasound. Certainly, gradual degeneration as observed biochemically or histologically is at a level that cannot be detected by the resolution of ultrasound, and recent studies have failed to identify prodromal changes ultrasonographically, even though some subtle heterogeneity is sometimes interpreted as signs of aging change (Figure 3.10). However, the detection of previous injury, which may have been missed clinically, is

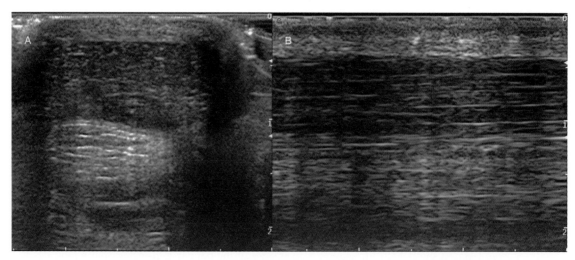

Figure 3.8 Transverse (A) and sagittal (B) ultrasound scan images of the palmar mid-metacarpal region (zone 3). The SDFT is generally enlarged, hypoechogenic without a discrete lesion being visible. The striation is poorly organized and uneven on the sagittal scan.

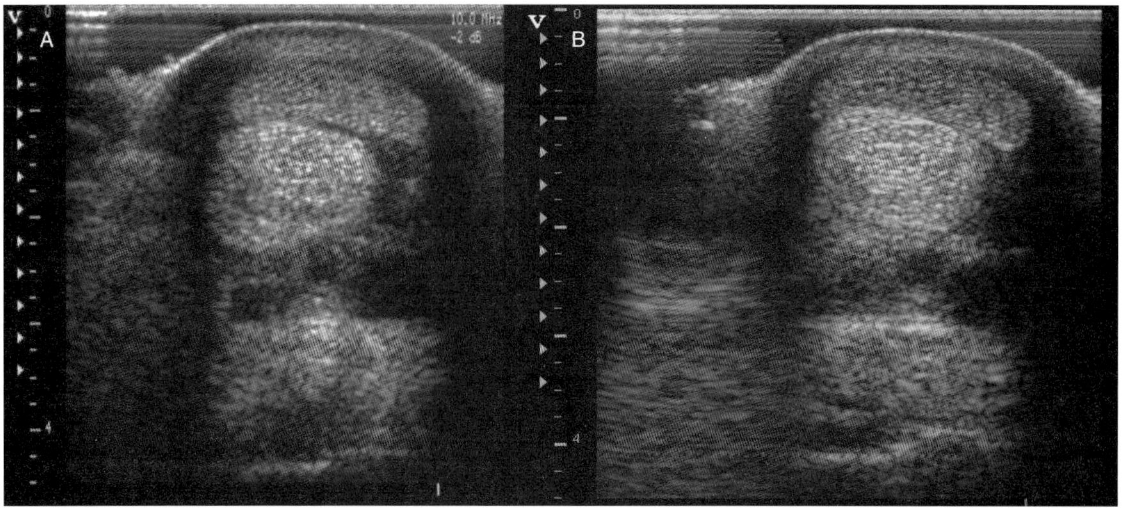

Figure 3.9 Transverse ultrasonographs from the mid-metacarpal region (level 4) showing peritendinous edema but without any tendon enlargement (A) when compared to the contralateral limb (B). This can either be a sign of mild local trauma or early overstrain injury. The limb should be re-examined ultrasonographically if the edema does not spontaneously resolve within a few days.

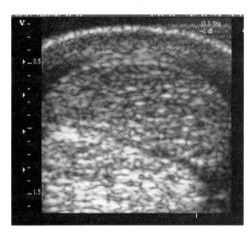

Figure 3.10 Transverse ultrasonograph from the proximal metacarpal region showing scattered hyperechoic foci within the superficial digital flexor tendon without any alteration in longitudinal pattern, characteristic of aging degeneration but not always associated with active or chronic clinical tendon disease.

a recognized risk for re-injury. Therefore, with increasing use of ultrasonography as a preventive means, the identification of chronic pathology or very mild injuries will increase. Subclinical tears or degeneration are represented by slightly hypoechogenic foci or diffuse areas, without overt signs of tendinitis (Figure 3.11).

Injury can also occur to the SDFT either proximally or distally and should not be overlooked. Distally in the fetlock ("low bow") and pastern regions, they can be associated with variable amounts of digital sheath effusion. These injuries are addressed in Chapters 1 and 2. However, occasionally lesions may occur in the distal metacarpal area and extend into the sheathed portion of the tendon without concurrent sheath effusion or inflammation. There is usually secondary subcutaneous fibrosis with these injuries, in contrast to those affecting the SDFT more proximally. Proximal SDFT tendinitis can extend to within the carpal sheath region, again with or without associated tenosynovitis (Figure 3.12). All injuries occurring within an intrathecal portion of the tendon tend to carry a graver prognosis because of the absence of a paratenon within these regions and, if confluent with the cavity of the tendon sheath, synovial fluid inhibits tendon healing and subsequent adhesions can prevent restoration of normal function. Often these are recurring injuries occurring distal or proximal to the previous scar. One should therefore look for evidence of previous injury to the mid-metacarpal region.

Complete rupture of the SDFT is the most severe extreme of an over-strain injury and often results in an almost totally anechoic region of the SDFT surrounded by a thin echogenic line (the paratenon, which usually remains intact unless the injury has been caused by percutaneous trauma) (Figure 3.13). Evidence of damage will also be apparent proximal and distal to the rupture. If the tendon ends have retracted, the outline of the paratenon at the site of the rupture may not be particularly enlarged but bunched-up, retracted fibers will be identifiable proximal and distal to the rupture site, giving the tendon a "cauliflower"-like

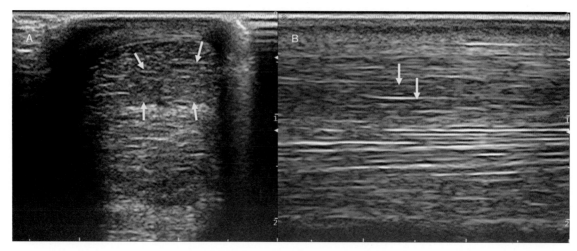

Figure 3.11 Transverse (A) and sagittal (B) ultrasound scan images of the palmar metacarpal region (zone 3). Despite this horse having no known history of previous or current tendon injury, the SDFT is heterogeneous with iso- to hypoechogenic areas within the tendon. On longitudinal images, these areas present with finer, less organized striation and decreased echogenicity. These were interpreted as subclinical, chronic lesions.

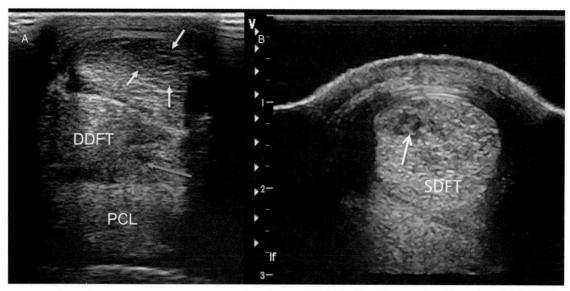

Figure 3.12 Proximal metacarpal superficial digital flexor tendinopathy. (A) Transverse image obtained palmar to the proximal metacarpal area. There is a diffuse hypoechogenic lesion in the palmaromedial aspect of the superficial digital flexor tendon (SDFT; yellow arrows) associated with diffuse thickening of the carpal flexor tendon sheath synovial membrane (red arrow), a sign of tenosynovitis. The lesion extended proximad from a metacarpal SDFT tear. PCL: palmar carpal ligaments. (B) Transverse image obtained at the level of carpometacarpal joint showing a hypoechogenic "core" lesion that spans the carpal and metacarpal regions. This lesion did not communicate with the carpal sheath and there was minimal associated tenosynovitis. While marked distension of the tendon sheath occurs when the lesion communicates with the tendon sheath cavity, its presence is not unique to surface disruption. DDFT: deep digital flexor tendon; SDFT: superficial digital flexor tendon.

appearance. The SDFT also becomes medially displaced because of lengthening of the tendon. Subcutaneous thickening is usually marked in these cases. Complete rupture of the SDFT may occur spontaneously in the carpal sheath in older horses (Figure 3.14). This is usually combined with massive sheath distension and intrathecal bleeding.

Semi-Objective Assessment of Severity

Objective measurements potentially allow better determination of prognosis and assessment of healing. The percentage ratio of damaged tendon can be calculated for discrete lesions by summing the CSA for the focal lesion and total tendon CSA at each individual level

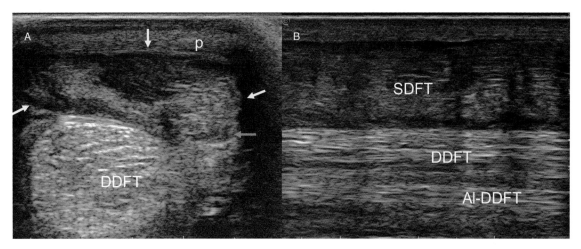

Figure 3.13 Transverse (A) and sagittal (B) ultrasound images of the palmar metacarpal region (zone 4). The SDFT is very enlarged and hypoechogenic with no evidence of normal striations over most of its cross-section (yellow arrows). Some remaining fibers are seen medially (red arrow), and amorphous tissue strands are mixed with the hypoechogenic material. This was an acute, spontaneous rupture following recurrence of a severe tendinitis lesion in a French trotter racehorse. Al-DDFT: accessory ligament of the deep digital flexor tendon; DDFT: deep digital flexor tendon; p: paratenon; SDFT: superficial digital flexor tendon.

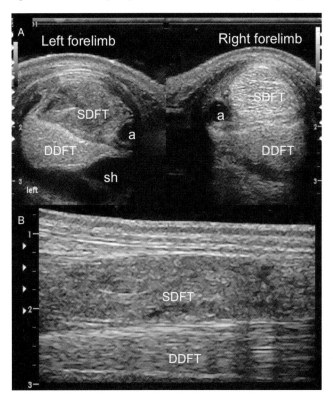

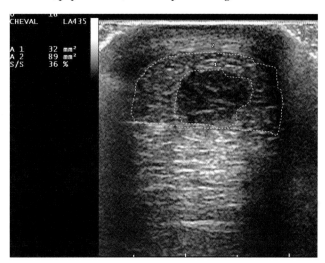

Figure 3.15 Transverse image at level 3, showing trace measurements of the ratio of the lesion to total cross-sectional area of the SDFT. This is repeated at each standard level from proximal to distal and either the greatest ratio, or the average of all measured ratios is used to assess severity.

Figure 3.14 Transverse (A) and longitudinal (B) images obtained at the level of the carpal canal with comparison between right and left transverse plane images. The right SDFT is minimally enlarged but hypoechogenic and devoid of any normal longitudinal striation because the tendon fascicles have been pulled apart. This appearance is typical of spontaneous rupture where the tendon parenchyma is replaced by hemorrhage and granulation tissue, contained within the visceral synovial layer. The common medial palmar arteries (a) are normal in this case, and there is marked carpal sheath effusion (sh). DDFT: deep digital flexor tendon; SDFT: superficial digital flexor tendon.

for all seven zones (Ia to IIIc) to give an approximation of the "volume" ratio of the lesion over the whole tendon (Figure 3.15). This has been used to objectively assess severity: injuries are considered to be mild if the ratio is in the 0–15% range, moderate for 16–25% ratios, and severe if >25%. An alternative and simpler method is to consider the maximum injury zone only: mild injuries involve <10% of the cross-sectional area; moderate 10–40%; and severe >40%. This obviously does not take into account the length of the lesion, although, even with short, discrete lesions, the pathology usually extends further than the visible lesion, throughout most of the metacarpal region. Combining these measurements provides a fairly reliable assessment of the severity. It is generally recognized that the severity of the lesion is related to the prognosis for return to work at the same level; the larger the lesion, the greater the loss of alignment and the lower the echogenicity of the lesion, the poorer the chances for return to work at the same level as prior to injury. This, together with the fiber alignment at the time the horse returns to work, provides the best assessment of prognosis, although the relationship is not strong and outcome is still variable. Thus small lesions can fail to heal adequately, while larger lesions can heal well.

Assessment of Healing

Evaluating the progression of healing over time requires a great deal of experience and is somewhat subjective. There is a lot of variation depending on many factors, including severity of the initial lesion, individual factors, occurrence of small recurrent lesions etc. However, it is generally accepted that ultrasonography will help monitor the progress and quality of the healing process to some extent (Figure 3.16). There is a relatively poor correlation between the ultrasonographic image and molecular composition but there are definite features that are believed to relate to histological stages of healing. Initial hypoechogenicity is induced by a mixture of fluid infiltration (edema) and cellular infiltrates that decrease the number of detectable interfaces. Both the initial thrombus and early granulation tissue contain cells, microscopic debris, poorly organized matrix, and microvascular struc-

tures, all of which are below the definition of ultrasound. They appear therefore hypoechogenic.

Gradual increase in echogenicity occurs because newly formed collagen fibers aggregate to form more organized bundles and thus create detectable interfaces. Peritendinous swelling resolves after a few weeks. With time, in the absence of recurrence or chronic evolution, the immature scar tissue is gradually replaced by more mature tissue, which usually manifests itself as a more echogenic and homogeneous tissue containing finely striated longitudinal interfaces. These initially form dots or small dashes, giving the scar an even, grainy appearance. As fibers form larger bundles, linear interfaces become visible but until these are longitudinally aligned the striation is irregular and very short. An adequately remodeled scar forms a rough striated pattern in longitudinal scans and a fairly homogeneous, grainy image on transverse ultrasound scans.

All tendon injuries should ideally be monitored ultrasonographically at up to 3-monthly intervals or less, and/or after any change in the exercise level. At each examination, the following factors indicate good progress.

1. A stable or decreasing cross-sectional area: sequential CSA measurements provide the most sensitive indicator of adequacy or mismatch between exercise intensity and tendon healing during the rehabilitation phase. If the CSA at any level increases by more than 10% compared to the previous examination, it is advisable to lower the exercise level.
2. An increase in the lesion echogenicity and an increasingly homogeneous texture. A subjective type score of the relative echogenicity of the lesion

Figure 3.16 Combined evaluation of transverse and longitudinal plane images allows us to subjectively assess the stage and quality of healing. (A) At the acute stage (the first few days), fibrinous clots and debris fill the lesion creating a heterogeneous, poorly defined, and variably hypoechogenic area, with a more echogenic halo often visible (yellow arrows). Longitudinal images show loss of fiber continuity, with normal fibers being visible at the extremities of the lesion (red arrow). Note the marked peritendinous soft tissue swelling (white arrow). (B) After a few days, the clot becomes invaded by cellular infiltrates and eventually immature granulation tissue. In the absence of organized fibers creating interfaces, this tissue is very hypoechogenic, although remaining matrix may create slightly more echogenic foci. (C) During the fibroblastic stage (2 weeks until 3–6 months) the lesion gradually increases in echogenicity and decreases in cross-sectional area. The overall tendon surface area decreases slightly and the peritendinous swelling resolves. (D) With time and tissue remodeling, the lesion regains an echogenicity similar to that of normal tendon tissue on transverse scans; however, long-axis images still show a lack of adequate fiber realignment. Horses may resume training at this stage but should still be monitored closely for re-injury. (E) The tendon can be considered to be healed and sufficiently remodeled to sustain return to exercise when its cross-section has reduced to near its original size, the lesion is isoechogenic to the rest of the parenchyma, and a linear pattern can be seen within it. The tendon, however, will never return to normal, with an abnormally short, coarse pattern usually noted in the scar tissue.

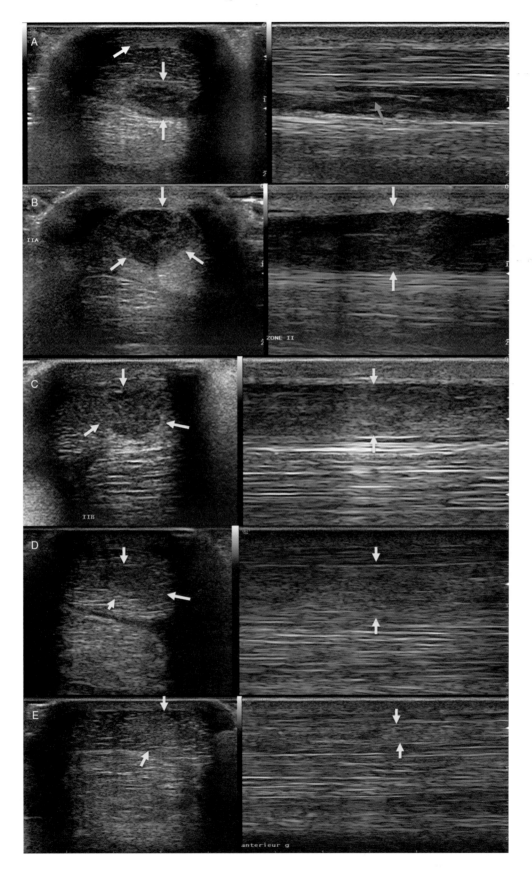

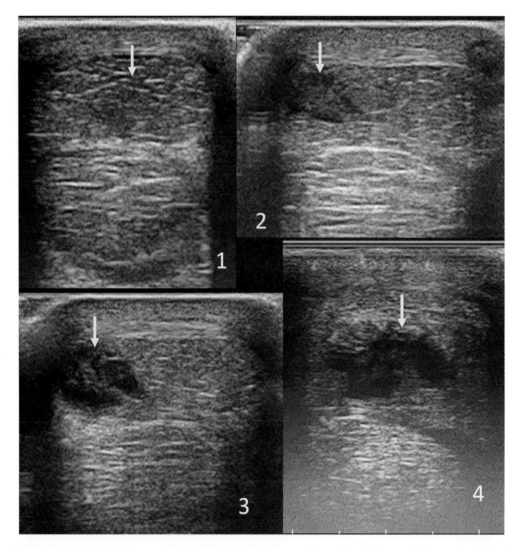

Figure 3.17   Subjective echogenicity score: depending on the echogenicity of the lesion relative to the normal parenchyma, the lesion may be subjectively graded from 1 (slight hypoechogenicity) to 4 (anechogenic). However, echogenicity cannot be quantified as it depends on many factors including beam frequency, gain, contrast and brightness settings, and subjective factors such as "echogenicity" of the skin and tissues.

has been proposed compared to that of the surrounding, intact parenchyma (Figure 3.17): type 1 lesions are only slightly hypoechoic (more white than black); type 2 lesions are moderately hypoechoic (same amounts of white and black); type 3 lesions are very hypoechoic (more black than white); and type 4 lesions are anechoic (totally black).

3. An improvement in the striated pattern seen longitudinally (Figure 3.16). A subjective fiber alignment score can be used to monitor the improvement in the longitudinally aligned interfaces in the lesion on sagittal or frontal plane images – varying from 0 (76–100% parallel fibers considered normal) to 3 (0–25% of parallel fibers).

4. Absence of peritendinous fibrosis and adhesions.

5. Blood flow within healing digital flexor tendons has been assessed with the limb raised using colour flow Doppler imaging. Normal digital flexor tendons usually have minimal discernible blood flow while, after injury, a pronounced vascular pattern is usually visible (Figure 3.18). Hypervascularity is normal in the healing process but should subside as healing progresses (normally between 3 and 6 months after injury) and its re-appearance can be an indication of re-injury.

Chronic Tendinopathy

Horses suffering from tendinitis are constantly at risk of re-injury. Complete healing, determined histologi-

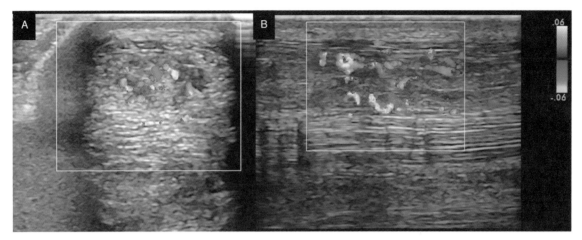

Figure 3.18 Transverse (A) and longitudinal (B) images obtained from a subacute case of superficial digital flexor tendinopathy. These images are obtained in the **non-weightbearing limb** and the presence of a positive Doppler signal, while subjective, is indicative of an active healing lesion (normal tendon has no Doppler signal). The reappearance of a positive Doppler signal after it has disappeared during the chronic stages of healing is strongly suggestive of re-injury.

cally, takes at least 15–18 months. The mean interval between injury and return to training in racehorses is dependent on the severity of the initial injury and varies between 9 and 18 months. Sports horses may be able to return to full work in a shorter time but even the mildest ultrasonographically detectable injuries should entail at least 6 months off work. Occasionally horses are successfully returned to full work prior to full resolution of the ultrasonographic lesion, however, this success may be due to the horse being capable of sustaining work in spite of the presence of a tendon injury.

Chronic tendinitis refers to either an end-stage tendinopathy or recurring and/or ongoing tearing and inflammation, generally caused by poor healing of the initial, acute injury or premature return to work before the scar tissue has sufficiently matured. True recurrence should be differentiated from chronic tendinopathy, as there is usually an acute lesion, most commonly located at one extremity of a previous scar. Nevertheless, recurring lesions are often associated with a chronic progressive tendon damage.

Ultrasonographic characteristics of chronic tendinopathy are variable and can be subtle. The tendon is often enlarged and this tends to be rather diffuse (Figure 3.19). Its echogenicity varies from hypoechogenic through normoechogenic to hyperechogenic, if the injury was severe and substantial fibrosis has occurred. The parenchymal pattern is usually coarser, heterogeneous, with a lack of striations in longitudinal images. In some cases, the outline of the original core lesion can still be seen. Mineralization may occur, causing discrete, hyperechoic interfaces casting acoustic shadowing. If calcification is florid, previous intra-

tendinous injection of depot corticosteroids should be suspected. Off-incidence transducer orientation can help to define areas of disorganized scar tissue in chronic injury, because it retains its echogenicity at greater transducer angles than normal tendon (Figure 3.20).

Recurrence is common after tendon injury. The presentation is very variable, from a mottled, diffuse hypoechogenicity superimposed on the repair tissue, to discrete tearing elsewhere in the tendon. The most common site of re-injury is one extremity of the scar after the tendon has healed. If the horse is exercised maximally too early, then re-injury can occur at the same site. In this case, the scar seems to be detached from the rest of the tendon by a conical hypoechogenic area (Figure 3.21).

Local Trauma

Spontaneous, over-strain injuries need to be distinguished from local trauma. These injuries may be caused by a slipped or over-tight bandage ("bandage bow"), hitting obstacles or loose objects, or percutaneous trauma, particularly from interference with another limb, most frequently a hind foot. If trauma occurs through bandages or boots, the skin may not be breached or damaged, and contusion and bleeding occur deeper, at the tendon interface. The effects of local trauma can vary from localized subcutaneous or peritendinous edema with no evidence of intratendinous damage through localized hypoechoic/anechoic lesions on the palmar surface of the tendon to partial or complete transection of the SDFT (Figure 3.22), sometimes extending to the deeper tendons. Local

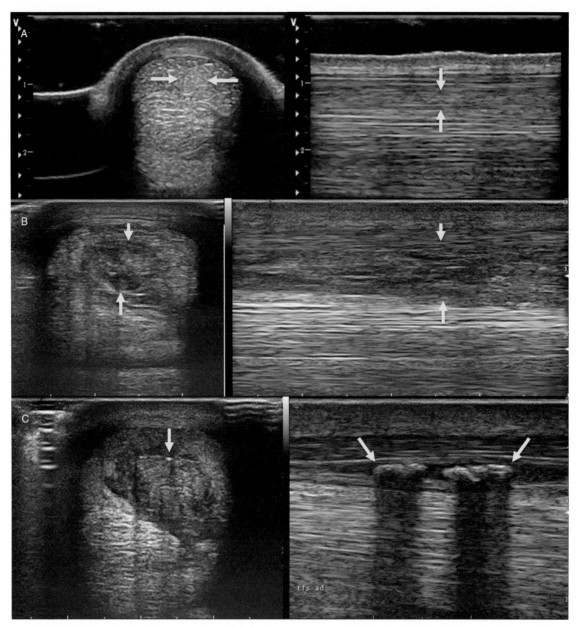

Figure 3.19 Chronic superficial digital flexor tendinopathy showing different qualities of healing. (A) A well healed lesion showing good incorporation of the scar tissue within the tendon. Note the persistent poor longitudinal pattern that remains. (B) Chronic tendinopathy characterized by a heterogeneous tissue with mixtures of echogenic scar tissue and hypoechogenic areas representing either recurring tears or amorphous connective tissue. (C) Calcification is rare in the SDFT, being more common in the DDFT. It may be subtle as in the left transverse image, or more florid as in the right longitudinal image. The latter had received previous intratendinous injections with neat bone marrow.

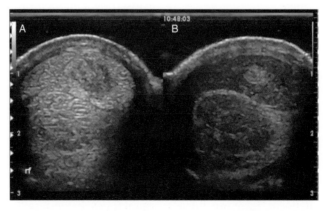

Figure 3.20 Using an off-incidence (non-orthogonal) imaging artifact can help highlight poorly organized scar tissue within a tendon, as the normal parenchyma (A) will become hypoechogenic, whereas the scar tissue, being devoid of longitudinal arrangement, usually remains echogenic (B).

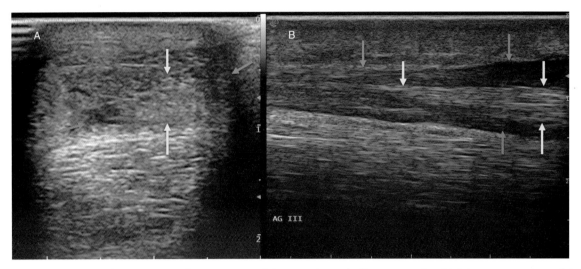

Figure 3.21 Recurrence often occurs at the extremity of the scar tissue (yellow arrows), which becomes separated from the normal tendon tissue by an ill defined, hypoechogenic area (red arrows).

traumatic injuries are, at least in the acute stage, very localized. They rarely extend far proximodistally. However, partial lacerations can be associated with longitudinal splits in the tendon, extending proximally or distally, and resulting from shear stresses (Figure 3.23). Partial lacerations can be easily missed if the examination is restricted to the site of the wound as they often occur when the tendon is fully loaded, so that the site of injury moves more proximally in the resting limb. Ultrasound is therefore very useful to identify these sites of injuries not visible through the wound.

Sepsis following a penetrating injury (or occasionally, hematogenous spread) of the SDFT is rare and usually gives an anechoic lesion, often with a communicating tract to the periphery of the tendon (Figure 3.24). It may occasionally be very extensive and diffuse. Aspiration of the lesion will yield an exudate containing large numbers of degenerate neutrophils. These lesions do not usually cause gross enlargement of the affected tendon and change rapidly in time in comparison to core lesions in a tendon strain. If the lesion is present within a tendon sheath, there will usually be an accompanying septic tenosynovitis.

"Bandage bows" may be subtle with only focal thickening of the skin, subcutaneous tissue, and paratenon. If the latter is involved, the condition should really be termed paratendinitis. Typically, this richly vascularized tissue surrounding the tendon is slightly hypoechogenic to the parenchyma and measures 1–2 mm. Injury will present either as diffuse thickening with decreased echogenicity, or as focal hypo- to hyperechogenic tissue lifting the paratenon and over-

lying fascia. This represents hemorrhage, often with a fusiform appearance in longitudinal scans. Blood collection is most often seen at the lateral or medial borders of the tendon, in the space between the edges of the SDFT and DDFT or between the DDFT and ALDDFT (Figure 3.25). The lesion occasionally extends over the whole length of the metacarpus/metatarsus. It should be noted that the majority of curb deformities of the plantar aspect of the hock are due to focal contusion and paratendinitis (Figure 3.26).

In some cases, the lesion extends into the periphery of the tendon, forming variably large, discrete, and hypoechogenic peripheral lesions with a large base facing eccentrically toward the paratenon. Although these may be caused by the initial trauma, they are often seen to occur gradually over sequential examinations. They may be due to the release of collagenase induced by the initial hemorrhage.

Paratendinitis rarely affects the integrity of the tendon parenchyma and therefore carries a better prognosis than tendinitis. However, the owners should be warned that resolution may take 3–12 weeks and that recurrent bleeding can create severe tendon defects that carry a poorer prognosis (E. Cauvin personal data).

Deep Digital Flexor Tendinopathy

Deep digital flexor tendon injuries are extremely rare in the extrathecal regions of the metacarpus, as they nearly always occur within the confines of the digital sheath or navicular bursa (i.e. intrathecally). They will therefore be addressed in the section on the pastern.

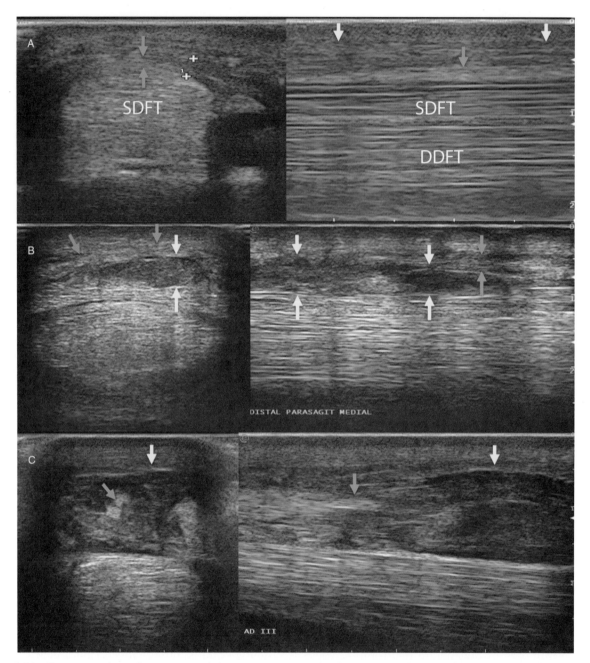

Figure 3.22 Trauma to the palmar aspect of the metacarpus can lead to varying degrees of injury. A superficial contusion (A) extends to the subcutaneous and peritendinous tissue (yellow arrow), with thickening of the paratenon (red arrow). In some cases (B), the contusion will affect the palmar surface of the tendon, causing a hypoechogenic, superficial lesion (yellow arrows) and elevating the paratenon (red arrow). When the skin is breached, the lesion may extend any distance down to the bone. (C) Transection of the SDFT will cause the torn ends to retract proximally and distally (red arrows). The gap becomes filled with hemorrhage and debris (yellow arrow). DDFT: deep digital flexor tendon; SDFT: superficial digital flexor tendon.

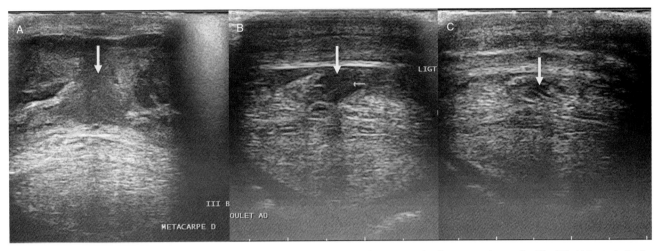

Figure 3.23   (A) This horse sustained a laceration proximal to the palmar annular ligament (zone 6). (B), (C) Although fairly superficial at the level of the wound, a longitudinal tear extended distally into the parenchyma (arrows).

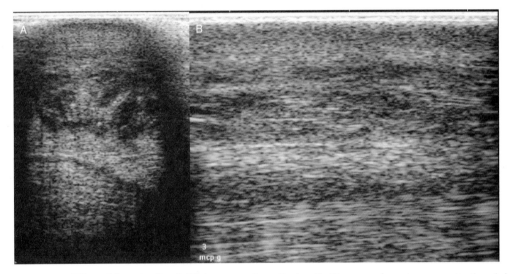

Figure 3.24   Transverse (A) and longitudinal (B) images of septic tendinitis secondary to a penetrating injury. Note the mottled, moth-eaten appearance of the SDFT and severe, peritendinous swelling.

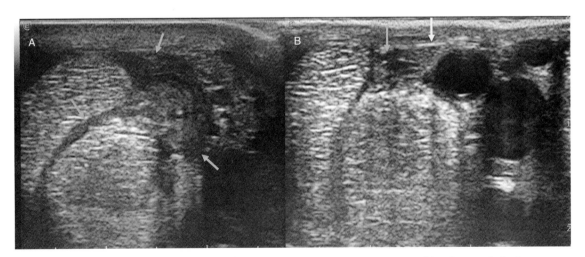

Figure 3.25   Transverse images of percutaneous injury which can cause peritendinous bleeding with the hematoma spreading around and between the tendons (A). Although usually benign, these lesions can be painful, especially when associated with palmar nerve compression (B).

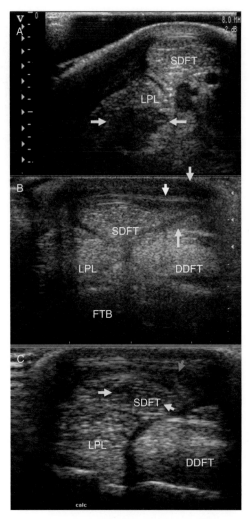

Figure 3.26 "Curb" deformity has long been associated with injury to the long plantar ligament of the tarsus (A; arrows). (B), (C) This is in fact extremely rare and curb is most often caused by subcutaneous and peritendinous thickening (yellow arrows) and/or injury to the SDFT (red arrow). DDFT: deep digital flexor tendon; p: paratenon; FTB: fibular tarsal bone; LPL: long plantar ligament; SDFT: superficial digital flexor tendon. The white arrow points to the superficial fascia.

They have also been described in the metatarsal region although care should be taken to avoid confusing DDF tendinopathy and desmitis of the ALDDFT in the hind limb which appear very similar.

Suspensory Desmopathy

"Suspensory desmitis" should in fact be called "tendinitis", since the suspensory ligament (SL) is actually the tendon of the interosseous III muscle. However the term "desmitis" is more generally accepted because of the relative scarcity of muscular tissue in this structure. It is the second most common site for injury in this region. Although it is encountered in all breeds, it is most common in the fore limbs of Thoroughbred racehorses and in the fore and hind limbs of Standardbreds and other trotters. The etiology is believed to be similar to that of SDF tendinitis. Proximal suspensory desmitis is a very common diagnosis in the hind limbs of sports horses but may not always involve the ligament as the primary pathology and hence should probably be regarded as a different condition.

The features differ depending on the level of the lesion. Desmitis is therefore divided into proximal desmitis, desmopathy of the body, and desmopathy of the branches.

Proximal Suspensory Desmitis Also called high suspensory disease, this refers to injury to the origin, or proximal enthesis, of the SL. It is encountered in most breeds but is particularly prominent in the fore and hind limbs of trotters and Standardbreds and in the hind limbs of dressage, eventing, and show jumping horses. Horses with straight hock and low metatarsophalangeal joint (hyperextension) conformations may be predisposed to SL injuries, particularly proximal desmitis. Conversely this deformity may be a consequence of SL injury.

The ultrasonographic appearance of this injury has considerable overlap with the normal appearance because of the heterogeneous echogenicity of this region. The ultrasonographic features must therefore be interpreted with great caution. The appearance of the SL at any given level is bilaterally symmetrical in normal horses and so comparison between right and left limbs is recommended to assist with diagnosis. Bear in mind, however, that SL injuries are commonly bilateral, although rarely symmetrical. More than for any other condition, proximal SL ultrasonography must be interpreted in the light of clinical findings (swelling, pain on palpation) and diagnostic local analgesia. The use of other diagnostic techniques, including radiography, scintigraphy, and magnetic resonance imaging (MRI), may be useful in some cases but is beyond the scope of this chapter. However, it is highly recommended that a good quality radiographic examination be performed to look for plantar fissure fractures, avulsion fragments, injury to the splint bones, and sclerosis of the proximopalmar/plantar third metacarpus/metatarsus.

Ultrasonographic features of proximal SL injury are similar to those of other tendons but may be very subtle. Changes are usually more easily identified in the fore limbs. Diffuse enlargement of the suspensory ligament is common but may be difficult to ascertain, unless severe. On long-axis scans, the palmar or plantar

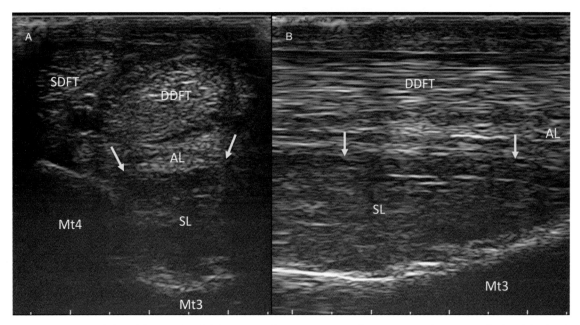

Figure 3.27 Transverse (A) and longitudinal (B) images of severe, proximal suspensory desmitis in the hind limb of a French trotter racehorse. A common feature is loss of the sharp margins of the suspensory ligament (SL): it is thickened, bulging plantarly, and displacing the soft tissue structures (arrows), here the DDFT and its accessory ligament (AL). There is diffuse thickening of the peritendinous and periligamentous tissues, and the outline of the SL is poorly defined, especially dorsally. DDFT: deep digital flexor tendon; Mt4: fourth metatarsal bone; Mt3: third metatarsal bone; SDFT: superficial digital flexor tendon.

border of the ligament may appear convex. However, sagittal images can be difficult to obtain in the hind limb and obliquity can distort the shape of the SL. A very consistent feature is poor definition to the margins, especially dorsal, of the SL, which seems to blend into the peripheral inflammatory tissue (Figure 3.27). The deep fascia becomes indistinguishable from the ligament and may be pushed palmarly/plantarly until the SL, fascia, accessory ligament of the DDFT, and DDFT are difficult to differentiate. In the acute stage this is caused by hypoechogenic edema and bleeding in and around the ligament. In chronic cases, echogenic fibrous tissue is isoechogenic to the injured ligament.

Discrete, hypoechogenic core lesions are unusual in proximal SL injuries unless they extend from more distal body injuries (especially in Standardbreds). Single or multiple poorly defined focal areas of hypoechogenicity, or diffuse, mottled hypoechogenicity are more frequent features (Figure 3.28), whose identification can be improved in the hind limb by moving the transducer medially to avoid the large head of the lateral splint bone (Figure 3.29) or by using off-incidence views in a non-weightbearing limb where the normal connective tissue within the proximal SL can be identified and differentiated from pathology. In chronic cases, the ligament appears more diffusely enlarged and heterogeneous but remains fairly echogenic (Figure 3.30). Ectopic calcifications are extremely

rare in this area unless intralesional injections have been previously performed. Sagittal/parasagittal plane images typically show a diffuse loss of longitudinally arranged striation at any stage; in chronic or long-standing cases, the long-axis sections show a granular, either mottled or densely packed appearance with ill defined, hyperechogenic areas (Figure 3.31).

Irregularity of the palmar/plantar surface of the proximal metacarpus/metatarsus is indicative of enthesophytosis or simply bony reaction to chronic inflammation. It gives a spiky or irregular appearance to the normally smooth bone surface (Figure 3.31). Larger enthesophytes can mimic "avulsion" fragments.

Avulsed fragments of the palmar/plantar cortex occur at the SL origin, usually 1–3 cm distal to the carpometacarpal or tarsometatarsal joint but they may be displaced 1 cm (or more) distally. The fragments may be quite large but never seem to involve the whole enthesis. They appear as flat, discrete hyperechogenic images casting a strong acoustic shadow, 1–3 mm palmar/plantar to the surface of the third metacarpal/metatarsal bone (Figure 3.32). Fibers are seen in continuity with the ligament and there is usually an area of ligament disruption around the lesion, with focal to more diffuse desmitis usually present. Avulsions appear to be most common in racehorses, particularly Standardbreds. The lesion may be more clearly visible on longitudinal images.

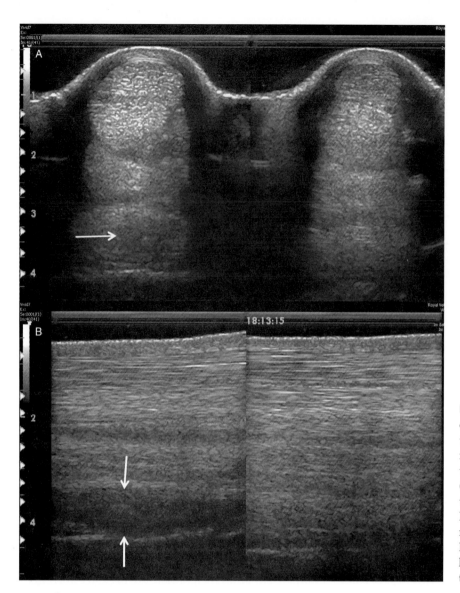

Figure 3.28 Proximal suspensory desmitis of the fore limb. Desmitis of the proximal suspensory ligament is more readily identified in the fore limb than its counterpart in the hind limb. (A) Transverse ultrasonographs from the left and right fore limbs showing a lesion in the proximal suspensory ligament of the left fore limb (arrow). The lesion can be seen as a corresponding hypoechoic area (arrows) in the longitudinal images (B).

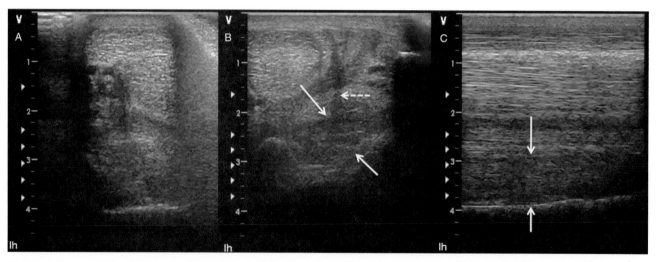

Figure 3.29 Proximal suspensory desmitis of the hind limb. (A) shows the standard transverse image from the plantar aspect of the limb showing diffuse hypoechogenicity of the proximal suspensory ligament. The lesion is more clearly observed (arrows) by moving the probe to the plantaromedial aspect (B), utilizing the "medial window" associated with the smaller head of the medial splint bone. Note, however, that edge refraction artifacts from the tendon borders and blood vessels can still compromise the image (dashed arrow) and so longitudinal views (C) should always be used in conjunction to confirm the presence of pathology (arrows).

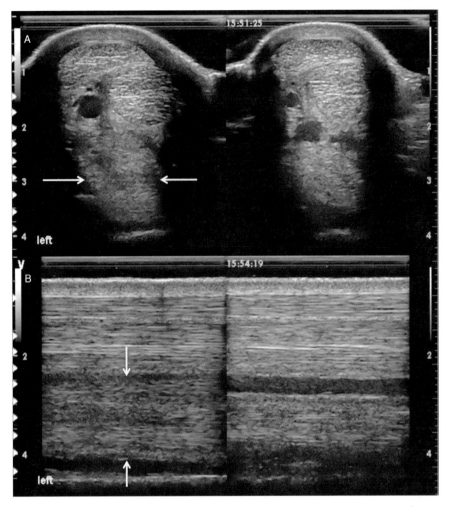

Figure 3.30 Transverse (A) and longitudinal (B) images from a case of chronic proximal suspensory desmitis in the left hind limb. The left hind limb images are on the left and the right hind limb images on the right. Note the enlarged but echogenic ligament on the left (arrows).

Spontaneous, non-displaced unicortical fatigue fractures of the palmar or plantar cortex may be seen on ultrasound scans as a focal, longitudinal defect in the palmar/plantar cortex of the third metacarpus/ metatarsus (Figure 3.33). There is usually no evidence of SL desmitis, and there does not seem to be a direct link between these conditions. Focal hypoechogenic reaction is occasionally noted between the dorsal surface of the SL and the bone around the lesion, representing hematoma, granulation tissue, or early callus. In more chronic cases, irregular new bone is visible. Radiography remains the technique of choice to visualize these, although scintigraphy and MRI may be useful in some cases.

Desmitis of the Body of the SL Injuries to the body portion of the SL usually present with generalized hypoechogenicity and enlargement of the ligament (Figure 3.34). Although diffuse lesions are most frequent, core lesions are also encountered and may extend proximally to the origin and distally into one or both branches (Figure 3.35). As an isolated lesion, it is rare in disciplines other than racehorses, especially in Standardbreds. Chronic desmitis is common because of recurrent injury and leads to very marked enlargement and periligamentous fibrosis. Percutaneous trauma can damage the borders of the body of the ligament while the proximal part of the ligament is protected by the splint bones. Such trauma is best identified with an abaxially positioned transducer (Figure 3.36). Intraparenchymal, ectopic mineralization, forming discrete hyperechogenic foci casting an acoustic shadow, may rarely be observed in long-standing cases. Previous corticosteroid injections have been incriminated.

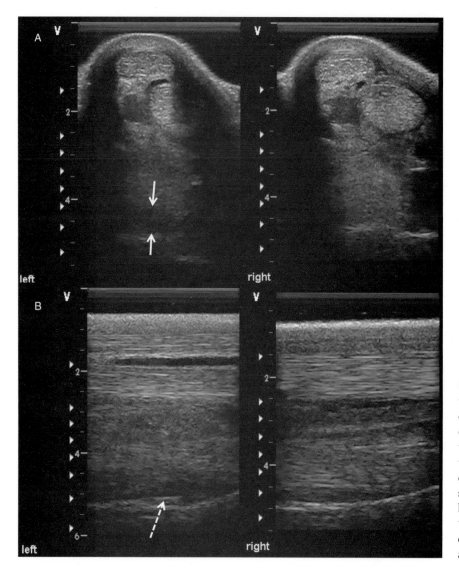

Figure 3.31 Transverse (A) and longitudinal (B) images from a case of chronic bilateral proximal suspensory desmitis in both hind limbs, but with the left hind limb more severely affected than the right. Note the more hypoechoic dorsal border of the left proximal suspensory ligament (arrows) although both ligaments are enlarged with a "ground glass" texture. There is also evidence of enthesopathy (dashed arrow).

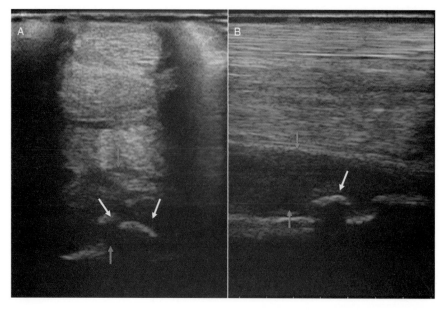

Figure 3.32 Transverse (A) and longitudinal (B) images of avulsion of the origin of the suspensory ligament. The SL is very enlarged, hypoechogenic and devoid of normal linear striation on the sagittal image (red arrows) (B). A hyperechogenic interface, casting a strong acoustic shadow is visible within the dorsal portion of the SL and represents an avulsed fragment of the palmar cortex of the third metacarpal bone (yellow arrow). This injury appears to be more common in Standardbreds.

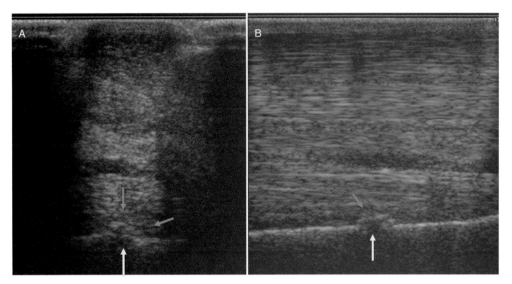

Figure 3.33 Transverse (A) and longitudinal (B) unicortical "fissure" fractures of the palmar cortex of the third metacarpal bone – a rare condition usually unrelated to SL desmitis. Ultrasonographically, focal irregularity of the palmar cortex interface (yellow arrow) represents new bone formation around the fracture line. There is no obvious damage to the SL, except a slight hypoechogenic halo at the interface between the bone spikes and the ligament (red arrows).

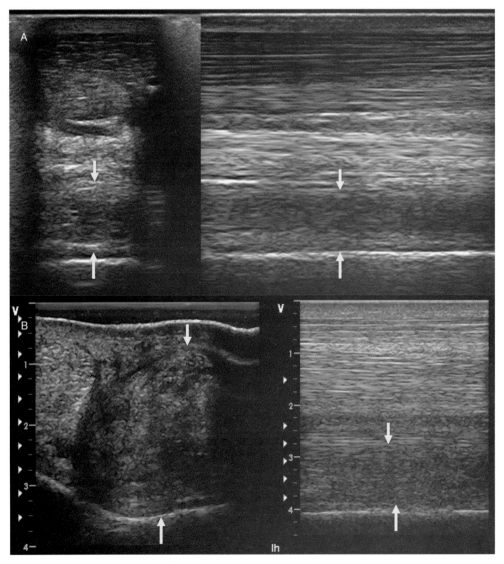

Figure 3.34 (A) Diffuse, subacute lesion in the body of the SL in a 3-year-old French trotter: the SL body (arrows) is moderately enlarged with poorly defined contours and a mottled, hypoechogenic parenchyma. There is obvious loss of striation on the sagittal image. (B) In this horse, the lesion is very mottled and diffuse, with severe enlargement of the ligament.

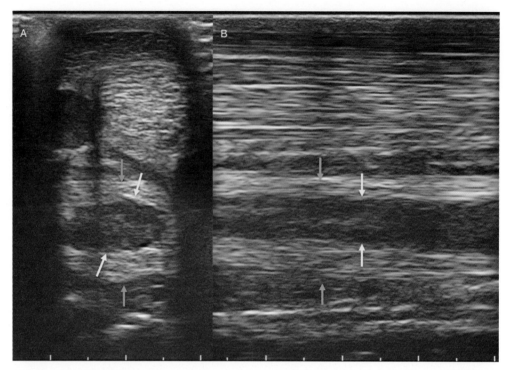

Figure 3.35 (A) Transverse and (B) sagittal images of acute SL body desmitis in a French trotter: a discrete "core" lesion (yellow arrows) is present in the center of the body of the SL. The SL is only slightly enlarged at this stage (red arrows). This presentation is more frequently encountered in racehorses.

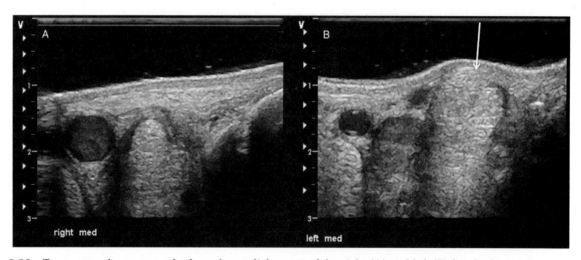

Figure 3.36 Transverse ultrasonographs from the medial aspect of the right (A) and left (B) fore limbs in a horse which has suffered trauma to the medial aspect of the left suspensory ligament body, characterized by enlargement and altered skin contour (arrow).

Body SL desmitis may be associated with second and fourth metacarpal/metatarsal bone periostitis ("splints") and fractures. There is some controversy over the link between these two conditions. Aggressive exostoses may mechanically impinge on the SL and cause focal, hypoechogenic lesions centered on the new bone (Figure 3.37). This, however, probably occurs in only the minority of cases. Most exostoses grow abaxially, rather than into the SL. Nevertheless splints are often associated with focal or more diffuse SL body or branch injuries. Careful assessment by oblique positioning of the ultrasound transducer from the opposite side of the limb can help to visualize focal SL lesions. A curved array probe occasionally improves imaging. The encroachment may be better assessed by lifting the limb while scanning and gently flexing/extending the

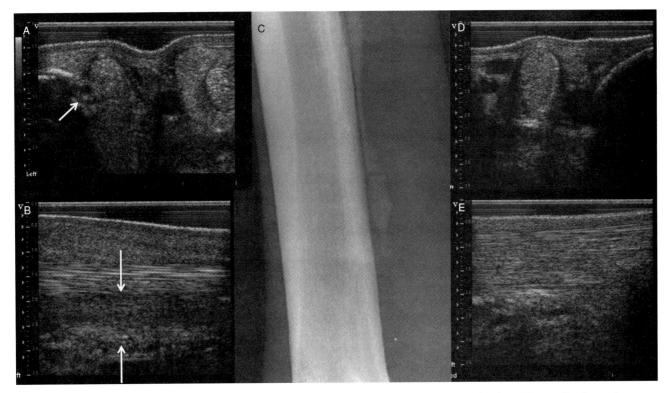

Figure 3.37 Damage to the adjacent suspensory ligament branch caused by a fractured splint. Most splint bone fractures do not cause irritation of the adjacent suspensory ligament but in this case the fracture (seen radiographically in (C)) has resulted in callus that is impinging on the suspensory ligament branch (A; arrow) and causing disruption of the branch seen in the longitudinal view (B; arrows) compared to the contralateral limb (D and E).

fetlock. Adhesions between the fibrous tissue and periosteum may thus be visualized. Pre-existing desmitis may lead to splints because of adhesion formation or increased tension on the fascia that attaches to the palmar/plantar surface of the splint bone. The distal third of the splint bones is anatomically related to the suspensory apparatus, as there are ligamentous connections to the sesamoid bones and the periosteum blends into the deep fascia that is tightly adherent to the SL paratenon.

Desmitis of the Suspensory Ligament Branches

This is the most common SL injury in sports and pleasure horses but it is encountered in all breeds and is also very common in racehorses. It occurs in both fore and hind limbs affecting any of the branches or both. The prognosis appears to be significantly worse when both branches are affected. In all cases, injury to associated structures of the suspensory apparatus, including the distal sesamoidean ligaments, should be ruled out. A core lesion or generalized involvement of the branch together with very marked enlargement are seen ultrasonographically (Figure 3.38). Longitudinal images from the abaxial aspect give an excellent assessment of the abaxial surface of the proximal sesamoid bones,

where associated enthesopathy ("sesamoiditis") is demonstrated by spikes or steps in the S-shaped surface of the bone ("ski jump" image), extending into or between the ligament fibers (Figure 3.39).

Desmitis is associated with enlargement, and the size of the suspensory ligament branches should be compared with both contra-axial and contralateral branches at the same level. One of the most sensitive indicators of suspensory branch desmitis is periligamentar fibrosis, common after all ligament injuries, although rarer with tendon pathology. This has the effect of displacing the abaxial surface of the suspensory ligament branch away from the skin surface (Figure 3.38). This periligamentous fibrosis is characteristic of ligament healing, while rarer with tendon pathology. SL injuries may heal in a similar way to SDFT injuries, although usually with a shorter (6–9 months) time course, or else result in persistent painful lesions causing long-term lameness (chronic desmitis) (Figure 3.40). New lesions often occur proximal or distal to the previous scar, creating overlapping areas of hyperechogenic and hypoechogenic areas. Ectopic mineralization foci may also be encountered in the branches in chronic cases. The recurrence rate is high for these injuries.

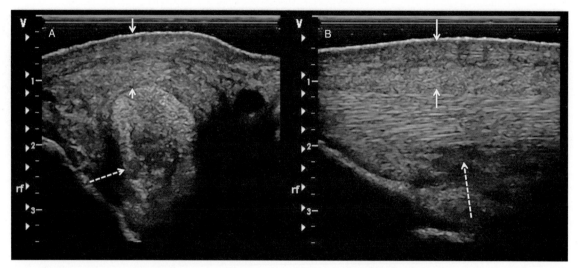

Figure 3.38   Desmitis of the medial suspensory ligament branch. Note the hypoechoic lesion seen in both the transverse (A) and longitudinal (B) images which appears to have a defect at its articular margin (dashed arrow). It is not uncommon for such suspensory branch lesions to tear into the palmar pouch of the metacarpophalangeal joint, thereby causing an inflamed joint, justifying arthroscopic debridement. Note also the periligamentar fibrosis which commonly accompanies these injuries (solid arrows).

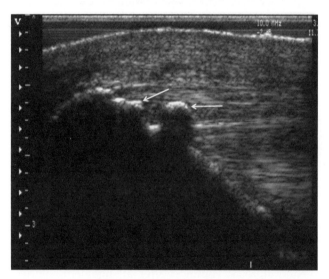

Figure 3.39   Longitudinal ultrasonograph directly over the insertion of the suspensory branch onto the abaxial surface of the proximal sesamoid bone. There is enthesophytosis at the attachment site characterized by irregular bone protruding along the suspensory ligament fibers (arrows).

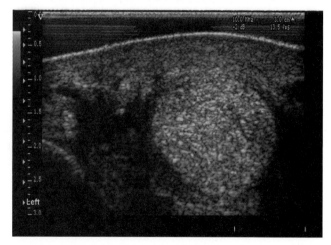

Figure 3.40   Transverse ultrasonograph over the lateral suspensory ligament of the left fore limb showing chronic desmitis characterized by branch enlargement and periligamentous fibrosis.

It should be noted that irregular, mottled, or heterogeneous areas are occasionally seen within the SL branches in horses that are apparently sound and without clinical evidence of focal pain or swelling. The ligament may be of normal size or slightly enlarged and longitudinal images show core-like areas devoid of normal fiber alignment. Some of these horses will

also present with enthesophyte formation on the sesamoidean insertion site. The significance of these is unclear but they may in fact represent subclinical lesions that may or may not evolve to overt strain injury.

Another feature that is occasionally observed as an incidental finding in horses, especially trotters, is diffuse soft tissue thickening over the abaxial aspect of the distal branch, often extending over the abaxial aspect of the sesamoid bone distal to the SL insertion.

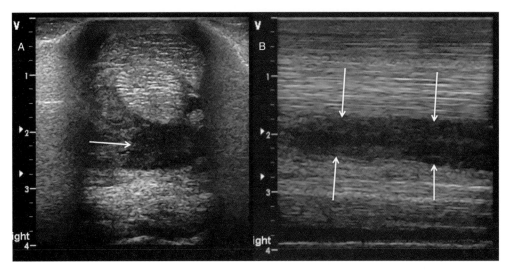

Figure 3.41 Transverse (A) and longitudinal (B) ultrasound images of desmitis of the accessory ligament of the deep digital flexor tendon. Note the hypoechoic ligament (arrows) fills the space between the flexor tendons and the suspensory ligament.

There may be mild, irregular new bone formation on the sesamoid bone palmar or distal to the enthesis. This is currently of unclear significance.

Desmitis of the Accessory Ligament of the Deep Digital Flexor Tendon (ALDDFT)

The ALDDFT can suffer a variety of ultrasonographic pathologies – from generalized enlargement and hypoechogenicity of the whole ligament (Figure 3.41) to, less commonly, more focal areas of involvement (Figure 3.42). The swelling of the ligament results in obliteration of the space between the ALDDFT and the underlying suspensory ligament. Some focal lesions, including those rare cases caused by percutaneous trauma to the lateral aspect of the metacarpal region, will only be visible if the transducer is moved over the palmarolateral aspect of the limb (Figure 3.42). This action is also important to detect adhesion formation between the lateral (usually) and medial (less commonly) borders of the ALDDFT and the SDFT, which can be responsible for flexural deformities and persistent lameness in chronic, unresponsive cases. Careful concurrent assessment of the SDFT should also be performed because concurrent injuries to the SDFT are not uncommon in horses, while ALDDFT desmitis alone is the most common palmar metacarpal soft tissue injury in ponies.

ALDDFT Desmitis of the Hind Limb

The equivalent ligament in the hind limb, the subtarsal check ligament, is a thin structure lying on the dorsal

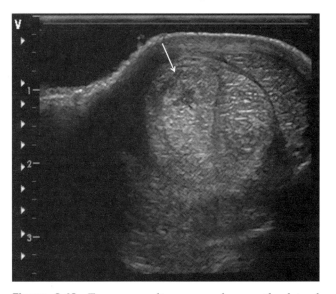

Figure 3.42 Transverse ultrasonograph over the lateral aspect of the proximal metacarpal region showing a focal lesion (arrow) in the accessory ligament of the deep digital flexor tendon, not visible from a standard palmar view.

surface of the distal limit of the tarsal sheath. In normal animals it is poorly visible although always present (Figure 3.43). Desmitis of this ligament can manifest in two forms – as an acute desmitis causing lameness or as chronic disease with a distal interphalangeal joint flexural deformity. In all these cases, the ligament has been grossly enlarged, resembling a fore limb ALDDFT (Figure 3.44). Interestingly, while most cases of fore limb ALDDFT desmitis are unilateral, these cases have been invariably bilateral.

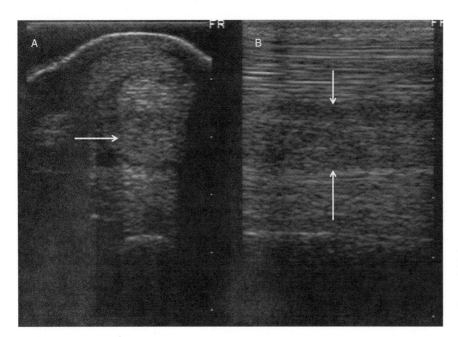

Figure 3.43 A diffusely enlarged ALDDFT in the hind limb (arrowed) in the standard plantar aspect transverse view (A) and with the transducer moved medially to the "medial window" (B). Note the filling of the space between the DDFT and the SL.

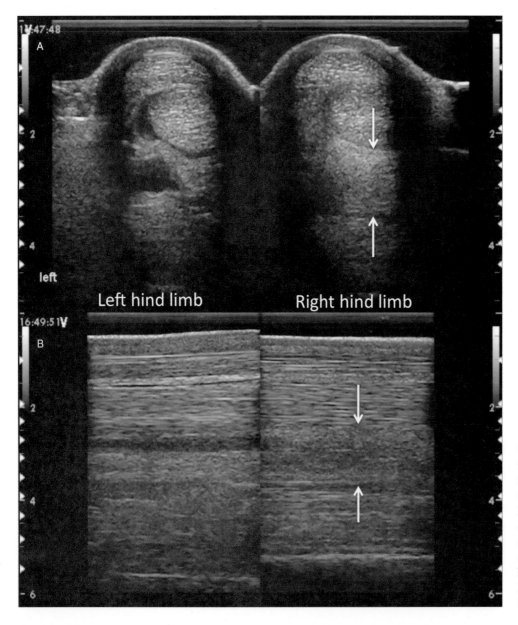

Left hind limb   Right hind limb

Figure 3.44 Desmitis of the accessory ligament of the deep digital flexor tendon in the right hind limb. Note the enlargement of the ligament on the dorsal surface of the deep digital flexor tendon in both transverse (A) and longitudinal (B) images (arrows).

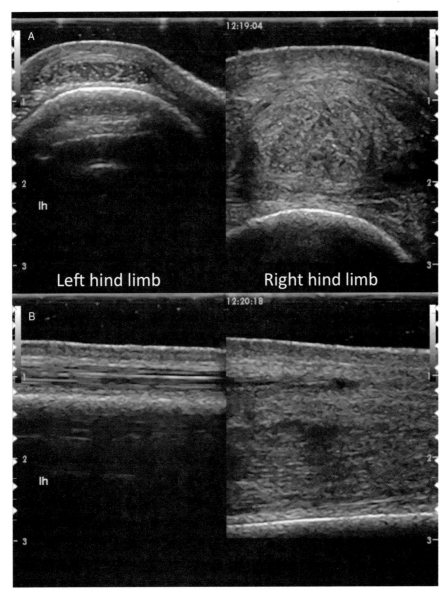

Figure 3.45 Long digital extensor tendinopathy. Transverse (A) and longitudinal (B) images of both the normal left hind limb and affected right hind limb. Note the considerable enlargement of the tendon with a completely disrupted longitudinal pattern. In spite of the severity of the pathology, these injuries rarely cause long-term problems.

Extensor Tendons

Percutaneous extensor tendon injuries are common, especially in the hind limb, through wounds to the dorsal aspect of the limb although they can occasionally be due to over-strain injuries (Figure 3.45). Although the diagnosis is usually obtained through clinical evaluation, and treatment usually unnecessary, ultrasonography can provide valuable information, such as the extent of the wound, involvement of part of the tendon or complete transection, and involvement of the tendon sheaths. The periosteum should be also assessed to look for evidence of severe stripping which may lead to sequestrum formation.

Spontaneous rupture of the common or long digital extensor tendon over the dorsal aspect of the carpus is observed in foals and can cause severe longitudinal swelling of the accompanying tendon sheath. In the acute stage, mottled, hypoechogenic tissue represents hematoma formation. The retracted ends of the torn tendon are seen proximal and distal to the rupture site, sometimes at a surprising distance.

Bony Injuries

While metacarpal bone fractures are most readily assessed radiographically, ultrasonography can occasionally provide additional useful information. The configuration of complex third metacarpal/metatarsal bone fractures may be difficult to ascertain radiographically. Ultrasonographic evaluation can help to localize more accurately the position of the fracture line around the bone (Figure 3.46). Associated periosteal lifting and hemorrhage can help to detect the fracture line.

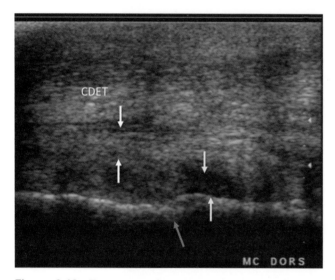

Figure 3.46 Transverse ultrasonographic image obtained over the dorsal aspect of the mid-metacarpus. The periosteum (white arrows) is thickened, hypoechogenic, and lifted from the cortical bone interface by hypoechogenic tissue (yellow arrows: edema and hemorrhage). An ill defined, focal irregularity and loss of continuity of the cortical surface is caused by a non-displaced longitudinal fracture. CDET: common digital extensor tendon.

Periostitis and fracture of the second and fourth metacarpal/metatarsal (splint) bones may not be visible radiographically initially. These can occur from trauma to the splint bones, to the third metacarpus/metatarsus or both, with the medial aspect being most commonly involved. The horses are generally very lame but focal swelling may be subtle or, on the contrary, masked by diffuse edema. Ultrasonography is very useful to confirm the injury: the periosteum is thickened and hypoechogenic; subperiosteal hemorrhage is seen as a spindle-shaped, hypoechogenic tissue separating the hyperechoic bone interface from the lifted periosteum (Figure 3.47). In the subacute stage, early new bone formation can give a spiky or sunburst appearance on ultrasonography despite being barely visible on radiographs (Figure 3.48).

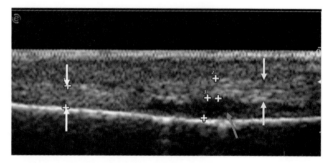

Figure 3.47 Acute trauma over the metacarpal bones can cause subperiosteal hemorrhage. This is characterized ultrasonographically (longitudinal/frontal plane image obtained over the second metacarpal bone) by lifting of the periosteum (yellow arrows) from the cortical bone interface by a spindle-shaped layer of hypoechoic material (blood) (red arrow). The surrounding, attached periosteum is abnormally thickened (white arrows).

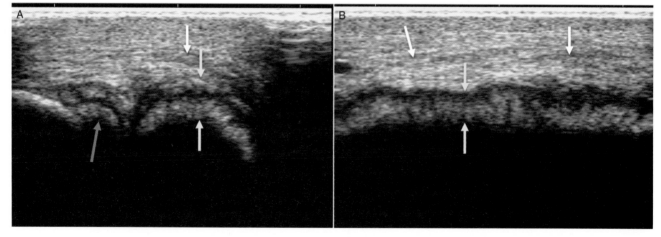

Figure 3.48 Transverse (A) and longitudinal (frontal plane – B) images over the second metacarpal bone. Subacute periostitis has a typical appearance: the bone interface is irregular and spiky, with a "sunburst" appearance highlighted by an ill defined hypoechogenic halo (yellow arrows). The fibrous layer of the periosteum is thickened and lifted, and poorly visualized because of peripheral soft tissue reaction (white arrows). This appearance is that of early periosteal new bone formation. Note the new bone production from the third metacarpal bone in the interosseous space (red arrow).

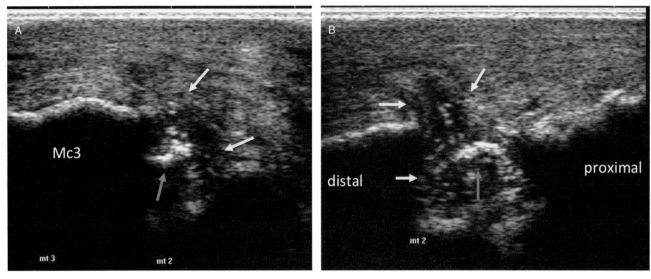

Figure 3.49   Transverse (A) and longitudinal (B) images obtained over the medial mid-metacarpal region. A fluid- and gas-filled fistula is seen (yellow arrows) to penetrate an irregular defect in the surface of the second metacarpal bone. A hyperechogenic, irregular interface represents a bony fragment sitting in the defect (red arrow). The fragment, surrounded by fluid, is most likely to be necrotic (sequestrum).

Finally, ultrasonography can be useful for monitoring the progression of bony fragments in terms of sequestrum formation. This is characterized by a thin but strongly echogenic bone interface casting a shadow, lying in a depression in the underlying bone and surrounded by anechoic fluid (Figure 3.49).

Recommended Reading

Avella, C.S., Ely, E.R., Verheyen, K.L., Price, J.S., Wood, J.L., & Smith, R.K.W. (2009) Ultrasonographic assessment of the superficial digital flexor tendons of National Hunt racehorses in training over two racing seasons. *Equine Veterinary Journal*, 41, 449–454.

Eliashar, E., Dyson, S.J., Archer, R.M., Singer, E.R., & Smith, R.K.W. (2005) Two clinical manifestations of desmopathy of the accessory ligament of the deep digital flexor tendon in the hindlimb of 23 horses. *Equine Veterinary Journal*, 37, 495–500.

Kristoffersen, M., Ohberg, L., Johnston, C., & Alfredson, H. (2005) Neovascularisation in chronic tendon injuries detected with colour Doppler ultrasound in horse and man: implications for research and treatment. *Knee Surgery, Sports Traumatology, Arthroscopy*, 13, 505–508.

Reef, V.B. (1998) *Equine Diagnostic Ultrasound*. W.B. Saunders Co, Philadelphia.

Reef, V.B. (2001) Superficial digital flexor tendon healing: ultrasonographic evaluation of therapies. *Veterinary Clinics of North America: Equine Practice*, 17(1), 159–178, vii-viii.

Smith, R.K.W., Jones, R., & Webbon, P.M. (1994) The cross-sectional areas of normal equine digital flexor tendons determined ultrasonographically. *Equine Veterinary Journal*, 26, 460–465.

Smith, R.K.W. (2011) Pathophysiology of tendon injury. In: *Diagnosis and Management of Lameness in the Horse*, 2nd edn. (eds M.W. Ross & S.J. Dyson). W.B. Saunders Co, St. Louis.

Van Schie, H.T., Bakker, E.M., Jonker, A.M., & Van Weeren, P.R. (2003) Computerized ultrasonographic tissue characterization of equine superficial digital flexor tendons by means of stability quantification of echo patterns in contiguous transverse ultrasonographic images. *American Journal of Veterinary Research*, 64, 366–375.

CHAPTER FOUR

ULTRASONOGRAPHY OF THE CARPUS

Ann Carstens

University of Pretoria, Onderstepoort, South Africa

INTRODUCTION

Radiography is the modality most often used to evaluate the equine carpus, since most lesions in this area are bony in nature; however, radiologically evident soft tissue swelling is often associated with, and secondary to, bony carpal pathology, i.e. a mid-carpal joint effusion secondary to a distal radiocarpal chip fracture. Additionally, there is also often no radiological evidence of bony changes in the carpus, and ultrasonography lends itself to evaluate soft tissue changes. Cortical abnormalities are also amenable to ultrasonographic evaluation and particularly useful as a preliminary evaluation if radiological equipment is not handy.

Inspection, palpation, and flexion of the carpus are usually adequate to determine the anatomic structure/s affected in the presence of a pericarpal swelling, but perineural or intra-articular blocks may be required if the above are negative or equivocal. The carpus is a complex joint with multiple bones, ligaments, tendons, tendon sheaths, bursae, and three joints with recesses. To scan the entire carpus may be time consuming, and it is suggested that the area or areas identified clinically or with other modalities, such as radiography or scintigraphy, be ultrasonographically evaluated in detail and the rest of the carpus scanned in a more cursory manner if time is not available.

Carpal anatomy should be revised prior to ultrasonographic evaluation, if the ultrasonographer is unfamiliar with the area to be scanned.

A 7.5–13 MHz linear transducer is advised for evaluating the carpus, with or without a standoff pad, depending on the depth of the area to be evaluated. A split screen or C-scape modality can be used to make a composite image on the screen. The figures in this chapter include a view of the joint to show where the transducer is positioned.

ANATOMY AND SCANNING TECHNIQUE

Dorsal Carpus

The transducer is placed sagittally at the distal aspect of the radius cranially and moved distally, respectively evaluating the bones and superficial structures of the distal radius, the antebrachiocarpal joint (ACJ), the proximal row of carpal bones, the middle carpal joint (MCJ), the distal row of carpal bones, the carpometacarpal joint (CMCJ) and the proximal aspect of metacarpus 3 (MC3) (Figure 4.1). The surface of the bones should be smooth hyperechoic lines with elevations at the dorsal tubercles at implantation of the dorsal intercarpal ligaments. The hyperechoic cortical line will have a distinct interruption where the joint margin starts; angling the transducer will allow visualization of the most dorsal part of the articular surface. The approximately 1 mm thick dorsal intercarpal ligaments can be noted, running transversely immediately deep to the skin surface. Hereafter the transducer can be moved again to the distal aspect of the radius laterally or medially and the movement repeated until the entire dorsum is scanned. This is repeated with the transducer held in a transverse plane. In this way the distal cranial radius, dorsal aspect of the radial (RCB), intermediate (ICB), ulnar (UCB), second (C2), third (C3), and fourth (C4) carpal bones, the third metacarpal bone (MC3) and the three joints can be visualized. The tendons of the common digital extensor (CDET), extensor carpi radialis (ECRT), lateral digital

Atlas of Equine Ultrasonography, First Edition. Edited by Jessica A. Kidd, Kristina G. Lu, and Michele L. Frazer.
© 2014 John Wiley & Sons, Ltd. Published 2014 by John Wiley & Sons, Ltd.
Companion Website: www.wiley.com/go/kidd/equine-ultrasonography

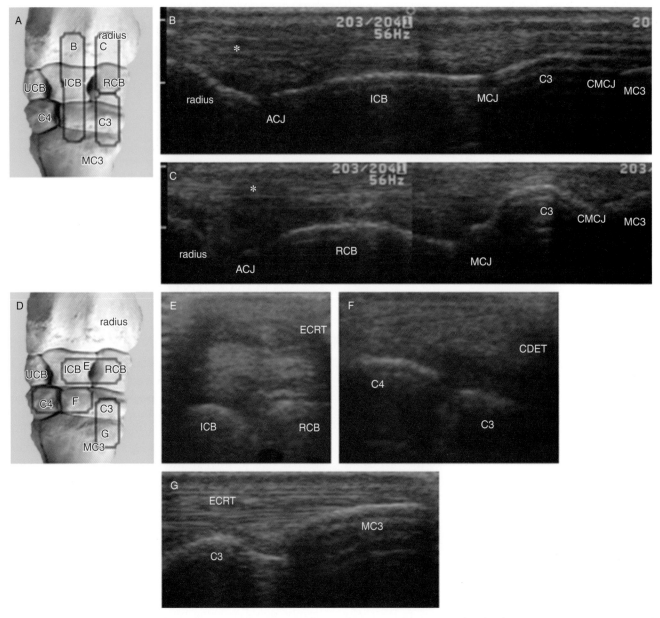

Figure 4.1   (A,D) Anatomical specimens indicating transducer placement. (B) Longitudinal split screen composite image of the mid-carpus showing the antebrachiocarpal joint (ACJ), the middle carpal joint (MCJ), the carpometacarpal joint (CMCJ), and the tendon of the common digital extensor (CDET)(*); note the hypoechoic fluid within the dorsal ACJ and MCJ; proximal is to the left. (C) Longitudinal split screen composite image of the mid-lateral aspect of the carpus showing the ACJ, the MCJ, and the CMCJ and the tendon of the extensor carpi radialis (ECR)(*); note the hypoechoic villous structures within the dorsal ACJ; proximal is to the left. (E) Transverse image showing the dorsal hyperechoic surfaces of the intermediate carpal bone (ICB) and the radiocarpal bone (RCB) and transverse section through the ECR tendon (ECRT); the hyperechoic structure deep to the ECRT is thickened joint capsule; lateral is to the left. (F) Transverse image showing the dorsal hyperechoic surfaces of fourth and third carpal bones (C4 and C3) and transverse section through the CDE tendon; lateral is to the left. (G) Longitudinal image showing the dorsal hyperechoic surfaces of C3 and third metacarpal bone (MC3) and the implantation of the ECRT on the proximodorsomedial MC3 tuberosity; proximal is to the left. UCB: ulnar carpal bone.

extensor (LDET), and the abductor digiti longus (ADL) must also be examined, noting the size, echogenicity, and fiber alignment. A bursa (ECRB) is present under the implantation of the ECRT, but usually only visible when more than normal synovial fluid is present within. The tendon sheaths and joints are evaluated for the presence, echogenicity, and amount of fluid within and the joint capsule, the synovial membrane, and sheaths themselves are evaluated for thickening, abnormal echogenicity, or abnormal tissue.

A specific structure such as a single tendon and its sheath should be evaluated in full, noting the muscular portion as well as the implantation, if pathology in this structure is suspected.

Lateral Carpus

Again using a sequential sagittal and transverse scanning technique, starting slightly dorsolaterally, the lateral aspect of the carpus is evaluated, identifying the lateral styloid process, the lateral aspects of the ACJ, C4, MCJ, UCB, CMCJ, and MC4 (Figure 4.2). The CDET can be visualized and also the very thin muscle body. The hypoechoic cartilaginous or partially mineralized C5 may be noted although uncommonly seen. Further palmarly, the lateral collateral ligament provides passage for the LDET, between its long superficial and short deep parts. The main insertion of the ulnaris lateralis tendon (ULT) is on the proximal aspect of the accessory carpal bone (ACB). The long part of the ULT can be visualized where it inserts on proximal MC4 after running through a groove on the lateral part of the ACB. Again the size, echogenicity, and fiber align-

ment and sheaths of the tendons are examined. Further palmarly and proximal to the ACB, the musculotendinous junction of the deep digital flexor tendon (DDFT) can be seen next to the distocaudal radius. If there is an effusion in the palmar recess of the ACJ or very marked effusion in the carpal canal (CC), this may be seen between the radius and the DDFT.

Medial Carpus

Again using a sequential sagittal and transverse scanning technique, starting slightly dorsomedially, the medial aspect of the carpus is evaluated, identifying the medial styloid process, the medial aspects of the ACJ, RCB, MCJ, C2 (possibly also C1), CMCJ, MC2, both the long and short segments of the medial collateral ligament (MCL), and the flexor carpi radialis tendon (FCRT) (Figure 4.3).

The bellies and tendons of the superficial digital flexor muscle (tendon – SDFT) and DDFT can be seen best on the palmar view. The palmar proximal recess of the ACJ as well as the carpal canal may be visualized adjacent to the distal medial radius caudally if there is synovial distension.

Palmar Carpus

This aspect is actually approached as the mediopalmar to palmar aspect since the ACB curves around on the most lateropalmar aspect of the carpus providing the lateral border of the CC and partially providing the insertion of the retinaculum of the carpus (RetC)

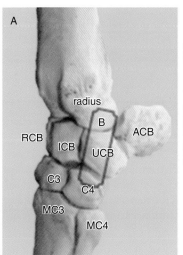
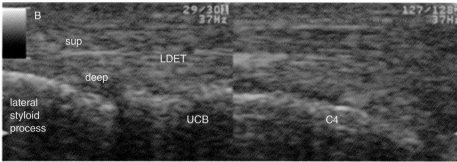

Figure 4.2 (A) Anatomical specimen indicating transducer placement. (B) Longitudinal image of the lateral carpus with the superficial (sup) and deep parts of the lateral collateral ligament and the lateral digital extensor tendon (LDET) between them; proximal is to the left. ACB: accessory carpal bone; C: carpal bone; ICB: intermediate carpal bone; MC: metacarpal bone; RCB: radiocarpal bone; UCB: ulnar carpal bone.

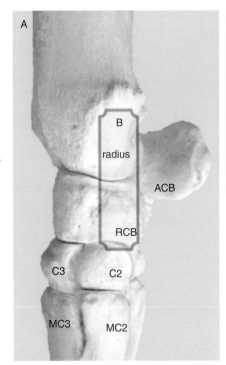

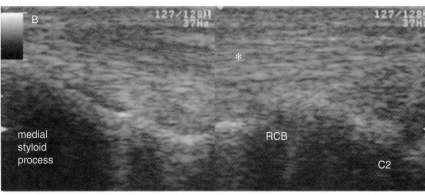

Figure 4.3 (A) Anatomical specimen indicating transducer placement. (B) Longitudinal image of the medial carpus with the superficial part of the medial collateral ligament marked (*); proximal is to the left. ACB: accessory carpal bone; C: carpal bone; MC: metacarpal bone; RCB: radiocarpal bone.

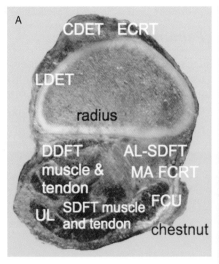

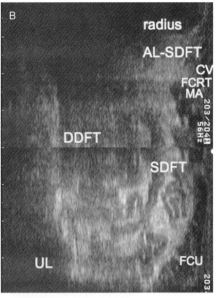

Figure 4.4 (A) Anatomical specimen indicating transducer placement. (B) Palmar transverse split screen ultrasound image at level of distal chestnut; medial is to the right. AL-SDFT: accessory ligament of the superficial digital flexor tendon; CDET: common digital extensor tendon; CV: cephalic vein; DDFT: deep digital flexor tendon; ECRT: extensor carpi radialis tendon; FCRT: flexor carpi radialis tendon; FCU: flexor carpi ulnaris; LDET: lateral digital extensor tendon; MA: median artery; SDFT: superficial digital flexor tendon; UL: ulnaris lateralis.

(Figure 4.4 and palmar images Figures 4.5 and 4.6). The CC extends from approximately 20 cm proximal to the ABCJ and to approximately 10 cm distal to the CMJ. The ULT can be viewed inserting on the proximal aspect of the accessory carpal bone (ACB). Within the

carpal canal the muscular bodies of the tendons of the DDFT and SDFT are visualized from the level of the chestnut where they start becoming tendinous. Immediately proximal to the carpus the MA sends off the distal radial artery (DRA) and then enters the carpal

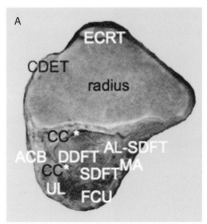
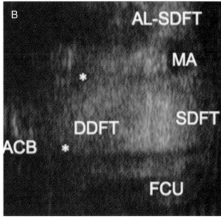

Figure 4.5 (A) Anatomical specimen indicating transducer placement. (B) Palmar transverse ultrasound image at level of distal radius; medial is to the right. ACB: accessory carpal bone; AL-SDFT: accessory ligament of the superficial digital flexor tendon; CC (*): carpal canal; CDET: common digital extensor tendon; DDFT: deep digital flexor tendon; ECRT: extensor carpi radialis tendon; FCU: flexor carpi ulnaris; MA: median artery; SDFT: superficial digital flexor tendon; UL: ulnaris lateralis.

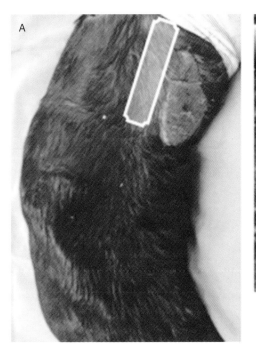
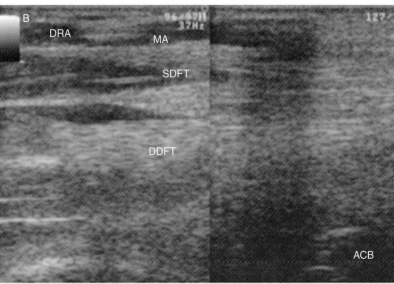

Figure 4.6 (A) Anatomical specimen indicating transducer placement. (B) Palmaromedial longitudinal ultrasound image showing superficial and deep digital flexor tendon musculotendinous junctions immediately proximal to the accessory carpal bone (ACB). Proximal is to the left. DDFT: deep digital flexor tendon; DRA: distal radial artery; MA: median artery; SDFT: superficial digital flexor tendon.

canal, seen as an anechoic tubular structure. The accessory ligament of the SDFT (AL-SDFT) is seen as a homogeneous hyperechoic trapezoid structure (in the transverse plane) originating from the caudomedio-distal aspect of the radius dorsomedial to the SDFT, thinning further distally and fusing to the SDFT tendon. The AL-SDFT is bordered medially by the FCRT, palmaromedially by the median artery (MA),

vein, and nerve. Mediopalmar to the MA and the AL-SDFT is the flexor carpi ulnaris muscle (FCU). Medially to the SDFT is the muscle belly of the ulnar carpal flexor (tendon – FCUT) and caudolaterally to the DDFT is the UL muscle. The cephalic vein (CV) is situated medial to the RetC. The palmar carpal canal should be evaluated transversely and longitudinally. See Figures 4.4, 4.5, 4.6, 4.7, 4.8, 4.9, 4.10.

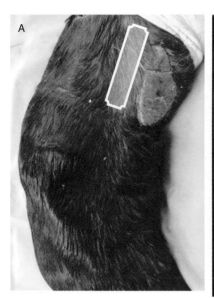

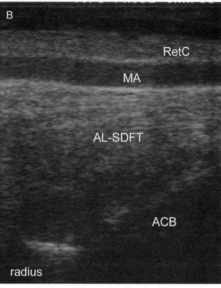

Figure 4.7 (A) Anatomical specimen indicating transducer placement. (B) Medial longitudinal ultrasound image showing the median artery and accessory ligament of the superficial digital flexor tendon (AL-SDFT). Proximal is to the left. ACB: accessory carpal bone; MA: median artery; RetC: retinaculum of the carpal canal.

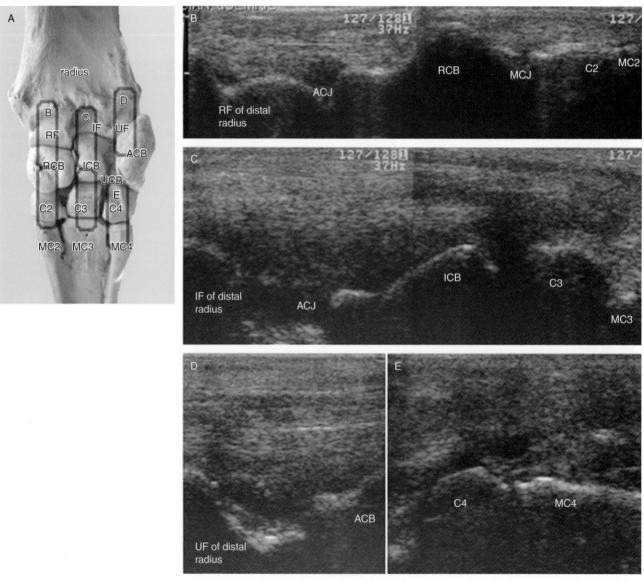

Figure 4.8 (A) Anatomical specimen indicating transducer placement. (B,C,D,E) Longitudinal split screen composite image of the palmar aspect of the right carpus showing the hyperechoic palmar surfaces of the carpal and metacarpal bones and the palmar aspect of the carpal joint spaces. Proximal is to the left. ACB: accessory carpal bone; ACJ: antebrachiocarpal joint; C: carpal bone; ICB: intermediate carpal bone; IF: intermediate facet; MC: metacarpal bone; MCJ: middle carpal joint; RCB: radiocarpal bone; RF: radial facet; UCB: ulnar carpal bone; UF: ulnar facet.

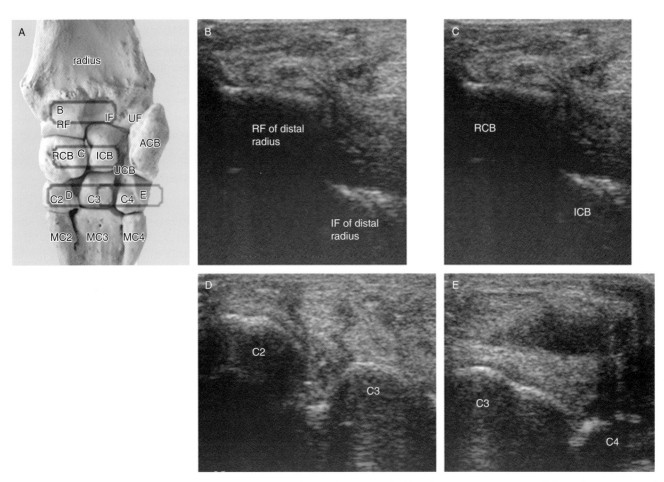

Figure 4.9   (A) Anatomical specimen indicating transducer placement. (B,C,D,E) Transverse images of the palmar aspect of the right carpus showing the hyperechoic palmar surfaces of the carpal bones and the palmar aspect of the carpal joint spaces. Medial is to the left. ACB: accessory carpal bone; ACJ: antebrachiocarpal joint; C: carpal bone; ICB: intermediate carpal bone; IF: intermediate facet; MC: metacarpal bone; MCJ: middle carpal joint; RCB: radiocarpal bone; RF: radial facet; UCB: ulnar carpal bone; UF: ulnar facet.

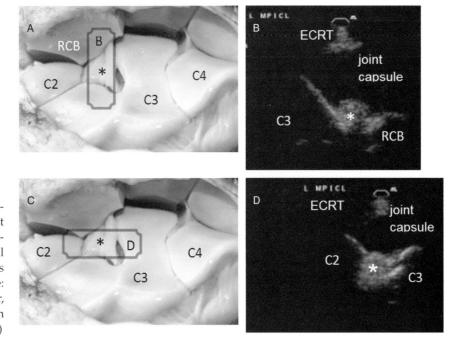

Figure 4.10   Sagittal (A,B) and transverse (C,D) images of the palmar aspect of the medial palmar intercarpal ligament (*); medial is to the left. C: carpal bone; ECRT: extensor carpi radialis tendon; RCB: radiocarpal bone. (Source: Parts B and D – Adapted from Driver, A.J. *et al.* (2004) [1]. Reproduced with permission of John Wiley & Sons Ltd.)

The palmar aspects of all the carpal bones can be visualized to a greater or lesser degree; again use a sequential approach to evaluate them from either medially to laterally or *vice versa* from proximally to distally. Proximally the distal radius condyle is divided into the lateral ulnar facet (UF), the more medial intermediate facet (IF), and the medial radial facet (RF). Similarly the palmar aspect of the carpal joint spaces can be seen (Figure 4.8).

JOINTS AND BONE

Higher-frequency transducers can optimize evaluation of the articular cartilage and subchondral bone. Normal cartilage should be anechoic, with a smooth surface and in the case of the carpus be approximately 1 mm thick. The subchondral bone of the adult horse should be relatively smooth. Flexing the joint and using a curvilinear or micro-convex transducer will allow visualization of the deeper (more palmar) joint surfaces. Interarticular ligaments, such as the medial palmar intercarpal ligament, extending from between palmar C2 and RCB distally extending to palmar proximally, has been described and other intercarpal ligaments may also be visualized. (See Recommended Reading.) Ultrasonography of the intercarpal ligaments such as the medial palmar intercarpal ligament (MPaICL) is performed with the carpus in flexion and the MCJ imaged through the ECRT.

In the immature horse the distal radial epiphysis can be seen as a gap in the distal radius cortex. In young foals the carpal bones have a thicker anechoic cartilage with the underlying mineralized bone having a slightly less regular surface. In the premature animal the cartilage is particularly thick and the hyperechoic bony center small or absent (Figure 4.11A).

ULTRASONOGRAPHIC ABNORMALITIES

Ultrasonographically pathology can be suspected when the normal ultrasonographic anatomy is not appreciated. Comparison with the opposite limb is encouraged to compare between the pathological limb and the normal limb. Be aware, however, that the contralateral limb may itself have ultrasonographically visible pathology, particularly since some injuries may occur simultaneously bilaterally. See Figures 4.11, 4.12, 4.13, 4.14, 4.15, 4.16, 4.17, 4.18, 4.19, 4.20, 4.21.

Superficial Soft Tissues

Skin may be thicker than normal due to fibrosis (hyperechoic) or granulomatous (hypoechoic) or neoplastic (mixed echogenicity) tissue, e.g. sarcoids or squamous cell carcinoma. Subcutaneous tissue may be deeper than normal due to edema, hemorrhage or contusion which often gives a heterogeneous hypoechoic appearance.

Tendons and Ligaments

Inflammation or partial tearing of these structures is seen as enlargement with loss of echogenicity and loss of normal fiber alignment. Complete disruption of the structure is seen as a complete loss of anatomic detail in the affected area with intervening heterogeneous echogenicities consistent with the stage of the condition, whether acute, subacute, or chronic. Healed tendons/ligaments are usually hyperechoic and fiber alignment is usually haphazard.

Tendon Sheaths, Bursae, Joint Spaces

Usually there is little to no free fluid within tendon sheaths and bursae, and little in the joints, and if present, as in cases of stable edema of the carpal canal, is anechoic in nature. If fluid is excessive and anechoic it is usually a transudate and unlikely to be of major concern. If fluid is excessive and hypo- to hyperchoic, increased cellularity and increased protein content is likely, and a modified transudate or exudate should be suspected. The latter is often indicative of a septic process. If there are also very hyperechoic multifocal single specks that tend to move proximally within the fluid, the presence of gas is likely and indicative of an open wound and/or gas-producing bacteria.

Bones

If the normal smooth hyperechoic cortex is disrupted, a fracture should be considered. New bone can be seen as irregular hyperechoic extensions of the subchondral bone (osteophytic), or source or implantations of ligaments, or joint capsules (enthesophytic) or on the bone surface (periosteal). Hypo- to anechoic fluid accumulation between the periosteum and cortical bone is highly indicative of osteomyelitis.

Joint Surfaces

Although challenging, and more clearly visualized by means of arthroscopy, the keen ultrasonographer may

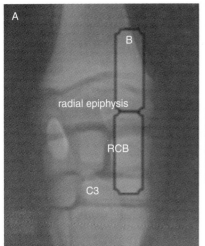

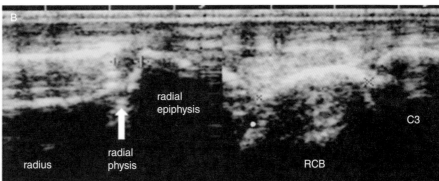

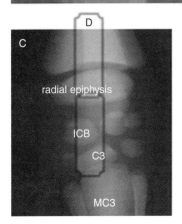

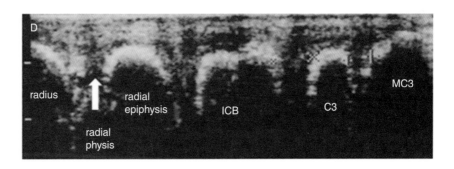

Figure 4.11 Incomplete ossification of the cuboidal bones of the carpus. (A) 2-day-old term donkey foal carpus. Dorsal palmar radiographic view showing normal ossification expected for this age animal. The Skeletal Ossification Index (SOI) [2] is Grade 4 (the cuboidal bones are appropriately ossified, with an adult appearance, and the joint spaces are of an expected width. (B) Split screen dorsal image of distal radius and carpal bones. (C) 303 days gestation twin filly. Dorsal palmar radiograph showing incomplete ossification of carpal bones, apparent widened joint spaces, and irregular endochondral ossification. SOI is Grade 2 (All cuboidal bones show some radiographic evidence of ossification except first carpal and tarsal bones; proximal epiphysis of the third metacarpal/metatarsal bones is present; styloid processes and malleoli absent). (D) Split screen dorsal image of distal radius and carpal bones; note the rounded carpal bone edges, the apparent widened joint spaces and distal radial physis; proximal is to the left. C: carpal bone; ICB: intermediate carpal bone; MC: metacarpal bone; RCB: radio-carpal bone. (Source: Images courtesy of Dr SM Higgerty, Crowthorne Veterinary Clinic, Johannesburg, South Africa.)

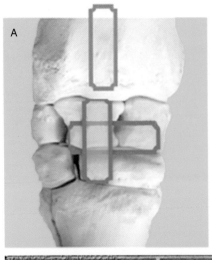
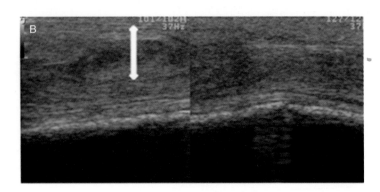
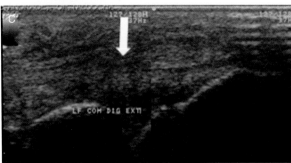
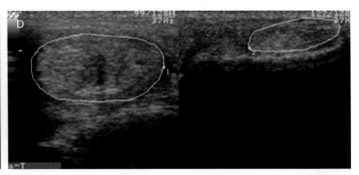

Figure 4.12   Common digital extensor tendon (CDET) rupture. (A) Anatomical specimen indicating transducer placement. Longitudinal (B,C) and transverse (D) images of the dorsal aspect of the left carpus showing partial rupture of the CDE tendon. (B) Split screen image with mildly thickened subcutaneous tissues and marked disruption of the tendon fibres of the CDET (double headed arrow) with focal hypoechoic areas within. Proximal is to the left. (C) Split screen image with mildly thickened subcutaneous tissues and marked disruption of the tendon fibers of the CDE (arrow) with hypoechoic striations within and mild amount of hypoechoic fluid within the tendon sheath. Proximal is to the left. (D): Abnormal left and comparative normal right carpus showing marked enlargement and inhomogeneously hypoechoic left CDE tendon and increased distance between the skin surface and underlying bone. Medial of the left carpus is to the right. C: carpal bone; ICB: intermediate carpal bone; Le: left; MC: metacarpal bone; RCB: radiocarpal bone; Rt: right; UCB: ulnar carpal bone.

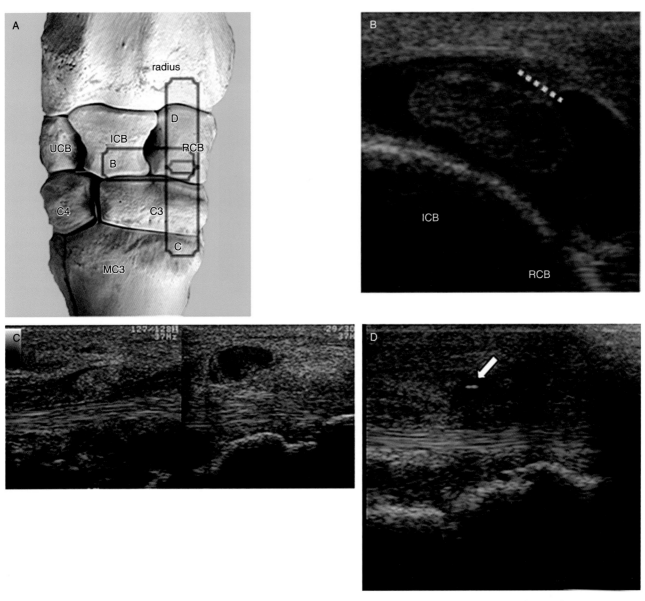

Figure 4.13 Septic extensor carpi radialis tenosynovitis. (A) Anatomical specimen indicating transducer placement. Transverse (B) and longitudinal (C,D) images of the dorsal aspect of the carpus showing a septic extensor carpi radialis (ECR) tenosynovitis as result of a penetrating foreign body. (B) Marked distension of the ECR sheath with anechoic as well as hypoechoic fluid therein with a few criss-crossing hyperechoic fibrin-like bands. The tendon itself appears slightly swollen and more hypoechoic than normal. Note the widened hypoechoic mesotendon (stippled line). Medial is to the right. (C) Marked distension of the ECR sheath with hypoechoic and hyperechoic fluid therein with a few hyperechoic fibrin-like bands and formation of some inhomogeneous pockets of fluid. The ECR tendon is slightly swollen with some decrease in fiber alignment. Proximal is to the left. (D) Thickened subcutaneous tissues with a focal poorly marginated hypoechoic area with a hyperechoic structure (arrow) within this with mild acoustic shadowing distally consistent with a foreign body. The ECRT periphery is irregular. Note the irregular cortical margin of C3. Proximal is to the left. C: carpal bone; ICB: intermediate carpal bone; MC: metacarpal bone; RCB: radiocarpal bone; UCB: ulnar carpal bone.

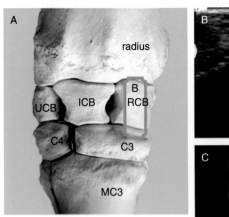
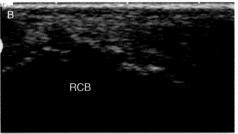
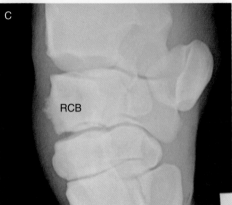

Figure 4.14 (A) Anatomical specimen indicating transducer placement. Periosteal new bone formation. (B) Longitudinal image of the dorsum of the carpus with marked irregular cortical margins of the radiocarpal bone (RCB), either as result of traumatic periostitis or enthesopathy of the dorsal intercarpal ligaments. Proximal is to the left. (C) DLPaMO view of the carpus with periosteal new bone of the dorsomedial aspect of the RCB. C: carpal bone; ICB: intermediate carpal bone; MC: metacarpal bone; UCB: ulnar carpal bone.

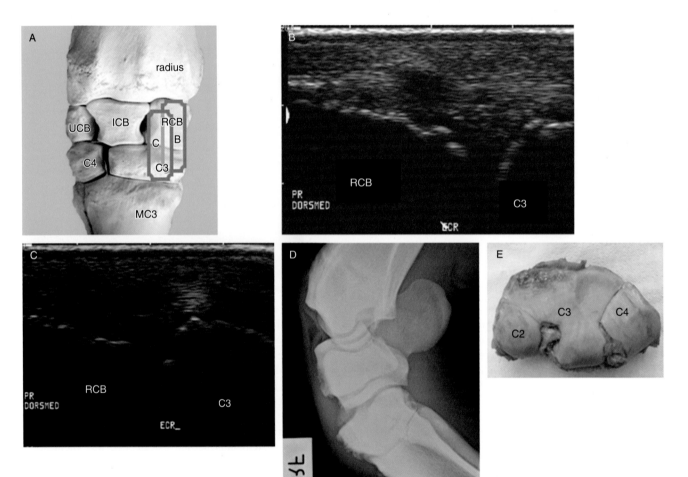

Figure 4.15 Osteochondral fragmentation. (A) Anatomical specimen indicating transducer placement. (B) Longitudinal image of the dorsum of the carpus with marked irregular cortical margins of the radiocarpal bone (RCB), consistent with chip fracture/osteophyte and mildly irregular proximodorsal margin of C3. Note the hyperechoic parallel orientated fibers of the extensor carpi radialis tendon superficially with focal loss of echogenicity due to off-incidence artifact. Proximal is to the left. (C) Marked irregular proximodorsal margin of C3, likely a chip fracture or osteophyte. Proximal is to the left. (D) Flexed LM view of the carpus in C with a chip fracture dorsodistal RCB, suspect chip fracture dorsoproximal C3 and dorsal periosteal reaction C3. (E) Macerated postmortem specimen of proximal joint surfaces of C2, C3, C4. Note the marked articular cartilage destruction of dorsoproximal C3. Medial is to the left. C: carpal bone; ICB: intermediate carpal bone; MC: metacarpal bone; RCB: radial carpal bone; UCB: ulnar carpal bone.

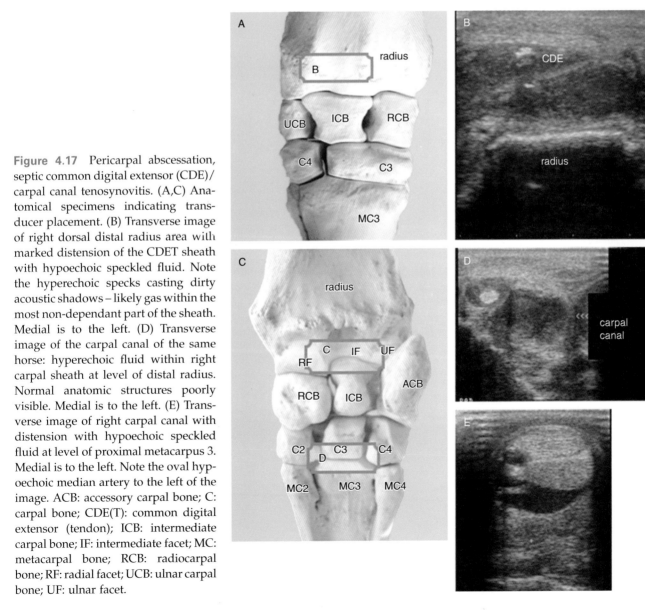

Figure 4.16 Sagittal slab fracture of C3. (A) Anatomical specimen indicating transducer placement. (B) Transverse image of the dorsum of C3 and C2 (transducer positioned more obliquely dorsomedially than depicted in guide image). A 5.4 mm wide hyperechoic structure with distal acoustic shadowing is depicted separate from and slightly dorsal to the parent C3 with a few smaller hyperechoic structures in the vicinity. Medial is to the left. C: D35°PrDDiO radiographic view of carpus, showing a focal area of multiple fragments off the medial aspect of the radial facet of C3. C: carpal bone; ICB: intermediate carpal bone; MC: metacarpal bone; RCB: radiocarpal bone; UCB: ulnar carpal bone.

Figure 4.17 Pericarpal abscessation, septic common digital extensor (CDE)/ carpal canal tenosynovitis. (A,C) Anatomical specimens indicating transducer placement. (B) Transverse image of right dorsal distal radius area with marked distension of the CDET sheath with hypoechoic speckled fluid. Note the hyperechoic specks casting dirty acoustic shadows – likely gas within the most non-dependant part of the sheath. Medial is to the left. (D) Transverse image of the carpal canal of the same horse: hyperechoic fluid within right carpal sheath at level of distal radius. Normal anatomic structures poorly visible. Medial is to the left. (E) Transverse image of right carpal canal with distension with hypoechoic speckled fluid at level of proximal metacarpus 3. Medial is to the left. Note the oval hypoechoic median artery to the left of the image. ACB: accessory carpal bone; C: carpal bone; CDE(T): common digital extensor (tendon); ICB: intermediate carpal bone; IF: intermediate facet; MC: metacarpal bone; RCB: radiocarpal bone; RF: radial facet; UCB: ulnar carpal bone; UF: ulnar facet.

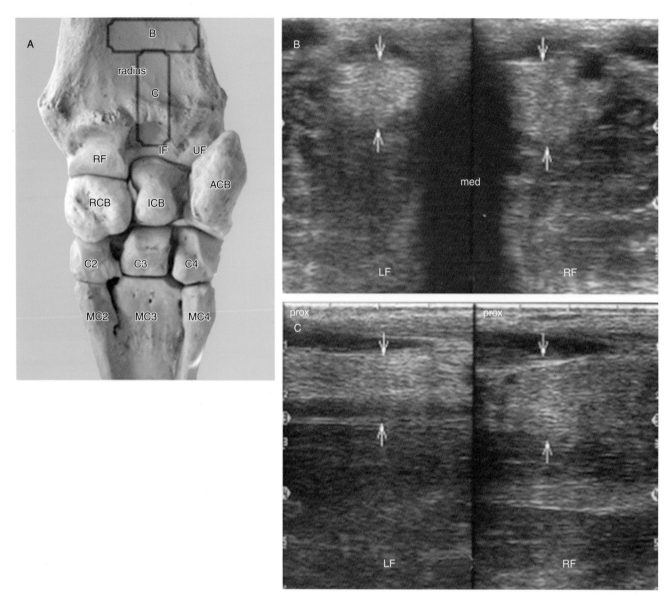

Figure 4.18   Desmitis of the right accessory ligament of the superficial digital flexor tendon (AL-SDFT). C: carpal bone; ICB: intermediate carpal bone; IF: intermediate facet; MC: metacarpal bone; RCB: radiocarpal bone; RF: radial facet; UCB: ulnar carpal bone; UF: ulnar facet. (A) Anatomical specimen indicating transducer placement. (B,C) Transverse images of the AL-SDFT of the left (LF) and right fore limbs (RF). An injury to the RF AL-SDFT at level 2A (approximately 9–11 cm proximal to the accessory carpal bone (ACB)) is present illustrating enlargement and decreased echogenicity; medial sides of each limb marked (med). (Source: Parts B and C – Adapted from Jorgensen, J.S. *et al.* (2010) [3]. Reproduced with permission of John Wiley & Sons Ltd.)

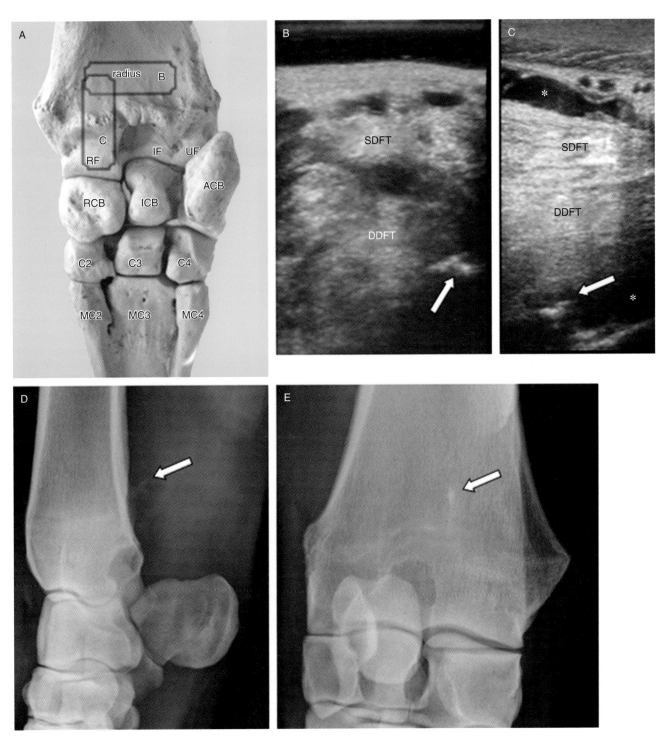

Figure 4.19 Osteochondroma distocaudomedial radius. (A) Anatomical specimen indicating transducer placement. (B) Transverse image of the distal radial metaphysis. Note the hyperechoic acoustic shadow-casting structure in the depth of the field (arrow). (C) Longitudinal image distal metaphysis radius. The irregular hyperechoic acoustic shadow-casting structure (arrow) is in the depth nearly adjacent to the radius. Note the anechoic fluid with a few hyperechoic fibrin-like strands in the near and far field within the carpal canal (*). Proximal is to the left. (D) Lateromedial radiograph of the carpus. Note the poorly mineralized spike extending from the caudodistal radius (arrow). There is also marked soft tissue swelling associated with carpal canal effusion. (E) Dorsopalmar radiograph of the same case: note the focal mineralized opacity superimposed over the caudodistal radius slightly medially. There is also marked soft tissue swelling associated with carpal canal effusion. ACB: accessory carpal bone; C: carpal bone; DDFT: deep digital flexor tendon; ICB: intermediate carpal bone; IF: intermediate facet; MC: metacarpal bone; RCB: radiocarpal bone; RF: radial facet; SDFT: superficial digital flexor tendon; UCB: ulnar carpal bone; UF: ulnar facet. (Source: Parts B, C and D – Images courtesy of Drs Baker and McVeigh and Associates, Summerveld, South Africa.)

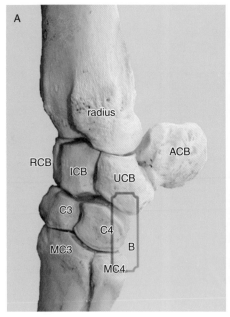

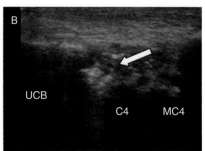

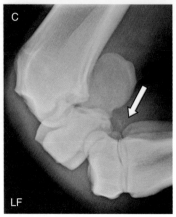

Figure 4.20 Multiple palmar chip fractures from the palmar distal aspects of the proximal row of carpal bones and/or the palmar proximal aspect of the distal row of carpal bones. (A) Anatomical specimen indicating transducer placement. (B) Longitudinal image, palmarolateral ulnar carpal bone (UCB), C4 and fourth metacarpal bone (MC4). Overlying the slightly recessed C4 there are multiple irregular small hyperechoic fragments consistent with small bony chip fractures (arrow). Proximal is to the left. (C) Lateromedial flexed view of the carpus illustrating multiple mineralized fragments in the palmar recess of the middle carpal joint (arrow). ACB: accessory carpal bone; C: carpal bone; ICB: intermediate carpal bone; MC: metacarpal bone; RCB: radiocarpal bone; UCB: ulnar carpal bone.

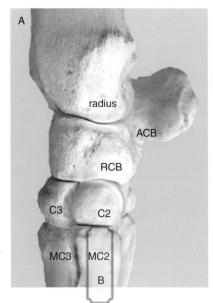

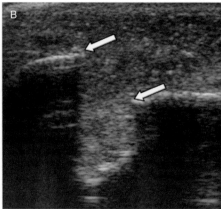

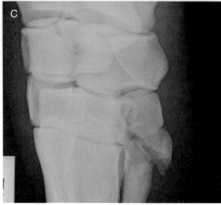

Figure 4.21 Recent moderately displaced fracture. (A) Anatomical specimen indicating transducer placement. (B) Longitudinal image, palmar proximolateral metacarpal (MC)4 showing marked disruption of the lateral cortex and separation of the fracture fragments (arrows) with inhomogeneously hypoechoic material between the fragments – likely hemorrhage. Proximal is to the left. (C) DMPaLO view left carpus illustrating recent moderately displaced fracture MC2. ACB: accessory carpal bone; C: carpal bone; RCB: radiocarpal bone.

be able to evaluate the joint surface for irregular thinned cartilage and irregular subchondral bone, indicative of possible osteoarthritis or developmental orthopedic disease.

SURGERY

Ultrasound-guided surgical procedures of the carpus have been described, such as removal of osteochondral fragments of carpal bones and foreign bodies and is perhaps an underutilized surgical tool.

RECOMMENDED READING

Denoix, J.-M. & Yousfi, S. (1996) Spontaneous injury of the accessory ligament of the superficial digital flexor tendon (proximal check ligament): a new ultrasonographic diagnosis. *Journal of Equine Veterinary Science*, 16, 191–194.

Denoix, J.M. & Busoni, V. (1999) Ultrasonographic anatomy of the accessory ligament of the superficial digital flexor tendon in horses. *Equine Veterinary Journal*, 31, 186–191.

Desmaizieres, L.M. & Cauvin, E.R. (2005) Carpal collateral ligament desmopathy in three horses. *Veterinary Record*, 157, 197–201.

Driver, A.J., Barr, F.J., Fuller, C.J., & Barr, A.R.S. (2004) Ultrasonography of the medial palmar intercarpal ligament in the Thoroughbred: technique and normal appearance. *Equine Veterinary Journal*, 36, 402–408.

Jorgensen, J.S., Stewart, A.A., Stewart, M.C., & Genovese, R.L. (2010) Ultrasonographic examination of the caudal structures of the distal antebrachium in the horse. *Equine Veterinary Education*, 22, 146–155.

Piccot-Crezollet, C. & Cauvin, E.R. (2005) Treatment of a second carpal bone fracture by removal under ultrasonographic guidance in a horse. *Veterinary Surgery*, 34, 662–667

Probst, A., Macher, R., Hinterhofer, C., Polsterer, E., Guarda, I.H., & König, H.E. (2008) Anatomical features of the carpal flexor retinaculum of the horse. *Anatomy, Histology, Embryology*, 37, 415–417.

Reef, V.R. (1998) *Equine Diagnostic Ultrasound*. WB Saunders Co, Philadelphia.

Reef, V.R., Whittier, M., Allam, L.G. (2004) Joint ultrasonography. *Clinical Techniques in Equine Practice*, 3, 256–267.

Smith, M. & Smith, R. (2008) Diagnostic ultrasound of the limb joints, muscle and bone in horses. *In Practice*, 30, 152–159.

Tnibar, M., Kaser-Hotz, B., & Auer, J.A. (1993) Ultrasonography of the dorsal and lateral aspects of the equine carpus: technique and normal appearance. *Veterinary Radiology and Ultrasound*, 34, 413–425.

REFERENCES

[1] Driver, A.J., Barr, F.J., Fuller, C.J., & Barr, A.R.S. (2004) Ultrasonography of the medial palmar intercarpal ligament in the Thoroughbred: technique and normal appearance. *Equine Veterinary Journal*, 36, 402–408.

[2] Adams, R. & Poulos, P. (1988) A skeletal ossification index for neonatal foals. *Veterinary Radiology*, 29, 217–222.

[3] Jorgensen, J.S., Stewart, A.A., Stewart, M.C., & Genovese, R.L. (2010) Ultrasonographic examination of the caudal structures of the distal antebrachium in the horse. *Equine Veterinary Education*, 22(3), 146–155.

CHAPTER FIVE

ULTRASONOGRAPHY OF THE ELBOW AND SHOULDER

Barbara Riccio

Studio Veterinario Associato Cascina Gufa, Merlino (LO), Italy

INTRODUCTION

Ultrasonographic examination of the elbow and shoulder yields information about the soft tissue structures of these joints, complementing the information that is obtained through radiography and nuclear scintigraphy. These areas have been traditionally difficult to examine properly in the field with radiography, and ultrasonographic examination can be helpful for the practitioner to obtain diagnostic information about conditions related to these areas. An upper limb lameness, a history of trauma, a swelling or local deformation, a hematoma, an abscess, a draining tract, or a lameness localized to the joint are all common indications for ultrasonography of the shoulder and elbow. In the latter case, ultrasonography is considered more sensitive than radiography for detection of early bone remodeling that is usually associated with osteoarthritis. As an ultrasound examination of the shoulder and the elbow is less commonly performed than in other regions, it is recommended to prepare both limbs in order to use the opposite limb for comparison. Sedation is usually not needed in adults while young animals usually require a low dose of sedation.

ELBOW

Preparation and Scanning Technique

Routine skin preparation is used. Diagnostic images can be obtained with high-frequency linear transducers (5–10 MHz), but a convex probe can be useful at the cranial aspect of the elbow to study the distal insertion of the biceps brachii tendon. In cases of ultrasound-guided injections, a micro-convex probe is suitable. A standoff pad is required to improve contact with the lateral aspect of the elbow during examination of the lateral collateral ligament of the elbow joint.

The elbow joint can be scanned from cranial, lateral, and medial approaches. Ultrasonography of the elbow is performed in the weightbearing position, but the evaluation of the medial aspect of the elbow joint is limited in this position. To allow better positioning of the transducer in this area the limb should be pulled forward, but nevertheless medial access is not easy.

A complete sonographic examination of the elbow should involve the lateral and medial collateral ligaments, the triceps brachii tendon, the proximal tendon of the ulnaris lateralis, the distal biceps brachii tendon, the joint space, and the articular cartilage. Examination of the lateral collateral ligament, the triceps brachii tendon, the proximal tendon of the ulnaris lateralis, and the articular cartilage of the humeral trochlea is straightforward. The medial collateral ligament and the distal biceps brachii tendon require more expertise to assess.

Ultrasonographic Anatomy and Ultrasonographic Abnormalities

Elbow Joint

The elbow joint is formed by the articulation of the distal humerus with the radius and ulna. The distal humerus has two condyles that are unequal in size, with the medial condyle being significantly larger. They are separated by a groove that sometimes contains a synovial fossa (Figure 5.1). The epicondyles sit proximal and caudal to the condyles, and between the epicondyles is the olecranon fossa which interdigitates with the anconeal process of the ulna. The joint

Atlas of Equine Ultrasonography, First Edition. Edited by Jessica A. Kidd, Kristina G. Lu, and Michele L. Frazer.
© 2014 John Wiley & Sons, Ltd. Published 2014 by John Wiley & Sons, Ltd.
Companion Website: www.wiley.com/go/kidd/equine-ultrasonography

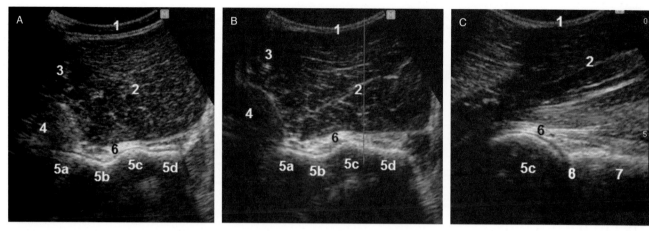

Figure 5.1   Normal images of the dorsal aspect of the elbow joint in transverse (A, B) (medial is to the left) and longitudinal (C) (proximal is to the left) sections. (A, B) The dorsal aspect of the elbow joint is characterized by a strong articular capsule with the attachment of the extensor carpi radialis tendon. By slightly changing the orientation of the probe, we can better visualize the articular cartilage and the biceps brachii becomes more echogenic as seen in (A). (C) Longitudinal section corresponding to the red line in fig 5.1B. 1: skin; 2: extensor carpi radialis muscle; 3: brachialis muscle; 4: biceps brachii muscle; 5: dorsal aspect of the humeral condyle: 5a: medial ridge of the trochlea, 5b: groove, 5c: lateral ridge of the trochlea, 5d: capitulum; 6: dorsal articular capsule; 7: dorsal aspect of the proximal radius; 8: joint space.

is supported medially and laterally by collateral ligaments and dorsally by a thick dorsal capsule, which includes the attachment of the proximal tendon of the extensor carpi radialis. At this level, the humeral condyle is covered by three muscles (from medial to lateral): the biceps brachii muscle belly and distal tendon, the brachialis muscle, and the extensor carpi radialis muscle. The biceps brachii tendon and the brachialis muscles may appear hypoechoic as a function of the orientation of the probe. In a normal joint, no synovial fluid is present on the cranial aspect of the joint. The amount of synovial fluid and the articular margins are better evaluated on the lateral aspect at the level of the collateral lateral ligament. In the lateral recess of normal horses, it is possible to find a small amount of synovial fluid. The best site to perform an ultrasound-guided injection is at the level of the joint space, immediately caudally to the lateral collateral ligament, in transverse section.

Abnormalities of the elbow joint other than septic arthritis are uncommon and septic arthritis is the most common abnormality seen. Septic arthritis is most common in foals, but occasionally is seen in older horses in association with trauma. The humerus, other than the deltoid tuberosity, is largely protected from the effects of direct trauma by muscles, but the olecranon of the ulna and the lateral aspect of the elbow are covered with minimal soft tissues and are therefore much more susceptible. With trauma to the lateral aspect of the elbow joint, wounds may easily extend

into the elbow joint and sepsis should be considered. Ultrasonographically, this condition is characterized by a large amount of synovial fluid, which can appear hypoechogenic or echogenic due to an increased cellularity and/or the presence of fibrin (Figure 5.2).

In horses, osteoarthritis of the elbow joint is relatively unusual but can be seen in older sport horses, often with a history of trauma. Osteoarthritis can also be secondary to collateral ligament desmitis, osseous cyst-like lesions of the proximal aspect of the radius, olecranon fractures, post-sepsis, or some other primary insult to the joint. Periarticular bone modeling, osteophytes, and an increased amount of synovial fluid with echogenic spots consistent with fibrin are the most likely ultrasonographic findings (Figure 5.3).

Collateral Ligaments of the Elbow Joint

The lateral collateral ligament of the elbow joint is short; it originates from the lateral humeral condyle and inserts distally on the lateral tuberosity of the radius just distal to the joint margin. The lateral collateral ligament is a strong ligament compared to the medial, which is thinner and weaker. The lateral collateral ligament is easily imaged under the lateral head of the triceps brachii muscle. This ligament is slightly heterogeneous because of its spiral fibers. The ligament has two portions with different fiber orientation: the deep portion, which is less echoic, and a superficial one. In a transverse section, it is possible to obtain

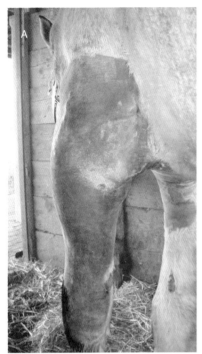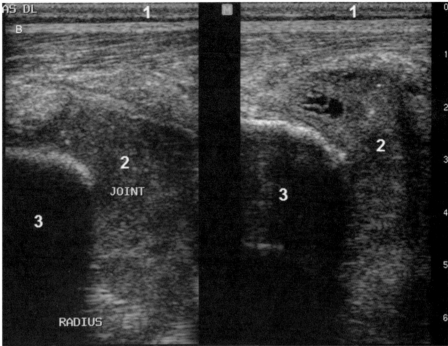

Figure 5.2 Septic arthritis of the elbow joint. (A) A 5-year-old draft horse with a severe swelling of the left elbow region caused by septic arthritis of the joint secondary to trauma. (B) Ultrasonogram of the lateral aspect of the left elbow. The lateral recess of the elbow joint is filled of a large amount of echogenic synovial fluid consistent with septic arthritis. The diagnosis was confirmed by synovial fluid analysis. 1: skin; 2: lateral recess of the elbow joint; 3: radius.

three different images of the collateral ligament: at its proximal humeral enthesis, at the joint space, and at its distal radial insertion. The proximal part of this ligament appears ovoid/elliptic shaped and appears less homogeneous than distally (Figures 5.4 and 5.5).

Compared to the lateral collateral ligament, the medial collateral ligament is longer and thinner so its ultrasonographic examination is more challenging. The muscular mass of the pectoralis muscles make its visualization more complicated. Pulling the limb forward and pushing back the pectoralis muscles may help in the examination of this area. The medial collateral ligament originates proximally from an eminence on the medial humeral epicondyle, and consists of a long superficial portion and a short deeper portion. The deep part inserts on the radial tuberosity; the longer branch ends more distally on the medial border of the radius, just distal to the interosseous space between the radius and the ulna. Figure 5.6 shows the medial collateral ligament at its proximal insertion and at the level of the joint space. The distal insertion can be more difficult to identify. The medial aspect of the radius is often irregular without clinical significance, and care should be taken in interpreting these findings. At the medial aspect of the elbow joint, superficially

and adjacent to the medial collateral ligament, there are large neurovascular structures: the median arteries and veins, and the median nerve (Figure 5.7).

Collateral ligament injuries are uncommon and usually the result of trauma. Lesions to the collateral ligaments result in an enlarged hypoechoic collateral ligament with disruption of the normal fiber pattern. Sometimes avulsion fractures of the collateral ligaments from the humeral condyle or the distal radial insertion are seen, or periosteal new bone can be associated with collateral ligament desmitis.

Ulnaris Lateralis Muscle

The ulnaris lateralis muscle originates proximal to the lateral epicondyle of the distal humerus, caudal and deep to the lateral collateral ligament; its tendon then courses caudal to the lateral collateral ligament. For this reason, an ultrasound examination of the ulnaris lateralis is easier if it begins with the transverse section of the lateral collateral ligament just proximal to the joint space, and then the probe is moved slightly caudally (Figure 5.8). In cases with synovial distension of this lateral articular recess, the ulnaris lateralis tendon

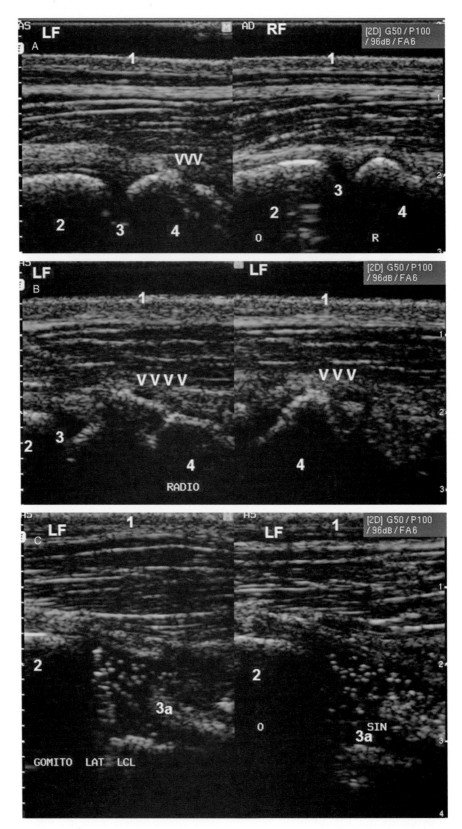

Figure 5.3 Osteoarthritis of the elbow joint. Ultrasonogram of the lateral aspect of the left elbow of a 10-year-old show jumper horse with a chronic intermittent left fore limb lameness. (A) Longitudinal sections of the joint slightly cranial to the lateral collateral ligament. The bone surface of the lateral aspect of the affected left radial condyle (LF) is irregular (arrows) compared to the unaffected contralateral right limb (RF). (B) Two longitudinal sections of the affected left fore limb showing similar abnormal findings to (A). (C) Two transverse images of the lateral recess of the elbow joint which is markedly distended. The synovial fluid contains multiple echogenic "spots", consistent with fibrin. These findings are indicative of osteoarthritis with chronic synovitis. 1: skin; 2: lateral humeral condyle; 3: joint space, 3a: lateral recess of the elbow joint; 4: lateral radial condyle.

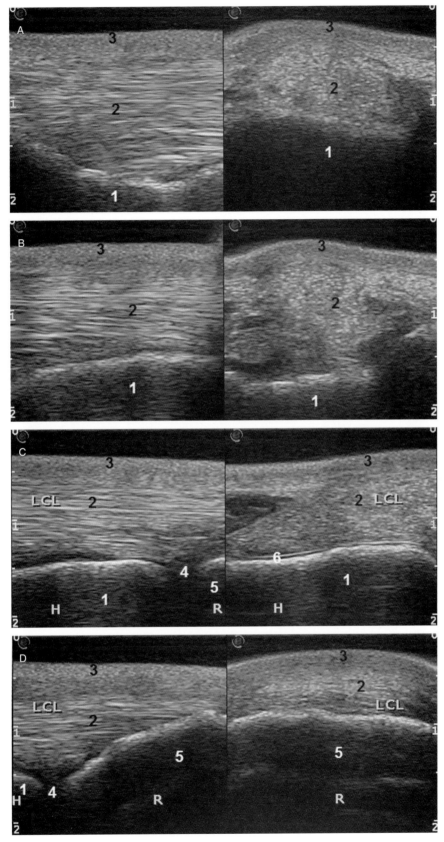

Figure 5.4 Normal longitudinal (left) and transverse (right) ultrasound scans of the lateral collateral ligament (LCL) of the elbow joint from its origin (A), just proximal to the joint space (B), at the level of the joint space (C) and at its distal insertion (D). The shape of the LCL is ovoid proximally and becomes more flat distally. In the transverse scan at the level of the joint space (C) it is possible to appreciate the articular cartilage layer (6). Longitudinal section: proximal is to the left, lateral is to top. Transverse section: cranial is to the left, lateral is to top. 1: lateral humeral condyle; 2: lateral collateral ligament; 3: skin; 4: joint space; 5: lateral radial tuberosity; 6: articular cartilage; R: radius.

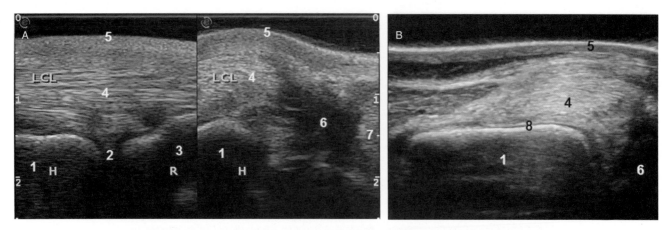

Figure 5.5 Normal longitudinal (left) and transverse (right) ultrasound scans of the lateral collateral ligament (LCL) of the elbow joint at the level of the joint space. (A) Longitudinal section (proximal is to the left, lateral is to top) and transverse section (cranial is to the left, lateral is to top). (B) Transverse section (cranial is to the left, lateral is to top). In transverse section, caudally to the LCL there is the lateral recess of the elbow joint which shows a small amount of anechoic synovial fluid. 1: lateral humeral condyle; 2: joint space; 3: lateral radial tuberosity; 4: lateral collateral ligament; 5: skin; 6: synovial fluid in the lateral recess of the elbow joint; 7: ulnaris lateralis tendon; 8: articular cartilage.

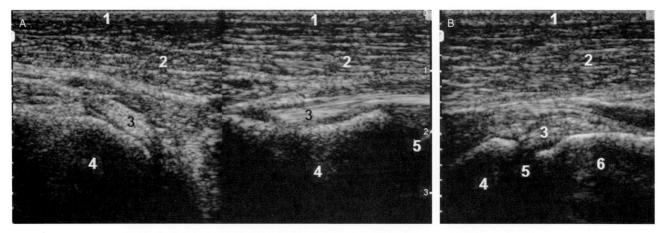

Figure 5.6 (A) Normal transverse ultrasound scan of the medial collateral ligament (MCL) of the elbow joint at the level of the joint space. When the transducer is perpendicular to the ligament fibers in transverse scans, the MCL looks homogeneous and echogenic. (B) In longitudinal section, the MCL can appear more or less flat depending on the position of the probe in the craniocaudal plane. Cranial is to the left, medial is to the top. 1: skin; 2: pectoralis transversus muscle; 3: MCL; 4: medial humeral condyle; 5: joint space; 6: medial aspect of the proximal radius.

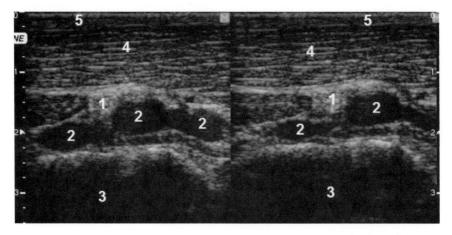

Figure 5.7 Normal transverse ultrasound scan of the medial aspect of the elbow joint at the level of the medial radial condyle showing the vessels and the median nerve. The irregularity of the radial bone surface is normal. 1: median nerve; 2: median arteries and veins; 3: medial radial condyle; 4: pectoralis transversus muscle; 5: antebrachial fascia.

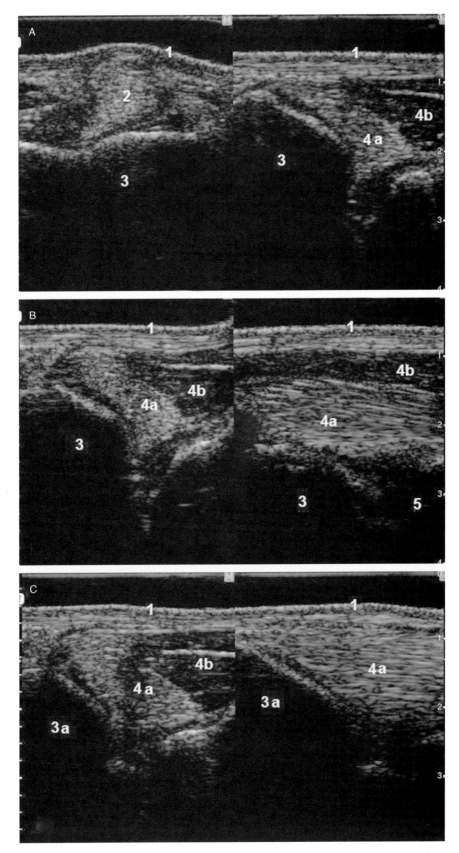

Figure 5.8 Normal ultrasound scans of the ulnaris lateralis (UL) at the lateral aspect of the elbow. (A) Transverse section of the lateral collateral ligament (left) and ulnaris lateralis tendon (right). (B) Transverse (left) and longitudinal (right) sections of the UL tendon. (C) Transverse (left) and longitudinal (right) sections of the UL tendon at the level of its enthesis on the lateral epicondyle. Longitudinal section: proximal is to the left, medial is to top. Transverse section: cranial is to the left, medial is to top. 1: skin; 2: lateral collateral ligament; 3: lateral aspect of the humerus, 3a: lateral humeral epicondyle; 4: ulnaris lateralis, 4a: tendon, 4b: muscle; 5: lateral recess of the cubital joint with a small amount of synovial fluid.

is separated from the lateral collateral ligament by a synovial fold.

Distal Insertion of the Biceps Brachii

In horses, the biceps brachii muscle is characterized by an intramuscular tendon continuing to its distal tendon. Because of the concave shape of this anatomical area, it is easier to examine the distal insertion of the biceps brachii with a convex transducer. To identify the biceps brachii enthesis, it is useful to begin with longitudinal scanning on the dorsal aspect of the elbow joint (see Figure 5.1) and then move the probe slightly medially to identify the insertion located at the craniomedial aspect of the elbow (Figure 5.9).

Enthesopathy of the biceps brachii insertion is caused by a tearing of its distal attachment on the cranioproximal aspect of the radius. In chronic cases, radiographic and ultrasonographic examination may identify periosteal new bone on the cranial tuberosity of the radius at the site of the insertion of the biceps brachii. Pathology of the biceps brachii is much more common in the shoulder region and will be discussed in the shoulder section.

Triceps Brachii Muscle and Distal Tendon

Situated at the caudolateral aspect of the elbow region, the triceps brachii muscle is one of the principal extensors of the elbow joint and inserts on the olecranon tuberosity of the ulna. Figure 5.10 shows the normal appearance of the distal triceps brachii tendon.

The muscle can be affected by a post-anesthetic myopathy. Sonographic findings of post-anesthetic myopathy consist of loss of normal muscle striations and an overall increased muscle echogenicity. Sometimes, an affected triceps brachii muscle can return to a normal ultrasonographic appearance, but in most

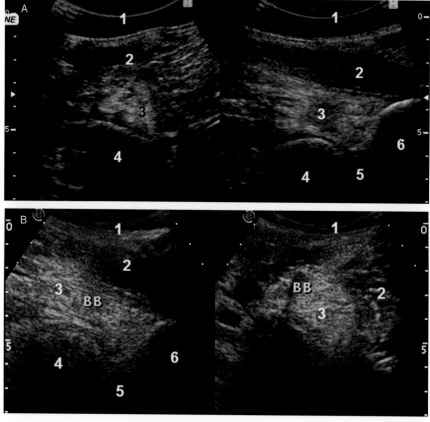

Figure 5.9 Normal ultrasonograms of the distal insertion of the biceps brachii tendon on the craniomedial aspect of the elbow. (A) Transverse (left: medial is to the left) and longitudinal (right: proximal is to the left) sections of the distal biceps brachii tendon. The hypoechoic area inside of the tendon in both scans is normal and it is due to the presence of hypoechoic muscle fibers. (B) Longitudinal (left: proximal is to the left) and transverse (right: medial is to the left) sections of the distal biceps brachii tendon. The shape of the distal tendon on transverse scans appears different according to the level of the section. 1: skin; 2: extensor carpi radialis muscle; 3: distal tendon of biceps brachii muscle; 4: dorsomedial aspect of the humeral condyle; 5: joint space; 6: radial tuberosity.

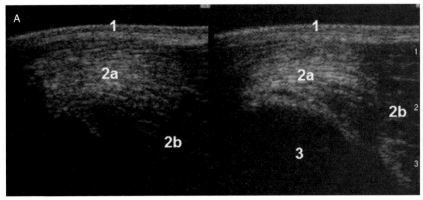
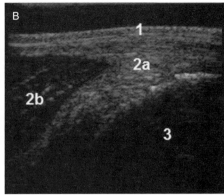

Figure 5.10 Normal ultrasonogram of the distal insertion of the triceps brachii tendon on the olecranon tuberosity of the ulna. (A) Transverse (medial is to the left) sections of the distal triceps brachii tendon just proximal to the olecranon tuberosity (left) and at the level of the olecranon (right). (B) Longitudinal (proximal is to the left) section of the distal enthesis of the triceps brachii tendon. The hypoechoic tissue proximal to the tendon is the muscle belly of the triceps brachii. 1: skin; 2: triceps brachii, 2a: distal tendon of triceps brachii muscle, 2b: triceps brachii muscle; 3: olecranon tuberosity.

cases it remains abnormal. A rare condition is a tendinopathy of the distal tendon of the triceps brachii muscle. In these cases, the tendon is enlarged and becomes heterogeneous; if there is also a damage of the enthesis, it is possible to find modeling of the olecranon surface with new bone formation.

SHOULDER

Scanning Technique

A standoff pad is usually not necessary because most anatomic structures are positioned relatively deeply, except at the point of the shoulder where a standoff is useful to improve the contact between the skin and the probe. The shoulder should be scanned from cranial to caudal with the horse fully weightbearing on the limb to avoid hypoechogenic artifacts. Diagnostic images are best obtained with medium- to high-frequency linear or curved transducers (5–10 MHz). Anatomic structures close to the skin surface are visualized with a high-frequency linear probe, but this can be inadequate to examine the scapulohumeral joint in large horses. The advantage of a convex probe is a larger acoustic window which is useful to visualize the entire biceps brachii tendon at the level of the humeral tubercles. A 5–7.5 MHz micro-convex transducer is useful in case of ultrasound-guided injection.

A complete sonographic examination of the shoulder should include the scapula, the supraglenoid tubercle, the biceps brachii tendon, the bicipital bursa, the humeral tubercles, the intertubercular groove, the supraspinatus and infraspinatus tendons, and the scapulohumeral joint.

Ultrasonographic Anatomy and Ultrasonographic Abnormalities

Scapula and Supraglenoid Tubercle

The equine shoulder is characterized by a simple scapulohumeral joint without collateral ligaments and a remarkable muscle mass providing stability to the joint. An ultrasound study of the scapula begins proximally at the level of the scapular cartilage, which is very superficial and covered by the trapezius muscle. This muscle appears hypoechogenic and attaches to the scapular spine. The scapula consists of a scapular spine and two fossae; the spine is identified as a regular hyperechoic line generating acoustic shadowing. The scapular spine becomes taller around the mid part of the scapula. At this level, the fossae are easily identified. The supraspinatus fossa is cranial to the scapular spine and houses the supraspinatus muscle (Figure 5.11). Caudally, the infraspinatus fossa, larger than the supraspinatus fossa, accommodates the origin of the infraspinatus muscle covered with the deltoideus muscle (Figure 5.11).

Fractures of the body of the scapula may be difficult to identify with a radiographic examination but they are more easily detected ultrasonographically. A fracture line appears as a hypoechoic to anechoic line through the cortical bone, allowing the ultrasound beam to penetrate through the bone for a certain distance. Distraction of the fracture fragment from the parent portion may occur and should be detected in two mutually perpendicular planes. In cases of chronic scapular fractures, ultrasonographic findings show an irregular bone surface consistent with a bone callus (Figure 5.12).

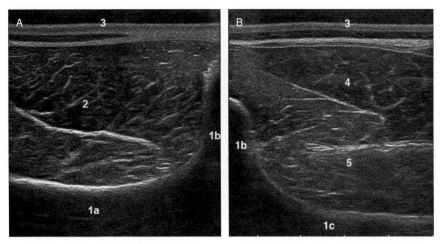

Figure 5.11 Normal transverse ultrasound scans of the mid-scapular spine (cranial to the left, caudal to the right). (A) The supraspinatus muscle originates from the supraspinatus fossa. (B) At this level, in the infraspinatus fossa the infraspinatus muscle is deep to the deltoideus muscle, 1: scapula, 1a: supraspinatus fossa, 1b: scapular spine, 1c: infraspinatus fossa; 2: supraspinatus muscle; 3: skin; 4: deltoideus muscle; 5: infraspinatus muscle.

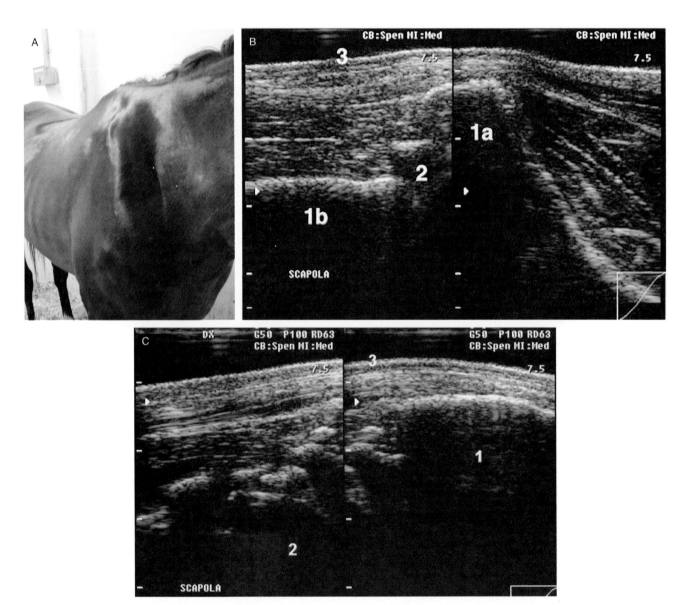

Figure 5.12 Chronic scapular fracture. (A) A 7-year-old Thoroughbred gelding with severe deformation of the right shoulder region caused by an old fracture of the body of the scapula. (B) Transverse scan of the right scapula (cranial is to the left). The scapular spine appears irregular in shape and enlarged. The suprascapular fossa also shows an abnormal convex shape. (C) Longitudinal scan of the right scapula. Bone remodeling is present at the cranial aspect of the scapular body. 1: scapula, 1a: scapular spine, 1b: suprascapular fossa; 2: bone remodeling; 3: skin.

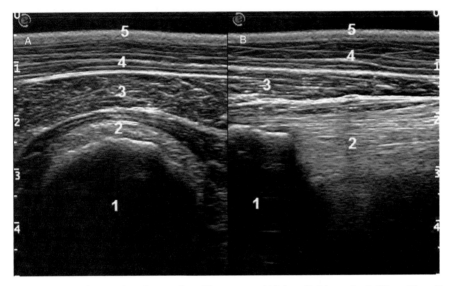

Figure 5.13 Normal origin of the biceps brachii tendon. Transverse (A) (medial is to the left) and longitudinal (B) (proximal is to the left) ultrasound scans of the origin of the biceps brachii tendon on the supraglenoid tubercle of the scapula. The tendon looks homogeneously echogenic in both sections. The bone surface of the supraglenoid tubercle should be smooth and regularly hyperechoic in both sections. 1: supraglenoid tubercle; 2: proximal tendon of the biceps brachii; 3: supraspinatus muscle; 4: brachiocephalicus muscle; 5: skin.

Fractures of the scapula most commonly involve the supraglenoid tubercle. Figure 5.13 shows the normal ultrasonographic appearance of the supraglenoid tubercle. These fractures are one of most common shoulder injuries, particularly in young horses. The fracture may be simple or comminuted and there is often an intra-articular component. In these cases, ultrasonographic findings are characterized by an irregular bone surface of the neck of the scapula with an irregular defect in the hyperechogenic bone line and distal displacement of the bony fragment, as the fracture is distracted by the pull of the biceps brachii tendon (Figure 5.14). This lesion is therefore often associated with relaxation of the proximal insertion of the biceps brachii muscle along with scapulohumeral synovitis and bicipital bursitis.

Intertubercular Sulcus and Humeral Tubercles

In a normal horse, the bone surface of the intertubercular sulcus (also called the intertubercular groove) is visualized as a smooth hyperechoic W-shaped line, which corresponds to the medial (lesser), intermediate, and lateral (greater) humeral tubercles (Figure 5.15). The greater tubercle has two eminences: cranial (the point of the shoulder) and caudal. Between these two landmarks is the site for intra-articular injection of the shoulder joint. In foals, there are two separate centers of ossification of the proximal humeral epiphysis: one

for the greater tubercle and one for the humeral head and lesser tubercle. The cartilage skeleton of the tubercles is still very large and anechoic and should not be mistaken for fluid (Figure 5.16). In yearlings, because of the on-going ossification process, the intermediate tubercle has an irregular contour which is normal in this age group (Figure 5.17). The proximal humeral physis closes between 24 and 36 months of age. In some mature horses, a notch over the intermediate tubercle can be seen as a result of incomplete ossification and represents a normal variant. The contour of demarcation between cartilage and subchondral bone can normally be quite irregular.

Osseous lesions, including osteomyelitis, osseous cyst-like lesions, and penetrating tracts, can involve these structures. In most cases of osseous lesions there is a cortical defect with underlying abnormal architecture of the subchondral bone. It is often useful to examine the opposite limb to determine if a lesion truly exists. Malformation of the intertubercular sulcus has been reported in four adult horses and in a Welsh pony.

Biceps Brachii Tendon

Bicipital tendinitis and bursitis are uncommon but, nonetheless, pathology in these structures is a significant cause of lameness referable to the shoulder. The biceps brachii tendon should be scanned in transverse

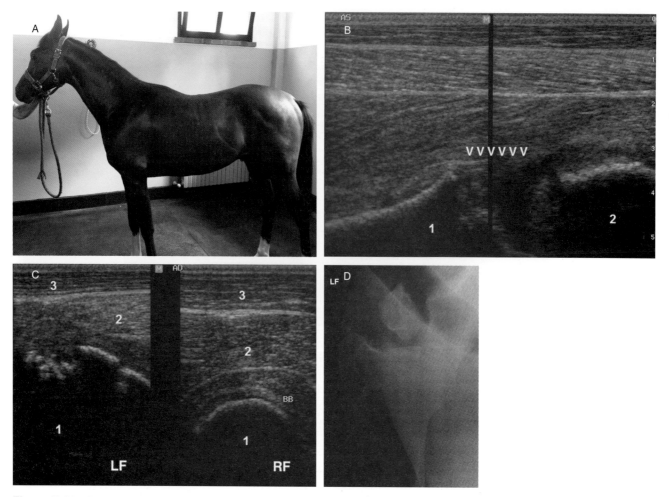

Figure 5.14 Supraglenoid tubercle fracture. (A) An Arabian yearling with an acute-onset severe left fore limb lameness caused by a fracture of the supraglenoid tubercle (photo). (B) Longitudinal ultrasound scan of the scapular neck. The bony fragment (2) is displaced distally and a large anechoic space (arrows) is visible between the fragment and the scapular neck (1) (proximal is to the left). (C) Transverse (medial is to the left) ultrasound scans of the supraglenoid tubercle in the same horse showing the fracture of the supraglenoid tubercle (LF) compared with the normal opposite limb (RF). The fracture fragment shows extensive bone remodeling. (D) Mediolateral radiographic view of the left scapulohumeral joint confirming the intra-articular fracture of the supraglenoid tubercle with distal displacement of the bony fragment. 1: supraglenoid tubercle of the scapula; 2: supraspinatus muscle; 3: brachiocephalicus muscle; BB: proximal biceps brachii tendon.

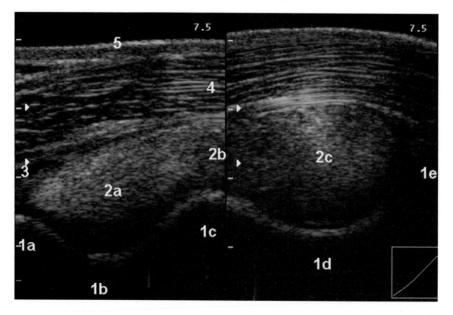

Figure 5.15 Normal proximal biceps brachii tendon. Transverse ultrasound scans (medial is to the left) of the proximal tendon of the biceps brachii over the intertubercular sulcus in a normal horse. The bicipital bursa lies between the tendon and the intertubercular sulcus. Normally the bicipital bursa is a virtual cavity and no fluid is visible. 1: intertubercular humeral sulcus, 1a: lesser tubercle, 1b: medial groove, 1c: intermediate tubercle, 1d: lateral groove, 1e: greater tubercle; 2: proximal tendon of the biceps brachii, 2a: medial lobe, 2b: isthmus, 2c: lateral lobe; 3: supraspinatus muscle; 4: brachiocephalicus muscle; 5: skin.

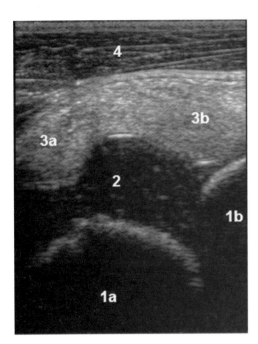

Figure 5.16 Normal point of the shoulder in a foal. Transverse ultrasound scan (medial is to the left) of the cranial aspect of the point of the shoulder in a normal foal. Because of the age of the subject, in this image the separation between the two ossification centers (1a and 1b) is still visible. 1: intertubercular humeral sulcus, 1a: intermediate tubercle, 1b: greater tubercle; 2: cartilage; 3: proximal tendon of the biceps brachii, 3a: medial lobe, 3b: lateral lobe; 4: brachiocephalicus muscle.

and longitudinal sections from its origin on the supraglenoid tubercle of the scapula (Figure 5.13) to its distal insertion on the proximal tuberosity of the radius (see Elbow). In a normal horse, the origin of the tendon of the biceps brachii appears as an echogenic crescent-shaped convex structure in cross-sectional scans. Just proximal to the intertubercular sulcus, the tendon becomes bilobed and shows a linear fibrillar echogenic pattern with a thin hypoechoic layer over its cranial border, corresponding to the muscular fibers of the biceps brachii (Figure 5.18). Coursing distally from the supraglenoid tubercle, the tendon becomes irregularly elliptic in shape and heterogeneous because it is infiltrated by hypoechogenic fatty connective tissue (Figure 5.19). Some of these muscular fibers are sometimes also visible at the level of the intertubercular sulcus (Figure 5.20). Over the point of the shoulder, the tendon is molded to the intertubercular sulcus, which is covered with fibrocartilage; the bicipital bursa is interposed between the bone surface and the tendon (Figure 5.15). The tendon is bilobed in shape, with a larger lateral lobe and a smaller medial lobe connected by an isthmus. The isthmus lies cranial to the intermediate humeral tubercle. The lateral lobe runs in the intertubercular groove between the greater and the intermediate tubercles of the humerus, and the medial between the intermediate and the lesser humeral tubercles. At

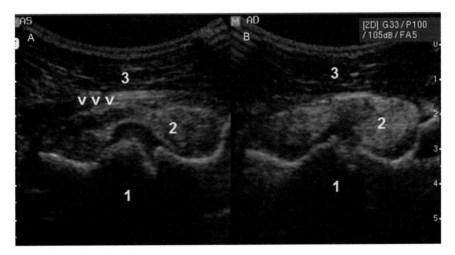

Figure 5.17 Point of the shoulder in a yearling. Transverse (medial is to the left) ultrasound scans, obtained with a convex probe, of the proximal biceps brachii tendon at the level of the intertubercular sulcus in a yearling. (A) The medial lobe has a large anechoic lesion (arrows) without enlargement of the tendon. This image is indicative of an acute tendinitis of the biceps brachii tendon. This yearling had a supraglenoid tubercle fracture the month before. The irregularity of the contour of the intermediate tubercle present in both limbs is normal. At this age there is a partial degree of ossification of the two ossification centers. (B) Normal opposite limb. 1: intermediate tubercle; 2: proximal tendon of the biceps brachii (lateral lobe); 3: brachiocephalicus muscle; arrows: lesion of the medial lobe of the biceps brachii tendon.

this level, the tendon is so large that it is almost impossible to visualize the entire tendon in one transverse image using most linear transducers. A convex probe can provide a better representation of the entire tendon on a transverse scan. When using a linear transducer, an independent evaluation of each lobe is often required. Figure 5.21 shows a longitudinal scan of the proximal bicipital tendon from its origin; the probe should be moved medially and laterally to examine the

medial and lateral lobes. Distal to the intertubercular groove, the proximal tendon of the biceps brachii merges progressively into the muscle belly. On a transverse section, the tendon is now oval and heterogeneous, due to the presence of hypoechogenic striated

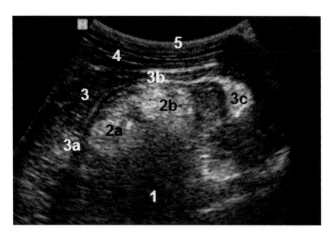

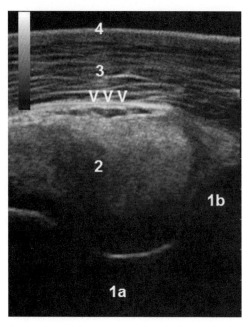

Figure 5.18 Normal transverse image (medial is to the left) of the cranial aspect of the shoulder, just distal to the supraglenoid tubercle and proximal to the intertubercular sulcus. 1: scapulohumeral fat pad; 2: proximal biceps brachii tendon, 2a: medial lobe, 2b: lateral lobe; 3: supraspinatus muscle, 3a: medial tendon, 3b: aponeurosis of the supraspinatus muscle, 3c: lateral tendon; 4: brachiocephalicus muscle; 5: skin.

Figure 5.20 Normal transverse (medial is to the left) ultrasound scan of the lateral lobe of the proximal tendon of the biceps brachii over the intertubercular sulcus in a normal horse. 1: intertubercular sulcus, 1a: lateral groove, 1b: greater tubercle; 2: lateral lobe of proximal bicipital tendon; 3: brachiocephalicus muscle; 4: skin; arrows: cranial muscle fibers of the biceps brachii.

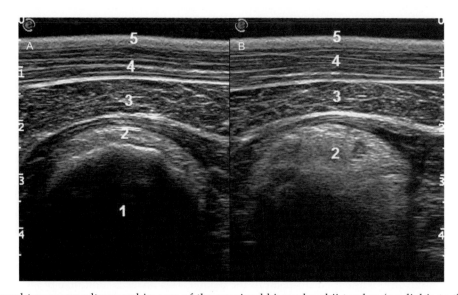

Figure 5.19 Normal transverse ultrasound images of the proximal biceps brachii tendon (medial is to the left). (A) At the level of the supraglenoid tubercle, the tendon is homogeneously echogenic. (B) Just distal to the supraglenoid tubercle, the proximal biceps brachii tendon has a heterogeneous echogenicity because of the presence of fat connective tissue areas. 1: supraglenoid tubercle; 2: proximal tendon of the biceps brachii; 3: supraspinatus muscle; 4: brachiocephalicus muscle; 5: skin.

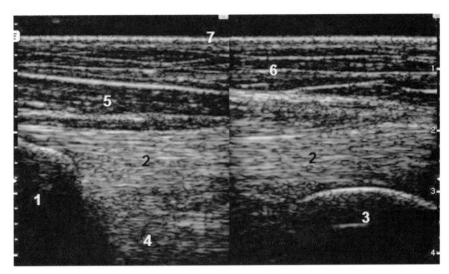

Figure 5.21 Normal sagittal (proximal is to the left) ultrasound scans of the proximal tendon of the biceps brachii from the supraglenoid tubercle to the intertubercular sulcus. The tendon shows parallel echogenic fibers deep to the supraspinatus and brachiocephalicus muscles. 1: supraglenoid tubercle of the scapula; 2: proximal tendon of the biceps brachii; 3: intertubercular sulcus (sagittal ridge); 4: fat; 5: supraspinatus muscle; 6: brachiocephalicus muscle; 7: skin.

fibers in its center. The distal recess of the bicipital bursa and fat are interposed between the biceps brachii tendon and the proximal humerus.

Injuries of the biceps brachii tendon itself consist of enlargement of the tendon, presence of hypoechoic–anechoic areas, and loss of the normal fiber pattern. Artifactual hypoechoic areas in the bicipital tendon are easily created because its fibers do not lie all in the same scan plane due to its curved contour. Changing the orientation of the probe is useful and lesions should be identified in both the transverse and longitudinal scan to be sure that the hypoechoic area is not an artifact (Figures 5.17 and 5.22). In chronic cases, distrophic mineralization or calcification of the biceps brachii tendon may occur. A case of rupture of the biceps tendon in a Thoroughbred steeplechaser has also been described.

Bicipital Bursa

The bicipital bursa is a potential space between the biceps brachii tendon and the proximal humerus. In normal horses, this bursa is not clearly visible because no or very little fluid is discernible (Figure 5.15). The small anechoic space between the humeral tubercles and the biceps brachii tendon is fibrocartilage and should not be confused with fluid. Bicipital bursitis can be found alone or secondary to bony lesions or bicipital tendinitis. Distension of the bicipital bursa is seen as fluid accumulation around the medial and lateral sides of the biceps brachii tendon (Figure 5.23). In normal

horses, a small amount of synovial fluid can be found at the lateral aspect of the bicipital bursa slightly distal to the greater tubercle. However, when the distension is severe, anechoic synovial fluid causes cranial protrusion of the tendon and the mesotendon becomes visible. In most chronic cases of bicipital bursitis, sonographic findings include an increased volume of hypoechoic fluid, and fibrin and synovial proliferation within the bursa (Figure 5.24). In most cases of septic bursitis, the synovial fluid becomes echogenic, although when anechoic synovial fluid distension is seen, a recent-onset septic process cannot be ruled out without bursocentesis. The underlying bone should also be carefully examined for lytic areas of the intertubercular groove, particularly in cases of septic bursitis.

Supraspinatus Muscle and Tendons

The supraspinatus muscle originates from the homonymous fossa of the scapula (Figure 5.25) and splits at the neck of the scapula into two branches each with an intramuscular tendon. The tendons can be identified as echogenic structures within the less echoic supraspinatus muscle. They run superficially, one laterally and the other medially, to the biceps brachii tendon. The two tendons are connected by an aponeurosis of the supraspinatus muscle (Figure 5.18). The lateral tendon, bigger and roughly triangular in shape, is easier to identify and follow to its insertion on the cranial part of the greater humeral tubercle, where it is in close proximity to the lateral lobe of the biceps brachii

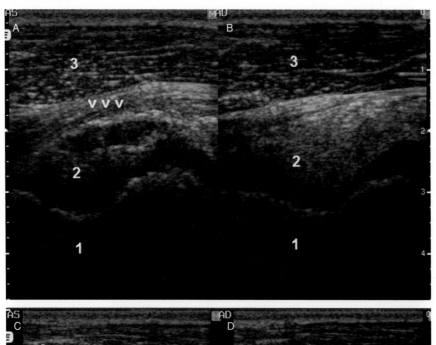

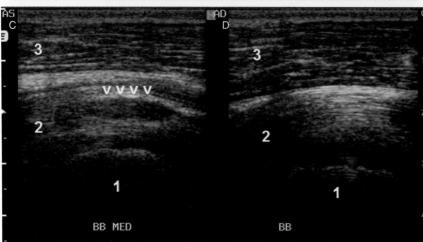

Figure 5.22 Acute tendinitis of the biceps brachii tendon in a yearling associated with a recent fracture of the supraglenoid tubercle. Transverse (A, B, medial is to the left) and longitudinal (C, D, proximal is to the left) ultrasound scans of the medial lobe of the proximal biceps brachii tendon. (A) The medial lobe (2) is not enlarged compared to the opposite limb but a large oval anechoic lesion (arrows) is present within the tendon. (B) Normal medial lobe on the opposite limb. (C) A large oval anechoic lesion (arrows) is present within the medial lobe of the biceps brachii tendon. This image, also visualized in cross-section, is typical of an acute tendinitis. (D) Normal medial lobe on the opposite limb. 1: medial groove of the intertubercular sulcus; 2: medial lobe of the proximal tendon of the biceps brachii muscle; 3: brachiocephalicus muscle.

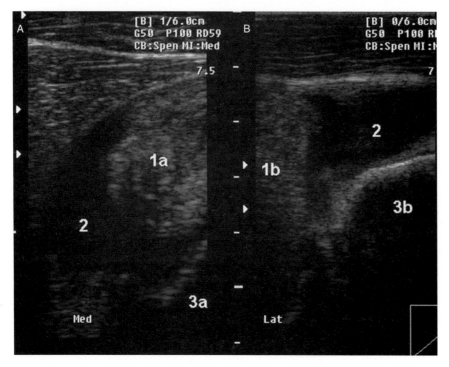

Figure 5.23 Chronic bicipital bursitis secondary to a supraglenoid tubercle fracture. Transverse (medial is to the left) ultrasound scans of the cranial aspect of the shoulder in a young horse. (A) The medial lobe of the bicipital tendon (1a) looks hypoechoic and is surrounded by an anechoic space (2) compatible with a fluid effusion. (B) On the lateral side of the biceps brachii tendon (1b) there is anechogenic fluid distension (2). These abnormal findings are consistent with a chronic bicipital bursitis. 1: proximal tendon of the biceps brachii, 1a: medial lobe of the proximal tendon of the biceps brachii, 1b: lateral lobe of the proximal tendon of the biceps brachii; 2: synovial distension of the bicipital bursa; 3: intertuberculus humeral sulcus, 3a: medial groove, 3b: greater tubercle.

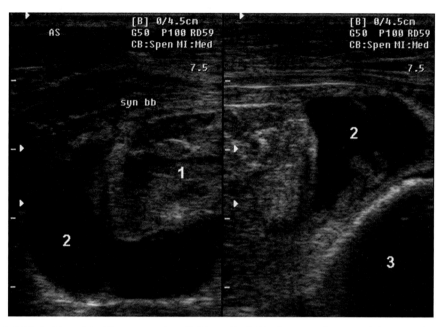

Figure 5.24 Chronic bicipital bursitis. Transverse (medial is to the left) ultrasound scans of the cranial aspect of the shoulder in a colt with a chronic left fore limb lameness. The probe is slightly distal to the point of the shoulder. The biceps brachii tendon (1) is imaged just distal to the intertubercular sulcus. Its heterogeneous pattern is due to a tendon lesion but also the presence of hypoechogenic striated fibers of the muscle body. The distal recess of the bicipital bursa (2) is well visualized because of the extensive synovial fluid distension. Synovial membrane thickening and proliferation are also seen. 1: proximal tendon of the biceps brachii; 2: synovial distension of the bicipital bursa; 3: proximal humerus.

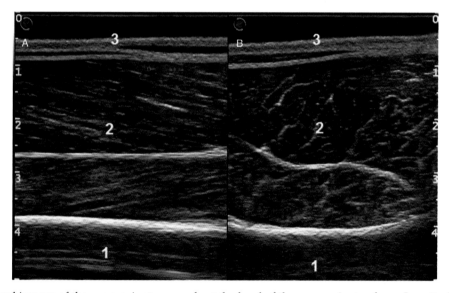

Figure 5.25 Normal images of the supraspinatus muscle at the level of the supraspinatus fossa. Longitudinal (A) and transverse (B) ultrasound scans. 1: supraspinatus fossa; 2: supraspinatus muscle; 3: skin.

tendon (Figure 5.26). The medial tendon, smaller and flatter, is more difficult to scan (Figure 5.18). It attaches on the cranial part of the lesser tubercle of the humerus in a position close to the medial lobe of the biceps brachii tendon. The bicipital bursa is interposed between these two structures. At this level, the lateral tendon is covered with the hypoechoic brachiocephalicus muscle.

Infraspinatus Muscle and Tendon

At the lateral aspect of the shoulder, the infraspinatus muscle originates from the infraspinatus fossa of the

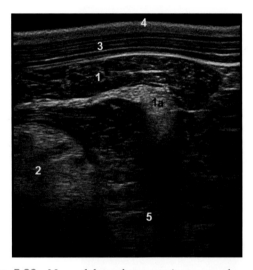

Figure 5.26 Normal lateral supraspinatus tendon at the level of the scapulohumeral joint. Transverse (medial is to the left) ultrasound scan proximal to the intertubercular sulcus. 1: supraspinatus muscle, 1a: lateral supraspinatus tendon; 2: biceps brachii tendon; 3: brachiocephalicus muscle; 4: skin; 5: scapulohumeral fat pad.

scapula (Figure 5.27). Its distal tendon slides over the convexity of the greater tubercle of the humerus and inserts on the caudal eminence of the tuberosity. The intramuscular tendon looks echoic within the infraspinatus muscle (Figure 5.28). Distally, as it approaches its humeral insertion, it becomes wider and heterogeneous because of its lobulated structure. In fact, over the caudal part of the greater tubercle, it appears as first three and then further distally two superimposed portions. There is a bursa located between this tendon and the caudal part of the greater humeral tubercle, which can be visualized as an anechoic space deep to the infraspinatus tendon. A small amount of synovial fluid in the infraspinatus bursa is also visible in normal horses (Figure 5.29).

Traumatic injury of the lateral aspect of the shoulder can cause infraspinatus bursitis, associated with fracture of the greater tubercle. In horses with suprascapular nerve paralysis, the infraspinatus muscle is more echogenic than normal as the muscle atrophies leaving the connective tissue surrounding the muscle fascicles, and consequently its tendon becomes less visible.

Scapulohumeral Joint

The scapulohumeral joint is composed of two bones: the distal end of the scapula (glenoid cavity) and the proximal humerus (humeral head). Because no collateral ligaments are present, the thick surrounding musculature provides stability to the joint. The glenoid labrum sits around the margins of the glenoid cavity and is a fibrous pad which enlarges the contact between the two articular surfaces. A large portion of the scapulohumeral joint space is hidden from view. Only the craniolateral, lateral, and caudolateral aspects of the

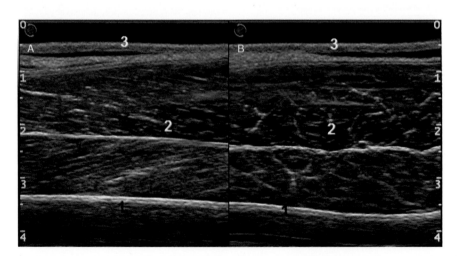

Figure 5.27 Normal infraspinatus muscle. Longitudinal (A) and transverse (B) ultrasound scans of the infraspinatus muscle at the level of the infraspinatus fossa. 1: infraspinatus fossa; 2: infraspinatus muscle; 3: skin.

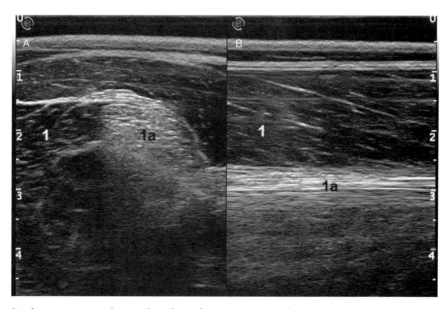

Figure 5.28 Normal infraspinatus tendon within the infraspinatus muscle. Transverse (A) and longitudinal (B) ultrasound scans of the infraspinatus muscle at the lateral aspect of the shoulder distal to the infraspinatus fossa. 1: infraspinatus muscle; 2: infraspinatus tendon.

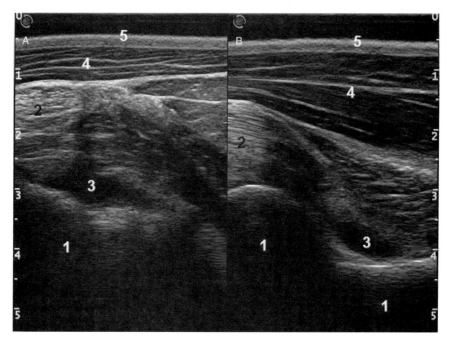

Figure 5.29 The infraspinatus bursa containing a small amount of synovial fluid. (A) Transverse ultrasound scan (cranial is to the left); (B) Longitudinal ultrasound scan (proximal is to the left). 1: caudal part (crest) of the major humeral tubercle; 2: infraspinatus tendon; 3: infraspinatus bursa (mild synovial distension); 4: omotransverse muscle; 5: skin.

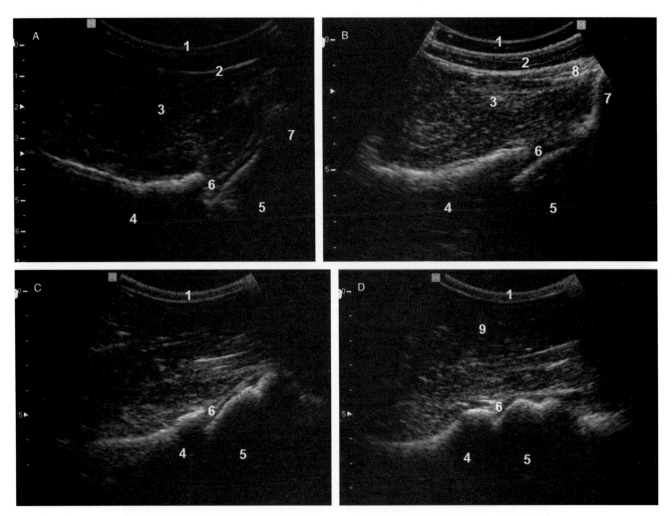

Figure 5.30 Normal proximodistal ultrasound scans of the scapulohumeral joint (SHJ) (proximal is to the left). The convex probe is held vertically and moved cranial to caudal. (A) Craniolateral aspect of the SHJ: the probe is positioned between the supraspinatus and infraspinatus muscles. (B) Lateral aspect of the SHJ: the probe is positioned at the level of the infraspinatus intramuscular tendon. (C, D) Caudolateral aspect of the SHJ: the probe is positioned caudal to the infraspinatus tendon. The humeral head always has a bilobed shape. 1: skin; 2: omotransverse muscle; 3: infraspinatus muscle; 4: scapula; 5: humeral head; 6: joint space; 7: major tubercle; 8: infraspinatus tendon; 9: triceps brachii muscle.

shoulder joint can be scanned in a longitudinal plane using a linear or convex 5–7.5 MHz probe without a standoff pad. All three approaches to the scapulohumeral joint in longitudinal section allow detection of the presence of a synovial effusion and periarticular bony proliferation. Conversely, ultrasound can only provide a limited examination of the humeral head using a caudolateral approach. A normal joint has smooth articular margins and little or no synovial fluid (Figures 5.30 and 5.31). Transverse images are more useful in cases of ultrasonographic-guided injection of this joint.

In adult horses, synovial fluid distension and articular margin modeling are indicative of osteoarthrosis of the scapulohumeral joint. In young horses, a diagnosis of scapulohumeral osteochondrosis, with osteochondral fragmentation of the humeral head, may be made with a caudolateral approach. Septic synovitis of the shoulder joint occurs more frequently in foals than in adults. In yearlings and adults, injuries to this joint are infrequent and are more likely to occur secondary to trauma such as a fracture of the supraglenoid tubercle (Figure 5.32 and Figure 5.33). In cases of supraglenoid tubercle fractures, ultrasonographically there is synovial fluid distension causing the joint capsule to bulge. The echogenicity of the synovial fluid may be increased because of the presence of blood or fibrin.

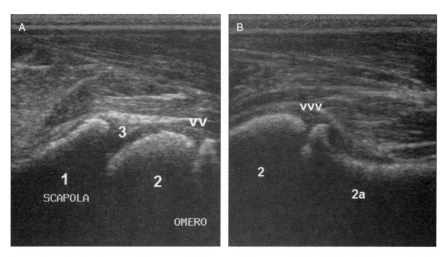

Figure 5.31 Normal proximodistal ultrasound scans of the scapulohumeral joint (A) and the proximal aspect of the humerus (B) in a 7-month-old foal (proximal is to the left). At this age, the proximal humeral epiphysis (arrows) is not closed and should not be mistaken for a fracture line. 1: scapula; 2: humeral head, 2a: humeral neck; 3: joint space.

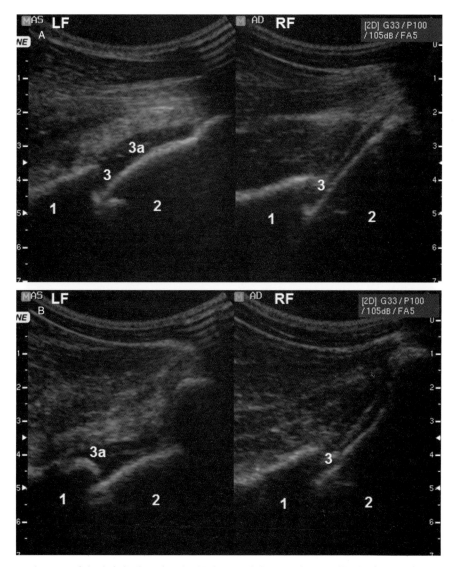

Figure 5.32 Ultrasound scans of the left (LF) and right (RF) scapulohumeral joints (SHJ) of an Arabian yearling who suffered an acute intra-articular supraglenoid fracture of the left shoulder (Figure 5.14). These scans have been obtained with a convex probe. In both images (A and B) the left SHJ has synovial fluid distension which is raising the articular capsule. The echogenicity of the synovial fluid is increased because of the presence of fibrin. There is no synovial fluid evident in the contralateral SHJ (RF). 1: scapula; 2: humeral head; 3: SHJ space, 3a: synovial fluid.

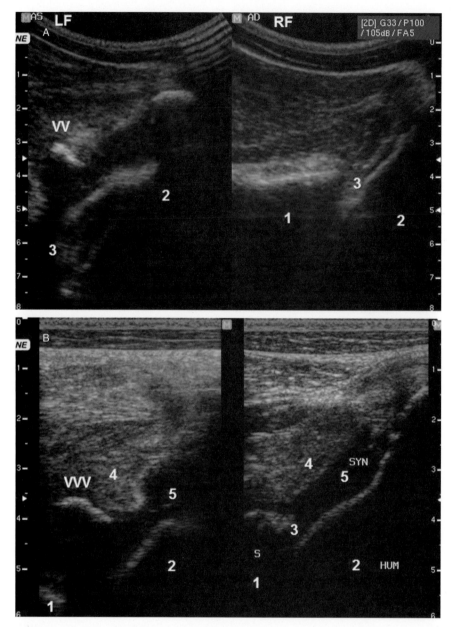

Figure 5.33   Ultrasound scans of the left (LF) and right (RF) scapulohumeral joints (SHJ) of the same Arabian yearling in Fig. 5.14 and Fig. 5.32. (A) On the abnormal left fore limb, the synovial recess is markedly distended and a bony fragment (arrows) is present in the synovial fluid. There is no synovial fluid evident in the contralateral normal SHJ (RF). (B) The same images as A obtained with a linear transducer. The images obtained with a convex probe (A) show a larger view of the SHJ but with less detail. In B it is possible to appreciate the thickening and the heterogeneous pattern of the synovial membrane, which are underestimated in A. 1: scapula; 2: humeral head; 3: SHJ space; 4: synovial membrane; 5: synovial fluid.

RECOMMENDED READING

Carnicer, D., Coudry, V., & Denoix, J.-M. (2008) Ultrasonographic guided injection of the scapulohumeral joint in horses. *Equine Veterinary Education*, 20(2), 103–106.

Cauvin, E.R.J. (1998) Soft tissue injuries of the equine shoulder region: a systematic approach to differential diagnosis. *Equine Veterinary Education*, 10(2), 70–74.

Coudry, V., Allen A.K., & Denoix, J.-M. (2005) Congenital abnormalities of the bicipital apparatus in four mature horses. *Equine Veterinary Journal*, 37(3), 272–275.

Gough, M.R. & McDiarmid, A.M. (1998) Septic intertuberal (bicipital) bursitis in a horse *Equine Veterinary Education*, 10(2), 66–69.

Little, D., Redding, W.R., & Gerard, M.P. (2009) Osseous cyst-like lesions of the lateral intertubercular groove of the proximal humerus: a report of 5 cases. *Equine Veterinary Education*, 21(2), 60–66.

McDiarmid, A.M. (1999) The equine bicipital apparatus – review of anatomy, function, diagnostic investigative techniques and clinical conditions. *Equine Veterinary Education*, 11(2), 63–68.

Pasquet, H., Coudry, V., & Denoix, J.-M. (2008) Ultrasonographic examination of the proximal tendon of the *biceps brachii*: technique and reference images. *Equine Veterinary Education*, 20(6), 331–336.

Redding, W.R. & Pease, A.P. (2010) Imaging of the shoulder. *Equine Veterinary Education*, 22(4), 199–209.

Tnibar, M.A., Auer, J.A., & Bakkali, S. (1999) Ultrasonography of the equine shoulder: technique and normal appearance. *Veterinary Radiology & Ultrasound*, 40(1), 44–57.

Tnibar, M.A., Auer, J.A., & Bakkali, S. (2001) Ultrasonography of the equine elbow: technique and normal appearance. *Journal of Equine Veterinary Science*, 21(4), 177–187.

CHAPTER SIX

ULTRASONOGRAPHY OF THE HOCK

Katherine S. Garrett

Rood and Riddle Equine Hospital, Lexington, KY, USA

INTRODUCTION

Ultrasonography of the tarsus can be challenging, but it is an important part of a complete diagnostic evaluation of tarsal disease. As with other body regions, a thorough understanding of normal anatomy is essential. Comparison with magnetic resonance images, radiographs, and dissected specimens can be helpful in understanding the anatomic relationships and the precise locations and paths of the tendinous and ligamentous structures.

Excellent reviews of scanning techniques for the tarsal region have been published. Regardless of the particular approach chosen, a systematic method for evaluation of this complex structure is helpful. The structures to be examined include the tendons and ligaments, the synovial structures, the bony surfaces, and the subcutis. Comparison with the opposite limb can be extremely helpful in determining if an unusual abnormality is present or in cases of mild disease.

A linear transducer (8–12 MHz) is generally most useful, but a micro-convex transducer (7–10 MHz) can be helpful in some situations. Sedation is often necessary to ensure patient compliance and sonographer safety.

TENDONS AND LIGAMENTS

The tarsal region contains many tendons and ligaments, some of which have complex attachments or insertions distant from the tarsus itself. The lateral and medial collateral ligaments both have two major components, a long superficial component and a short deeper component.

The long portion of the lateral collateral ligament originates on the caudal portion of the lateral malleolus of the distal tibia and has insertions on the calcaneus, fourth tarsal bone, and third and fourth metatarsal bone. The tripartite short portion originates on the cranial portion of the lateral malleolus and extends in a nearly transverse plane to the lateral aspect of the talus and calcaneus.

The long medial collateral ligament originates on the medial malleolus of the distal tibia and extends distally, inserting on the distal talus, central, fused first and second, and third tarsal bones, and second and third metatarsal bones. The short portion of the ligament originates on the medial malleolus and has three subsections that travel in a more transverse plane than the long portion and insert on the proximal medial talus and the sustentaculum tali.

During ultrasonographic examination, the lateral and medial collateral ligaments can be located most easily in the longitudinal plane. The short components lie in a more transverse plane than the long components. An image in the transverse plane can then be obtained by rotating the transducer 90°. In addition, some of the short portions are in partial relaxation when the horse is weightbearing, so imaging these ligaments when the horse is not fully weightbearing may aid in identification of pathology.

Desmitis of any of the collateral ligaments can occur, but is more commonly seen in the long medial collateral ligament. Horses with collateral ligament desmitis typically demonstrate moderate to severe lameness and synovial effusion. Ultrasonographic signs of desmitis are similar to those in any ligament and include increased size, decreased echogenicity, and abnormal fiber pattern (Figure 6.1). If the insertion of

Atlas of Equine Ultrasonography, First Edition. Edited by Jessica A. Kidd, Kristina G. Lu, and Michele L. Frazer.
© 2014 John Wiley & Sons, Ltd. Published 2014 by John Wiley & Sons, Ltd.
Companion Website: www.wiley.com/go/kidd/equine-ultrasonography

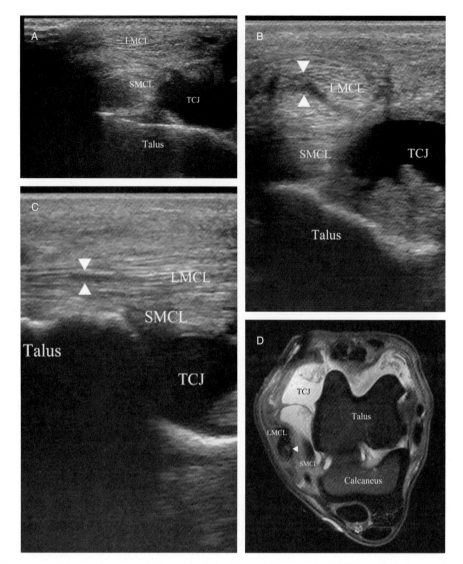

Figure 6.1 (A) Transverse image of a normal long medial collateral ligament (LMCL) and short medial collateral ligament (SMCL). TCJ: tarsocrural joint. Dorsal is to the right of the image. B and C: Transverse (B) and longitudinal (C) plane images of an abnormal LMCL. The ligament is enlarged with a focal region of marked hypoechogenicity and fiber disruption (arrowheads). Synovial effusion is present in the TCJ. Dorsal and proximal are to the right of the images. (D) Transverse plane magnetic resonance image of the same horse. Note the marked synovial effusion in the TCJ and focal region of increased signal (arrowhead) in the LMCL. Dorsal is to the top of the image, medial is to the left of the image.

the ligament is involved, bony irregularity or avulsion fragments may be imaged (Figure 6.2).

The short lateral collateral ligament is invariably involved in fractures of the lateral malleolus of the distal tibia while the long lateral collateral ligament is less commonly affected (Figure 6.3). These fractures are usually caused by external trauma. Ultrasonography can be useful to assess the degree of involvement of the collateral ligaments and potential for instability of the joint.

The common calcaneal tendon/gastrocnemius tendon, superficial digital flexor tendon, and long

plantar ligament are found on the plantar aspect of the tarsus. The gastrocnemius tendon inserts on the proximal surface of the tuber calcanei. The long plantar ligament originates on the plantar surface of the proximal tuber calcanei and inserts on the fourth tarsal and fourth metatarsal bones. The superficial digital flexor tendon largely passes over the surface of the tuber calcanei, but the medial and lateral aspects insert on the proximal aspect of this bone.

Soft tissue swelling of the plantar aspect of the tarsus ("curb") may be caused by injury to the long plantar ligament or superficial digital flexor tendon.

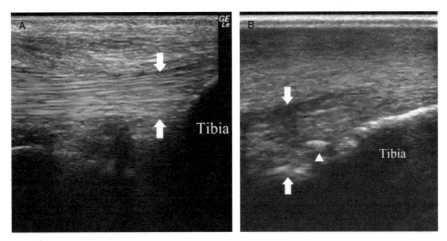

Figure 6.2 Longitudinal plane images of the proximal insertion on the medial malleolus of a normal (A) and abnormal (B) medial collateral ligament (arrows). In B, there are areas of hypoechogenicity within the ligament as well as small avulsion fragments (arrowhead) and thickening of the subcutis. Proximal is to the right of the images.

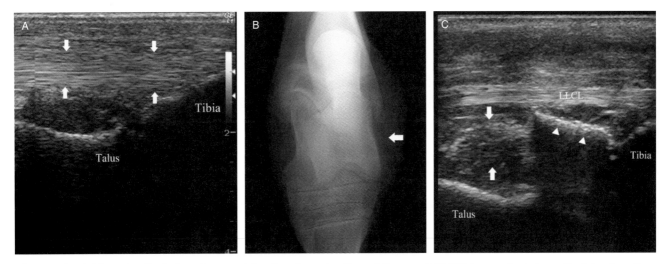

Figure 6.3 (A) Longitudinal plane image of the short lateral collateral ligament (SLCL) (arrows) origin on the lateral malleolus. Proximal is to the right of the image. (B) Dorsoplantar radiographic image of a horse with a lateral malleolus fracture (arrow). Note the distal displacement of the fragment. Lateral is to the right of the image. (C) Longitudinal plane image of the lateral malleolus fragment (arrowheads) and involvement of the SLCL (arrows) of the horse in B. The fragment has displaced distally and plantarly along the course of the SLCL to lie deep to the long lateral collateral ligament (LLCL). Short collateral ligament association with the fragment was confirmed arthroscopically. Thickening of the subcutaneous tissue is evident. Proximal is to the right of the image.

Subcutaneous edema or thickening may give a similar external appearance. Desmitis of the long plantar ligament is characterized by enlargement and hypoechogenicity of the ligament (Figure 6.4).

The deep digital flexor tendon is located on the plantaromedial aspect of the tarsus, passing over the sustentaculum tali within the tarsal sheath. The smaller medial head of the tendon is contained within its own synovial sheath and joins the main body of the tendon in the proximal metatarsal region. In the absence of

soft tissue swelling of the plantaromedial aspect of the tarsus, an image of the deep digital flexor tendon can often be more easily obtained with a micro-convex probe due to its smaller footprint.

The peroneus tertius and the tendons of the cranial tibial muscle have complex insertions on dorsal aspect of the distal tarsal region. The distal peroneus tertius forms a tunnel through which the distal cranial tibial tendon emerges. The dorsal tendon of the peroneus tertius then inserts on the central and third tarsal and

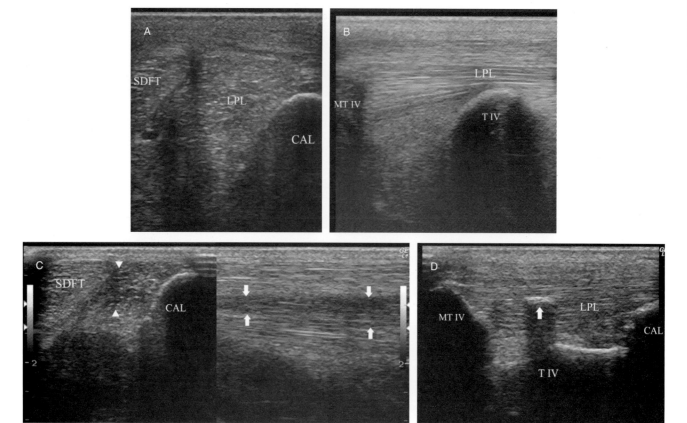

Figure 6.4 (A) Transverse plane image of the long plantar ligament (LPL). CAL: calcaneus; SDFT: superficial digital flexor tendon. Lateral is to the right of the image. (B) Longitudinal plane image of the LPL distal insertion on the fourth tarsal bone (T IV) and fourth metatarsal bone (MT IV). Proximal is to the right of the image. (C) Transverse (left image) and longitudinal (right image) images of a horse with LPL desmitis. Hypoechogenicity of the ligament is apparent (arrowheads and arrows). SDFT: superficial digital flexor tendon. Lateral and proximal are to the right of the images. (D) Longitudinal plane image of an LPL with focal mineralization within the ligament (arrow). Proximal is to the right of the image.

third metatarsal bones. The lateral tendon inserts on the fourth tarsal bone and the distolateral calcaneus and talus. The dorsal tendon of insertion of the cranial tibial muscle inserts on the third tarsal and third metatarsal bones. The cunean tendon is the medial tendon of insertion of the cranial tibial muscle. It passes medially across the central tarsal bone, inserting on the fused first and second tarsal bone, central tarsal bone, and second metatarsal bone. The tendons of insertion of the cranial tibial and peroneus tertius can be identified by following each of the tendons individually from their origins in the distal tibia.

Diagnosis of peroneus tertius rupture can generally be made on physical examination by extending the tarsus while the stifle is flexed. Ultrasonography shows a discontinuity in the tendon with edema and disrupted muscle architecture of the cranial tibial muscle (Figure 6.5).

Two extensor tendons cross the tarsal region, both within a separate synovial sheath. The long digital extensor tendon is located on the dorsolateral aspect of the limb. The lateral digital extensor tendon is located on the lateral aspect of the tarsus and is closely related to the long portion of the lateral collateral ligament. Tendinitis of these structures is characterized by enlargement, hypoechogenicity, and abnormal fiber pattern of the tendons with effusion of the synovial sheath or bursa (Figure 6.6).

SYNOVIAL STRUCTURES

The tarsus contains multiple synovial structures, including joints, bursae, and tendon sheaths. Ultrasonography is useful in differentiating potential causes of tarsal region swelling, allowing differentiation of cellulitis, synovitis, or abscessation. In cases of synovitis or bursitis, ultrasonography can assist with determination of which synovial structures may be involved. Penetrating wound tracts can also be followed to assess possible synovial structure involvement.

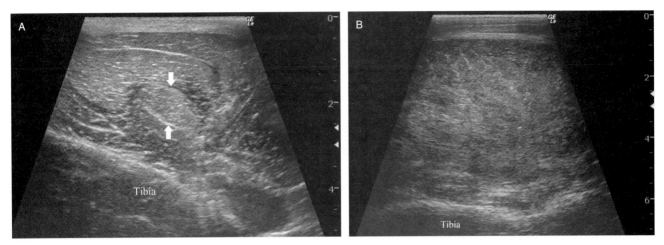

Figure 6.5 (A) Transverse plane image of normal peroneus tertius tendon (arrows) surrounded by muscle. (B) Transverse plane image of disrupted peroneus tertius tendon showing loss of the normal muscle and tendon architecture. Lateral is to the right of the images.

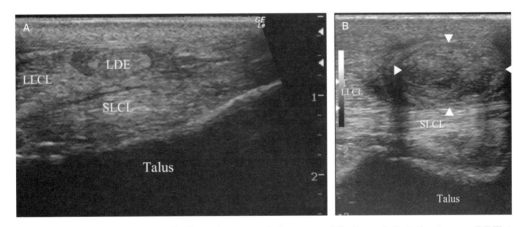

Figure 6.6 (A) Transverse plane image at the lateral aspect of the tarsus. The lateral digital extensor (LDE) tendon (LDET) is immediately dorsal to the long lateral collateral ligament (LLCL) and superficial to the short lateral collateral ligament (SLCL). (B) Tendinitis of the LDET (arrowheads). Note enlargement of the tendon and heterogeneous echogenicity. Dorsal is to the right of the images.

In general, the synovial structures should be evaluated for the amount and character of the synovial fluid and synovial membrane thickness. Normal synovial fluid is anechogenic. In cases of synovitis, the synovial fluid may appear more echogenic than normal and may contain hyperechogenic strands or clumps consistent with fibrin accumulation. The synovial membrane may be thickened, especially in cases of septic synovitis (Figure 6.7). While assessment of the character of the synovial fluid may provide some information on the degree of cellularity of the fluid, it is important to note that ultrasonography is not a substitute for synoviocentesis and fluid analysis when determining the nature of an effusion.

The tarsus is composed of four joints: the communicating tarsocrural and proximal intertarsal joints, the distal intertarsal joint, and the tarsometatarsal joint. The dorsolateral, dorsomedial, plantarolateral, and plantaromedial portions of the tarsocrural joint should all be examined as they may contain varying amounts of synovial fluid, fibrin, or synovial membrane proliferation. This information can assist in determining an appropriate site for arthrocentesis of the tarsocrural joint. The distal intertarsal joint is most easily assessed on the medial and dorsal aspects of the joint (Figure 6.8), while the tarsometatarsal joint is most easily assessed on the plantarolateral aspect of the joint in the typical site for arthrocentesis (Figure 6.9).

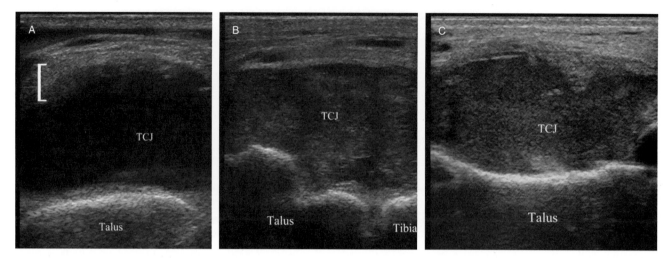

Figure 6.7 Dorsomedial pouch of the tarsocrural joint (TCJ). (A) Anechogenic effusion of the TCJ with synovial membrane thickening (bracket). The synovial fluid analysis of this joint was within normal limits. (B, C) Similar appearance of heterogeneous echogenic effusions of the TCJ. The horse in B was confirmed to have septic arthritis of the TCJ, while the horse in C had a non-septic hemarthrosis. Proximal is to the right of the images.

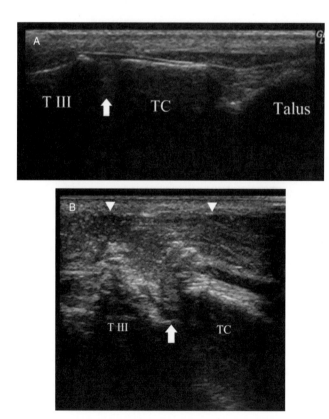

Figure 6.8 Normal (A) and abnormal (B) distal intertarsal joint (arrow) imaged from the medial aspect of the tarsus. The horse in B has a marked echogenic effusion of the joint (arrowheads) as well as irregularity of the third tarsal bone (T III) consistent with osteomyelitis. Purulent material was obtained from this joint. TC: central tarsal bone. Proximal is to the right of the images.

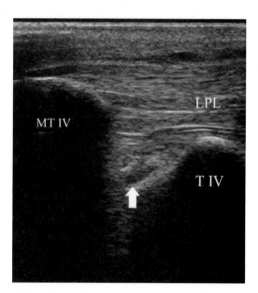

Figure 6.9 Normal tarsometatarsal joint (TMTJ) (arrow) imaged from the plantarolateral aspect of the tarsus. LPL: long plantar ligament; MT IV: fourth metatarsal bone; T IV: fourth tarsal bone. Proximal is to the right of the image.

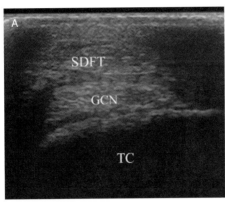
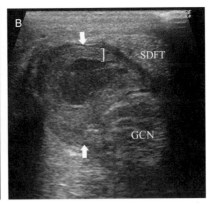

Figure 6.10 (A) Transverse plane image of a normal superficial digital flexor tendon (SDFT) and gastrocnemius tendon (GCN) at the proximal aspect of the tuber calcanei (TC) obtained from the plantar aspect of the limb. (B) Effusion of the calcaneal bursa (arrows) imaged from a slightly plantaromedial aspect immediately proximal to the TC. Note the degree of synovial membrane thickening (bracket). This horse was confirmed to have septic synovitis of the calcaneal bursa. Lateral is to the right of the images.

There are two consistent bursae present on the plantar aspect of the proximal tarsus, the gastrocnemius bursa, deep to the distal aspect of the gastrocnemius tendon, and the calcaneal bursa, between the gastrocnemius tendon and the superficial digital flexor tendon (Figure 6.10). A subcutaneous bursa ("capped hock") may be present between the superficial digital flexor tendon and the skin in some horses. This bursa may develop in response to local trauma and can be quite large in the initial stages (Figure 6.11). When evaluating penetrating wounds or potentially septic bursitis, it should be kept in mind that the gastrocnemius bursa and the calcaneal bursa consistently communicate and communication between the subcutaneous bursa and calcaneal bursa is present in approximately 40% of horses. The cunean bursa is deep to the cunean tendon on the dorsomedial aspect of the limb and is generally not imaged unless it is distended (Figure 6.12).

Multiple synovial sheaths surround tendons and ligaments of the tarsal region. The deep digital flexor tendon is contained within the tarsal sheath while the medial head of the deep digital flexor tendon is contained within its own sheath. Effusion of the tarsal sheath ("thoroughpin") may be confused with effusion of the plantar pouches of the tarsocrural joint. The tarsal sheath is also susceptible to septic tenosynovitis, which should be suspected if moderate–severe lameness, tarsal sheath effusion, synovial membrane thickening, and fibrin accumulation are present. In more severe cases, regions of hypoechogenicity may be seen within the deep digital flexor tendon itself and the bony contour of the sustentaculum tali may be irregular, suggestive of osteomyelitis (Figure 6.13). The

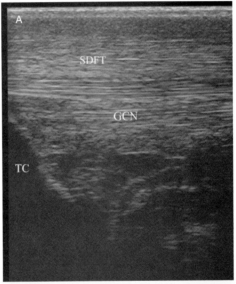
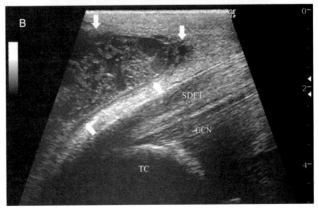

Figure 6.11 (A) Normal longitudinal images of the superficial digital flexor tendon (SDFT) and gastrocnemius tendon (GCN) at the insertion of the GCN on the tuber calcanei (TC). The horse in B has a large heterogeneous mass in the subcutaneous space (arrows) consistent with subcutaneous bursitis. Relaxation artifact is present in the SDFT and GCN. Proximal is to the right of the images.

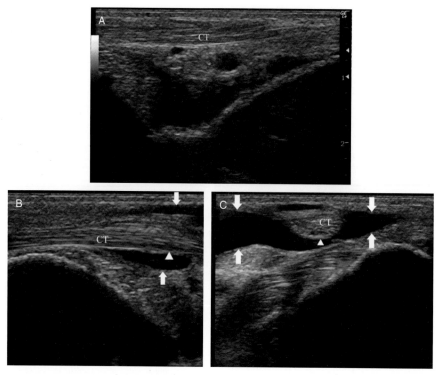

Figure 6.12 (A) Longitudinal image of a normal cunean tendon (CT). The cunean bursa surrounding the cunean tendon is not imaged distinctly due to the small amount of fluid in the normal bursa. Dorsoproximal is to the right of the image. (B) Longitudinal image of the cunean tendon in a horse with cunean bursitis and cunean tendonitis. There is an increase in ane-chogenic fluid (arrows) within the cunean bursa as well as hypoechogenicity in the cunean tendon on the right side of the image (arrowhead). Dorsoproximal is to the right of the image. (C) Transverse image of the CT and effusion of the cunean bursa (arrows) of the same horse as in B. The area of hypoechogenicity in the deep aspect of the cunean tendon is visible (arrowheads). Plantaroproximal is to the right of the image.

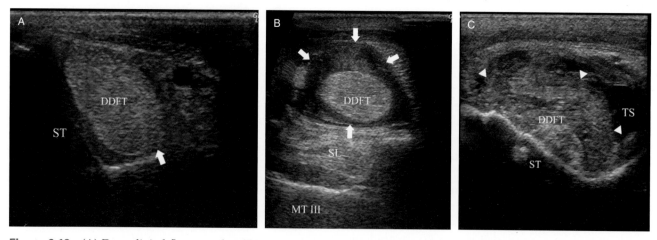

Figure 6.13 (A) Deep digital flexor tendon (DDFT) within the tarsal sheath at the level of the sustentaculum tali (ST) in a normal horse. Due to the DDFT curving over the ST, some fibers of the DDFT appear hypoechogenic to the remainder of the tendon (arrow). (B) Echogenic effusion of the tarsal sheath (arrows) surrounding the DDFT in the proximal metatarsal region in a horse with septic synovitis of the tarsal sheath, distal to the image in A. MT III: third metatarsal bone; SL: suspensory ligament. (C) DDFT within the tarsal sheath at the level of the ST (at the same level as the image in A) in a horse with septic tenosynovitis. The tendon has decreased echogenicity and its margins are irregular and difficult to define (arrowheads). Mild irregularity of the ST margin is present. Lateral is to the right of the images.

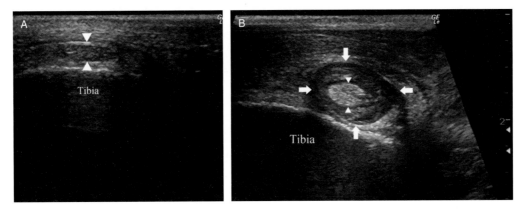

Figure 6.14 Transverse images of the medial head of the deep digital flexor tendon (DDFT) (arrowheads) in its synovial sheath at the level of the distal tibia in a normal horse (A) and in a horse with septic tenosynovitis (B). In B, an echogenic effusion (arrows) is present within the sheath and mild irregularity of the tendon margin is present. Plantar is to the right of the images. These images were obtained at the level of the tuber calcanei immediately plantar to the medial malleolus of the tibia.

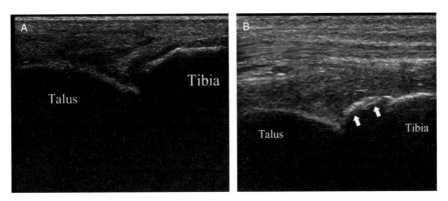

Figure 6.15 Longitudinal image of the distal intermediate ridge of the tibia in a normal horse (A) and in a horse with an osteochondrosis fragment (arrows) (B) and synovial membrane thickening. This fragment was removed arthroscopically. Proximal is to the right of the images.

medial head of the deep digital flexor tendon and its sheath may be affected as well (Figure 6.14).

The long and lateral digital extensor tendons also cross the tarsal region within synovial sheaths. If abnormalities of these tendon sheaths (e.g. increased synovial fluid) are present, the tendon within the sheath should be carefully assessed for abnormalities.

BONY STRUCTURES

The bony structures of the tarsal region should be evaluated critically because ultrasonography may reveal subtle bony surface changes at an earlier stage than radiography. Assessment can be challenging due to the many contours of the tarsal bones, particularly the talus, calcaneus, and distal tibia. Bony margins should

be smooth and regular. Areas of irregularity may represent sites of osteomyelitis, osteophyte formation, fracture, osteochondrosis, or sequestrum formation.

Osteochondrosis and osteochondrosis dessicans are typically diagnosed using radiography. However, ultrasonography has been shown to be more sensitive than radiography for lesions of the medial malleolus and distal intermediate tibial ridge (Figure 6.15). Areas of abnormal bony contour consistent with osteitis, osteomyelitis, or sequestrum formation can be identified using ultrasonography (Figures 6.16 and 6.17).

In young horses, the physes of the distal tibia and the tuber calcanei should be examined. The physis is normally a thin structure with well defined, crisp margins. Widening, irregularity, or increased echogenicity of the physeal region are indicative of septic or traumatic physitis (Figure 6.18).

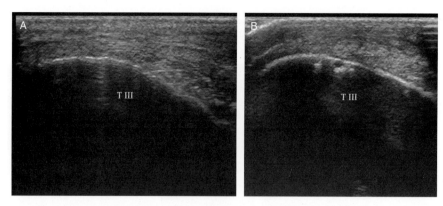

Figure 6.16 Transverse plane image of the dorsal aspect of the third tarsal bone (T III) in a normal horse (A) and in a horse with osteomyelitis (B) where irregularity of the bony margin is present. Lateral is to the right of the images.

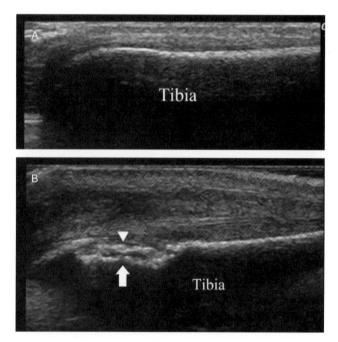

Figure 6.17 Longitudinal images of the distal medial tibia in a normal horse (A) and in a horse with a draining tract (B). A sequestrum is indicated by the arrowhead and the involucrum is indicated by the arrow. Subcutaneous thickening and edema are present. Proximal is to the right of the images.

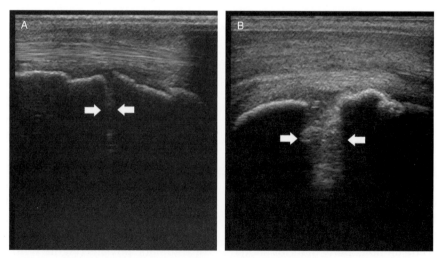

Figure 6.18 Longitudinal images of the distal tibial physis (arrows) in a normal horse (A) and in a horse with septic tibial physitis (B) with widening and irregularity of the physis as well as subcutaneous thickening.

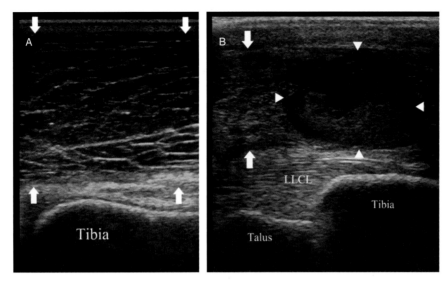

Figure 6.19 Longitudinal images of the lateral distal tibia and proximal tarsus. (A) A horse with subcutaneous cellulitis. The thickened, edematous subcutaneous tissues are indicated by the arrows. (B) A horse with a subcutaneous abscess and cellulitis. The abscess is indicated by the arrowheads and the thickened subcutaneous tissues are indicated by the arrows. LLCL: long lateral collateral ligament.

SUBCUTIS

In cases with profound soft tissue swelling of the tarsal region, it can be difficult to determine the nature and location of the swelling or effusion. Ultrasonography can assist with differentiation of cellulitis or abscessation from synovial sepsis (Figure 6.19).

CONCLUSION

Although the tarsus region is anatomically challenging, ultrasonography provides important information that assists with prompt diagnosis and institution of appropriate treatment.

RECOMMENDED READING

Dik, K.J. (1993) Ultrasonography of the equine tarsus. *Veterinary Radiology*, 34, 36–43.

Post, E.M., Singer, E.R., & Clegg, P.D. (2007) An anatomic study of the calcaneal bursae in the horse. *Veterinary Surgery*, 36, 3–9.

Raes, E.V., Vanderperren, K., Pille, F., *et al.* (2010) Ultrasonographic findings in 100 horses with tarsal region disorders. *Veterinary Journal*, 186, 201–209.

Relave, F., Meulyzer, M., Alexander, K., *et al.* (2009) Comparison of radiography and ultrasonography to detect osteochondrosis lesions in the tarsocrural joint: a prospective study. *Equine Veterinary Journal*, 41, 34–40.

Smith, M.R.W. & Wright, I.M. (2010) Arthroscopic treatment of fractures of the lateral malleolus of the tibia: 26 cases. *Equine Veterinary Journal*, 43, 280–287.

Updike, S.J. (1984) Functional anatomy of the equine tarsocrural collateral ligaments. *American Journal of Veterinary Research*, 45, 867–874.

Vanderperren, K., Raes, E., Bree, H.V., *et al.* (2009) Diagnostic imaging of the equine tarsal region using radiography and ultrasonography. Part 2: bony disorders. *Veterinary Journal*, 179, 188–196.

Vanderperren, K., Raes, E., Hoegaerts, M., *et al.* (2009) Diagnostic imaging of the equine tarsal region using radiography and ultrasonography. Part 1: the soft tissues. *Veterinary Journal*, 179, 179–187.

Whitcomb, M.B. (2006) Ultrasonography of the equine tarsus. *Proceedings of the American Association of Equine Practitioners*, 52, 13–30.

Young, A., Whitcomb, M.B., Vaughan, B., *et al.* (2010) Ultrasonographic Features of Septic Synovial Structures in 62 Horses (2004–2009). *Proceedings of the American Association of Equine Practitioners*, 56, 238.

CHAPTER SEVEN

ULTRASONOGRAPHY OF THE STIFLE

Eddy R.J. Cauvin

AZURVET Referral Veterinary Centre, Cagnes sur Mer, France

Stifle injuries are increasingly recognized as a major cause of hind limb lameness. Ultrasonography has tremendously improved our ability to confirm or rule out stifle lesions, which primarily involve soft tissue structures. Radiography is often disappointing or inaccurate, and it will only allow us to detect late degenerative changes. The equine stifle is a large, complex region and its ultrasonographic examination requires a thorough knowledge of the anatomy.

PREPARATION AND SCANNING TECHNIQUE

The stifle region should be finely clipped from distal to the tibial tuberosity up to the stifle skin fold, and all around the limb, then prepared as usual. Most of the examination is performed with the limb weight bearing, although, in very lame horses, examination can be adequately performed with the limb partially flexed. To scan the cranial aspect of the femorotibial joints, however, the limb must be flexed. It may be useful to use a wooden block to stabilize the foot. It is not necessary to achieve full flexion, which is often not tolerated by the injured horse. Intra-articular analgesia will dramatically interfere with evaluation of the joint, as it causes hemorrhage, inflammation, and effusion, and because air may be introduced into the joint space or periarticular soft tissues. Gas can persist in the joint for up to 2 weeks, so it is therefore preferable to perform an ultrasonographic examination prior to diagnostic intra-articular analgesia whenever possible.

A high-frequency (7–15 MHz) linear probe is best to evaluate the femoropatellar joint and the medial aspect of the stifle. A standoff pad may be used but can be fiddly and is not necessary. To examine the cranial, lateral, and caudal aspects of the stifle, a 6–12 MHz micro-convex, curved array transducer is preferred.

ULTRASONOGRAPHIC ANATOMY

The anatomy of the stifle region has been described elsewhere and the reader is encouraged to study anatomy texts in detail to better understand the three-dimensional arrangement of this complex joint.

Femoropatellar Joint

The femoropatellar joint is best imaged with the joint extended, as most of the trochlea is hidden by the patella when the limb is flexed. In the extended position the patella points craniolaterally, and the large medial trochlear ridge is palpable under the skin cranially. Starting in transverse planes, the probe is placed cranioproximally over the quadriceps muscles and examination is continued from proximal to distal, down to the tibial tuberosity. The quadriceps muscle is relatively homogeneous with a typical hypoechogenic muscular pattern. There is no insertion tendon as such, so that there is a sharp interface between the muscle belly and the proximal surface of the patella (Figure 7.1). The cranial surface of the patella forms a sharp, smooth hyperechogenic interface. Distally, it forms a shallow groove at the origin of the middle patellar ligament (PL) (see below). Medially, it is prolonged by the hypoechogenic, crescent-shaped parapatellar fibrocartilage, which curves around the medial

Atlas of Equine Ultrasonography, First Edition. Edited by Jessica A. Kidd, Kristina G. Lu, and Michele L. Frazer.
© 2014 John Wiley & Sons, Ltd. Published 2014 by John Wiley & Sons, Ltd.
Companion Website: www.wiley.com/go/kidd/equine-ultrasonography

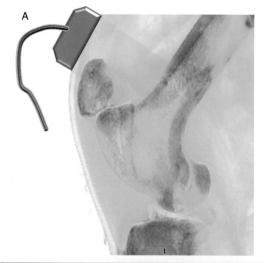

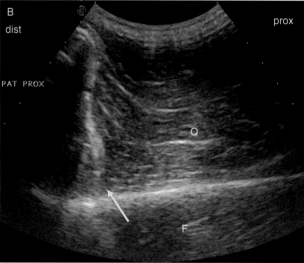

Figure 7.1 Normal proximal patella and distal crus. (A) Position of the transducer cranio-proximal to the patella (sagittal plane) and (B) corresponding ultrasonographic image. The arrow points to the virtual position of the suprapatellar pouch of the femoropatellar joint. F: femur; Q: quadriceps.

longitudinal sections (parasagittal), the ridges form a smooth, convex bone interface, topped by anechogenic cartilage, which should be perfectly regular in thickness. The lateral PL is seen as a striated structure lying directly over the lateral ridge. The capsule is tightly applied against the cartilage surface, and no fluid is normally visible over the trochlea.

The patellar ligaments actually anatomically correspond to the quadriceps tendon and are therefore similar in appearance to digital flexor tendons. Their borders are, however, ill defined due to poor contrast with the surrounding infrapatellar fat pad. The middle PL is round to oval in cross-section (Figure 7.3) and is the largest of the three PLs. It runs from the apex of the patella to the cranial-most part of the tibial tuberosity, within the fat pad and in the center of the trochlear groove. Distally, it becomes more triangular and often contains thin, hypoechogenic lines, giving it a webbed appearance. This should not be mistaken for a tear. Tilting of the probe to create an off-incidence artifact will cause the ligament to become hypoechogenic, enhancing its outline within the fat pad. The medial PL is triangular in cross-section and, in the extended limb, lies over the medial aspect of the medial trochlear ridge, 4 or 5 cm caudal to the apex of the ridge (Figure 7.4). Proximally it becomes more heterogeneous as its fibers spread out into the parapatellar fibrocartilage. Distally, it inserts approximately 2 cm medial to the middle PL and receives a tendinous branch from the sartorius muscle. The lateral PL is thinner and crescent shaped in cross-section (Figure 7.2). It caps the apex of the lateral trochlear ridge, outlining the cartilage. It inserts on the tibial tuberosity, immediately lateral to the middle PL's insertion. There is often a small to moderate amount of anechogenic synovial fluid in the lateral and medial joint recesses caudal to the respective PLs, over the surface of the lateral and medial trochlear ridges.

Medial Femorotibial Joint: Medial Aspect

A linear transducer is best, as the joint is very close to the skin. The topography of the medial aspect of the joint is reviewed in Figure 7.5. The proximal edge of the tibial condyle and the round, smooth surface of the medial femoral condyle form a triangular space filled by the echogenic medial meniscus (Figure 7.6). Linear, anechogenic artifacts are caused by refraction at the insertion of the capsule on the outer surface of the meniscus. These are easily mistaken for tears but they should remain perpendicular to the probe when the latter is tilted. The capsule inserts over the whole abaxial aspect of the meniscus, so that fluid can only

trochlear ridge and terminates via the thin medial collateral patellar ligament (Figure 7.2). It also gives rise to the medial PL (see below).

Distal to the apex of the patella, the trochlear groove appears as a wide, U-shaped bone interface covered by anechogenic cartilage (Figure 7.2). In many horses, the latter is irregular in the center of the groove, which is considered to be a normal feature. The medial trochlear ridge is broad, smooth, and rounded, and is covered by relatively thin cartilage (0.8–1 mm thickness). This becomes irregular medially. The lateral trochlear ridge is much narrower and triangular in cross-section. Its cartilage is thicker (2–2.5 mm). In

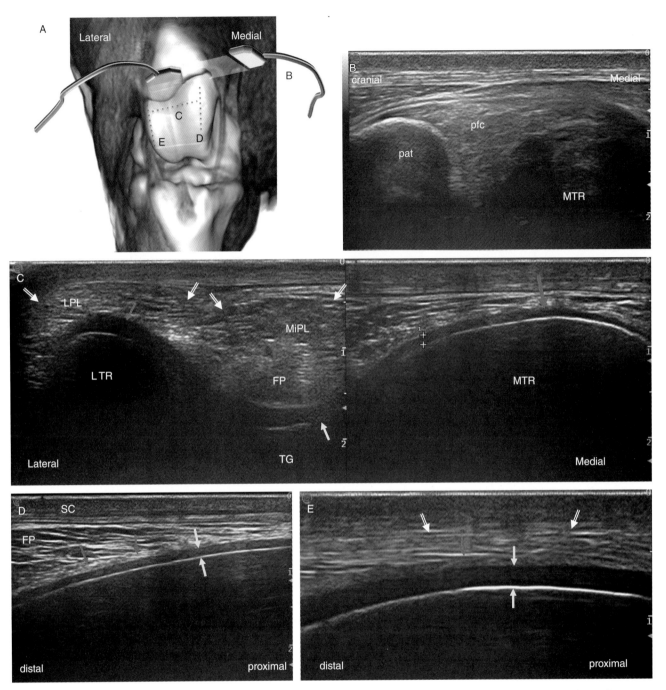

Figure 7.2 Cranial view of the normal femoropatellar joint. (A) Position of the transducer and corresponding ultrasonographic images in 7.2B–E. (B) Transverse plane image showing the medial aspect of the patella (pat) and parapatellar fibrocartilage (pfc). (C) Transverse plane image over the cranial aspect of the trochlea. The cartilage over the center of the trochlear groove (TG) is often irregular (yellow arrow), it is smooth over the ridges (red arrows). The fat pad (FP) is echogenic and heterogeneous. The middle patellar ligament (MiPL) is often difficult to discern from the fat pad in transverse images. The lateral patellar ligament (LPL) is flattened and curves over the sharp lateral trochlear ridge (LTR) (double arrows). (D) Longitudinal image of the medial trochlear ridge (MTR), showing the smooth subchondral bone outline and thin overlying cartilage (yellow arrows). The fibrous part of the capsule (red arrows) is tightly applied against the ridge surface. SC: subcutis. (E) Longitudinal plane image of the LTR. The cartilage (yellow arrows) is thicker than on the MTR and is thickest at the apex of the ridge. The capsule (red arrow) adheres to the LPL (white arrows).

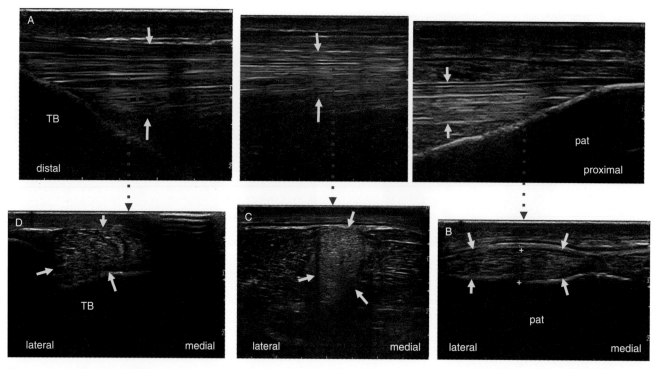

Figure 7.3   Normal middle patellar ligament (MiPL). Longitudinal (A) and transverse (B,C,D) ultrasonographic images. At the patellar origin (B) the cranial surface of the distal patella (pat) forms a trough. The MiPL is homogeneous and finely striated (arrows). (C) Central portion of the MiPL (yellow arrows): the edges contrast poorly with the surrounding FP. The two vertical anechogenic lines are edge refraction artifacts. (D) Distal insertion of the MiPL on the tibial tuberosity (TB): this portion is triangular and contains thin, hypoechogenic reticulations due to thicker endotendon tissue trabecula (red arrows).

accumulate proximal to it, over the abaxial surface of the medial femoral condyle. Discrete distension of the joint is common but the synovial membrane should remain very thin. Small villi may be seen in the pouch in normal horses. Transverse plane images of the menisci are obtained by rotating the probe 90°. These images are useful to better evaluate the configuration of certain tears.

The medial collateral ligament (MCL) is a strong, flattened structure, approximately 5–6 mm in thickness. As in most joints it is made up of two poorly differentiated branches (Figure 7.7). It is necessary to rotate the probe to image each branch individually, as they run obliquely to each other, crossing over the meniscus. The superficial branch runs vertically; it originates on the femoral epicondyle several centimeters proximal to the joint, and inserts on the abaxial surface of the tibia. It receives part of the insertion of the adductor muscle proximally. The deep branch originates caudal to it, and runs in a craniodistal direction to insert on the tibia, cranial to the superficial branch.

Lateral Femorotibial Joint: Lateral Aspect

The general topography is presented in Figure 7.8. The joint is covered by a thicker layer of muscle and the bone surfaces are very oblique to the skin. It is consequently difficult to obtain images using a linear transducer. A micro-convex probe provides better images. Craniolaterally, the tendon of origin of the long digital extensor and peroneus tertius muscles originates on the lateral femoral epicondyle and runs within the deep extensor groove of the proximal tibia (Figure 7.9). The groove is covered by cartilage and a synovial recess extends from the lateral femorotibial joint (LFT), between the bone surface and the tendon. Similarly to the MCL, the lateral collateral ligament (LCL) is divided into two branches, although they are more difficult to tell apart. They both insert on the tibia and fibular head. The popliteal tendon originates immediately cranial to the LCL. It runs obliquely in a caudodistal direction, over the meniscus and underneath the LCL. It is triangular in cross-section and should not be

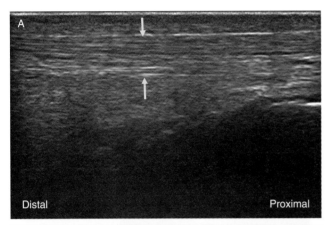

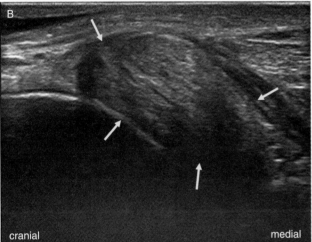

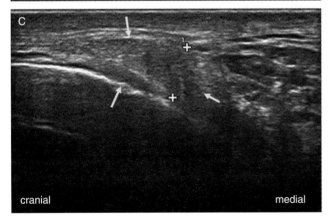

Figure 7.4 Normal medial patellar ligament (MPL). Longitudinal (A) and transverse (B,C) ultrasonographic images. A and C are obtained at mid-distance, caudomedial to the medial trochlear ridge. The ligament lies within the joint capsule, making its outline indistinct (yellow arrows). B is obtained just distal to the parapatellar fibrocartilage (pfc). The MPL (calipers) curves around the proximal prominence of the medial trochlear ridge (MTR), blending into the pfc. There it broadens and becomes more heterogeneous as the fibers spread into the thickness of the fibrocartilage. (C) Further distally, the MPL (calipers) is poorly defined from the fibrous capsule.

mistaken for a torn portion of the meniscus. It fans out over the caudal proximal tibia as a hypoechogenic muscle. Fluid may be seen proximal to the meniscus and cranial or caudal to the collateral ligament, but this is less common than in the medial compartment.

Cranial Aspect of the Femorotibial Joints

Imaging the cranial aspect of the femorotibial articulation requires that the stifle be flexed, in order to expose the intercondylar space and the cruciate ligaments (Figure 7.10). A micro-convex transducer must be used. The surface of the femoral condyles, overlying cartilage, and cranial horns of the menisci are easily visualized deep to the fat pad. The round condylar surfaces can be assessed for cartilage or subchondral defects.

The cranial cruciate ligament (CrX) can be identified with the ultrasound beam perpendicular to the ligament fibers (Figure 7.11): the probe is placed immediately distal to the patella, over or medial to the middle PL. The probe is angled downward in a sagittal plane to image the surface of the tibial eminence. The beam is then rotated 15–20° clockwise in the left limb and anticlockwise in the right limb until the linear pattern of the ligament is recognized. The CrX originates caudally on the axial (medial) aspect of the lateral femoral condyle, and inserts in a dip between the medial and lateral prominences of the tibial eminence. Cross-sectional images can be obtained by rotating the probe 90° in the same position. The CrX is hyperechogenic with a regular striated pattern.

The cranial (femoral) origin of the caudal cruciate ligament (CaX) is visualized by directing the beam upward, with the probe placed between the lateral and middle PLs, immediately proximal to the tibial tuberosity (Figure 7.12). The surface of the intercondylar space of the femur is identified between the condyles and distal to the trochlear groove. The CaX runs disto-caudally in a sagittal plane, directly over the bone surface. It crosses over the medial aspect of the cranial cruciate ligament within the intercondylar fossa.

Finally, the cranial tibial insertions of the menisci (cranial meniscotibial ligaments) are imaged from the craniolateral and craniomedial aspects respectively. The cranial horn of the meniscus is seen as a wedge-shaped structure between the femoral and tibial condyles and followed axially along the cranial aspect of the tibial eminence. To visualize the ligaments, the probe must be angled downward to keep the surface of the tibia perpendicular to the beam (Figure 7.13). Longitudinal images of the ligaments may be obtained from this position by rotating the transducer 90°.

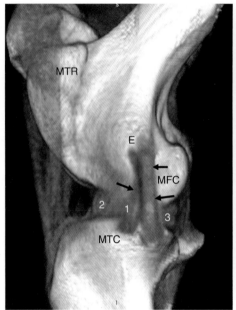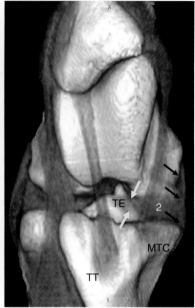

Figure 7.5 Computed tomography (CT) scan three-dimensional (3-D) reconstruct of the stifle showing the topography of the medial femorotibial joint. The medial femoral condyle (MFC) and medial tibial condyle (MTC) are separated by the wedge-shaped meniscus. The latter is topographically divided into body (1), at the level of the medial collateral ligament (black arrows), and cranial (2) and caudal (3) horns. The cranial horn inserts onto the craniomedial aspect of the tibial eminence (TE) via a cranial meniscotibial ligament (yellow arrows). A very short caudal meniscotibial ligament links the caudal horn to the caudomedial edge of the tibial plateau. The medial collateral ligament (MCL) is flat but strong and extends from the medial femoral epicondyle (E) to the medial aspect of the MTC and is divided into two distinct branches. MTR: medial trochlear ridge; TT: tibial tuberosity.

Caudal Aspect of the Femorotibial Joints

The topography is reviewed in Figure 7.14. The leg is examined extended and weightbearing. Because of the large caudal muscle mass, the depth of the joint varies from 5–20 cm. For this reason, 3.5–5 MHz transducers are best. Convex or micro-convex probes are necessary to angle the probe up or down in relation to the skin to image the various ligaments. Adequate images are obtained with the transducer placed 10–15 cm proximal to the junction thigh/leg, and angled downward at approximately 10° (i.e. perpendicular to the tibia). The condyles are round and smooth with an even anechoic cartilage, and the caudal meniscal horns are wedge shaped abaxially. The joint capsule is only obvious when highlighted by a joint effusion.

The CaX is imaged in the sagittal plane. It runs between the condyles and inserts on a sharp prominence on the caudal proximal border of the tibia, axial to the end of the medial meniscus. The probe must be oriented downward 30°. From this position, the transducer can then be rotated anticlockwise in the right stifle, clockwise in the left limb, by approximately 30° to the axial plane, to image the lateral meniscofemoral

ligament, which links the lateral meniscus to the femur immediately proximal to the medial condyle.

ULTRASONOGRAPHIC ABNORMALITIES

General principles applying to ultrasonographic signs of joint disorders are reviewed in detail in the fetlock joint chapter. The same basic signs should be looked for in the stifle, including inflammatory changes in the synovial membrane and capsule, cartilage and subchondral bone defects, fragmentation, etc. More specific conditions are reviewed here.

Femoropatellar Joint

Effusion

Effusion is the most common finding in this joint and may be encountered in sound horses without synovial thickening ("cold effusion") (Figure 7.15A). *Inflammatory changes (synovitis)* may be observed without identifiable causes, but a primary lesion should always be

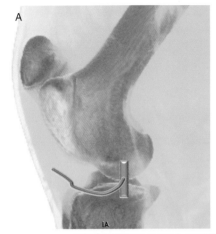

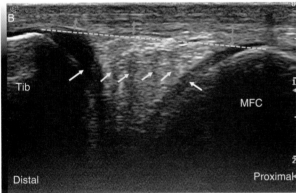

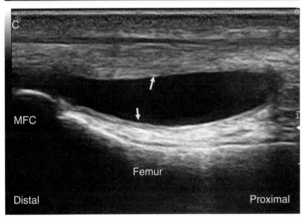

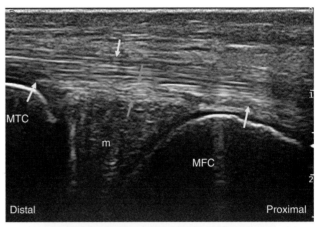

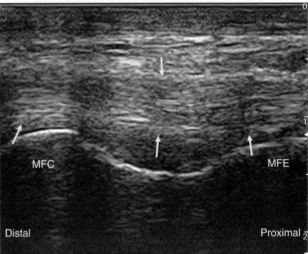

Figure 7.7 Longitudinal (frontal) plane ultrasonographic images over the medial aspect of the stifle showing the superficial branch of the collateral ligament (yellow arrows), recognized by its striated pattern. It runs from the medial femoral epicondyle (MFE) over the medial meniscus (m) and abaxial borders of the medial femoral condyle (MFC) and medial tibial condyle (MTC). The deep branch (red arrows) runs obliquely to it, hence a grainier pattern as the fibers are not aligned with the transducer. It separates the superficial branch from the meniscus to which it adheres. Note that the ligaments are poorly distinguished from the rest of the fibrous capsule.

Figure 7.6 (A) Position of the transducer over the medial aspect of the medial femorotibial joint. (B) Longitudinal (frontal) plane ultrasonographic image obtained cranial to the collateral ligament. The meniscus is echogenic, wedge shaped and amorphous. It sits axial to an imaginary line drawn between the edges of the condyles (dotted line). The underlying cartilage is smooth and even (white arrows) and the fibrous capsule (red double arrows) inserts over its abaxial border. Note the hypoechogenic artifacts running perpendicular to the transducer (yellow arrows. (C) Image obtained proximal to that in B. Note the mild distension of the joint pouch by anechogenic fluid. No fluid is seen over the meniscus (B). The membrane is thin and even (yellow arrows) in the absence of inflammation. MFC: medial femoral condyle; Tib: tibia.

investigated. *Synovial effusion* is most prominent in the abaxial recesses, lateral and medial to the trochlea. Large amounts of anechogenic fluid may be present, displacing the capsule and overlying muscles. Only in severe, chronic cases will the fluid accumulate in the trochlea, occasionally displacing the patella away from the femur. Signs of hemorrhage may be noted, although this appears to be rare in the stifle and is usually associated with trauma. As in other joints, the thickness of the synovial membrane can be assessed. Villous

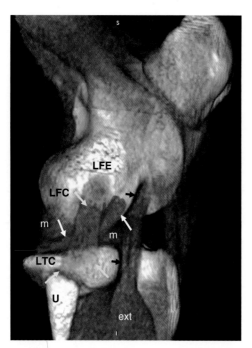

Figure 7.8 CT scan 3-D reconstruct showing the topography of the lateral femorotibial joint. The lateral femoral (LFC) and tibial (LTC) condyles are separated by the lateral meniscus (m). The lateral collateral ligament (yellow arrows), is made up of two closely related branched originating on the lateral femoral epicondyle (LFE) and inserting both on the tibia and fibula (yellow arrows). The common tendon of origin (black arrowheads) of the peroneus tertius and long digital extensor muscles (ext) originates on the abaxial aspect of the lateral trochlear ridge and runs over the cranial horn of the mm, within the extensor fossa of the tibia. The tendon of origin of the popliteus muscle originates on the femoral epicondyle, cranial to the collateral ligament and runs between the latter and the lateral meniscus in a caudodistal direction (white arrows). U: ulna.

proliferation may be seen as lollipop- or polyp-shaped images in the abaxial recesses (Figure 7.15B), and synovial masses are occasionally observed (Figure 7.15C). Osteoarthritis may be very subtle in this joint but significant, generalized cartilage thinning may be found in severe, long-standing cases. Osteophytes are visible at the apex of the patella and at the abaxial edges of the trochlear ridges.

Patellar Ligament Injuries

Patellar ligament injuries have been increasingly recognized. They may be due to direct trauma in many cases, although progressive degeneration through repeated strain injuries might be incriminated as for digital flexor tendons. The middle PL is most com-

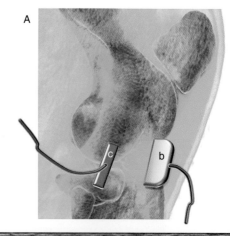

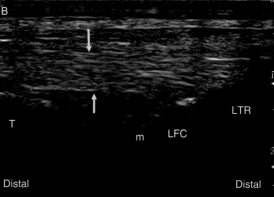

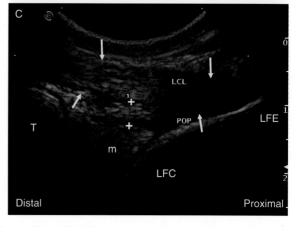

Figure 7.9 (A) 3-D reconstruct showing the position of the transducer in the two positions (B and C) corresponding to the ultrasound images over the extensor groove of the tibia (B) and lateral aspect of the lateral femorotibial joint (C). (B) Longitudinal (frontal) plane ultrasonographic image showing the common tendon of origin of the peroneus tertius and long digital extensor muscles (ext) (arrows) and extensor groove of the tibia (T). (C) Longitudinal (frontal) plane ultrasonographic image showing the lateral collateral ligament (LCL, yellow arrows). The striation is lost proximally because of the use of a curved array transducer inducing an off-incidence artifact. The hypoechogenic artifact helps, however, to better see the ligament contours. At this level the popliteus tendon (POP: calipers) is flat and located between the meniscus (m) and LCL. LFC: lateral femoral condyle; LFE: left femoral epicondyle; LTR: lateral trochlear ridge.

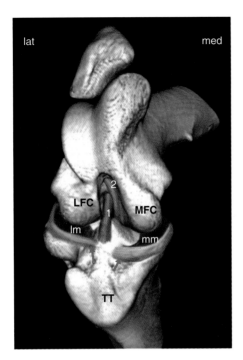

Figure 7.10 3-D CT-scan reconstructs showing the topographic anatomy of the femorotibial articulation. The stifle is fully flexed to expose the intercondylar space. The ligaments have been drawn to show their general topography. The cranial cruciate ligament (1) runs in a caudoproximolateral to distocraniomedial direction, between the axial surface of the lateral femoral condyle (LFC) and the tibial eminence; the caudal cruciate ligament (2) runs in the sagittal plane, in a cranioproximal to caudodistal direction, crossing its cranial counterpart medially between the two condyles. It originates distal to the trochlea and inserts on the caudal aspect of the tibial plateau; the two arrows indicate the cranial meniscotibial ligaments. lm: lateral meniscus; MFC: medial femoral condyle; mm: medial meniscus; TT: tibial tuberosity.

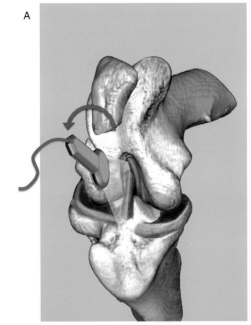

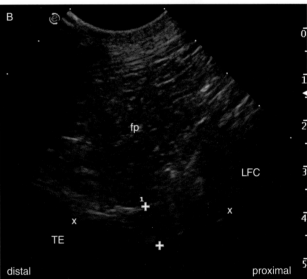

Figure 7.11 (A) Position of the transducer to image the cranial cruciate ligament; the stifle is partially flexed; the probe is applied distal to the patella, pushing it into the skin, and angled downward 20–30° in the sagittal plane; it is rotated anticlockwise (right stifle) to align the beam to the ligament fibers. (B) Corresponding longitudinal (sagittal) plane ultrasonographic image showing the cranial cruciate ligament (calipers) between the axial aspect of the lateral femoral condyle (LFC) and tibial eminence (TE). fp: fat pad.

monly affected although the medial PL may be primarily injured, particularly in trotters. This should not be mistaken for previous desmotomy of the medial PL, which can give rise to a very thickened, heterogeneous or hyperechogenic ligament.

"Core lesions", similar to those in the superficial digital flexor tendon, have been described, associated with enlargement and decreased echogenicity of the ligament (Figure 7.16A,B). In most cases, however, diffuse or reticulated anechoic areas are visible in the enlarged ligament (Figure 7.16C). Severe ligament tears cause them to appear grossly enlarged and poorly defined with a diffuse, hypoechogenic and mottled appearance (Figure 7.17). Spontaneous rupture or avulsion of the patellar origin or tibial insertion occur occasionally. Severe, complex PL injuries may be encountered, due in particular to high speed falls or road traffic accidents: these may be associated with patellar fracture or dislocation. PL injury may also occur in combination with fractures of the tibial tuberosity. This may have important repercussions when

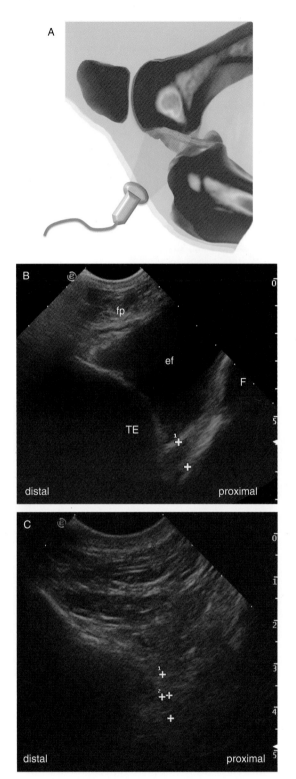

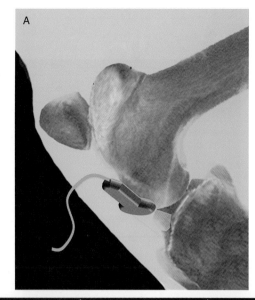

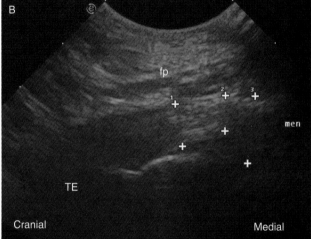

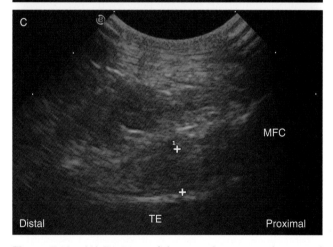

Figure 7.12 (A) Position of the transducer over the cranial aspect of the flexed stifle. The probe is placed distally close to the tibial tuberosity, the beam is directed in the sagittal plane, proximally, to visualize the intercondylar fossa of the femur. (B) Corresponding longitudinal (sagittal) plane ultrasonographic image showing the caudal cruciate ligament (calipers) running from just distal to the femoral trochlea (F) to the caudal aspect of the proximal tibia (TE: tibial eminence). Severe medial femorotibial effusion (ef) in this horse enhances the normal appearing ligament. fp: fat pad. (C) Slightly oblique view obtained half-way between those in Figures 11B and 12B, showing the crossing point between the cranial (calipers 1) and caudal (calipers 2) cruciate ligaments.

Figure 7.13 (A) Position of the transducer over the cranial aspect of the flexed stifle to image the cranial medial meniscotibial ligament. The probe is placed craniomedially in a transverse or longitudinal plane and the beam is directed downward in a caudolaterodistal direction. (B) Corresponding transverse plane ultrasonographic image showing the meniscotibial ligament (calipers) running across the image between the medial meniscus (men) and tibial eminence (TE). fp: fat pad. (C) Parasagittal plane image showing the same ligament in cross-section. MFC: medial femoral condyle.

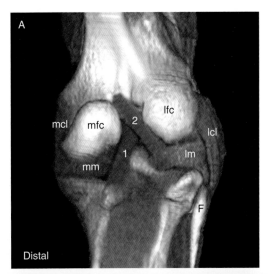

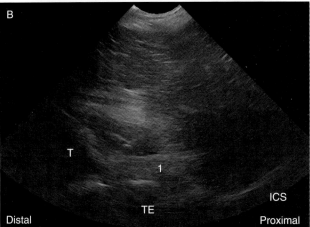

Figure 7.14 (A) 3-D CT scan reconstruct showing the topographic anatomy of the caudal aspect of the femorotibial articulation. F: fibular head; lcl: lateral collateral ligament; lfc: lateral femoral condyles; lm: lateral meniscus; mcl: medial collateral ligament; mfc: medial femoral condyles; mm: medial meniscus; 1: caudal cruciate ligament inserting on a sharp tibial tubercle on the caudal aspect of the tibial plateau; 2: meniscofemoral ligament. (B) Corresponding sagittal plane ultrasonographic image. 1: caudal cruciate ligament; ICS: femoral intercondylar space; T: tibial insertion; TE: tibial eminence (caudal aspect).

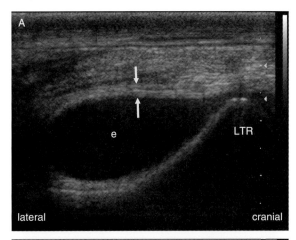

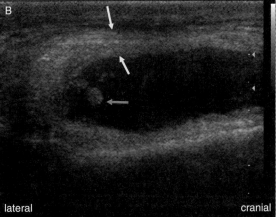

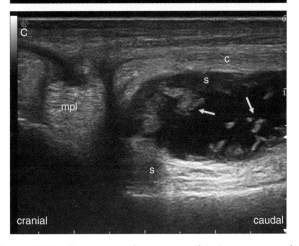

Figure 7.15 Transverse ultrasonographic images over the lateral aspect of the lateral trochlear ridge (LTR). (A) Idiopathic joint effusion (e) without inflammatory signs: the fluid is anechogenic and the synovial membrane is thin (yellow arrows). (B) The lateral recess of the femoropatellar joint is distended by anechogenic fluid. The synovial membrane is thickened and echogenic (yellow arrows) with small, hypertrophied synovial villi (red arrow) protruding into the space. (C) Medial recess (transverse image over the medial aspect of the medial trochlear ridge) with severe, hypertrophic synovitis: both capsule (c) and synovial membrane (s) are thickened, enlarged villi and synovial masses extend into the distended joint pouch (arrows). mpl: medial patellar ligament.

assessing the peroperative recovery risk or long-term prognosis.

Although ultrasonographic examination is often requested by trainers and veterinarians in cases of upward fixation of the patella, it is very unusual to observe any abnormality of the patellar ligaments in these cases. Desmitis of the medial PL usually occurs in combination with middle PL injury, although the author has encountered it as a primary entity in trotters, either as a result of previous surgery (longitudinal

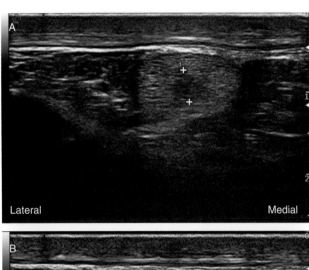

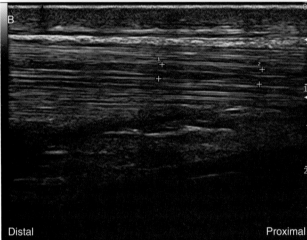

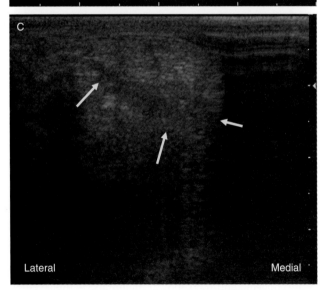

Figure 7.16 Transverse (A) and sagittal (B) images of the middle patellar ligament and trochlea. Although the ligament is little enlarged, there is a discrete, hypoechogenic core lesion in the center (calipers). (C) There is more diffuse fiber disruption, giving the ligament a reticulated appearance in the transverse image.

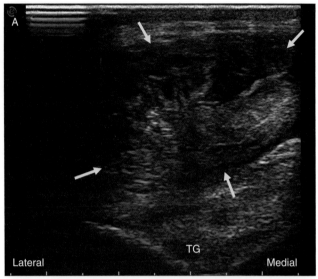

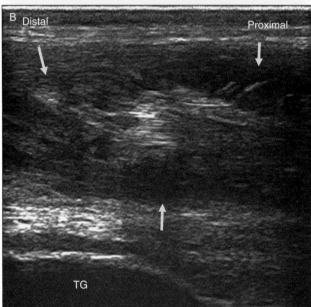

Figure 7.17 Transverse (A) and sagittal (B) images of the middle patellar ligament showing gross enlargement of the ligament (yellow arrows) which appears hypoechogenic, poorly defined, with complete loss of fiber pattern. The torn proximal stump (red arrowheads) is surrounded by hypoechogenic hemorrhagic tissue. TG: trochlear groove.

desmotomy, intraligamentous injections) or as a spontaneous injury (Figure 7.18). Ultrasonography may be useful in such cases, however, in order to rule out associated synovitis and trochlear or secondary patellar injuries.

Osteochondrosis

Ultrasonography is more sensitive than radiography to detect osteochondrosis (OC), especially of the troch-

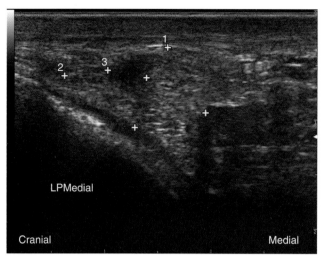

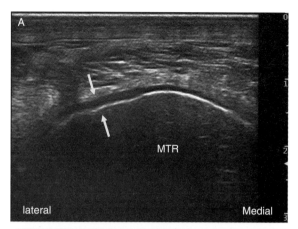

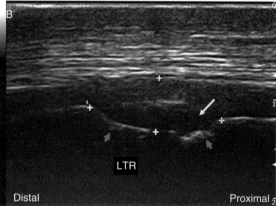

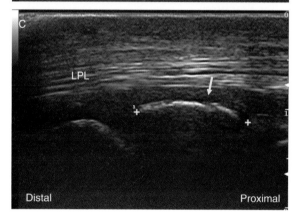

Figure 7.18 Transverse ultrasonographic image of the medial patellar ligament: the ligament (calipers 1 and 2) is moderately enlarged with a central, hypoechogenic area (calipers 3), itself surrounded by slightly hypoechogenic, poorly defined areas.

lear ridges. In one study comparing ultrasound with radiography and arthroscopy (Bourzac *et al.* 2009), ultrasonography provided a 94% sensitivity and 100% specificity. It is particularly helpful for accurately determining the extent of the lesions, which has been closely related to the prognosis after surgery. OC lesions of the trochlear ridges have been graded in relation to their proximodistal extent (McIlwraith & Martin 1985): grade I lesions are less than 2 cm in length, grade II measure 2–4 cm and grade III lesions are greater than 4 cm. The prognosis is closely related to the lesion size, with grade I, II, and III lesions carrying a 78, 63, and 54% chance of returning to the intended use, respectively.

In trochlear ridge OC the subchondral bone is flattened (Figure 7.19A) or irregular, forming a discrete defect (Figure 7.19B). The overlying cartilage is increased and irregular in thickness. It is often heterogeneous, with moderately to strongly echogenic areas. Occasionally, hyperechogenic areas casting an acoustic shadow represent mineralized flaps or fragments (Figure 7.19C). Both the proximodistal and lateromedial extent of the lesion should be evaluated as this may have important repercussions on the prognosis. Irregular areas in the centre of the trochlear groove should be considered as a normal feature. Ultrasound has also been found useful to confirm, prior to surgery, the location of free osteochondral fragments, which may detach and migrate proximally into the suprapatellar pouch, abaxially or distally into the corresponding joint recesses. Many fragments are enclosed in the

Figure 7.19 (A) Transverse ultrasonographic image of the medial trochlear ridge (MTR): the subchondral bone outline is flattened and slightly irregular. The overlying cartilage (arrows) is abnormally thick and echogenic. This is pathognomonic of osteochondrosis. There is no sign of cartilage dissection in this lesion. (B) Longitudinal image over the lateral trochlear ridge (LTR). There is a discrete defect within the subchondral bone (red arrowheads). The cartilage is echogenic and mottled and separated from the mineralized tissue by a hypoechogenic area (yellow arrow) representing necrotic tissue. This is a typical OCD lesion. (C) Longitudinal image over the LTR. A smooth, hyperechogenic interface casting a shadow is present within a subchondral bone defect, indicating a mineralized OC fragment. The fragment is covered by a layer of echogenic cartilage tissue (arrow). LPL: lateral patellar ligament.

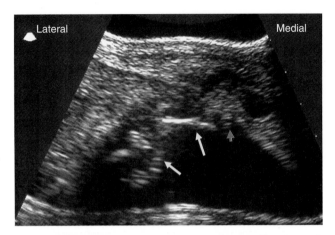

Figure 7.20 Transverse image over the patella. Several, irregular bony fragments are present (thin arrows). The main fracture line (red arrow) is surrounded by hypoechogenic tissue representing hemorrhage.

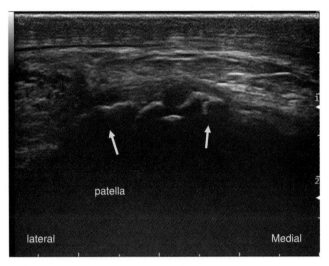

Figure 7.21 Transverse ultrasonographic image over the distal patella: multiple, coalescing fragments are present at the distal end of the patella (arrows).

synovial membrane and may therefore be more difficult to locate arthroscopically. OC of the patella is not visible ultrasonographically.

Patellar Fractures

Patellar fractures, sometimes difficult to visualize on radiographs, can be seen ultrasonographically as loss of continuity of the bone interface. Fragments may be visible and the fracture line(s) can usually be followed to assess the configuration (Figure 7.20). In early cases, large hematomas are usually present over the patella and within the quadriceps. In more chronic cases, a hyperechoic callus may be visible and irregular new bone is present around the fracture site. Joint involvement (articular fractures) leads to severe synovitis, and hemarthrosis may be obvious in the acute stage. Severe effusion, synovial thickening, and signs of osteoarthritis may be prominent in more chronic cases. *Apical patellar fragmentation* has been referred to as *chondromalacia patellae*, although the condition differs significantly from that described in man. Medial PL desmotomy has been incriminated as a possible cause of the fragmentation. Although this relationship has been questioned, the author has observed fragmentation in French trotters a few months after MPL desmotomy, whereas this condition is extremely rare as a spontaneous occurrence. Typically the apex of the patella is truncated and shortened, and multiple fragments are visible within a moderately echogenic tissue which extends to the joint surface (Figure 7.21). Effusion and chronic synovitis are always prominent.

Hematomas and Abscesses

Hematomas and abscesses are relatively common over the cranial stifle (Figure 7.22). Abscesses are characterized by echogenic, grainy, and heterogeneous fluid; they contain irregular echogenic clots and are surrounded by a thick, hyperechogenic capsule. Large hematomas are frequently encountered in the stifle region, especially over the quadriceps muscle or on the medial aspect of the joint, directly adjacent to the synovial membrane. They present with a honeycomb pattern, characteristic of organized hematomata, although they may initially present as poorly defined hypoechogenic areas, in the acute or subacute stages. They are often very painful initially and eventually form large fluid-filled pouches that can persist for significant amounts of times (seroma). The latter form anechogenic fluid-filled sacs with an obvious capsule. Quadriceps muscle tears can give rise to diffuse swelling or hematoma formation. They can cause persistent, severe lameness and should be ruled out in the present of a hematoma.

Femorotibial Joints

Ultrasonography is particularly valuable in the assessment of the lateral and medial femorotibial joints (LFT and MFT, respectively). Radiography is often disappointing because most injuries affect the soft tissues and because the large dimensions and complexity of the bone structures cause superimpositions which mask potential changes.

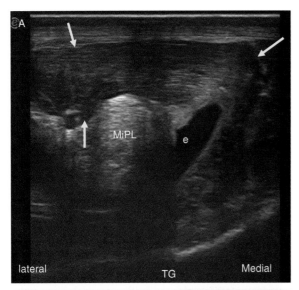

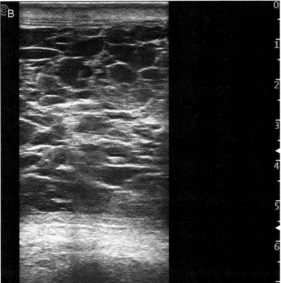

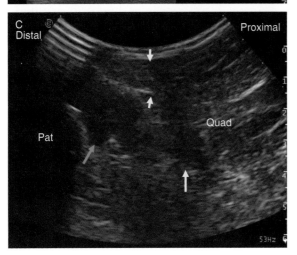

Figure 7.22 (A) Transverse scan over the trochlear groove (TG): echogenic fluid is present within the fat pad, superficial to the middle patellar ligament (MiPL), with an amorphous, heterogeneous appearance. There is marked synovial effusion, although the joint fluid remains anechogenic (e). This was an abscess due to a wound more proximally in the limb. (B) Sagittal image over the patella. A large, soft cavity is filled with anechogenic fluid separated into geometric cavities by thin, echogenic trabeculae. This is the typical appearance of an organized hematoma. (C) Sagittal plane image over the distal cranial thigh. The junction between the quadriceps muscle (Quad) and patella (pat) has a hypoechogenic, heterogeneous appearance (yellow arrow). Fluid is present over the proximal border of the patella (red arrow) and there is diffuse swelling between the muscle and fascia (short yellow arrows). This is a severe quadriceps tear.

Fluid effusion, visible as large, fluid-filled (anechogenic) pockets bulging proximal to the menisci, and cranial and caudal to the collateral ligaments, is a very common finding. However, marked distension may be encountered in clinically normal horses (see Figure 7.6C). It is therefore important to look for signs of synovial inflammation (see Chapter 2 for principles) or concurrent pathology and interpret the sonograms in the light of clinical findings.

A systematic approach to the joints is paramount to avoid overlooking subtle changes, which may have strong clinical repercussions, in particular meniscal tears or focal cartilage or subchondral trauma. Many artifacts can impair the sensitivity and specificity of the examination, so it is particularly important to acquire experience and a thorough knowledge of the gross and ultrasonographic anatomy for stifle ultrasonography.

Collateral Ligament (CL) Desmitis and Tears

CL lesions are rare in the author's experience and are always associated with severe injury to other stifle structures (meniscal tears, bone fractures, cruciate ligament damage). They cause severe joint instability and should not be overlooked, particularly in severe trauma cases. CL tears occasionally present as well defined, hypoechogenic "core" lesions within the ligament, representing fiber tearing and hemorrhage. In most cases, however, the affected ligament is enlarged with a diffuse decrease in echogenicity and loss of fiber pattern in long-axis planes (Figure 7.23). There is often marked periligamentous thickening.

Milder cases present with swelling around the ligament, thus forming a hypoechogenic halo, without obvious structural changes within the ligament. In complete rupture the affected CL cannot be visualized,

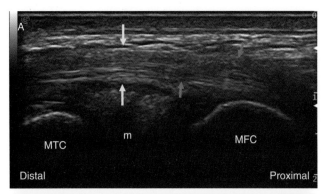

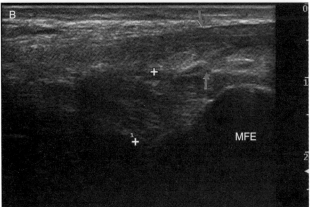

Figure 7.23 Longitudinal (frontal plane) images of the medial collateral ligament. (A) The superficial branch is enlarged (yellow arrows) and contains a poorly defined, hypoechogenic lesion with diffuse loss of fiber pattern (red arrows). (B) The ligament is grossly enlarged (calipers) and disorganized at its femoral origin on the MFE. There is marked periligamentous tissue thickening (red arrows). m: meniscus; MFE: medial femoral epicondyle; MTC: medial tibial condyle.

and it is usually replaced by a heterogeneous, hypoechogenic tissue or an organized hematoma. In chronic cases, organized fibrous tissue replaces the ligament and some partial fiber realignment may become evident after several months. There may be mineralization or fibrosis within and around the ligament (Figure 7.24).

Most commonly both superficial and deep branches are involved, although one of them may be more severely affected (Figure 7.24). Both lateral and medial CLs may be involved. The prognosis with stifle CL injury is generally poor because of the associated instability, involvement of other structures, and secondary degenerative joint disease.

Meniscal Injuries

Meniscal tears have been increasingly recognized since the advent of arthroscopy and ultrasonography. The first technique reveals fraying and linear tears at the

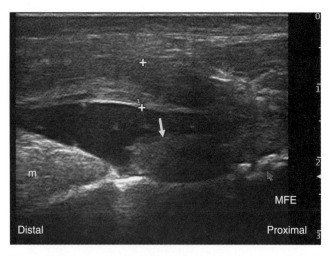

Figure 7.24 Longitudinal (frontal plane) image of a chronic injury to the medial collateral ligament. The superficial branch (calipers) is enlarged with an amorphous pattern. Intraligamentous mineralization and irregular entheseous new bone are present (red arrowheads). The deep branch has been completely torn, all that is left being a cauliflower-shaped fibrous mass (yellow arrow). m: meniscus; MFE: medial femoral epicondyle.

cranial horn of the menisci and their tibial attachment (cranial meniscotibial ligaments – CMTL). However, only a very small portion of the meniscus is visible through standard cranial portals. Ultrasonography is currently the technique of choice to examine the entire meniscus. Recent reviews suggest that meniscal injuries are a common cause of stifle lameness and probably the most common femorotibial abnormality encountered.

Meniscal tears are variable in appearance (Figure 7.25). Actual tears appear as hypo- to anechogenic areas or lines running through the thickness of the meniscus (Figure 7.25A,B). Tears most commonly run horizontally through the thickness of the meniscus (i.e. perpendicular to the skin surface), from the abaxial edge to exit on the proximal or distal surface. Therefore, in frontal plane images, they create a hypoechogenic line running nearly in the direction of the beam. These should not be mistaken for the common anechogenic artifact described previously. Real tears are often irregular and remain in the same position when the probe is tilted.

These so-called bucket-handle tears form an axial sliver, which may become detached and fold back cranially or abaxially (Figure 7.25C). Less frequently, sharp tears running in a frontal oblique plane divide the meniscus into cranial and caudal fragments. Tears can be imaged over the entire circumference of the meniscus to ascertain their configuration and extent.

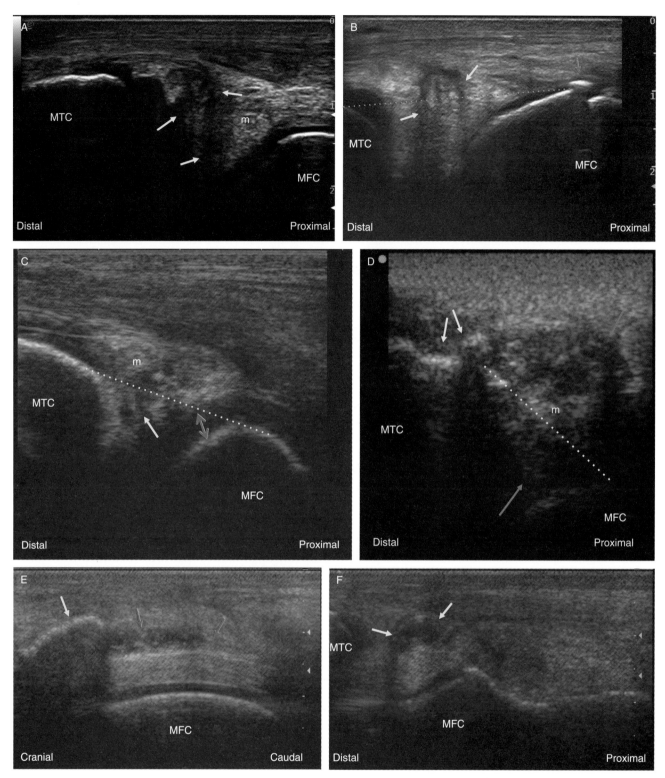

Figure 7.25 Various presentations of meniscal tears. (A) The yellow arrows delineate a hypoechogenic, horizontal (transverse) plane tear running through the entire thickness of the body of the medial meniscus (m). The distal fragment (to the left on the tibial side) is mottled and hypoechogenic. (B) This horizontal tear (yellow arrows) is filled with echogenic (fibrous) tissue. The meniscus is enlarged and protrudes abaxially well beyond a line drawn between the condyles (dotted line). Note the osteophyte on the medial femoral condyle (MFC) (red arrow). (C) Bucket handle type tear through the body of the medial meniscus. This image shows the cranial fragment, which also contains a horizontal tear (yellow arrow). It is split from the dorsocaudal fragment, allowing it to subluxate abaxially (dotted line), increasing the distance to the femur (double arrow). (D) Chronic medial meniscal injury with degenerative changes: the meniscus is heterogeneous with hypo- and hyperechogenic areas. It is deformed and enlarged (red arrows), protruding abaxial to the dotted line. Osteophytes (yellow arrows) are visible on the tibial condylar edge. (E) Chronic medial meniscal tear: this horizontal (transverse plane) image shows an abaxial degenerative lesion (red arrows) due to a sagittal tear. The cranial horn is mineralized, inducing an acoustic shadow (yellow arrow). (F) Cyst-like lesion within the disto-abaxial edge of the medial meniscus (yellow arrows). The latter is enlarged and deformed due to chronic degeneration. MFC: medial femoral condyle; MTC: medial tibial condyle.

Hypoechogenic areas or focal mottling within the meniscus probably represent degeneration secondary to chronic tears or degenerative joint disease. The meniscus may be distorted in outline, protruding outward of the joint space (Figure 7.25D). Normal menisci are bound by the capsule and should not extend more than 1 or 2mm beyond a line drawn between the edges of the tibial and femoral condyles. The capsule often appears be torn off the medial meniscus. Obvious collapse of the meniscus and joint space occur in most severe cases and direct contact between the joints surfaces of tibial and femoral condyles may be visualized. In such cases, the meniscus may become markedly hypoechogenic and appear like chewed gum extruded along the abaxial edge of the joint.

Mineralization of a meniscal fragment is uncommon but can be extensive (Figure 7.25E). Occasionally, cyst-like anechogenic structures develop with a damaged meniscus, resembling meniscal cysts described in man (Figure 7.25F).

Fraying and vertical tears of the CMTL have been extensively described based on arthroscopic findings. These are visible ultrasonographically (Figure 7.26), although the approach may be difficult because of the marked angle between the ligaments and the skin. The tears form irregular hypoechogenic areas within the striated ligament and there may be irregular new bone formation at the ligament insertion on the tibia (enthesophytes). Synovial proliferation and fraying of

the ligament, forming echogenic strands extending into the distended joint pouch(es), is usually obvious.

Cruciate Ligament Injuries

Damage to the cruciate ligaments is rare in the author's experience. It is sometimes difficult to confirm. Injured ligaments are enlarged, heterogeneous, and generally hypoechogenic (Figure 7.27A). Fraying of the ligaments is usually obvious as strands of tissue floating in the joint pouch cranially (Figure 7.27B). It is commonly accompanied by marked joint distension and thickening of the synovial membrane. Complete rupture is rare, but is evidenced by the inability to image the ligament (Figure 7.27C). The torn ends are visible at the insertion sites and often form cauliflower-like masses. Avulsion of either insertion or fracture of the tibial eminence is commonly encountered and is evidenced as large fragments protruding into the intercondylar space. Flexing the joint can be painful with cruciate ligament injury, so adequate analgesia and tranquilization is warranted.

Subchondral Cyst-like Lesions

Subchondral cyst-like lesions are usually fairly obvious on radiographs. Ultrasonography, however, is useful to determine more precisely the extent of the articular defect, to look for the presence of communication between the cyst cavity and joint space, and to allow standing injection of the cyst (Figure 7.28). This is achieved from a cranial distal approach with the stifle in full flexion. Associated cartilage, soft tissue damage and osteoarthritis should be evaluated.

Osteoarthritis

Joint disease is characterized by chronic synovial changes (membrane thickening, effusion, villous hypertrophy) and remodeling of the bone edges. Radiography is very insensitive to look for osteoarthritic changes in the stifle and ultrasonography will frequently reveal marked changes in radiologically normal joints (Figure 7.29): osteophytosis causes spike or spur-like deformity of the abaxial borders of the femoral and tibial condyles, and enthesophytosis induces irregular bone production at the insertions of the capsule and collateral ligaments (see Figure 7.24). Cartilage damage may be visible in advanced cases as irregular, echogenic areas. It may be secondary to any of the above and most commonly due to joint instability or osteochondrosis. Osteoarthritis is most often a consequence of chronic instability, as in meniscal tears and complex ligament injuries, or osteochondrosis.

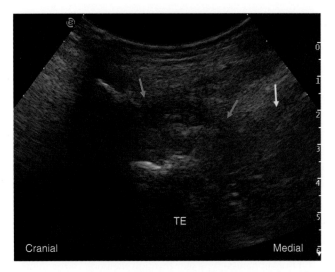

Figure 7.26 Transverse plane image of the cranial medial meniscotibial ligament. The ligament (red arrows) is enlarged, hypoechogenic, and heterogeneous. The cranial horn of the meniscus is of similar appearance, with poorly defined borders and a mottled, hypoechogenic appearance. This is a grade 4 tear. TE: tibial eminence.

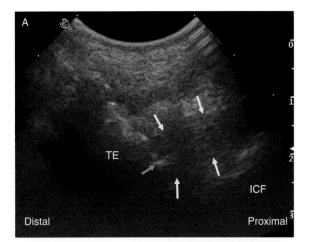

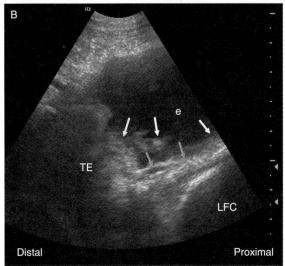

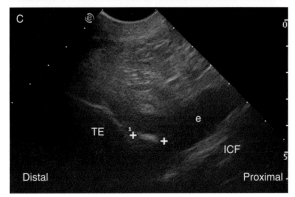

Figure 7.27 Cranial cruciate ligament injuries may be difficult to ascertain. (A) In partial tears (compare to Figure 7.11), the ligament is grossly enlarged (yellow arrows), hypoechogenic with partial to complete loss of fiber alignment. In chronic cases, there may be entheseous new bone at the tibial insertion (red arrow). Note the hyperechogenic, thickened synovial tissue around the ligament. (B) Severe tears lead to loss of definition of the ligament. Frayed fibers (white arrows) float in the effused joint space (e). The torn end of the ligament forms a cauliflower-like mass over the tibial eminence (yellow arrow). Some of the ligament fibres remain unruptured (red arrows). (C) In complete rupture, the ligament is impossible to visualize. Negative identification is made easier by the effusion (e). Note a large bony fragment off the tibial intercondylar eminence (calipers). ICF: intercondylar fossa; LFC: lateral femoral condyle; TE: tibial eminence.

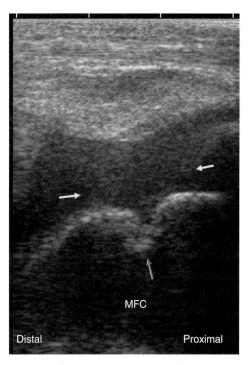

Figure 7.28 Longitudinal (parasagittal) image with the stifle in forced flexion showing the distal aspect of the medial femoral condyle (MFC). A cone-shaped defect is present in the subchondral bone surface (red arrow). It is filled by moderately echogenic tissue continuous with the thickened synovial membrane, representing a large adhesion (yellow arrows). This is consistent with a cyst-like lesion opening into the joint space.

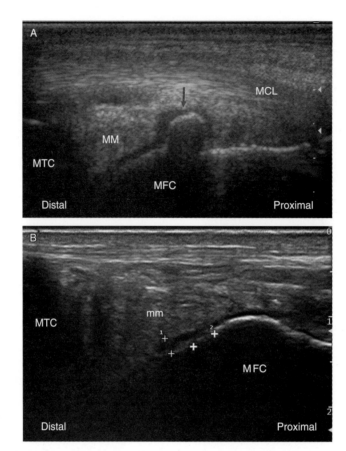

Figure 7.29 The two main ultrasonographic signs of osteoarthritis are periarticular new bone production and cartilage erosion. (A) Large, spur-like osteophyte (red arrow) on the medial aspect of the medial femoral condyle (MFC). The medial meniscus (MM) is deformed, heterogeneous and hypoechogenic. This is as much a result of degeneration as a tear and may be due to chronic instability. (B) The calipers show cartilage degeneration and sloughing over the MFC. The subchondral bone is relatively smooth but the cartilage is echogenic and irregular. MCL: medial collateral ligament; MTC: medial tibial condyle.

However, osteoarthritis may be encountered without other primary lesions detectable, both in older animals and in sports horses, presumably as a result of overuse, cyclic trauma, or age-related degeneration.

Septic Arthritis

The stifle may be infected through hematogenous spread in foals, or in adult horses via puncture wounds or iatrogenically as a complication of intra-articular medication or joint surgery.

The joint fluid can remain fairly anechoic, especially in foals with hematogenous infectious arthritis. However, in most cases, debris, hemorrhage and exudate cause the joint fluid to become echogenic and granular in appearance within hours of injury. Severe synovial proliferation is always present and fibrin clots may form strands or whorl-like masses in the fluid. Fibrin often clings to the joint surface to form an echo-

genic tissue overlying the cartilage. Cartilage or subchondral bone defects may develop in advanced or chronic cases over the condyles and trochlear ridges and bone, meniscus or cartilage fragments may be visible in the joint recesses.

Wounds over the stifle area should be examined thoroughly to look for evidence of joint sepsis or overt communications with the joint (Figure 7.30A) before the joint is tapped for synovial fluid analysis, in order to avoid inserting a needle through septic material into a non-infected joint.

In normal young foals less than 8 months old, the cartilage is very thick and the immature subchondral bone very irregular. The incompletely mineralized trochlear ridges have a "sunburst" appearance, due to centripetal ossification of the trochlear ridge ossification centers (Figure 7.30B). This should not be mistaken for infection. In these animals, however, the bone is very soft and prone to early defect formation or even joint surface destruction (Figure 7.30B).

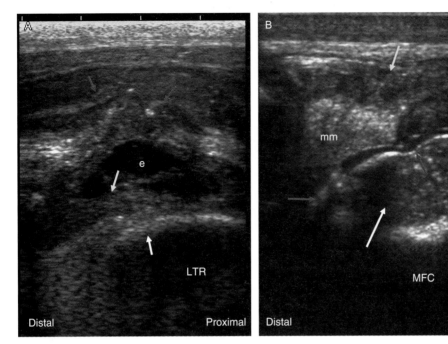

Figure 7.30   Septic arthritis. (A) Longitudinal (parasagittal) image over the lateral trochlear ridge (LTR) in an adult horse with a puncture wound. The tract is visible through the capsule (red arrows) and contains echogenic debris and hypoechogenic material. The soft tissues are grossly thickened. Heterogeneous "cellular" effusion is present (e). Pannus deposits form a thick echogenic layer over the joint surfaces (yellow arrow). Note a defect in the underlying bone (white arrow). (B) Longitudinal image over the medial aspect of the medial femorotibial joint of a 4-month-old foal with hematogenous septic arthritis. The medial meniscus (mm) is bulging and displaced medially. The capsule and synovium (yellow arrow) are severely thickened. Echogenic and grainy exudate (e) distends the joint pouch. Erosions are present in the subchondral bone (red arrows). Note that in this very young foal the condyles are not completely ossified, so that the sound beam penetrates some way into the cartilage template of the bone, which is a normal feature (white arrow). MFC: medial femoral condyle.

RECOMMENDED READING

Bourzac, C., Alexander, K., Rossier, Y., & Laverty, S. (2009) Comparison of radiography and ultrasonography for the diagnosis of osteochondritis dissecans in the equine femoropatellar joint. *Equine Veterinary Journal*, 41, 685–692.

Cauvin, E.R.J., Munroe, G.A., Boyd, J.S., & Paterson, C. (1996) Ultrasonographic examination of the femorotibial articulation in horses: imaging of the cranial and caudal aspects. *Equine Veterinary Journal*, 28, 285–296.

Denoix, J.M., Crevier, N., Perrot, P., & Bousseau, B. (1994) Ultrasound examination of the femorotibial joint in horses. *Proceedings of the American Association of Equine Practitioners*, 41, 57–58.

Dyson, S.J. (2002) Normal ultrasonographic anatomy and injury of the patellar ligaments in the horse. *Equine Veterinary Journal*, 34, 258–264.

Flynn, K.A. & Whitcomb, M.B. (2002) Equine meniscal injuries: A retrospective study. *Proceedings of the American Association of Equine Practitioners*, 48, 249–254.

Hoegaerts, M., Nicaise, M., Van Bree, H., & Saunders, J.H. (2005) Cross-sectional anatomy and comparative ultrasonography of the equine medial femorotibial joint and its related structures. *Equine Veterinary Journal*, 37, 520–529.

Labens, R., Busoni, V., Peters, F., & Serteyn, D. (2005) Ultrasonographic and radiographic diagnosis of patellar fragmentation secondary to bilateral medial patellar ligament desmotomy in a Warmblood gelding. *Equine Veterinary Education*, 17(4), 201–206.

McIlwraith, C.W. (1990) Osteochondral fragmentation of the distal aspect of the patella in horses. *Equine Veterinary Journal*, 22, 157–163.

Penninck, D.G., Nyland, T.G., O'Brien, T.R., Wheat, J.D., & Berry, C.R. (1990) Ultrasonography of the equine stifle. *Veterinary Radiology*, 31, 293–298.

Sanders-Shamis, M., Bukowiecki, C.F., & Biller, D.S. (1998) Cruciate and collateral ligament failure in the equine stifle: seven cases (1975–1985). *Journal of the American Veterinary Medical Association*, 193, 573–576.

Walmsley, J.P. (2005) Diagnosis and treatment of ligamentous and meniscal injuries in the equine stifle. *Veterinary Clinics of North America: Equine Practice*, 21, 651–672.

CHAPTER EIGHT

ULTRASONOGRAPHY OF THE PELVIS

Marcus Head

Rossdales Equine Hospital and Diagnostic Centre, Newmarket, UK

Ultrasonography is an extremely useful tool in the diagnosis and management of a number of conditions affecting the pelvis of horses, augmenting and, in some instances, replacing the established techniques of radiography and scintigraphy. The pelvis can be imaged percutaneously from the dorsal aspect, but also *per rectum*. Ultrasonographic assessment is useful in a wide variety of investigations, from subtle performance-limiting problems in sports horses to severe lameness in racehorses.

EQUIPMENT

Clipping is often necessary, although not in fine-coated horses. A high-frequency linear probe is the most useful for superficial structures but imaging the pelvis also requires a lower-frequency curvilinear or sector probe. Imaging can be difficult in patients with significant subcutaneous fat or thick skin. A rectal probe is necessary for internal examinations.

INDICATIONS

Reasons for performing an ultrasound assessment of the pelvis are varied but the commonest indication in non-Thoroughbred practice is evaluation of reduced performance. As for examination of the back and neck, these investigations can be time consuming and frustrating, but the use of ultrasonography enables a greater number of differential diagnoses to be considered. Other indications include lameness suspected to arise from the upper limb that has eluded diagnosis by distal anesthesia or is known to have been associated with a fall or other trauma. In Thoroughbred race-

horses, indications also include evaluation of stress fractures known to occur in the pelvis.

The main areas of interest in the pelvis are:

- ilial wings and shafts;
- tubera sacrale, tubera ischii, third trochanters, and tubera coxae;
- hip joints;
- the lumbosacral intercentral and intertransverse joints and sacroiliac joints;
- internal bony structures (*per rectum*).

THE ILIUM

The most important reason for imaging the ilium is the detection of fractures. In racehorses, these occur most frequently as fatigue injuries (stress fractures) caused by the accumulation of damage with cyclical loading and the vast majority originate on the caudal aspect of the ilial wing, close to the sacroiliac joint and the junction of the wing and shaft of the ilium. As they are caused by cumulative damage, horses often show extensive signs of injury on ultrasonography by the time they are presented for lameness examination or poor performance. However, while ultrasonography is very useful in the detection of these injuries, a normal ultrasound scan does not rule out injury to this region – some horses have "hotspots" on a bone scan that have no abnormalities ultrasonographically. In other types of horse, the most common reason for imaging the ilium is because of lameness thought to be caused by trauma to the pelvis – displacement of the tuber coxa or "knocked down hip" being the most common.

Figure 8.1 shows the technique described by Shepherd and Pilsworth to map the ilial wing by imagining

Atlas of Equine Ultrasonography, First Edition. Edited by Jessica A. Kidd, Kristina G. Lu, and Michele L. Frazer.
© 2014 John Wiley & Sons, Ltd. Published 2014 by John Wiley & Sons, Ltd.
Companion Website: www.wiley.com/go/kidd/equine-ultrasonography

four lines superimposed on the pelvis. The transducer is placed just off midline, holding the probe at 90° to the midline on the side of interest, and moved towards the tuber coxa slowly maintaining the image of the bone surface as a smooth, continuous echogenic line (Figure 8.2). It appears as a sweeping curve running from the tuber sacrale to the tuber coxa. It is important that the examination should cover the entire surface of the ilial wing, as stress fractures may produce pathology in a localized region – typically the caudal aspect – so that a single image may miss these injuries. The

operator must ensure that, particularly at the cranial and caudal sites (lines 1 and 3 in the illustration), the edges of the bone are imaged. This can be achieved by tilting the probe forwards and backwards so that the bone surface temporarily disappears from view at these sites.

By following a systematic approach, incomplete fractures will not be missed. Be aware of edge artifacts produced by the many large vessels and fascial planes between the muscles – these can give the impression that there is discontinuity in the surface of the bone. Subtle injuries may present with only minor changes to the contour of the bone surface (Figure 8.3) and in some cases it is possible to identify pathology of different ages – recent, sharply defined fracture lines cranially and more longstanding callus caudally (Figure 8.4). Immature callus will appear irregular and allow some of the ultrasound beam to pass through. Mature callus is smooth and of equal echogenicity to the adjacent, normal bone. As fractures heal the development of callus can be followed, as its contour changes from convex to concave and it becomes more echogenic with maturation. This is useful as fractures are monitored during recuperation.

Rotating the probe to image the ilial wing in a parasagittal plane is sometimes interesting, but its main use is to identify the ilial shaft easily – the smooth caudal edge of the wing becomes the long smooth surface of the shaft and can be followed down to the hip joint. Ilial shaft fractures can be difficult to diagnose unless they are complete – unlike ilial wing fractures, early changes to the bone that precede complete failure are

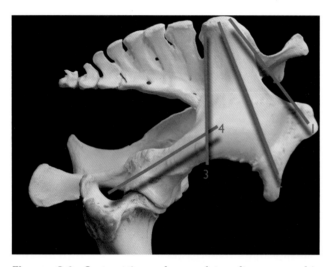

Figure 8.1 Systematic and complete ultrasonographic assessment of the ilium is best achieved by visualizing four planes – three running from the tuber sacrale to the tuber coxa and one following the ilial shaft.

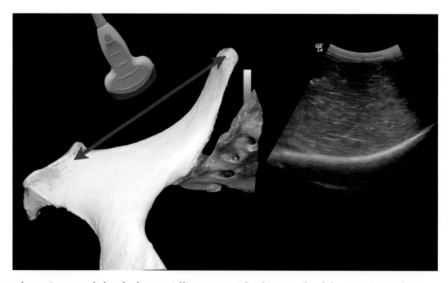

Figure 8.2 The transducer is moved slowly from midline outwards along each of the imaginary lines running from the tuber sacrale to the tuber coxa, imaging the smooth concave surface of the ilial wing.

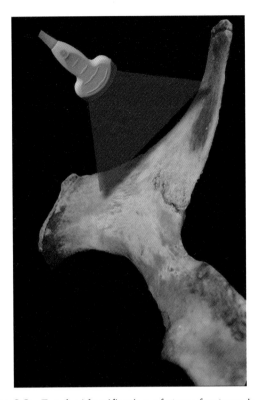

Figure 8.3 For the identification of stress fractures in race-horses (the commonest indication for this technique) care should be taken to assess the full width of the bone; almost all injuries of this kind begin caudally and propagate cranially, perhaps over a period of weeks. In this specimen, the cranial edge of the ilium would appear normal, while pathology can be seen clearly at the caudal aspect.

rarely detected. When complete, the normal linear contour to the bone surface that is visualized by running the transducer from cranial to caudal is interrupted, often with a step in the surface evident. This is frequently accompanied by significant hemorrhage. Young animals can suffer "green stick" fractures of the ilial shaft.

TUBERA SACRALE, ISCHII, AND COXAE

Imaging the bony prominences of the pelvis is best done with a combination of linear high frequency and lower frequency curvilinear transducers.

The tubera sacrale can be identified, along with the dorsal parts of the dorsal sacroiliac ligaments, in transverse and longitudinal planes. Asymmetry of these structures is quite common and does not correlate well with clinical disease.

Serving as the attachment for the large biceps femoris, semimembranosus, and semitendinosus muscles (all of which can be imaged), the tuber ischium can be injured as a result of direct trauma (frequently a fall) or as an avulsion injury in athletic horses. The bony prominences are easily palpated either side of the tail head and can be imaged horizontally and vertically. Although they have a certain degree of roughening in normal horses, they present a continuous surface

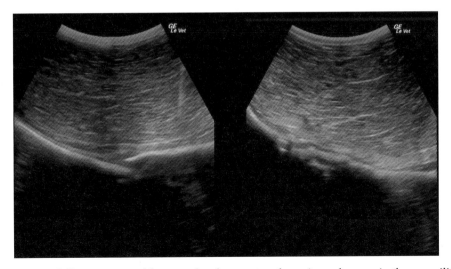

Figure 8.4 In some horses, different stages of fracture development and repair can be seen in the same ilial wing. The image on the left was obtained cranially (line 1 in Figure 8.1) while the image on the right was obtained caudally (line 3). The cranial image shows acute changes with separation of the fracture and relatively sharp bone edges. Caudally, however, there is clear evidence of callus formation with incompletely mineralized bone only partially attenuating the ultrasound beam.

readily amenable to ultrasound imaging. Careful comparison with the opposite side is useful – most injuries seem to involve displacement of bone, so roughening is rarely the only sign. Injury usually results in significant disruption to the normal bone contour and in some cases clear fragmentation (Figure 8.5).

Fractures to the tuber coxa also occur as a result of direct trauma or as an exercise-induced avulsion injury. They result in the typical "knocked down hip" appearance, and the sharp edge of the parent bone may, rarely, erode through the skin. Although not usually a

challenge to diagnose clinically, information regarding fracture configuration can be obtained through ultrasonography (Figures 8.6 and 8.7). It is also useful to scan from the fracture towards midline and attempt to reconstruct a mental map of the fracture configuration, particularly with regard as to whether the injury affects the shaft of the ilium. Some racehorses will suffer severe lameness caused by avulsion injury of the tuber coxa, but the typical clinical appearance associated with displacement of the fragment may not become evident for several days after the onset of lameness.

THIRD TROCHANTER

A much more common site of injury than is widely recognized, the third trochanter serves as the insertion for the superficial gluteal and its tendon which is easily visualized attaching to this bony prominence in the upper femur. Injuries typically occur in a fall but sometimes present as an avulsion. The area is easily palpated and amenable to percutaneous ultrasonography so do not forget to include this when assessing sudden-onset upper limb lameness (Figure 8.8). Once again, the structure can be imaged in orthogonal planes (Figure 8.9). Damage may consist of roughening or proceed to fracture, with or without displacement of the trochanter under the pull of the tendon (Figure 8.10).

Note that the ultrasonographic appearance of third trochanter, tuber coxa, and tuber ischium injuries may not alter significantly with time and it can be very

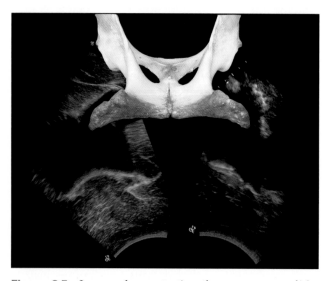

Figure 8.5 Images demonstrating the appearance of the normal (on the left) and injured tuber ischium, superimposed on a normal specimen.

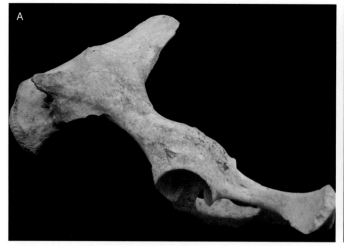
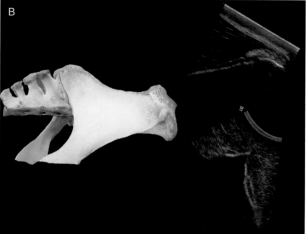

Figure 8.6 Anatomical specimen (A) and ultrasonographs (B) of "knocked down hip". In this injury, the tuber coxa is fractured and usually displaces cranioventrally. The normal smooth surface of the bone appears as a sharp point when damaged in this way (bottom right of B).

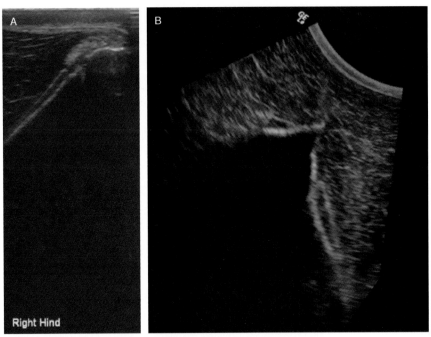

Figure 8.7 Fractures of the tuber coxa with a non-displaced fracture (A), and a complete fracture leaving a sharp bone point (B).

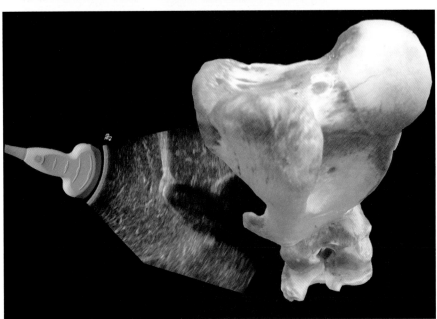

Figure 8.8 Transverse ultrasonograph of a normal third trochanter (note the tendon of insertion of the superficial gluteal and the use of the curvilinear transducer).

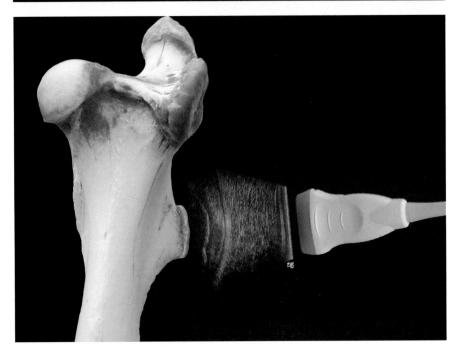

Figure 8.9 Longitudinal ultrasonograph of a normal third trochanter. Note the use of the linear transducer.

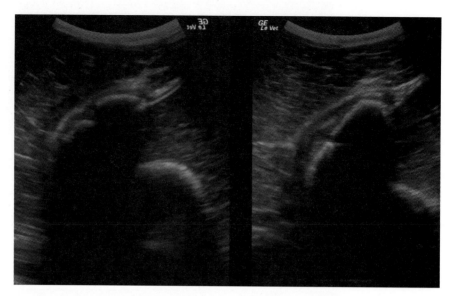

Figure 8.10   Two examples of injury to the third trochanter. In both, a fracture gap is visible on the caudal aspect of the bone surface. In the image on the right, the normal orientation of the trochanter to the femoral diaphysis is maintained, but in the image on the left the trochanter appears to have "fallen over", indicating displacement of the fracture.

difficult to age the lesion. This makes ultrasonography less useful in following these injuries during the healing process, and may lead to false positives if a horse has sustained an injury to these areas previously that may no longer be relevant clinically.

The Dorsal Sacroiliac Ligaments

Divided into dorsal and lateral parts, the dorsal ligaments connect the tubera sacrale and ilial wing to the sacrum. The dorsal parts are thin and crescent shaped cranially, becoming more "apostrophe shaped" caudally. The two separate parts of each left and right ligament can be appreciated in transverse and longitudinal images (Figure 8.11). The position of these parts relative to each other varies slightly from horse to horse and even from side to side in the same horse (often associated with clinically insignificant asymmetry of the tubera sacrale) so these "changes" need to be interpreted carefully (Figure 8.12). Care should be taken in interpretation as, like the supraspinous ligament (SSpL – Chapter 9), hypoechogenic areas can be seen in normal horses (Figure 8.13). Long-axis scans allow evaluation of longitudinal fiber pattern and assessment of the integrity of the entheses. As with the SSpL, a degree of off-incidence artifact and age-related change can cause false positives. Interpret changes with care as injury here is rare and artifact more common.

The lateral parts of the dorsal sacroiliac ligaments can be seen as thin echogenic structures attaching to the lateral border of the sacrum but clinically significant changes are rarely detected here.

Hip Joints

The hip joint is identified most easily by following the ilial shaft in a caudoventral direction. The transducer can then be rotated slowly to improve the image and identify the curved acetabulum, the smooth, convex femoral head, and the large greater trochanter (Figure 8.14 A and C). By rocking the transducer backwards and forwards, it should be possible to appreciate the relation between the closely apposed bone surfaces of the acetabulum and femoral head, and gain information regarding the health of the joint (Figure 8.15). Altering the orientation of the probe allows evaluation of the joint edges more easily. In a normal horse, the acetabulum and femoral head have a smooth appearance and there is only a narrow "gap" between them. In younger horses, the edges of the acetabulum are often rounded and the joint space is wider. The presence of the symphysis between the bones that form the acetabulum (ilium, ischium, and pubis) could be misinterpreted as a fracture. This fuses at approximately 1 year of age, and up to this time the appearance of the hip joint changes considerably, so comparisons with the contralateral limb are invaluable.

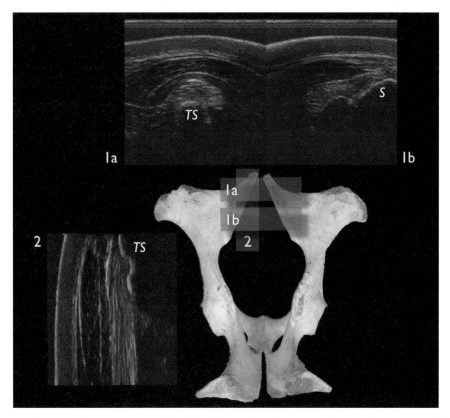

Figure 8.11   The normal appearance of the dorsal sacroiliac ligaments. S: sacral spine; TS: tuber sacrale.

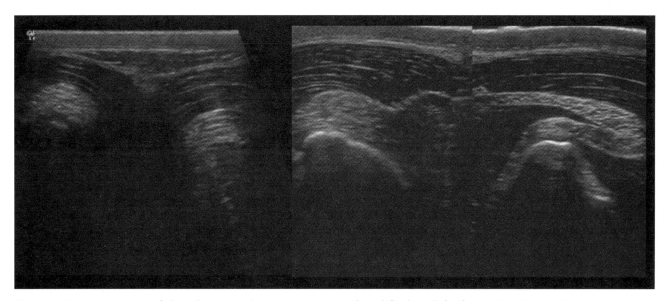

Figure 8.12   Asymmetry of the tubera sacrale is a common incidental finding (left of image) and normal variations in the appearance of the dorsal sacroiliac ligaments should not be interpreted as lesions (right of image).

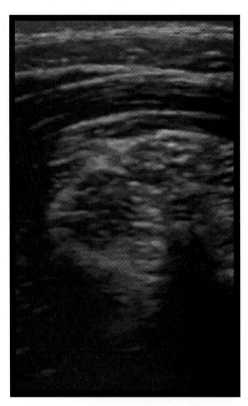

Figure 8.13 Central hypoechogenic regions within the dorsal sacroiliac ligaments should be interpreted with care, particularly when not accompanied by other signs such as an increase in cross-sectional area, as they are frequently artifactual.

In foals, the joint space also appears wider because of the increased thickness of articular cartilage. The normal discontinuity seen in foals should not be mistaken for a fracture, although it can be a site for injury (Figure 8.16). Again, comparison with the contralateral joint is useful.

Additional information can be obtained by rotating the probe through ninety degrees so that the transducer is perpendicular to the edge of the acetabulum (Figure 8.14 B and D). This approach allows further evaluation of the acetabulum, in particular, which should appear as a sharp, clearly delineated edge. The joint capsule can also be identified, permitting assessment of distension and the congruity of the joint. This is also the view that is used when performing ultrasound-guided injection of the hip joint [1].

It is fair to say that the assessment of the hip is limited because only a small portion of the joint can be imaged and pathology must be advanced or severe to be appreciated. However, it is probably also fair to say that, although hip joint injury is uncommon, it is frequently advanced when cases do present for investigation and ultrasonography can play a very useful role

as an adjunct to the clinical assessment, radiography, and scintigraphy.

Osteoarthritis (OA) will cause new bone production around the joint and roughening of the bone surfaces. This can be subtle, or more obvious if the inciting cause of OA were more dramatic (Figure 8.17). Through a dynamic assessment of the joint, by rocking the transducer back and forth, it may be possible to confirm flattening of the femoral head and incongruity of the normally narrow joint space. Be aware that the joint space will appear wider in a horse that is not weight-bearing properly, possibly leading to the false impression of subluxation.

In some cases of severe trauma, the normal alignment of the joint will be completely destroyed. Figure 8.18 shows images from a horse that suffered a complete fracture of the femoral neck. Although the primary injury could not be identified accurately, it was clear immediately that the normal joint architecture had been severely compromised.

PER RECTUM EVALUATION

Assessment of the internal surface of the pelvic bones is an important part of the examination, particularly in sudden onset severe lameness thought to be originating from the proximal limb. Palpation should be performed first, without ultrasound, but lack of abnormalities during palpation should not preclude scanning – fractures or callus can be missed with palpation alone and in some acute or subacute cases, hemorrhage can make direct manipulation of bone surfaces impossible. When palpated in acute injuries there may a feeling that there is swelling of the region, when compared to the other side. This often gives way to a sense that the bone is much more prominent, because muscle atrophy occurs, during the subacute and chronic stages.

Figure 8.19 highlights the common sites for injury that can be diagnosed during *per rectum* scanning. The normal medial acetabulum can be imaged with a linear rectal probe and seen as a smooth contour. Early in the injury this may become stepped or fragmented. Callus appears during the later stages (Figure 8.20). In some cases, the only findings are soft tissue swelling and hemorrhage and a definitive bone injury cannot be identified. This is still highly significant. In other cases, a step in the bone surface can be seen, but might only be appreciated with careful placement of the probe (Figure 8.21): a slow methodical approach is required. In cases with more longstanding pathology, callus may be evident as the injury repairs. In acute cases,

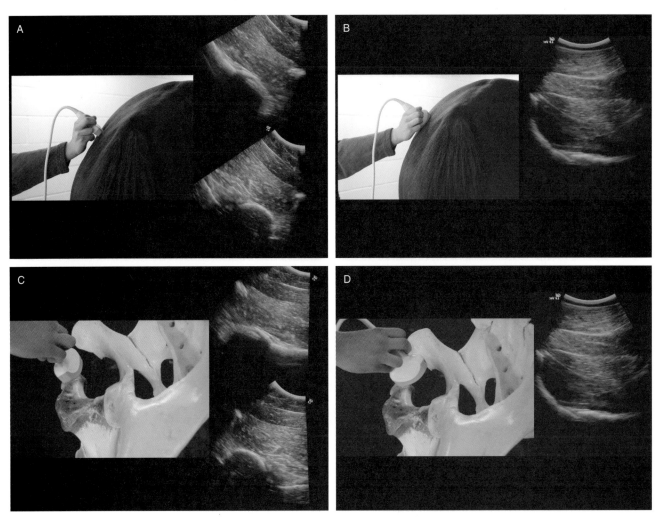

Figure 8.14   (A) The initial position of the transducer for imaging of the coxofemoral joint, having followed the line of the ilial shaft caudally. By tilting the probe, it is possible to image the acetabulum (top right) and the femoral head (bottom right). (B) The transducer is rotated to evaluate the edge of the acetabulum, the joint capsule and the femoral head. (C) The transducer and anatomical specimen illustrating the orientation of the transducer in (A). (D) The transducer and anatomical specimen illustrating the orientation of the transducer in (B).

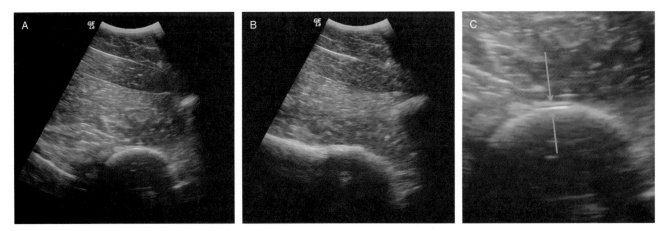

Figure 8.15   Hip joint: normal appearance of the femoral head (A) and acetabulum (B). Note that it is not possible to image both simultaneously – the transducer must be tilted back and forth to appreciate both structures separately. In some horses, the thickness of the articular cartilage on the femoral head can be assessed (C).

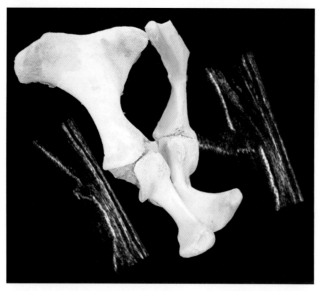

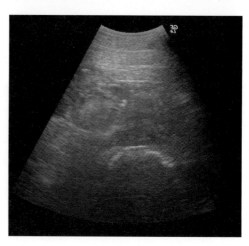

Figure 8.17 Ultrasonograph from a horse with chronic hip joint OA. The contour of the femoral head is irregular and roughened.

Figure 8.16 The physes forming the acetabulum close at around 1 year of age. Before then, disruption can occur through them. The image bottom left shows the normal appearance in a young foal while the image on the right shows a displaced fracture. A normal anatomical specimen is also seen, for reference.

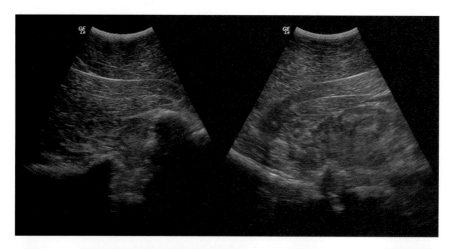

Figure 8.18 In these examples, from a horse that sustained a fracture of the femoral neck, the normal architecture of the joint has been severely disrupted. Note the abnormal proximity of the greater trochanter to the acetabulum (left image) and the hemorrhage into the periarticular tissues along with fragmentation seen around the hip joint (right image).

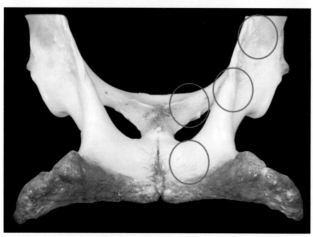

Figure 8.19 *Per rectum* palpation and ultrasonography can be very useful for detection of pelvic fractures. The sites circled on the right of the image are the areas injured most frequently, usually by trauma.

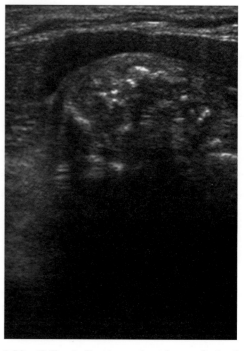

Figure 8.20 Callus indicating a chronic acetabular fracture.

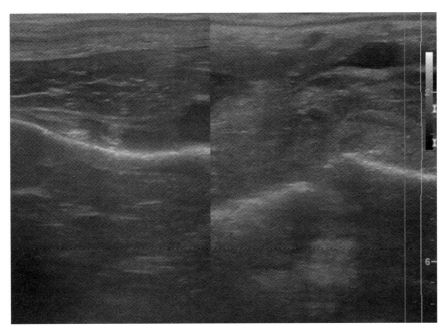

Figure 8.21 Ultrasonographs from a horse that had recently sustained a fracture of the pubis (*per rectum* examination; normal on the left, injured on the right). Note the discontinuity of the bone surface associated with soft tissue swelling and hemorrhage.

particularly ones in which hemorrhage could be seen but no primary bone injury, the ultrasound examination should be repeated 10–14 days later as the damage may become more evident with time.

THE LUMBOSACRAL AND SACROILIAC JOINTS

Much of the information we have on the imaging of these areas comes from the work of Jean-Marie Denoix and it is a region that we are still learning much about. Suffice to say, ultrasonography of this area must be interpreted with caution and with the knowledge that, although we can document several new disease processes, our view is restricted and the correlation with clinical syndromes is still, in some cases, vague.

Lumbosacral Joint

The lumbosacral joint consists of five articulations: the left and right intervertebral joints dorsally; left and right intertransverse joints (between the transverse processes of the last lumbar and first sacral vertebrae); and the intercentral joint with its large fibrocartilaginous disc. It is the intercentral joint that is usually being referred to when imaging of "the lumbosacral joint" is being discussed. The junction between the last lumbar vertebra and the sacrum contains a large fibro-

cartilaginous disc, which experiences significant movement during exercise. Almost all of the flexion/ extension of the caudal spine occurs at the lumbosacral junction and damage to the disc in this region can be associated with discomfort and performance-limiting problems. Although horses do not suffer from disc disease in the same way that humans and other species do, there is evidence that this disc can suffer degeneration and cause problems.

It is easily located by palpating the ventral spine *per rectum*: the joint is the prominent ventral midline bulge felt caudal to the terminal aorta and branching vessels when the fingers are run cranial to caudal along the underside of the caudal spine.

The lumbosacral joint can be imaged *per rectum* and is easily recognized, being larger than the adjacent intervertebral spaces (Figure 8.22). A linear rectal probe is placed midline and faced upwards, so that the ventral aspect of the joint is seen. The disc should not bulge out past the limits of the adjacent bone, the space should be even, and it should be possible to visualize the disc for its full depth, although sacralization may prevent this and does not necessarily indicate pathology. Ultrasonographically, it appears not dissimilar to the medial meniscus of the stifle (Figure 8.23). By examining further cranially, the next junction between L5/6 can be seen. Again, occasionally sacralization may occur so that the L6/S1 disc is reduced in size or absent, with the L5/6 disc often larger to compensate.

As well as being an important structure in its own right, the lumbosacral joint provides the main anatomic landmark to locate the other adjacent joints. In young horses, the irregularity caused by the presence of open physes in the vertebral bodies should not be confused with new bone formation.

Extreme pathology can be observed (Figure 8.24) and is likely to be significant if clinical evidence and the results of other techniques back this conclusion. Minor pathology in the form of uneven echogenicity or changes in shape of the disc require cautious interpretation.

Sacroiliac Joints

Only a very small part of the sacroiliac joint can be imaged *per rectum* and this is an important limitation of the technique. It is also unclear in many cases just how significant changes in this area are. The joint can

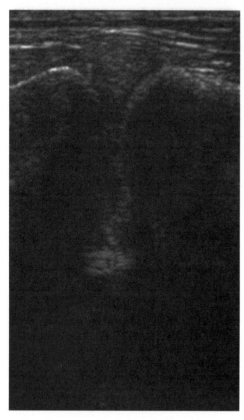

Figure 8.22 A normal lumbosacral junction obtained by scanning *per rectum*.

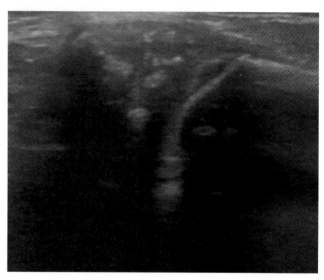

Figure 8.24 Image of a diseased lumbosacral junction disc showing severe disruption to the substance of the disc and the overlying ligament, and irregularity of the caudal aspect of L6.

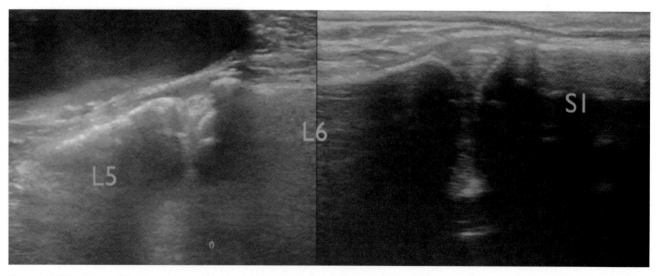

Figure 8.23 Composite *per rectum* ultrasonograph of the lumbosacral region. The transducer is imaging the ventral aspect of the caudal spine. The large intervertebral disc between L6 and S1 can be seen (lumbosacral junction) and the smaller disc between L5/6. The entire depth of the L6/S1 disc can be viewed down to the vertebral canal.

be visualized by starting from the lumbosacral joint, moving caudally one sacral vertebra's length and then swinging the transducer to the left, or right. In normal horses, a clear space can be identified (Figure 8.25). New bone production is seen in some horses. Widening of the sacroiliac joint is considered a normal variation, particularly in geldings.

INTERTRANSVERSE JOINTS

The horse is unusual in having normal articulations between the transverse processes of the last lumbar and first sacral vertebrae. They are easily identified by locating the intercentral joint and moving the probe a short distance to the left or right (Figure 8.26). The

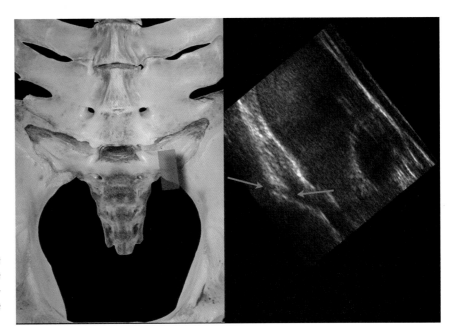

Figure 8.25 The caudal aspect of the sacroiliac joint imaged *per rectum*. The red area superimposed on the specimen demonstrates the position of the transducer to obtain this image.

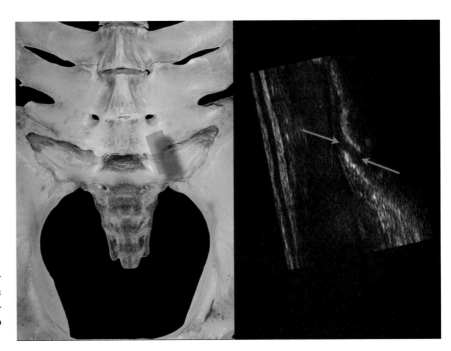

Figure 8.26 Imaging the normal intertransverse joint *per rectum*. The red area superimposed on the specimen demonstrates the position of the transducer to obtain this image.

normal intertransverse joints present a sharp, clearly demarcated joint space. Although disease of these joints can cause discomfort or reduced mobility, it is their proximity to the lumbosacral nerves that may be more important. New bone formation and soft tissue swelling may cause impingement of the lumbosacral nerves (especially that of L6) causing neuralgia and lower motor nerve signs (Figure 8.27). The author has seen several cases of what appeared to be equine "sciatica", responsive to anti-inflammatory medication of the region.

SACRUM

The ventral aspect of the sacrum can be assessed *per rectum*, simply by following the smooth bony surface caudally from the lumbosacral joint (Figure 8.28). Pathology needs to be extreme to be easily identified – complete fractures in racehorses may occur as the end stage of fatigue injuries or may be the result of trauma in all types of horses. In such cases, a step in the bone contour can be seen where the fracture displaces, often associated with significant hemorrhage (Figure 8.29).

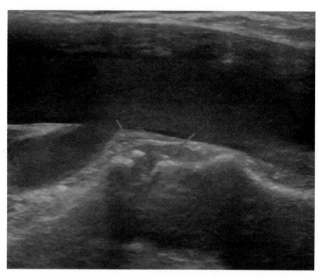

Figure 8.27 Irregular new bone formation (arrows) around the intertransverse joint. Abnormalities in this region can cause discomfort and neurologic signs if there is impingement on the L6 nerve.

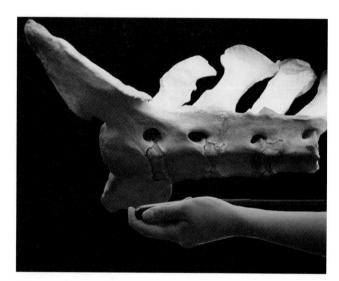

Figure 8.28 Position of the transducer to image the ventral sacrum *per rectum*. Note that this is a specimen from a young horse where fusion of the vertebral bodies is incomplete, however the ventral aspect presents a relatively flat surface.

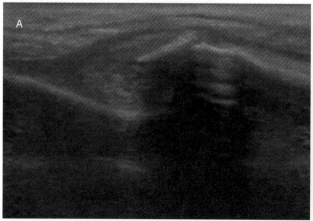

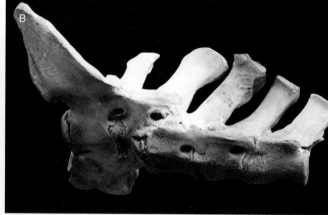

Figure 8.29 Ultrasonograph (A) and isolated sacrum (B) from a horse that had suffered a complete fracture through the caudal part of S2. In A note the displacement and comminution evident – this image was obtained soon after injury, before signs of repair such as new bone production became evident. In (B) the repair process is more advanced.

RECOMMENDED READING

Powell, S. (2011) Equine practice: investigation of pelvic problems in horses. *In Practice*, 33, 518–524.

Shepherd, M. & Pilsworth, R. (1994) The use of ultrasound in the diagnosis of pelvic fractures. *Equine Veterinary Education*, 6(4), 223–227.

REFERENCE

[1] David, F., Rougier, M., Alexander, K., & Morisset, S. (2007) Ultrasound-guided coxofemoral arthrocentesis in horses. *Equine Veterinary Journal*, 39, 79–83.

CHAPTER NINE

ULTRASONOGRAPHY OF THE NECK AND BACK

Marcus Head

Rossdales Equine Hospital and Diagnostic Centre, Newmarket, UK

Ultrasonographic assessment of the back and neck has added significantly to our ability to clinically evaluate these areas and provides imaging of the axial skeleton which complements radiography and scintigraphy. It also has the advantage that, in the axial skeleton, ultrasonography can be accomplished with most if not all ultrasound machines, compared to scintigraphy and the majority of axial skeleton radiography which can only be accomplished in a hospital setting. Although ultrasound examination of the back is limited to the epaxial structures, ultrasonographic assessment is useful in a wide variety of investigations, from trauma to poor performance.

INDICATIONS

Reasons for performing ultrasound assessment of the back and neck are varied but the commonest indication in non-Thoroughbred practice is evaluation of reduced performance due to suspected back or neck pain. These investigations can be time consuming and frustrating, but the use of ultrasonography enables a greater number of differential diagnoses to be considered. Lower motor nerve signs, such as muscle atrophy or abnormal "stringhalt-like" gaits, which may be caused by lumbosacral nerve compression, can also be evaluated. In Thoroughbred racehorses, indications also include evaluation of stress fractures known to occur in the back.

EQUIPMENT

Clipping is often necessary, although not in fine-coated horses – a 5 cm wide strip extending from the withers to behind the tubera sacrale should be prepared. It should be widened over the caudal thoracic and lumbar regions to allow imaging of the facet joints.

A high-frequency linear probe is the most useful for superficial structures but imaging the facet joints requires a lower-frequency curvilinear or sector probe. Imaging can be difficult in patients with significant subcutaneous fat or thick skin.

BACK

The main areas that can be imaged are:

- supraspinous (SSpL) and interspinous ligaments along with the dorsal aspects of the spinous processes;
- caudal thoracic and lumbar intervertebral (facet) joints;
- epaxial musculature.

Supraspinous and Interspinous Ligaments

The tough, fibrous SSpL connects the summits of the dorsal spinous processes (DSPs) and is easily visualized using a linear transducer. Its appearance is similar to that of other ligaments or tendons, with a striated fiber pattern evident when viewed longitudinally. The ligament lies in close apposition to the interspinous ligaments, whose fibers may run at a different angle, and this can cause off-incidence artifacts if care is not taken. The correct technique involves dynamic assessment of the ligament, tilting the probe forwards and backwards along its long axis to appreciate the slight

Atlas of Equine Ultrasonography, First Edition. Edited by Jessica A. Kidd, Kristina G. Lu, and Michele L. Frazer.
Companion Website: www.wiley.com/go/kidd/equine-ultrasonography

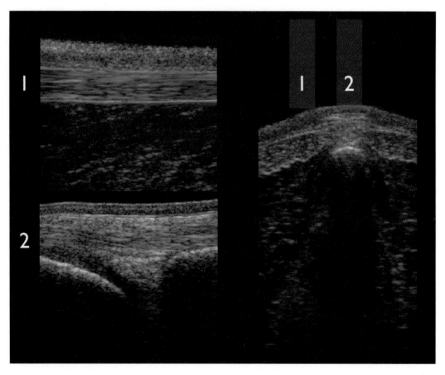

Figure 9.1 Care should be taken when imaging the supraspinous ligament that the transducer is midline (position 2). The aponeurosis of the longissimus muscles will appear as a striated, fibrous structure mimicking the ligament if the transducer is positioned to the left or right (position 1).

curve/angle change of the fibers as they insert onto the DSPs (a standoff pad is therefore very useful). In addition, care should be taken that it is the SSpL being imaged, as the strong aponeurosis of the longissimus muscle has a prominent tendon-like appearance just to the left and right of midline (Figure 9.1). Transverse images of the ligament can be obtained simply by rotating the probe and are useful to corroborate potential injury identified longitudinally.

The supraspinous ligament often appears hyperechogenic relative to the interspinous ligament and this can lead to errors in concluding that there is damage to the SSpL, when in fact it is normal interspinous ligament tissue. As well as this, the fibers of the SSpL alter their angle of orientation slightly as they insert upon the oblique dorsal surfaces of the DSPs. This can lead to misinterpretation due to off-incidence artifacts. The SSpL is larger and more fibrous as it progresses caudally – images in the lumbar region are generally more consistent between individuals but there is a wide variation in "normal" appearance. This may be due to operator factors, anatomic idiosyncrasy, or previous but currently insignificant injury.

Interpretation of potential lesions follows the same basic principles as with other ligaments or tendons,

with attention paid to size, echogenicity, and fiber pattern particularly (Figure 9.2). A certain degree of caution needs to be exercised when interpreting the appearance of the SSpL: it seems that a degree of dystrophic, possibly age-related change is evident in some horses and not necessarily indicative of disease. In addition, sites of injury rarely recover a normal appearance and regions of hypoechogenicity may not relate to current pathology. In almost all cases, evidence of injury will need to be confirmed with other techniques, such as diagnostic anesthesia.

It is easy enough to infiltrate local anesthetic around the "injury" and ascertain whether this alters the horse's movement/behavior, although there can be difficulties in reproducing that behavior consistently enough to allow this. Bear in mind that the ultrasonographic appearance of most SSpL injuries changes little with time and false positives can be a problem. This also makes follow-up of genuine lesions difficult. SSpL abnormalities are common in areas of significant impingement of the DSPs.

An assessment of the health of the DSPs is also possible during examination of the SSpL, in relation to their dorsal bony contour (well spaced or close, smooth or roughened, presence of osteophytes, etc.). However,

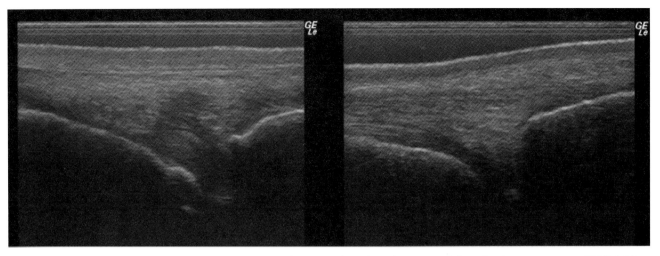

Figure 9.2 Longitudinal images of the supraspinous ligament (SSpL) and associated dorsal spinous processes (DSPs). Note the disruption to the longitudinal fiber pattern of the ligament, the close apposition of the DSPs, and the new bone production on the image to the left. Comparison with the adjacent interspinous region (to the right) can be helpful.

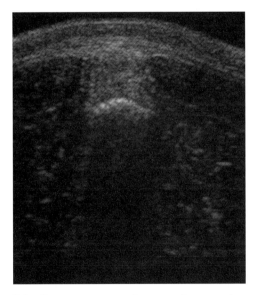

Figure 9.3 Transverse scan of a normal supraspinous ligament (SSpL) as an adjunct to longitudinal scans to ascertain the significance of changes seen on longitudinal images.

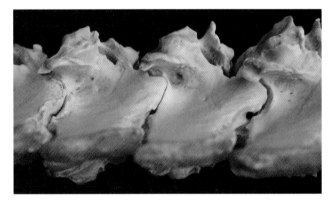

Figure 9.4 Post-mortem specimen of the caudal thoracic intervertebral articulations (IVAs) viewed dorsally – note their proximity to the dorsal spinous processes.

as only the very superficial part of these structures can be visualized, the technique is only supplementary to radiography and scintigraphy.

It is practical begin by performing a rapid, general appraisal of the ligament, running from cranial to caudal in the longitudinal plane. After this, move back to the cranial extent of the prepared area and scan longitudinally, identifying and recording areas of interest. If pathology is suspected, transverse scans (Figure 9.3) are used to try to ascertain the significance of changes. Suspicious areas should be marked, most

easily by a short clip in the coat, to allow subsequent diagnostic anesthesia.

The Caudal Thoracic and Lumbar Facet Joints

The anatomy of the thoracic and lumbar joints differs, making imaging of the more cranial thoracic joints more difficult due to their proximity to the dorsal spinous processes (Figure 9.4). Fortunately most pathology occurs in the last thoracic and cranial lumbar joints, which are easily imaged in horses without excessive subcutaneous fat or thick skin. The technique is compromised severely in patients with these last factors and in some horses it is impossible to obtain diagnostic images.

The technique aims to identify the articulation of the cranial articular process of one vertebra as it interdigitates with the caudal (and medial) process of the vertebra ahead of it (Figures 9.5, 9.6). The first image to acquire is with the probe (a lower-frequency curvilin-

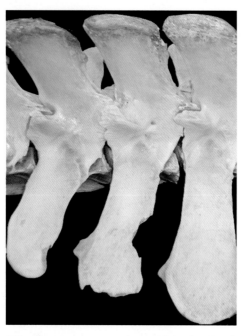

Figure 9.5 Post-mortem specimen of the lumbar intervertebral articulations (IVAs) viewed dorsolaterally. Note they are more easily discernible than the thoracic IVAs.

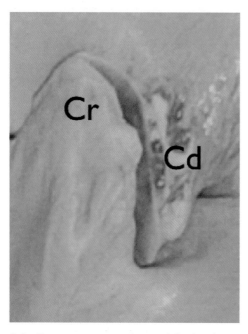

Figure 9.6 Post-mortem specimen of the lumbar intervertebral articulations (IVAs) with their finger-like cranial (Cr) and caudal (Cd) projections interlocking.

ear, ideally) at right angles to and just to the side of midline (Figure 9.7). By counting the ribs and following them up the operator can get an idea of the vertebrae being imaged. Moving the probe backwards (and, therefore, with the haircoat) the joints will appear and disappear from the field of view as the transducer heads caudally. Normal joints appear as the corner of a box, close to the junction of dorsal and transverse processes. In thin-skinned horses and with high-quality equipment, it is common to be able to identify the individual cranial and caudal processes of each joint as well as the joint space. Disease of the intervertebral articulations (IVAs) results, regardless of the inciting cause being a stress fracture or osteoarthritis, in enlargement of the joint and the loss of this definition, with new bone production, which may progress to joint ankylosis (Figure 9.8). The ultrasound appearance is as if someone has stuck a ball onto the corner of the box, which takes on a rounded shape. It is important to compare adjacent joints on the same side of the horse to establish the validity of changes and also to compare the left and right sides.

Longitudinal images, obtained by placing the transducer parallel to and just to the side of midline, can enable adjacent joints to be imaged in the same field of view (Figure 9.9). It should be remembered that it is not uncommon for pathology to affect more than one joint, either on the same side or opposite sides of the horse, although it is very rare for this pathology to be symmetric, so even horses affected in several locations will have noticeable discrepancies in joint size and shape. Note also that low-grade disease affecting several joints is common in racehorses and an abnormal ultrasound appearance does not necessarily indicate that the joint is a current concern – scintigraphy should be considered to evaluate the significance of lesions further. Ultrasound-guided injection of affected joints can be useful. Once the affected joints have been identified a curvilinear transducer is placed at right angles to the midline and the joint localized. Two techniques are available but with similar results – the aim is to guide the 3.5-inch 18-gauge spinal needle through the epaxial musculature and deposit the medication into, or close to, the joint. Whether the probe is positioned close to midline and the needle is directed from lateral or *vice versa*, the aim is to inject into multifidus close to the joint. A skin bleb of local anesthetic reduces the discomfort to the patient. The author would typically use 5 mg of triamcinolone acetonide diluted in 1.5 ml of sterile saline, per joint. In many cases, there is evidence of disease at multiple sites and even if only one joint seems to be affected, consideration should be given to treating the contralateral or neighboring

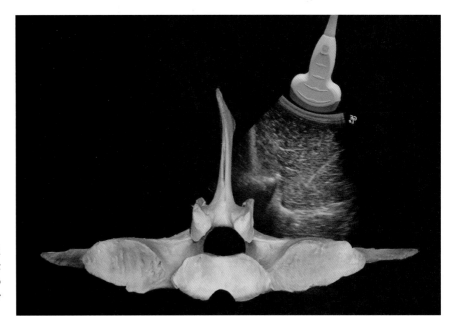

Figure 9.7 A frontal plane ultrasound image superimposed on an anatomic specimen showing the technique to image the caudal thoracic and lumbar IVAs.

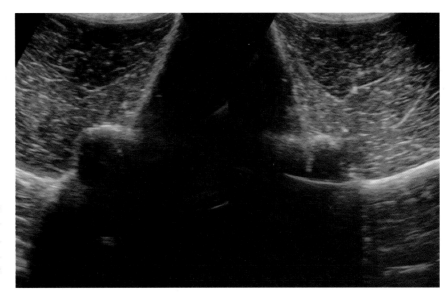

Figure 9.8 Osteoarthritis (OA) can be identified as enlargement and rounding of the IVA. The diseased joint is on the left of this image and is compared to the normal contralateral joint on the right.

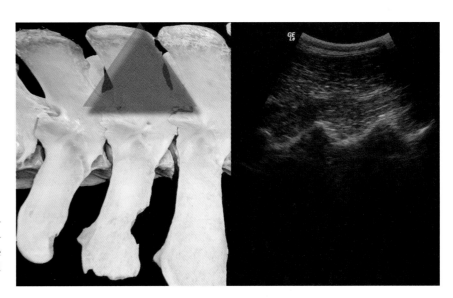

Figure 9.9 A sagittal plane ultrasound image superimposed on an anatomic specimen showing the technique to image the caudal thoracic and lumbar IVAs.

joints, as it is likely that these will have been under abnormal loading. The author prefers to place the needle very close to midline and direct it vertically downwards, being guided by the ultrasound transducer positioned a little further towards him. The joints are very close to the base of the dorsal spinous processes and it sometimes surprises people how close to the midline the needle needs to be. If the site of insertion is correct, the needle should advance onto or into the joint, ideally inside the fascia of multifidus. The transducer will need to be tilted towards the operator to allow room for the needle to be maneuvered and for the needle to be visualized.

The Epaxial Musculature

Views of the epaxial musculature of the thoracic and lumbar regions are easy to obtain at the same time as those of the SSpL. The longissimus and multifidus are particularly satisfying to image and, although clinical disease is rare, they are important during ultrasound-guided injection of the facet joints. Muscle atrophy can be appreciated and documented. Atrophy due to denervation injury is rare but an important differential diagnosis when cases present with muscle asymmetry. The characteristic marked increase in echogenicity throughout the affected muscle due to retention of connective tissue over muscle fibers, along with being able to rule out structural damage to the associated bony structures, may encourage an earlier return to exercise and the use of physiotherapy when prolonged rest is contraindicated.

Neck

Soft Tissues

The ligamentum nuchae can be imaged at its attachment on the occipital bone, most readily in the longitudinal plane, and appears as other ligamentous structures, with a strong fiber pattern, which stands out from the less echogenic muscle tissue surrounding it. Mineralization of the ligament close to its cranial attachment (Figure 9.10) is a reasonably common finding and of uncertain significance in most horses.

In some cases, trauma to the occipital region can result in new bone formation and damage to the tendon of insertion of the semispinalis capitis (Figure 9.11). While undoubtedly painful and restricting in the acute and subacute phases, the cases seen in the author's clinic have returned to full function in the

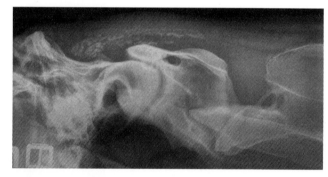

Figure 9.10 Lateral radiograph of the cranial cervical region showing dystrophic mineralization within the soft tissues.

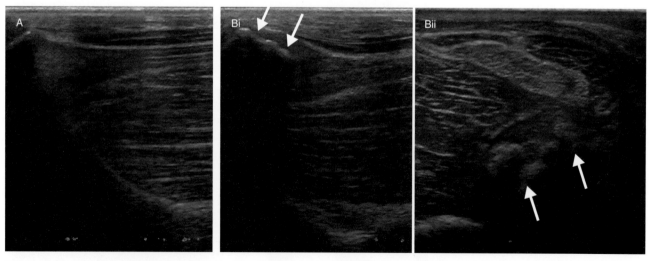

Figure 9.11 (A) Longitudinal image of the soft tissue attachments onto the squamous part of the occipital crest – normal side (rostral to the left). Note the smooth, concave bone surface and the longitudinal fibers of the semispinalis capitis tendon. (B) Abnormal side in longitudinal (Bi) and transverse (Bii) planes. Note irregular new bone formation in the attachment of the semispinalis capitis tendon (arrows).

long term. In chronic cases, it can be useful to try to desensitize the region using local anesthetic in order to assess the significance of changes (Figure 9.12).

The muscles of the neck are a common site for post-injection abscesses (Figure 9.13). Muscle soreness may precede ultrasonographic abnormalities, but if an abscess forms it produces the typical ultrasound appearance with a relatively uniform fluid-filled structure surrounded by a usually clearly defined boundary or capsule within the muscle tissue. The echogenicity of the abscess will be similar in whichever plane the transducer is positioned, unlike the muscle around it, helping to delineate its borders; it is usually somewhere between fluid and soft tissue in its appearance (Figure 9.14). The ultrasonographic appearance of a longstanding abscess is shown in Figure 9.15.

In some cases, swelling and infection may result from foreign body penetration. Ultrasonography can be invaluable in assessing the presence and nature of such objects (Figure 9.16).

Bones and Joints

The atlanto-occiptal (AO) joint is an occasional site of synovial sepsis secondary to osteomyelitis (most commonly, in the UK, caused by *Rhodococcus equi* infection – Figure 9.17). The left and right joints have separate joint capsules, but are said to communicate occasionally, particularly in older horses. Longitudinal and

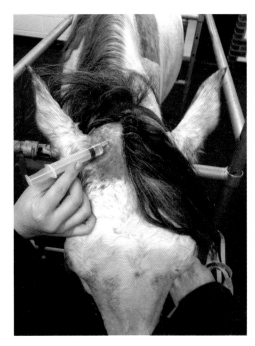

Figure 9.12 Local anesthetic is injected around an area of soft tissue damage so that the significance of the ultrasonographic changes could be assessed – this horse displayed consistent signs of head shaking which were not alleviated by this procedure.

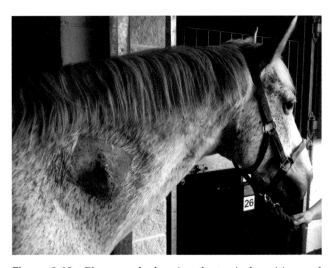

Figure 9.13 Photograph showing the typical position and appearance of a post-injection neck abscess.

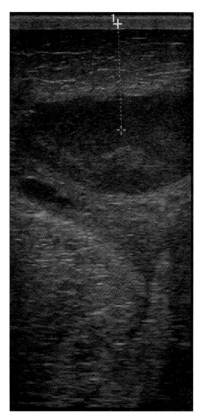

Figure 9.14 Typical ultrasonographic appearance of such an abscess – the calipers are used to aid the surgical approach for drainage (Source: Image courtesy of Rob Pilsworth MRCVS).

transverse images of the joint can be obtained by placing the transducer to each side of midline (Figure 9.18).

The easiest landmark to identify on the scans beginning in the longitudinal plane is the smooth convex surface of the occipital bone with its thin layer of hypoechogenic cartilage. The joint space can be identified beneath a thin joint capsule that bridges the space to the atlas (Figures 9.19, 9.20). In cases with synovial sepsis, the joint will be distended and the normally

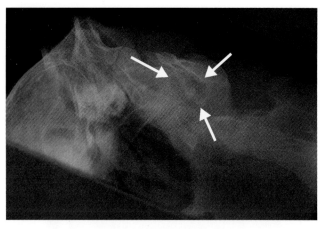

Figure 9.17 Lateral radiograph of the cranial cervical region of a Thoroughbred foal with bone lysis caused by osteomyelitis affecting the first cervical vertebra (arrows).

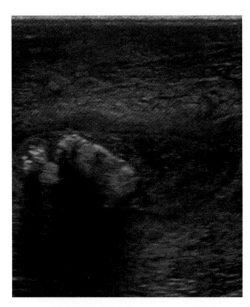

Figure 9.15 Ultrasonograph of a longstanding neck abscess. There is dystrophic mineralization of the soft tissues, which casts an acoustic shadow. More aggressive debridement was necessary in this case because of the extensive fibrosis and mineralized tissue.

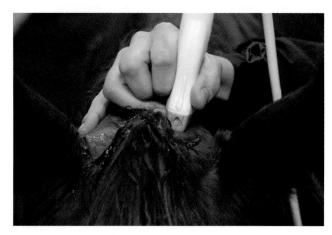

Figure 9.18 Photograph demonstrating the position of the transducer to obtain a longitudinal image of the atlanto-occipital (AO) joint.

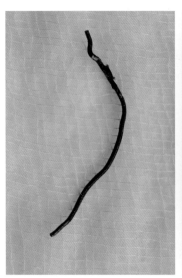
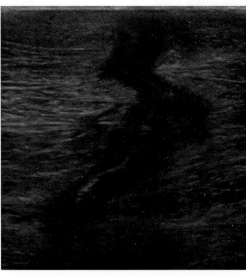

Figure 9.16 A wire embedded in the neck muscle caused a chronic, intermittently draining wound in this horse. The small skin lesion belied the size of the object buried within.

anechogenic fluid will often contain echogenic material, typical of an infected joint, or thickening of the joint capsule (Figure 9.21).

In two cases seen by the author, the infection was resolved with systemic antimicrobials and repeated to and fro lavage of the joint under sedation using ultrasound guidance, followed by injection of antimicrobials into the joint space.

Assessment of the AO region can also be used to facilitate cerebrospinal fluid (CSF) collection and, in neonates, it has been used to estimate CSF pressure in dysmature or premature foals (Figure 9.22).

Ultrasonography is now used commonly for the assessment of the caudal cervical IVAs and, in particular, to facilitate ultrasound-guided injection of the C5/6 and C6/7 joints. Occasionally, trauma will result in fractures involving the joints, the secondary effects of which can be assessed (Figure 9.23). Caudal cervical osteoarthritis (OA) has been described as a cause of forelimb lameness and is recognized increasingly as a factor in poor performance cases. Although radiography is still the standard imaging modality for assessment of these joints, ultrasonography can assist radiological interpretation and is invaluable for treating this region. Either linear or micro-convex transducers can be used, although the smaller footprint of the latter makes ultrasound-guided injection easier (Figures 9.24, 9.25).

For ultrasound-guided injection, the horse should be sedated reasonably heavily and made to stand squarely, preferably in stocks. It can be very useful to use a head rest, so that the head and neck remain in the same position throughout the procedure. Two techniques are described, varying in their ultrasonographic approach to the joints. In one, the transducer is positioned along the long axis of the neck (see Reef *et al.* 2004), but the author prefers to image perpendicular to this.

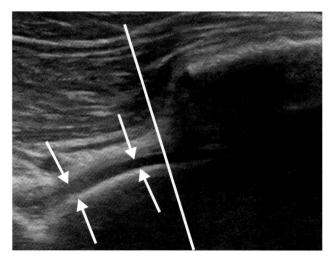

Figure 9.19 Longitudinal image of a normal AO joint. The cartilage overlying the occipital condyles can be seen as a thick anechogenic line (arrows). The cranial aspect of the atlas is the linear echogenic surface to the top right. Rostral is to the left.

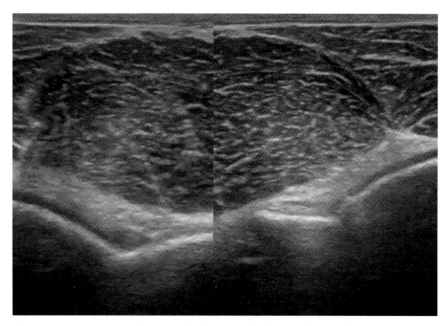

Figure 9.20 Composite transverse image of a normal AO joint – the bar on Figure 9.19 indicates the position of this image on the longitudinal scan.

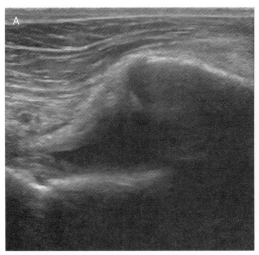
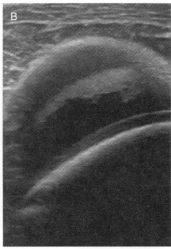

Figure 9.21 Ultrasonographs of the AO joint of the foal shown in Figure 9.17. (A) Longitudinal image. There is distension of the joint and thickening of the synovial lining and joint capsule. The cartilage cannot be seen clearly in this image – this is due to off-incidence artifact and not cartilage loss (compare with B). (B) Transverse image, once more showing joint distension and synovial hypertrophy. The cartilage is clearly delineated to the right of the picture, but less clear to the left side. Again, this is an artifact and not due to cartilage disease.

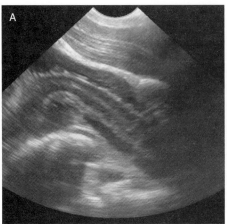
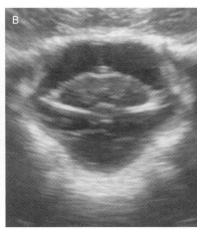

Figure 9.22 Longitudinal (A) and transverse (B) images of the AO region in a neonatal foal illustrating the normal position of the spinal cord within the vertebral canal.

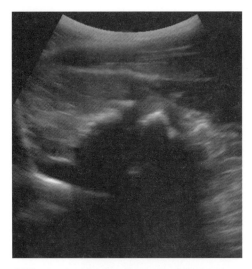

Figure 9.23 In this image, the normal architecture of the intervertebral articulation (IVA) has been severely disrupted due to prolific new bone formation secondary to a fracture of the articular process.

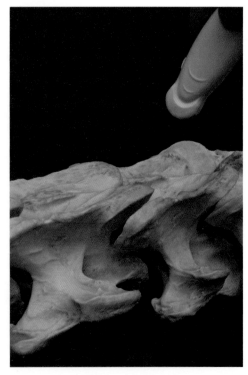

Figure 9.24 Photograph demonstrating the position of a micro-convex transducer to obtain an image of the C5/6 caudal cervical intervertebral articulation.

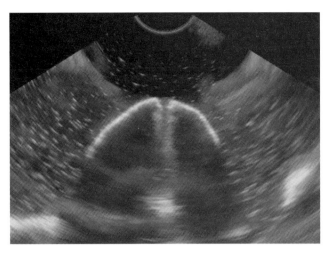

Figure 9.25 This image was acquired with a micro-convex transducer scanning a specimen in a water bath. Note the regular, clearly demarcated edges of the articular processes forming the borders of an easily recognisable joint space.

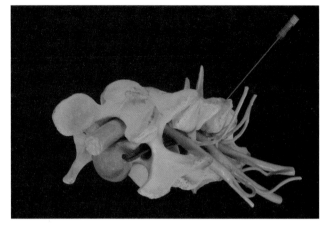

Figure 9.26 Photograph showing the correct orientation for placement of a spinal needle into the left C6/7 IVA. Note the steep angle of approach that follows the angle of the joint, maximising the chances of successful centesis.

The joints to be treated are imaged before clipping the hair, using liberal application of surgical spirit. The C5/6, C6/7, and C7/T1 joints appear similar and are most easily assessed with a micro-convex transducer, although it is possible to proceed with a high-frequency linear probe. In most horses, the musculature of the scapula/shoulder prevents imaging further back than C6/7 but in some patients the C7/T1 articulation can be seen. This should be borne in mind; it is often assumed that the most caudal joint imaged is always C6/7 but this may not be the case. If in doubt, a marker placed on the skin during radiographic assessment can be useful. The transverse processes of the caudal cervical vertebrae are palpated and the transducer placed above these, just in front of the shoulder musculature, oriented vertically to produce a transverse image of the joints. Once the joints have been identified, the hair can be clipped so that the site of injection and contact area for the transducer can be prepared. Once clipped and after a short scrub, a small bleb of local anesthetic is placed at the site of needle placement. The site for insertion of the needle is above (dorsal to) the contact point for the transducer and is estimated by imagining the course of the needle into the joint. However, the main rule is to start high as the angle of the needle direction should be steep to facilitate entry into the joint space which is angled sharply from laterodorsal to medioventral (Figure 9.26).

After placing the bleb, the site is prepared thoroughly. Usually, as it is most common to inject C5/6 and C6/7 on both sides of the neck, both joints on the left side can be prepared first so that they can be

scrubbed together and then injected in one sterile procedure; one can then proceed to the right side.

The author injects 5 mg of triamcinolone acetonide into each joint, drawn up into 1.5 ml sterile saline. Some clinicians prefer to use methylprednisolone but withdrawal times must be taken into consideration in competition horses. A separate 18-gauge 3.5-inch spinal needle is used for each joint. The transducer is covered with a large sterile glove or a sterile probe sleeve, which is held open by the operator while a colleague fills the bottom with sterile ultrasound couplant gel, before the transducer is dropped into the glove or sleeve. A micro-convex probe easily fits down one of the fingers of the glove. Sterile couplant gel is applied to the gloved end of the probe and the joint to be injected is visualized; surgical spirit between the skin and probe can also be used. For right-handed clinicians, the probe can be held in the left hand and the needle placed with the right; for the left side it is easier to face towards the rear of the horse (and towards the front of the horse for the right-side joints). The transducer is positioned so that the joint space is seen at the side of the image, allowing more space to visualize the needle approaching the joint. The needle is pushed through the skin bleb and advanced towards the joint. As mentioned previously, the angle of approach should be steep, mimicking the angle of the joint, to maximize the chance of successful entry (Figure 9.27).

The most important thing to remember during any ultrasound-guided technique is to be *guided by the ultrasound*. Take time to ensure that the needle follows the path of the ultrasound beam – failures are often attributable to the path of the needle diverging from

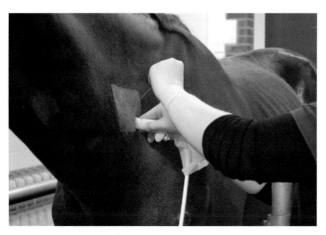

Figure 9.27 Photograph showing correct starting positions for the spinal needle and transducer prior to ultrasound-guided injection of the left C6/7 IVA.

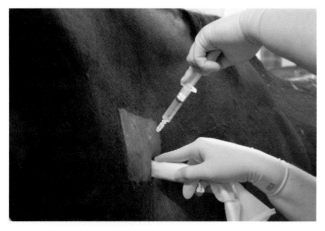

Figure 9.28 Photograph showing ultrasound-guided placement of a spinal needle into the left C6/7 IVA and successful aspiration of joint fluid, prior to medication.

the ultrasound. In some cases, the needle advances easily through the joint capsule and a distinct change in resistance indicates successful centesis. In other cases, the needle encounters bone. If the ultrasound image indicates that the tip of the needle is close to the joint, it is usually possible to "walk" the needle into the joint. Once into the joint space, avoid advancing the needle too far as it is, in theory, possible to enter the vertebral canal. Removal of the stilette occasionally prompts spontaneous flow of synovial fluid but more commonly aspiration with a syringe is necessary to confirm correct placement (Figure 9.28). Synovial fluid should be aspirated in all cases but, as with other joints, there are occasions when the needle is correctly placed but fluid cannot be obtained. Repeated placements of the needle (without coming back out through

the skin – if this is necessary a new needle should be used) should be kept to a minimum, and if the clinician is confident about the position, the joint can be injected without obtaining fluid. Of course, it gets easier with practice. The transducer can be removed while the injection is performed, to allow the hub of the needle to be held with one hand and the syringe with the other during the injection. If the injection is visualized with ultrasound, injection of fluid creates a stream of bubbles which appear as moving hyperechogenic areas. The procedure is repeated for the next joint on the same side, before moving equipment to the other side of the horse and starting again.

The horse is treated with a single dose of intravenous non-steroidal anti-inflammatory (usually phenylbutazone or firocoxib). The author usually advises 3 weeks of restricted turnout following treatment before any further exercise or physiotherapy. In many cases it is useful to suggest that the horse is fed from a height for this 3-week period – attaching hay nets to the fencing or similar. This is based on the observation that most affected horses display difficulty/discomfort when reaching to the floor; several cases displayed acute episodes of either severe pain or neurologic signs after grazing. It seems logical therefore to limit this (admittedly very normal activity!) for a short time after treatment.

Recommended Reading

Berg, L.C., Nielsen, J.V., Thoefner, M.B., *et al.* (2003) Ultrasonography of the equine cervical region: a descriptive study in eight horses. *Equine Veterinary Journal*, 35(7), 647–655.

Bucca, S., Fogarty, U., & Farelly, B.T. (2008) Ultrasound examination of the atlanto-occipital space. In: *Color Atlas of Diseases and Disorders of the Foal* (eds S.B. McAuliffe & N.M. Slovis). Saunders Elsevier, Philadelphia.

Cousty, M., Firidolfi, C., Geffroy O., & David, F. (2011) Comparison of medial and lateral ultrasound-guided approaches for periarticular injection of the thoracolumbar intervertebral facet joints in horses. *Veterinary Surgery*, 40(4), 494–499.

Denoix, J.M. (1999) Spinal biomechanics and functional anatomy. *Veterinary Clinics of North America: Equine Practice*, 15(1), 27–60.

Fuglbjerg, V., Nielsen, J.V., Thomsen, P.D., & Berg, L.C. (2010) Accuracy of ultrasound-guided injections of thoracolumbar articular process joints in horses: a cadaveric study. *Equine Veterinary Journal*, 42(1), 18–22.

Girodoux, M., Dyson, S., & Murray, R. (2009) Osteoarthritis of the thoracolumbar synovial intervertebral articulations: clinical and radiographic features in 77 horses with poor performance and back pain. *Equine Veterinary Journal*, 41, 130–138.

Nielsen, J.V., Berg, L.C., Thoefner, M.B., *et al.* (2003) Accuracy of ultrasound-guided intra-articular injection of cervical facet joints in horses: a cadaveric study. *Equine Veterinary Journal*, 35, 657–661.

Reef, V.B., Whittier, M., & Allam, L.G. (2004) Joint ultra-sonography. *Clinical Techniques in Equine Practice*, 3, 256–267.

Ricardi, G. & Dyson, S. (1993) Forelimb lameness associated with radiographic abnormalities of the cervical vertebrae. *Equine Veterinary Journal*, 25, 422–426.

Sgorbini, M., Marmorini, P., Rota, A., *et al.* (2011) Ultrasound measurements of the dorsal subarachnoid space depth in healthy trotter foals during the first week of life. *Journal of Equine Veterinary Science*, 31, 41–43.

Sisson, S. & Grossman, J.D. (1948) *The Anatomy of the Domestic Animals*. W.B. Saunders, Philadelphia.

CHAPTER TEN

ULTRASONOGRAPHY OF THE HEAD

Debra Archer
University of Liverpool, Wirral, UK

INTRODUCTION

Ultrasonographic assessment of the head has most frequently been utilized to image the ocular and peri-ocular structures (see Chapter 25). Imaging modalities such as radiography, endoscopy, and, increasingly, computed tomography are more commonly utilized to image other structures of the head. This is largely due to the fact that a number of anatomic areas of interest, such as the nasal passages, paranasal sinuses, and cranium, are encased within bone, precluding ultrasonographic assessment of these structures. In addition, soft tissue structures, such as the guttural pouch, are air filled in the normal horse, which limits ultrasonographic assessment of them. Bony structures such as the rami of the mandible may impede access when attempting to image soft tissue structures located in the caudal and more ventral regions of the head. However, ultrasonography has been shown to be a useful imaging modality in assessment of the temporomandibular joint and as an adjunctive technique for assessing the larynx and adjacent structures. Superficially located and other accessible soft tissue structures, such as salivary glands, masseter muscle, and tongue, can also be assessed ultrasonographically, as can the surface of the thin bones of the skull. Therefore, whilst its applications may be relatively limited in imaging of the non-ocular structures of the head, ultrasonography can provide valuable adjunctive information when assessing a variety of structures.

Sedation may not be required in all horses but may improve image acquisition, particularly where the larynx is being assessed, to avoid movement artifact and improve patient compliance.

TEMPOROMANDIBULAR JOINT

Normal Anatomy and Scanning Technique

Scanning the temporomandibular joint requires a 7.5–10 MHz linear or convex transducer and a standoff may be required in thin horses with little periarticular fat. The standard views are caudolateral, lateral, and rostrolateral. Structures that can be visualized include all or part of the temporal bone, including the retro-articular process (on the caudolateral view), the mandibular fossa (on the lateral view), and the articular tubercle (on the rostrolateral view). Additionally, the condylar process of the mandible and the articular disc, cartilage, and fluid, as well as the joint capsule can be seen, along with the parotid salivary gland, parotidoauricularis muscle, and the transverse facial vein (on the rostrolateral view).

For the caudolateral view, place the transducer (with or without a standoff) over the dorsal aspect of the vertical ramus of the mandible centered over the temporomandibular joint (TMJ) in a transverse position (Figure 10.1). The long axis of the transducer should be positioned in a rostroventral to dorsocaudal direction so that it is oriented parallel to the frontal and nasal bones. The condylar process of the mandible and retro-articular process of the temporal bone can be visualized as thin hyperechoic lines (Figure 10.2). Sandwiched between these two bones is the fibrocartilaginous intra-articular disc, which has a homogeneous, moderate echogenicity, similar to that of the menisci in the stifle joint (i.e. midway between muscle and fascial echogenicity). The base of this triangular-shaped structure is abaxial and approximately 2 cm wide in the adult horse; the disc

Atlas of Equine Ultrasonography, First Edition. Edited by Jessica A. Kidd, Kristina G. Lu, and Michele L. Frazer.
© 2014 John Wiley & Sons, Ltd. Published 2014 by John Wiley & Sons, Ltd.
Companion Website: www.wiley.com/go/kidd/equine-ultrasonography

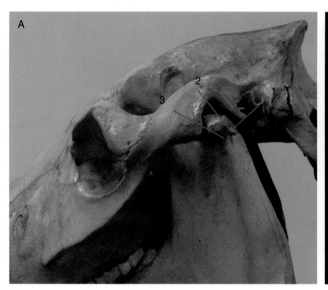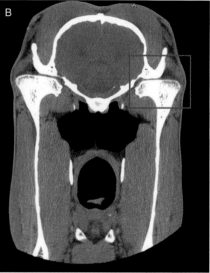

Figure 10.1 (A) Image of a cadaver skull of a horse demonstrating the position of the transducer over the temporomandibular joint in order to obtain caudolateral (1), lateral (2), and craniolateral (3) images. (B) Computed tomography cross-sectional image of a horse's head. The red box denotes the temporomandibular joint region; ultrasonographic assessment is limited to the lateral (abaxial) portions of the joint.

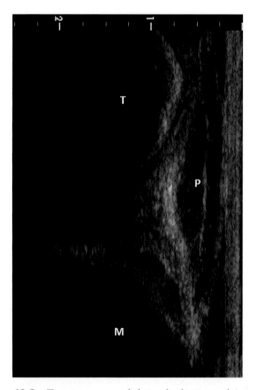

Figure 10.2 Transverse caudolateral ultrasound image of the temporomandibular joint in a normal adult horse obtained using a linear transducer operating at 10 MHz. The retroarticular process of the temporal bone (T), mandibular condyle (M), and overlying parotid salivary gland (P) can be visualized. The intra-articular disc is triangular in shape and is sandwiched between these structures.

then narrows axially. The disc also narrows towards the rostral aspect of the joint. Articular cartilage can be visualized as a hypoechoic layer between the bone and the intra-articular disc; this may be up to 3 mm thick in foals and is often barely visible in adult horses. It is uncommon to visualize any articular fluid. The parotid salivary gland lies superficial to these structures and the more hyperechoic TMJ capsule fibers can be seen to merge with this structure. The parotidoauricularis muscle can also be imaged on this view.

For the lateral view, rotate the dorsal aspect of the probe by 90° (Figure 10.1). The same structures can be visualized, with the mandibular fossa of the temporal bone now being visualized dorsally and the intra-articular disc again having a triangular shape (Figure 10.3). The parotidoauricularis muscle can sometimes be imaged on this view.

For the rostrolateral view, the whole probe should be moved rostrally by 1–2 cm and the dorsal tip rotated a further 30° in a rostral direction (Figure 10.1). The articular tubercle of the temporal bone is visible dorsally and the mandibular condyle ventrally. The intra-articular disc now appears as a thin wedge sandwiched between these two structures, and there is little in the way of soft tissue structures overlying this aspect of the joint (Figure 10.4). The transverse facial vein can often be visualized ventrally on this view.

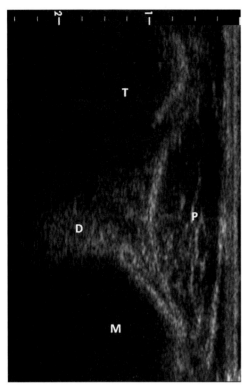

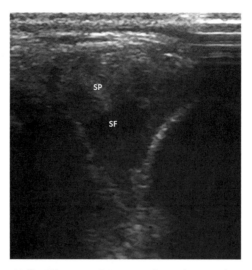

Figure 10.5 Ultrasound image of an abnormal temporomandibular joint with dorsal to the right and ventral to the left of the image. There is increased synovial fluid (SF) within the joint and evidence of synovial membrane proliferation (SP). (Source: Image courtesy of Katie Garrett.)

Figure 10.3 Transverse lateral ultrasound image of the temporomandibular joint in a normal adult horse. The superficial bone and thin layer of cartilage of the mandibular fossa of the temporal bone (T) and mandibular condyle (M) can be visualized together with the triangular-shaped intra-articular disc (D) and the more superficially positioned parotid salivary gland (P).

Ultrasonographic Abnormalities

Any disruption to the normal, smooth periarticular outline of the mandibular condyle or temporal bone or disruption to the substance of the intra-articular disc, for example tears or focal hypoechogenicity, is considered to be highly indicative of pathology within the TMJ (Figure 10.5).

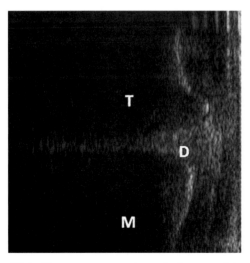

Figure 10.4 Transverse rostrolateral ultrasound image of the temporomandibular joint in a normal adult horse. The intra-articular disc (D) is more flattened in appearance and is positioned between the articular tubercle of the temporal bone (T) and the mandibular condyle (M).

LARYNX

Normal Anatomy and Scanning Technique

Ultrasonography of the larynx requires an 8.5–12.5 MHz linear array or convex transducer. The standard views are rostroventral, midventral, caudoventral, and caudolateral. Structures that can be visualized include parts of the basihyoid bone including the lingual process, portions of the ceratohyoid and thyrohyoid bones, the base of the tongue, the insertion of the thyrohyoid muscles, the ventral and abaxial aspects of the thyroid and cricoid cartilages, portions of the cricoarytenoideus lateralis, cricoarytenoideus dorsalis, and vocalis muscles, the vocal cords, and the abaxial aspects of the arytenoid cartilages.

To image the larynx, the horse's head should be held in a slightly extended position and the transducer initially positioned over the ventral aspect of the larynx. For the rostroventral view, the transducer should be placed in a transverse position immediately rostral to the base of the basihyoid bone between the rami of the mandible (Figure 10.6). The lingual process of the basihyoid bone can be identified (Figure 10.7). In some horses, narrow width of the intermandibular space may prevent this view from

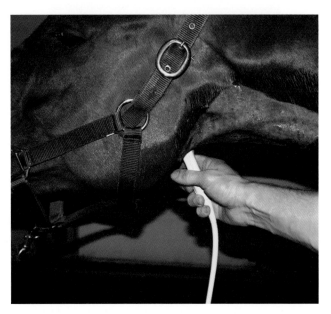

Figure 10.6   Positioning of the transducer in order to obtain the ventral transverse view of the larynx. This is facilitated by positioning the patient's head in a slightly extended position in order to position the larynx more caudally in relation to the mandible.

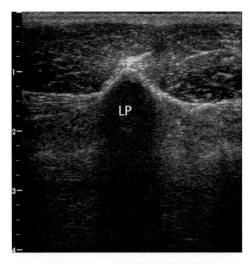

Figure 10.7   Transverse ventral ultrasound image obtained at the rostroventral window (just rostral to the base of the basihyoid bone) of the larynx in a normal adult horse using a linear transducer operating at 10 MHz. The surface of the lingual process of the basihyoid bone (LP) is identified as a semicircular hyperechoic line.

being obtained if a linear transducer is used. The lingual process can be followed caudally to the body of the basihyoid bone and, by rotating the transducer in a more rostral orientation, the ceratohyoid bones may be visualized as two, flat hyperechoic structures that course in a dorsal direction (Figure 10.8). The base of the tongue can be visualized but may require use of a lower-frequency transducer (2–5 MHz) to assess its full depth. The same structures can be visualized on the ventral midline (median) and just off the midline (paramedian) in a longitudinal view.

To obtain the midventral view, keep the transducer oriented longitudinally on the ventral midline, and by moving caudally the transducer should be positioned over the space between the basihyoid bone and thyroid cartilage. The caudal part of the basihyoid bone and rostral tip of the thyroid cartilage can be visualized at this location (Figure 10.9). Moving the transducer off midline (paramedian) allows the insertion of the thyrohyoid muscles onto the abaxial aspect of the thyroid cartilage to be visualized (Figure 10.10), and the thyrohyoid bones can be seen to course in a dorsocaudal direction.

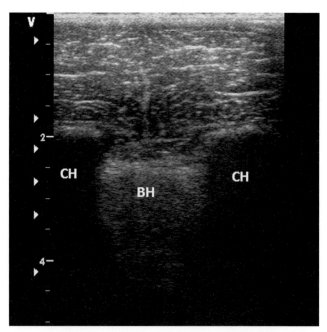

Figure   10.8   Transverse   ventral   ultrasound   image obtained at the rostroventral window of the larynx in a normal adult horse with the transducer angled more rostrally. The base of the basihyoid bone (BH) appears as a linear hyperechoic line, and the ventral surface of the paired ceratohyoid bones (CH) can be seen as smaller linear hyperechoic structures that can be followed as they course in a dorsal direction.

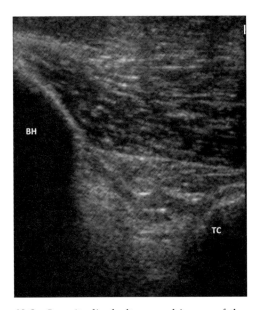

Figure 10.9 Longitudinal ultrasound image of the ventral midline of the larynx at the mid-ventral window. The caudal aspect of the basihyoid bone (BH) and cranial aspect of the thyroid cartilage (TC) can be visualized. Cranial is to the left of this image.

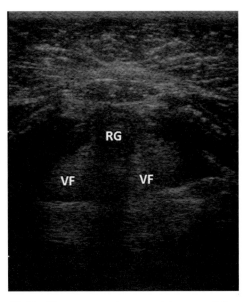

Figure 10.11 Transverse ultrasound image of the ventral aspect of the larynx at the cricothyroid notch (caudoventral window). Ventral is to the top of this image. Left and right vocal folds (VF) can be visualized in cross-section, with the rima glottidis (RG) imaged between the two structures.

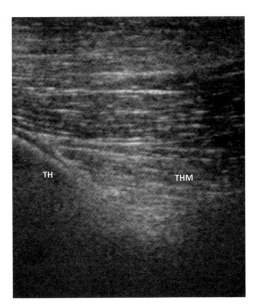

Figure 10.10 Longitudinal ultrasound image of the ventrolateral larynx; the insertion of the thyrohyoid muscle (THM) onto the abaxial aspect of the thyrohyoid bone (TH) can be visualized.

To obtain the caudoventral view, move the transducer back into a transverse position on the ventral midline and move further caudally so that it overlies the cricothyroid notch: the vocal folds can be visualized as paired, hyperechoic, circular/triangular struc-tures (Figure 10.11). Air within the lumen of the rima glottidis casts an acoustic shadow between these structures. By temporarily occluding the horse's nostrils, the patient can be made to take deeper respirations, enabling the vocal cords to be assessed dynamically.

The caudolateral view can be more technically challenging to obtain. Keeping the horse's head slightly extended and flexing the neck laterally away from the side being imaged can assist visualization of this region. Rotating the transducer so that it is in a longitudinal position (Figure 10.12) and moving dorsolaterally over the abaxial aspect of the larynx, the abaxial portions of the thyroid, cricoid, and arytenoid cartilages can be imaged (Figure 10.13). The cricoarytenoideus lateralis and vocalis muscles can be seen as roughly ovoid structures that lie deep to the thyroid and cricoid cartilages but superficial to the arytenoid cartilage. In addition the cricothyroid articulation can be assessed. Rotating the transducer into a transverse plane (Figure 10.14), enables the attachments of the cricoarytenoideus lateralis and vocalis muscles onto the bell-shaped contour of the arytenoid cartilage to be visualized. By moving the transducer more dorsally and angling the transducer slightly ventrally, the muscular process of the arytenoid cartilage, cricoarytenoid articulation, and lateral portion of the cricoarytenoideus dorsalis muscle can be imaged in some individuals.

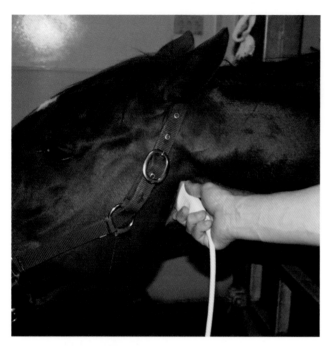

Figure 10.12 Positioning of the transducer in order to obtain the lateral transverse view of the larynx. This is facilitated by positioning the patient's head in a slightly extended position in order to position the larynx more caudally in relation to the mandible.

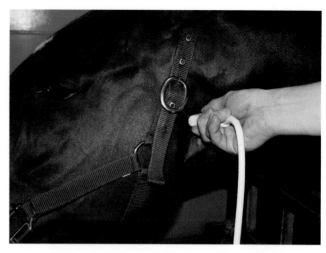

Figure 10.14 Positioning of the transducer in order to obtain the dorsal longitudinal view of the larynx. This is facilitated by positioning the patient's head in a slightly extended position in order to position the larynx more caudally in relation to the mandible.

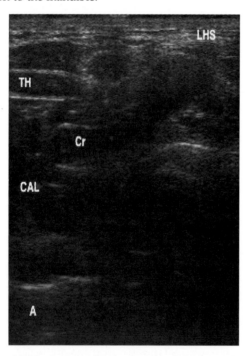

Figure 10.13 Longitudinal ultrasound image of the left lateral larynx centered over the abaxial aspects of the thyroid and cricoid cartilages. Cranial lies to the left and caudal to the right of this image. The caudodorsal abaxial portion of the thyroid cartilage (TH) and rostrodorsal abaxial portion of the cricoid cartilage (Cr) can be visualized, together with the cricoarytenoideus lateralis muscle (CAL) and ipsilateral arytenoid cartilage (A). (Source: Image courtesy of Neil Townsend.)

Ultrasonographic Abnormalities

Ultrasonographic examination of the larynx can provide important complementary or adjunctive information in a number of pathological conditions, including arytenoid chondritis (Figure 10.15), recurrent laryngeal neuropathy, congenital abnormalities such as fourth branchial arch defects (Figure 10.16), basihyoid bone malformation or cyst-like malformations of the laryngeal/tracheal cartilages, infection of the perilaryngeal soft tissue structures, or osteomyelitis of the basihyoid bone, and as a potential predictor of the likelihood of dorsal displacement of the soft palate (DDSP).

TONGUE

Normal Anatomy and Scanning Technique

The rostral and mid portions of the tongue can be imaged by placing a linear 5–7.5 MHz transducer directly onto its dorsal surface after placing a full mouth speculum and using an intra-oral approach, or by exteriorizing the rostral portion of the tongue. The mouth should be flushed with water to remove ingesta from the oral cavity and in order to reduce movement

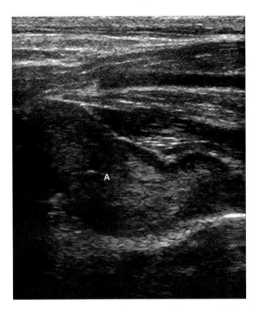

Figure 10.15 Transverse ultrasound image of the lateral aspect of the larynx in a horse with arytenoid chondritis. Dorsal lies to the left and ventral to the right of this image. The arytenoid cartilage (A) lies in the center of this image and is enlarged, has an irregular contour, and has increased echogenicity within its substance. (Source: Image courtesy of Katie Garrett.)

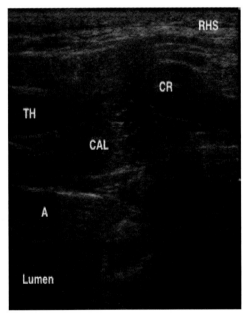

Figure 10.16 Longitudinal ultrasound image of the right lateral larynx in a horse with a fourth branchial arch deformity. The transducer is centered over the abaxial aspects of the thyroid (TH) and cricoid (CR) cartilages. The right cricothyroid articulation is absent and there is an abnormally wide space between the two cartilages in which the right cricoarytenoideus lateralis (CAL) muscle is visualized (in contrast to Figure 10.13). The ipsilateral arytenoid cartilage (A) lies abaxial to these structures. (Source: Image courtesy of Neil Townsend.)

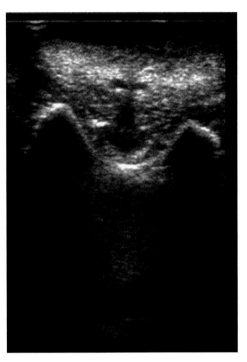

Figure 10.17 Transverse ultrasound image of the rostral portion of the tongue with a linear transducer operating at 7.5 MHz placed directly onto the dorsal aspect of the tongue. The tongue has a relatively homogeneous echogenic appearance and vascular structures appear as circular hypoechoic structures within its substance and on the ventral aspect of the tongue.

artifact; this is most easily performed following sedation of the horse. The tongue can be imaged in longitudinal and cross-sectional views (Figures 10.17, 10.18). The more caudal portions, base of the tongue, and sublingual musculature can be examined using a submandibular approach, placing the transducer between the mandibular rami. Transducer frequencies of 5–10 MHz are required depending on the size of the horse and depth required. The horse's head may be positioned in a neutral or slightly extended position and the tongue should be assessed in longitudinal and transverse planes (Figure 10.19). The transverse view may be impeded in smaller horses where a linear transducer is being used if the mandibular rami are positioned relatively closely together, thereby preventing physical contact of the probe with the soft tissues in this region.

The body of the tongue has a homogeneous, relatively hypoechoic appearance, and on transverse views, vascular structures can be imaged within its substance as circular hypoechoic structures. In a longitudinal view the muscle fibers have a more hyperechoic, slightly wave-like appearance. The genioglossus

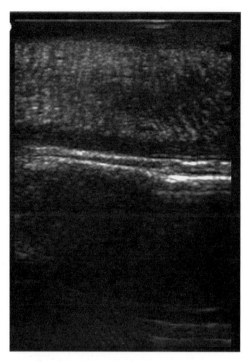

Figure 10.18 Longitudinal ultrasound image of the rostral portion of the tongue with a linear transducer operating at 7.5 MHz placed directly onto the dorsal aspect of the tongue. The muscle fibers have a slightly more echogenic, wave-like appearance.

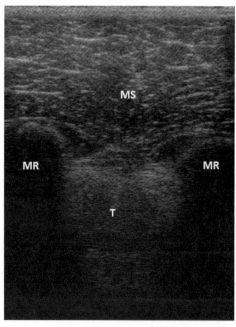

Figure 10.19 Transverse ultrasound image of the base of the tongue (T) and associated musculature (MS) obtained using a linear probe operating at 5 MHz positioned on the midline of the ventral aspect of the head between the rami of the mandible (MR) (submandibular view).

muscles can also be visualized as parallel structures with a similar echogenicity, that lie superficial to the base of the tongue.

Ultrasonographic Abnormalities

Ultrasonographic assessment of the tongue may be helpful in cases of suspected foreign body penetration (usually metallic or wood in nature) or abscess formation within the tongue and adjacent structures. Intraoperatively, ultrasonography may assist localization and removal of foreign bodies (particularly those that are radiolucent) within the tongue and adjacent soft tissue structures.

SALIVARY GLANDS

Normal Anatomy and Scanning Technique

The parotid gland and its duct can be imaged using a 6–10 MHz transducer set at a depth of around 4–8 cm. With the transducer in a dorsally oriented plane over the abaxial aspect of the cranial cervical region just caudal to the vertical ramus of the mandible and cranial to the wing of the atlas, the substance (parenchyma) of the gland has a relatively hypoechoic appearance and lobules can be seen enclosed within more hyperechoic fascial tissue (Figure 10.20). Axial to the parotid and mandibular

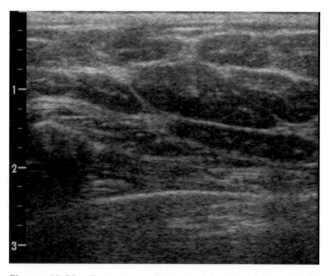

Figure 10.20 Transverse ultrasound image of the parotid salivary duct with a linear transducer operating at 10 MHz positioned vertically over the caudal aspect of the ventral ramus of the mandible. The substance of the gland is relatively hypoechoic and the lobules are enclosed within hyperechoic fascial tissues.

salivary glands lie the ipsilateral guttural pouch and retropharyngeal lymph nodes. The parotid salivary duct can be imaged as it courses across the ventral aspect of the mandible, and in a rostro-dorsal direction across the lateral aspect of the mandible alongside the facial artery and vein. Unless pathologic distension is present, this structure can be difficult to visualize. The mandibular salivary glands can be imaged axial to the parotid salivary gland and abaxial to the ipsilateral guttural pouch. The sublingual salivary glands lie superficial to the base and midbody of the tongue and can be imaged via a submandibular approach (see Tongue). Both are smaller than the parotid gland and are more difficult to visualize in the normal horse.

Ultrasonographic Abnormalities

Ultrasonography can assist diagnosis and assessment of obstructive sialolithiasis, foreign bodies, abscess formation, neoplastic infiltration, and generalized inflammation of the gland.

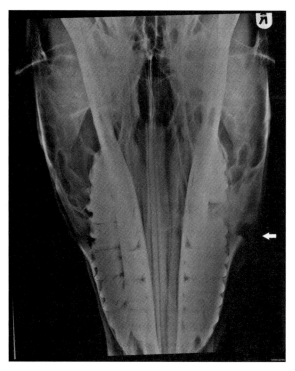

Figure 10.21 Dorsoventral radiograph obtained in a horse with a facial swelling associated with a draining tract where a portion of sequestered bone is evident (arrow).

ASSESSMENT OF OTHER STRUCTURES OF THE HEAD

The outline of the skull bones and normal foraminae can be visualized as a thin hyperechoic line. The normal vascular structures that run on the superficial aspect of the head, e.g. transverse facial vein and artery, are consistent in appearance with other vascular structures. Lymph nodes are visualized as ovoid, small structures with a homogeneous soft tissue echogenicity with a discrete more hyperechoic capsule. Ultrasonographic evaluation of pathological swellings of the head, particularly those of soft tissue density, can be particularly helpful. This may assist identification of abscesses, hematomas, dentigerous cysts, or soft tissue swellings, such as nasal atheromas or intra-oral masses. Ultrasonographic evaluation of swellings associated with draining tracts due to the presence of a foreign body or formation of a bony sequestrum (Figures 10.21, 10.22) can provide useful diagnostic information. Ultrasonography can also assist diagnosis and management of fractures to the thin bones of the skull, which may be difficult to visualize radiographically (Figures 10.23, 10.24), and can provide adjunctive information in the assessment of mandibular fractures (Figure 10.25, 10.26) and masses (Figures 10.27, 10.28).

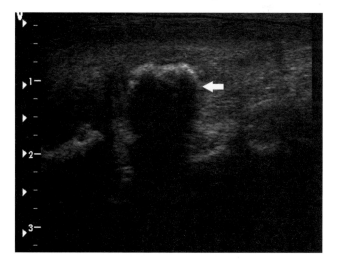

Figure 10.22 Ultrasound image of the same horse as in Figure 10.21. Discontinuity of the hyperechoic outline of the maxillary bone is evident on an ultrasound image of the site, consistent with a bone sequestrum (arrow). Ultrasonographic assessment assisted in more accurately localizing the site and assessing the depth and size of the sequestrum prior to surgical removal.

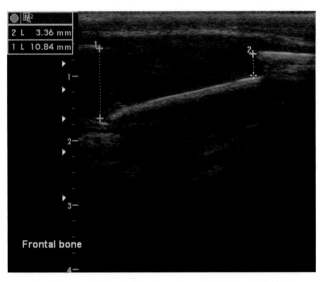

Figure 10.23 Ultrasound image of the frontal bone in a horse that sustained an open, depressed fracture of the skull. This enabled the size and shape of the fragment, together with the depth of depression into the paranasal sinuses to be accurately evaluated prior to surgical management (Figure 10.24).

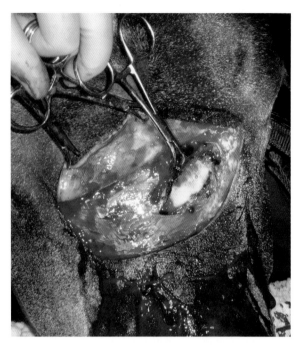

Figure 10.24 Surgical management of the depressed fracture of the skull of the horse in Figure 10.23.

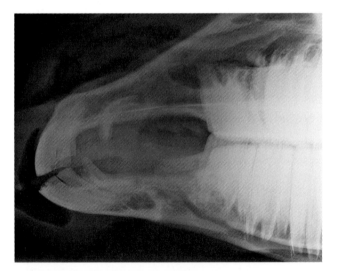

Figure 10.25 Latero-lateral radiograph of a horse that had sustained an open, oblique fracture of the horizontal ramus of the mandible.

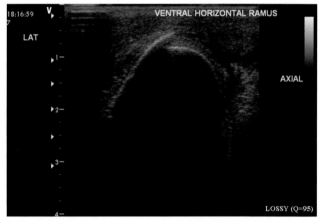

Figure 10.26 Ultrasonographic assessment of the mandible of the horse in Figure 10.25 demonstrates the discontinuity in the hyperechoic surface of the mandible consistent with a fracture.

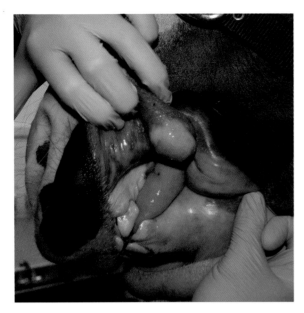

Figure 10.27   Assessment of a spherical mass in the oral cavity of a horse originating at the mucocutaneous junction of the upper lip.

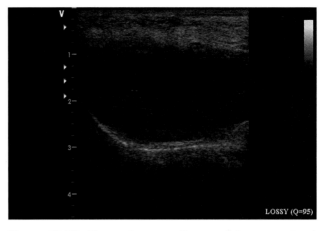

Figure 10.28   Transcutaneous ultrasound image centered over the mass in Figure 10.27, demonstrating a relatively hypoechoic appearance to the contents of the mass with some areas of slightly increased echogenicity consistent with mucoid contents (cyst). Ultrasonographic assessment enabled the presence of a foreign body to be ruled out.

RECOMMENDED READING

Chalmers, H.J., Cheetham, J., Yaeger, A.E., & Ducharme, N.D. (2006) Ultrasonography of the equine larynx. *Veterinary Radiology & Ultrasound*, 47, 476–481.

Chalmers, H.J., Yaeger, A.E., & Ducharme, N.D. (2009) Ultrasonographic assessment of laryngohyoid position as a predictor of dorsal displacement of the soft palate in horses. *Veterinary Radiology & Ultrasound*, 50, 91–96.

Garrett, K.S., Woodie, J.B., Cook, J.L., & Williams, N.M. (2010) Imaging diagnosis – nasal septal and laryngeal cyst-like malformations in a Thoroughbred weanling colt diagnosed using ultrasonography and magnetic resonance imaging. *Veterinary Radiology & Ultrasound*, 51, 504–507.

Garrett, K.S., Woodie, J.B., & Embertson, R.M. (2011) Association of treadmill upper airway endoscopic evaluation with results of ultrasonography and resting upper airway endoscopic evaluation. *Equine Veterinary Journal*, 43, 365–371.

Reef, V.B. (1998) Ultrasonographic evaluation of small parts. In: *Equine Diagnostic Ultrasound*. W.B. Saunders, Philadelphia, pp. 480–547.

Rodriguez, M.J., Soler, M., Latorre, R., Gil, F., & Agut, A. (2007) Ultrasonographic anatomy of the temporomandibular joint in healthy pure-bred Spanish horses. *Veterinary Radiology & Ultrasound*, 48, 149–154.

Solano, M. & Pennick, D. (1996) Ultrasonography of the canine, feline and equine tongue: normal findings and case history reports. *Veterinary Radiology & Ultrasound*, 37, 206–213.

Weller, R., Taylor, S., Maierl, J., Cauvin, E.R.J., & May, S.A. (1999) Ultrasonographic anatomy of the equine temporomandibular joint. *Equine Veterinary Journal*, 31, 529–532.

VIDEOS: DYNAMIC ULTRASONOGRAPHY OF MUSCULOSKELETAL REGIONS

Sarah Boys Smith

Rossdales Equine Hospital and Diagnostic Centre, Newmarket, UK

Unlike the other imaging modalities used in veterinary medicine, ultrasonography should be thought of as a "dynamic" form of imaging. As equipment and expertise advance, our ability to capture and then review multiple-frame ultrasound images in the form of videos is rapidly superseding the use of the one-off static image.

An ultrasonographical diagnosis is generally made at the time of the examination itself; that is, the diagnosis is made "dynamically". Being able to obtain, save, and then review these dynamic images allows more accurate record keeping of the patient's injury. There are many advantages to obtaining ultrasound videos and these are primarily centered around image review. In one static image, some of the structures will be off-incidence and can therefore not be assessed accurately. Taking a sequence of images in the form of a video allows all the structures to be assessed in detail. An ultrasound video enables the extent and severity of an injury to be more reliably reported upon and, in addition, follow-up ultrasonographic assessment is more straightforward.

This chapter illustrates a number of ultrasound videos. The chapter aims to give an overview of the use of dynamic ultrasonography but is by no means exclusive.

Unless otherwise stated, the following can be applied to the videos:

- transverse section: videos run in a proximal to distal direction;
- longitudinal sections: proximal is to the left of the image; videos run in a proximal to distal direction.

THE USE OF ULTRASONOGRAPHY IN ASSESSING ACUTE AND CHRONIC WOUNDS, TRAUMA, AND INJURY

Videos 1 and 2 Digital flexor tendon sheath: previous injury to the palmar aspect of the palmar annular ligament and the sheath wall

Transverse (Video 1) and longitudinal (Video 2) sections of the palmar aspect of the left fore digital flexor tendon sheath at the level of the fetlock joint. This horse had sustained an injury while hunting some months previously and had demonstrated an intermittent lameness since that time.

There are several focal areas of increased echogenicity, surrounded by well defined anechoic areas. These abnormal areas are located at different depths to each other: within the subcutaneous tissue, within the tendon sheath wall, within the paratenon of the superficial digital flexor tendon (SDFT), and on the palmar aspect of the SDFT itself. There appears to be mild disruption of the palmar aspect of the SDFT in the region of one of these abnormal ultrasonographic areas. Dynamic ultrasonographical assessment allows: the location of the foreign bodies to be more accurately defined, indicates the presence of ill defined acoustic shadows from some of these areas, and also allows a more accurate interpretation of the tendon margins to be made (which is often also easier in longitudinal section than in transverse section). There are no significant abnormalities of the deep digital flexor tendon, the palmar aspect of the proximal sesamoid bones, and the intersesamoidean ligament. A normal manica flexoria is also visible in transverse section.

Atlas of Equine Ultrasonography, First Edition. Edited by Jessica A. Kidd, Kristina G. Lu, and Michele L. Frazer.
Companion Website: www.wiley.com/go/kidd/equine-ultrasonography

Surgical removal confirmed these focal echogenic structures to be blackthorns encapsulated within pockets of fluid (represented by the surrounding areas of decreased echogenicity). The mild disruption to the palmar aspect of the SDFT was also confirmed. Ultrasonography was used at the time of surgery to aid in the location of the foreign bodies and to help direct the surgical procedure.

http://bit.ly/1feloKz

http://bit.ly/1h8hRfd

(This will take you directly to the video on Wiley Blackwell's companion website)

Video 3 Hock: blunt, traumatic injury of the lateral digital extensor tendon

Transverse section of the cranial aspect of the left hock, centered over the lateral digital extensor tendon (LaDET). This horse had been involved in a fall and had subsequently developed a marked effusion of the LaDET sheath.

There is moderate–severe disruption of the fiber pattern of the LaDET, particularly on its medial aspect. As expected, there is more synovial fluid evident within the distal aspect of the tendon sheath compared to further proximally. There is associated synovial proliferation, thickening of the synovial lining and the mesotenon. The underlying distocranial aspect of the tibia and the lateral trochlear ridge of the talus, with its overlying articular cartilage, are normal in appearance.

The horse was treated conservatively with rest, controlled exercise, and non-steroidal anti-inflammatory medication in the short term. The effusion has decreased (but by no means resolved) and the horse has remained sound with increasing exercise. There has been ultrasonographical improvement in the appearance of the LaDET.

http://bit.ly/NcLLFD

(This will take you directly to the video on Wiley Blackwell's companion website)

Video 4 Hock: kick injury to the sustentaculum tali, involving the tarsal sheath

Transverse section of the medial aspect of the right hock. This horse presented with a 3-week history of a moderate lameness and a draining wound on the medial aspect of the hock.

There is a significant effusion of the tarsal sheath with thickening of the synovial lining and mesotenon. The fluid is largely anechoic in nature. There is fragmentation of the sustentaculum tali adjacent to the deep digital flexor tendon (DDFT). The wound tract can be traced from the fragmented bone to the skin surface. The ability to follow a wound tract ultrasonographically is not only useful from a diagnostic view point but can also be used to aid surgical debridement. Debridement of the wound tract and the damaged sustentaculum tali was performed and there was a small communicating tract with the tarsal sheath which was flushed tenoscopically. There was no evidence of damage to the DDFT.

http://bit.ly/1nPjSz4

(This will take you directly to the video on Wiley Blackwell's companion website)

Video 5 Superficial digital flexor tendon: traumatic kick injury

Transverse section of the palmar aspect of the left fore metacarpus. This horse presented with a severe kick wound to the distal third of the palmar metacarpus and was non-weightbearing lame on initial assessment.

At the proximal and distal aspect of the superficial digital flexor tendon (SDFT), the tendon is enlarged with a generalized reduction in its echogenicity. At the level of the wound there appears to be a complete loss of the medial aspect of the SDFT. There are multiple small, focal and very echogenic artifacts at the level of the wound and also within the digital flexor tendon sheath (DFTS). These artifacts are caused by the presence of air and result in acoustic shadowing. In these types of cases, care must always be taken not to misinterpret the loss of image quality (due to the presence of air and the subsequent acoustic shadowing) as severe tendon damage. In this case digital palpation confirmed severe disruption to the SDFT.

http://bit.ly/MCsD3V

(This will take you directly to the video on Wiley Blackwell's companion website)

Video 6 Digital flexor tendon sheath: previous penetrating injury involving the superficial digital flexor tendon and the sheath wall

Transverse section of the palmar aspect of the right fore digital flexor tendon sheath (DFTS) at the level of the fetlock joint. This horse had sustained a wound to the palmar aspect of the left fore DFTS a few weeks previously. There had been associated effusion of the DFTS, a moderate but intermittent lameness, and an intermittently draining wound since that time. Repeat synoviocentesis of the DFTS, performed on several different occasions since the original injury, had not been consistent with infection and there had been no communication with the wound on distension of the DFTS with sterile saline.

An acoustic shadow from the skin surface is present in the first frame of the video and is caused by part of the wound. There is thickening of the tissues between the skin surface and the superficial digital flexor tendon (SDFT). The plica is evident with effusion of the DFTS on either side of this. Medial to the plica there is an area of increased echogenicity situated between the palmar wall of the DFTS and the palmar aspect of the SDFT. This tissue is of mixed echogenicity, and creates an acoustic shadow. There is apparent disruption of the palmar surface of the SDFT, but as in Video 5, it is important not to over-interpret areas of ultrasonographic "cut-off" as tissue damage. The thickened tissue can be traced ultrasonographically to the wound on the surface of the skin. Surgery confirmed the presence of an abscess within the thickened tissue present ultrasonographically. This tissue had formed an adhesion between the wound, the palmar DFTS wall, and the palmar aspect of the SDFT. This infected tissue had been walled off such that there was no associated infection of the DFTS. Surgery also confirmed a small longitudinal tear in the palmar aspect of the SFDT in the region of the adhesion.

http://bit.ly/1fiy3vC

(This will take you directly to the video on Wiley Blackwell's companion website)

Video 7 Digital flexor tendon sheath: penetrating injury involving the superficial digital flexor tendon and the sheath

Transverse section of the plantar aspect of the digital flexor tendon sheath (DFTS). This horse had sustained a penetrating injury to the plantar aspect of the DFTS and presented with a moderate hind limb lameness. Ultrasonographically there is a moderate amount of subcutaneous thickening, effusion of the DFTS, and thickening of the synovial lining on the plantar aspect of the superficial digital flexor tendon (SDFT). There is a linear tract of reduced echogenicity extending from the plantar to the dorsal aspects of the SDFT, which is consistent with a penetrating injury. Synoviocentesis confirmed sepsis of the DFTS. Surgical exploration confirmed that the penetrating injury had been caused by a blackthorn.

http://bit.ly/1mbQnbG

(This will take you directly to the video on Wiley Blackwell's companion website)

THE SUPERFICIAL DIGITAL FLEXOR TENDON (SDFT)

Video 8 Superficial digital flexor tendon: severe acute injury and re-injury lesions

Transverse section of a severely damaged superficial digital flexor tendon (SDFT). The tendon is grossly enlarged and is of mixed and irregular echogenicity. There is no normal fiber pattern present and the appearance of the tendon in this video is sometimes described as having an "open-weave" pattern. The outline of the tendon is not well defined throughout the duration of the video. Distally, there is the indication of a "halo" or ring of decreased echogenicity (giving a "donut" type of appearance), within the center of the tendon. This represents a re-injury lesion.

http://bit.ly/1c3K0Rq

(This will take you directly to the video on Wiley Blackwell's companion website)

Video 9 Superficial digital flexor tendon: acute injury and re-injury lesions

Transverse section of the superficial digital flexor tendon (SDFT). This tendon had initially been injured approximately 1 year before this ultrasonographical examination was performed. The old ("healed") tendon lesion is evident at the start of the video where there is a large central area of the tendon that is of increased echogenicity and of an abnormal fiber pattern, typical of a chronic injury. Further distally there are several small anechoic core lesions present within the center of the "healed" lesion. Further distally still there is a "halo" (ring of decreased echogenicity) present around the "healed" lesion giving a "donut" type of appearance. At the distal aspect of the tendon, just proximal to the level of the fetlock joint and within the digital flexor tendon sheath there is a large anechoic tendon lesion in the central and palmar aspect of the tendon, representing an acute lesion. This horse has re-injured the SDFT, at the distal junction between the initial tendon injury and the normal tendon distal to it. This junction is often the site of re-injury. The area of decreased echogenicity within the DDFT at the start of the video is due to the distal attachment of the accessory ligament of the DDFT and is normal.

http://bit.ly/1c3K1Vz

(This will take you directly to the video on Wiley Blackwell's companion website)

THE HIND LIMB SUSPENSORY APPARATUS

Video 10 Hind limb proximal suspensory ligament: normal

Longitudinal section of a normal hind limb proximal suspensory ligament. The dorsal and plantar borders of the ligament are clearly defined and there is a good fiber pattern of the ligament at its origin. There is a large anechoic oval structure present on the plantaroproximal aspect of the ligament which is a blood vessel. Blood vessels can cause edge artifacts (which are not that pronounced in this case), which can make ultrasonographical interpretation of the ligament difficult. Dynamic ultrasonography allows the probe angle to be constantly changed in order to evaluate the ligament as fully as possible, thereby reducing the "real effect" of these artifacts as much as possible. The plantaroproximal aspect of the third metatarsal bone is smooth in outline and echogenicity.

http://bit.ly/1kZHYdn

(This will take you directly to the video on Wiley Blackwell's companion website)

Video 11 Hind limb proximal suspensory ligament: abnormal

Longitudinal section of a right hind proximal suspensory ligament. There is a significant loss in the longitudinal fiber pattern (reduction in the echogenicity) of the origin of the ligament as well as significant disruption and irregularity of the plantaroproximal aspect of the third metatarsal bone.

http://bit.ly/1kZIb09

(This will take you directly to the video on Wiley Blackwell's companion website)

Video 12 Hind limb suspensory branch: abnormal

Transverse section of the lateral suspensory branch of the left hind limb. There is a loss in the fiber pattern of the axial (or deeper) aspect of the ligament as well as irregularity of the ligament–bone interface at the insertion of the ligament onto the lateral proximal sesamoid bone. There is also some thickening of the subcutaneous tissue overlying the suspensory branch.

http://bit.ly/1fB0QI5

(This will take you directly to the video on Wiley Blackwell's companion website)

Video 13 Hind limb suspensory branch: abnormal

Longitudinal section of the lateral suspensory branch of the right hind limb. There is mild irregularity and mild fragmentation of the lateral proximal sesamoid bone at the insertion of the ligament onto the bone. There is associated loss in the longitudinal fiber pattern of the ligament at the site of this irregularity. The changes in this video are mild and in similar cases the significance of these findings should be interpreted in light of the clinical and diagnostic findings. This video highlights the importance of examining the entire width of the ligament as the plantar aspect of the ligament is more affected than the dorsal aspect, which is often the case.

http://bit.ly/1eUILE0

(This will take you directly to the video on Wiley Blackwell's companion website)

Video 14 Oblique distal sesamoidean ligament: abnormal

Transverse section of the lateral oblique distal sesamoidean ligament (ODSL). The video starts over the distal aspect of the lateral suspensory branch, which appears normal, and the lateral attachment of the palmar annular ligament onto the lateral proximal sesamoid bone, which is demonstrating some mild irregularity. Distally, there is moderate damage to the lateral ODSL. The ligament is of mixed echogenicity, with some small focal areas of significantly increased echogenicity as well as more diffuse areas of reduced echogenicity. There are focal areas within the ODSL which represent fragmentation of the lateral proximal sesamoid bone at the attachment of the ligament onto the bone.

http://bit.ly/1muY7cn

(This will take you directly to the video on Wiley Blackwell's companion website)

Video 15 Oblique distal sesamoidean ligament: abnormal

Transverse section of the medial oblique distal sesamoidean ligament (ODSL) of the left hind limb. There is a focal area of decreased echogenicity on the dorsal aspect of the ligament but there is no apparent disruption to the bone–ligament interface.

http://bit.ly/MdSqP7

(This will take you directly to the video on Wiley Blackwell's companion website)

Video 16 Oblique distal sesamoidean ligament: normal

Longitudinal section of a normal oblique distal sesamoidean ligament (ODSL). The fiber pattern and the origin of the ligament from the base of the proximal sesamoid bone is normal. It is important to try to visualize the entire width of the ligament.

http://bit.ly/1gYxya1

(This will take you directly to the video on Wiley Blackwell's companion website)

THE DIGITAL FLEXOR TENDON SHEATH ((DFTS) AND PALMAR/PLANTAR ANNULAR LIGAMENT

Video 17 The digital flexor tendon sheath: normal

Transverse section of the plantar aspect of the left hind digital flexor tendon sheath (DFTS) illustrating the appearance of a normal plantar annular ligament (PAL). The PAL is traced from its lateral attachment onto the lateral proximal sesamoid bone (PSB) to its medial attachment onto the medial PSB. The ligament is of normal thickness and structure and there are no abnormalities at the ligament–bone interface. The palmar annular ligament of the fore limb would have a similar appearance. The superficial and deep digital flexor tendons (SDFT and DDFT) are normal. A small blood vessel on the plantar border of the DDFT (that is not ultrasonographically visible) causes the edge artifact within the lateral aspect of the tendon. This should not be confused with a tendon lesion. The PAL (both its fiber pattern as well as its dorsopalmar/dorsoplantar width) should be assessed from its most medial to its most lateral margins.

http://bit.ly/MdSyhy

(This will take you directly to the video on Wiley Blackwell's companion website)

Video 18 The digital flexor tendon sheath: effusion

Transverse section of the plantar aspect of the left hind digital flexor tendon sheath (DFTS) at the level of the fetlock joint. There is effusion of the DFTS, which highlights the vinculum on the palmar aspect of the SFDT. The video also highlights the effect on the image when the pressure of the probe is changed. This is important to realize when ultrasonography is being used to monitor the degree of effusion present within any tendon sheath or joint. The plantar annular ligament and the manica flexoria are normal.

http://bit.ly/1hx9rme

(This will take you directly to the video on Wiley Blackwell's companion website)

Video 19 Deep digital flexor tendon: core lesion

Transverse section of the distal flexor tendon sheath (DFTS) at the level of the proximal pouch. The area of decreased echogenicity within the DDFT at the start of the video is due to the distal attachment of the accessory ligament of the DDFT and is normal. Further distally, there is a small, mostly anechoic core/split-type lesion within the deep digital flexor tendon (DDFT).

http://bit.ly/1fB7BJV

(This will take you directly to the video on Wiley Blackwell's companion website)

Video 20 Deep digital flexor tendon (pastern): abnormal

Transverse section of the palmar pastern. There is enlargement of the deep digital flexor tendon (DDFT), a loss in the echogenicity and disruption of the fiber pattern, particularly on its palmar aspect. There is also irregularity of the outline of the palmar aspect of each tendon lobe with the lateral lobe being more severely affected. There is thickening of the palmar wall of the digital flexor tendon sheath (DFTS)/distal digital annular ligament, which is also of reduced echogenicity on the medial aspect. There are several focal linear echogenic structures, consistent with mineralization, within the palmar wall of the DFTS/distal digital annular ligament which are causing acoustic shadowing of the deeper structures. Altering the angle of the probe demonstrates the change in the echogenicity of the body of the tendon lobes which is normal and should be symmetrical in each lobe.

http://bit.ly/1gjmNgv

(This will take you directly to the video on Wiley Blackwell's companion website)

Video 21 Deep digital flexor tendon: abnormal

Transverse section of the plantar aspect of the digital flexor tendon sheath, at the level of the proximal pouch. There is an acute and significant tear of the palmaromedial aspect of the deep digital flexor tendon, represented by the anechoic lines, the disruption of the fiber pattern, and irregularity of the tendon outline.

http://bit.ly/NcTKCL

(This will take you directly to the video on Wiley Blackwell's companion website)

Video 22 Superficial digital flexor tendon: abnormal

Transverse section of the palmar aspect of the digital flexor tendon sheath (DFTS), proximal to the fetlock joint. There is effusion of the DFTS and at the start of the video there is the suggestion of an adhesion between the lateral margin of the superficial digital flexor tendon (SDFT) and the sheath wall. Further distally there is mild enlargement and disruption of the fiber pattern of the lateral margin of the SDFT. The mesotenon of the deep digital flexor tendon (DDFT) is thickened and of irregular echogenicity compared to normal. There is general thickening of the DFTS lining and some synovial proliferation evident. The adhesion between the SFDT and the tendon sheath wall was confirmed tenoscopically and there was also evidence of mild disruption of the lateral margin of the SDFT. The injury appeared chronic and the adhesion appeared well established, as expected from the ultrasonographic examination.

http://bit.ly/1oUD0it

(This will take you directly to the video on Wiley Blackwell's companion website)

Video 23 Manica flexoria: abnormal

Transverse section of the plantar aspect of the left hind digital flexor tendon sheath region (DFTS) just proximal to the fetlock joint. There is thickening of the manica flexoria, and the lateral attachment of the manica flexoria onto the lateral aspect of the superficial digital flexor tendon also appears to be disrupted. There is a significant degree of synovial proliferation in the lateral aspect of the DFTS and a mild irregularity in the contour of both the lateral aspect of the deep and superficial digital flexor tendons.

http://bit.ly/1h8LMnw

(This will take you directly to the video on Wiley Blackwell's companion website)

Video 24 Ganglion on the palmar aspect of the digital flexor tendon sheath

Transverse section of the palmar aspect of the digital flexor tendon sheath, at the level of the fetlock joint. There is a fluid-filled ganglion palmar to the superficial digital flexor tendon, situated palmar to the sheath wall. Ultrasonographically there is a strong suggestion that there is communication between the ganglion and the sheath; this information can only be gained from dynamic ultrasonography. The communication between the two structures was later confirmed using contrast radiography.

http://bit.ly/1mc7wBS

(This will take you directly to the video on Wiley Blackwell's companion website)

Video 25 Plantar annular ligament injury

Transverse section of the plantaromedial aspect of the digital flexor tendon sheath (DFTS) at the level of the fetlock joint. The attachment of the medial aspect of the plantar annular ligament onto the medial proximal sesamoid bone is abnormal. There is a moderate amount of disruption of the bone contour as well as of the ligament itself. There is a mild amount of effusion within the DFTS. This area is often overlooked when assessing the distal limbs.

http://bit.ly/1bNJPil

(This will take you directly to the video on Wiley Blackwell's companion website)

THE FETLOCK JOINT

Video 26 Collateral ligaments of the fetlock joint (normal)

Longitudinal section of the normal lateral collateral ligaments of the right hind fetlock joint (proximal to the left of the image). The entire ligament cannot be assessed using one static ultrasonographic view. Dynamic ultrasonography allows the proximal and distal attachments of both the superficial (long) and deep (short) collateral ligaments to be assessed fully. The superficial ligament runs perpendicular to the weightbearing surface of the joint in the standing horse. The deep ligament traverses the joint in a dorsoproximal-palmaro/plantarodistal direction. Only the section of the ligament that is perpendicular to the ultrasound beam should be assessed at any one time, meaning that artifacts within these ligaments can be easily created. The attachment of the ligaments onto the bone should also be carefully assessed.

http://bit.ly/1fiJUd3

(This will take you directly to the video on Wiley Blackwell's companion website)

Video 27 Fetlock joint: fragmentation and effusion

Transverse section of the lateral aspect of the left hind fetlock joint. The distolateral aspect of the third metatarsal bone is visualized on the left of the image. There is thickening of the synovial lining of the plantarolateral joint capsule with an associated effusion of the joint and synovial proliferation. There are several bone fragments present within the joint, which are represented by the focal areas of increased echogenicity. As expected, these cause acoustic shadows. There is also mild modeling of the distal aspect of the third metatarsal bone. The fragments were evident radiographically but ultrasonography allowed a more accurate assessment of their exact location. The video is not focused on the lateral suspensory branch but this ligament does demonstrate some mild changes in its fiber pattern/echogenicity.

http://bit.ly/NcUjwr

(This will take you directly to the video on Wiley Blackwell's companion website)

THE CARPUS

Video 28 The carpal joints and the extensor carpi radialis tendon: mild joint effusion

Longitudinal section of the extensor carpi radialis tendon (ECRT), which is normal in this case. The tendon is traced from the level of the proximal carpus to its distal attachment onto the dorsoproximal aspect of the third metatarsal bone. The radiocarpal (antebrachiocarpal), middle (inter-) carpal, and carpometacarpal joints are clearly evident in longitudinal section. There is some synovial effusion of the radiocarpal and middle carpal joints and some thickening of the synovial lining. Dynamic ultrasonography allows both the longitudinal fiber pattern as well as the tendon size to be easily assessed. When assessing a structure such as a tendon, in a longitudinal fashion, it is also important to assess its entire width.

http://bit.ly/1jexQdz

(This will take you directly to the video on Wiley Blackwell's companion website)

Video 29 The middle (inter-) carpal joint: osteochondral fragment, modeling, and effusion

Longitudinal section of the medial aspect of the middle carpal joint. The radiocarpal bone is to the left of the image and the third carpal bone is to the right. There is effusion of the joint and associated thickening of the synovial lining. There is a moderate degree of modeling associated with the bone margins of the radiocarpal and third carpal bones. There is also a suggestion of an osteochondral fragment associated with the dorsal aspect of the radiocarpal bone. This finding was confirmed radiographically, although ultrasonography provided a more accurate assessment of entire joint margin in this case and also allowed the joint abnormality to be more accurately located.

http://bit.ly/1glTtlT

(This will take you directly to the video on Wiley Blackwell's companion website)

Video 30 The radiocarpal (antebrachiocarpal) joint: osteochondral fragment, modeling, and effusion

Longitudinal section of the dorsal aspect of the radiocarpal joint. There is a much more obvious osteochondral fragment (compared to the case in Video 29 present within the joint, associated with the distolateral aspect of the radius. There is also an associated joint effusion, thickening of the synovial lining, synovial proliferation and modeling of the joint margins. As in Video 29, ultrasonography provides a more accurate assessment of the entire joint margin and also allows the exact location of any osteochondral fragment to be accurately located.

http://bit.ly/MCCBSZ

(This will take you directly to the video on Wiley Blackwell's companion website)

THE ELBOW JOINT

Video 31 Lateral collateral ligament injury

Longitudinal section of the lateral collateral ligament of the elbow joint (proximal to the left of the image). The video clip starts at the level of the distal insertion of the collateral ligament onto the radius and the joint space, before tracing the collateral ligament proximally. There is moderate disruption of the longitudinal fiber pattern (decreased echogenicity) with associated irregularity of the distal aspect of the lateral humerus at the origin of the ligament.

http://bit.ly/1gYzi2N

(This will take you directly to the video on Wiley Blackwell's companion website)

THE SHOULDER REGION

Video 32 Humeral tubercles and the biceps brachii tendon: irregularity of the bone and adjacent tendon

Transverse section of the cranial aspect of the shoulder region, centered over the biceps brachii tendon. There is a moderate amount of irregularity on the cranial aspect of the intermediate tubercle of the humerus and there is an associated loss in the echogenicity of the adjacent biceps brachii tendon. The tendon should be examined in its entirety in both length and width. The bone irregularity was only detected radiographically after taking multiple skyline projections of the cranial humerus.

http://bit.ly/1feNRBc

(This will take you directly to the video on Wiley Blackwell's companion website)

THE STIFLE

Video 33 Trochlear ridges of the femur: subchondral bone defect and disruption of the overlying cartilage on the lateral trochlear ridge

Transverse section of the lateral trochlear ridge (LTR) of the distal femur (medial to the left of the image; lateral to the right of the image). The contour of the trochlear ridge as well as the overlying cartilage is very irregular in outline compared to that in a normal horse (where both the bone and overlying cartilage contour should be smooth). The overlying cartilage is also thinner than in a normal stifle and even appears absent in some areas. There is also an increase in the echogenicity *within* the LTR. This is because the subchondral bone making up the cranial surface of the trochlear ridge is so abnormal with respect to its composition that it does not reflect all the ultrasound beams as it should do. The area of increased echogenicity within the LTR represents the area of abnormal bone. Distally there is an effusion of the femoropatellar joint on the lateral aspect of the LTR (right-hand side of the image). Ultrasonography of the trochlear ridges is often more sensitive in detecting subtle osteochondral irregularities and fragmentation than radiography.

http://bit.ly/1oUE6uy

(This will take you directly to the video on Wiley Blackwell's companion website)

Video 34 Trochlear ridges of the femur in a foal: normal

Transverse section of the medial and lateral trochlear ridges of a normal foal. The video depicts the medial trochlear ridge at the start, before traversing over the trochlear grove to the lateral trochlear ridge. The degree of cartilage thickness compared to that of an adult is clearly different. Also note the difference in the echogenicity of the subchondral bone compared to that in an adult. The use of ultrasonography can be used to assess skeletal maturity in the neonatal foal.

http://bit.ly/1h8N1CZ

(This will take you directly to the video on Wiley Blackwell's companion website)

Videos 35 and 36 Middle patella ligament: acute injury

Transverse (Video 35) and longitudinal (Video 36) sections of the middle patellar ligament (medial is to the left of the image). There is an area of decreased echogenicity within the ligament which is most obvious further distally at the distal insertion of the ligament onto the tibial tuberosity. Distally there are focal areas of increased echogenicity within the ligament itself, caused by bone fragmentation off the tibial tuberosity. These findings represent an acute tear of the middle patellar ligament with an associated avulsion fracture of the tibial tuberosity. On either side of the tear the ligament insertion is relatively normal. The length of the tear is more easily appreciated in longitudinal section. It is important to examine the entire width of the structure to avoid missing a lesion.

http://bit.ly/1muZl7v

http://bit.ly/1jeyAiO

(This will take you directly to the video on Wiley Blackwell's companion website)

Video 37 Medial femorotibial joint: normal medial meniscus, mild joint modeling, and effusion

Longitudinal section of the medial femorotibial joint. The medial meniscus is of a normal echogenicity and its capsular attachment is also clearly evident. There is a mild–moderate amount of effusion of the joint with some mild thickening of the synovial lining. There is also a mild amount of synovial proliferation present. There is very mild modeling of the distomedial aspect of the femur.

http://bit.ly/1e97QLt

(This will take you directly to the video on Wiley Blackwell's companion website)

Video 38 Medial femorotibial joint: damage of the medial meniscus, joint modeling, and effusion

Longitudinal section of the medial femorotibial joint. The degree of joint effusion, capsular thickening, and synovial proliferation is more marked in this case compared to the case in Video 37. The irregularity on the distomedial aspect of the femur is also much more marked and there is also modeling of the proximomedial aspect of the tibia. This modeling is consistent with osteophyte formation/osteoarthritis. The video 'runs' in a cranial to caudal direction. Further caudally there is considerable disruption of the medial meniscus, represented by the marked irregularity in the echogenicity of the meniscus. In addition, the medial meniscus appears to be prolapsing from the joint space and there is also apparent collapse of the medial femorotibial joint space.

http://bit.ly/1csnqFh

(This will take you directly to the video on Wiley Blackwell's companion website)

Video 39 Subchondral bone defect within the weightbearing surface of the medial femoral condyle

Longitudinal section of the weightbearing section of the medial femoral condyle, performed with the stifle in flexion. There is disruption of the surface of the condyle consistent with a subchondral bone defect (cyst). There is thinning of the overlying cartilage. Ultrasonography of this area is increasingly demonstrating the sensitivity of this imaging modality at detecting lesions within the medial femoral condyles compared to radiography.

http://bit.ly/1eV01ZK

(This will take you directly to the video on Wiley Blackwell's companion website)

ULTRASONOGRAPHY OF FRACTURES

Video 40 Ilial wing: fracture

Longitudinal section of an ilial wing fracture. There is an obvious anechoic line through the bone, representing the fracture. There is evidence of the displacement, overriding and comminution at the fracture site. Dynamic ultrasonography allows accurate assessment of the location and the severity of the fracture and is also important in monitoring the healing process.

http://bit.ly/1bNKQHw

(This will take you directly to the video on Wiley Blackwell's companion website)

Video 41 Third trochanter: fracture

Transverse section of a fractured third trochanter of the femur with evidence of fragment displacement and comminution. As with Video 40, dynamic ultrasonography allows accurate assessment of the location and the severity of the fracture and is also important in monitoring the healing process.

http://bit.ly/1bnOvv2

(This will take you directly to the video on Wiley Blackwell's companion website)

TRANSRECTAL ULTRASONOGRAPHY

Video 42 Lumbosacral disc: normal

Transrectal longitudinal section of a normal lumbosacral disc (ventral aspect). The probe is positioned in the midline, with the transducer pointed dorsally. The cranial aspect of the sacrum (on the right-hand side of the image) and the caudal aspect of the last lumbar vertebra (L6) (on the left-hand side of the image) should be smooth in outline and the disc itself should be of even echogenicity. The bright echogenic pattern evident deep to the disc is reverberation artifacts from the cerebrospinal fluid within the spinal canal. An inability to visualize these artifacts can indicate disruption of the lumbosacral region.

http://bit.ly/1fiQ251

(This will take you directly to the video on Wiley Blackwell's companion website)

Video 43 Lumbosacral disc: abnormal

Transrectal longitudinal section of an abnormal lumbosacral disc (ventral aspect; cranial to the left of the image). There is subtle irregularity of the cranial aspect of the sacrum and to a lesser degree of the caudal aspect of the sixth lumbar vertebra. There are several focal areas of increased echogenicity within the disc itself. The clinical significance of this finding must be taken in light of other clinical findings.

http://bit.ly/1h8NULZ

(This will take you directly to the video on Wiley Blackwell's companion website)

Video 44 Lumbosacral disc: abnormal

Transrectal longitudinal section of an abnormal lumbosacral disc (ventral aspect; cranial to the left of the image). There is marked disruption of the disc itself and the adjacent bone margins, in particular the caudal aspect of the sixth lumbar vertebra.

http://bit.ly/1d2P4pg

(This will take you directly to the video on Wiley Blackwell's companion website)

Video 45 Sacroiliac joint: normal

Transrectal longitudinal section of a normal sacroiliac joint (ventral aspect) and the ventral sacroiliac ligament. The sacroiliac joint is positioned caudal and abaxial to the lumbosacral disc. There should not be any significant irregularity of the bone contour. The probe angle should be manipulated to visualize as much of the ventral aspect of the joint as possible. The ligament in this video is of normal size and echogenicity.

http://bit.ly/MdU2s0

(This will take you directly to the video on Wiley Blackwell's companion website)

Video 46 Sacroiliac nerve root outlet and inter-transverse joint: normal

Transrectal longitudinal section of a normal sciatic nerve root outlet and inter-transverse joint (ventral aspect). These two structures are positioned abaxial to the lumbosacral disc. The bone surfaces should be smooth in outline. The inter-transverse joint should be traced as far as possible in an abaxial direction.

http://bit.ly/1feOmLq

(This will take you directly to the video on Wiley Blackwell's companion website)

Video 47 Sciatic nerve root outlet: abnormal

Transrectal longitudinal section of a sciatic nerve root outlet (ventral aspect), demonstrating mild irregularity. The true clinical significance of these findings is difficult to determine and must be taken in consideration with the clinical and dynamic examination of the horse, the results of nuclear scintigraphy, diagnostic analgesia, radiography, and ultrasonography to rule out alternative sites of pathology.

http://bit.ly/1fB9dTZ

(This will take you directly to the video on Wiley Blackwell's companion website)

Video 48 Inter-transverse joint: fracture

Transrectal longitudinal section of the lumbosacral disc, sciatic nerve root, and inter-transverse joint (ventral aspect). The video starts over the lumbosacral disc, which is normal, before imaging the right sciatic nerve root outlet and the inter-transverse joint. There is a severe fracture of the inter-transverse joint. This horse presented with a severe lameness and nuclear scintigraphy demonstrated a significant increase in the uptake of the radionucleotide in that region.

http://bit.ly/1csoklb

(This will take you directly to the video on Wiley Blackwell's companion website)

Video 49 First and second coccygeal junction: fracture

Transrectal longitudinal section of the disc between the first and second coccygeal vertebrae (ventral aspect). There is significant irregularity to the disc with disruption of the adjacent bone margins. The horse presented with swelling and pain, and on nuclear scintigraphy there was a significant increase in the uptake of the radionucleotide in this area. The findings are consistent with a fracture of the first and second coccygeal junction.

http://bit.ly/1jS7K2l

(This will take you directly to the video on Wiley Blackwell's companion website)

ULTRASONOGRAPHIC-GUIDED INJECTIONS

Video 50 Stifle: medial femoral condylar defect

Ultrasound-guided injection into a subchondral bone defect (cyst) in the medial femoral condyle, performed under standing sedation. The needle is visualized, being directed into the subchondral bone defect.

http://bit.ly/1c3R28K

(This will take you directly to the video on Wiley Blackwell's companion website)

Video 51 Neck: caudal articular process joint

Ultrasound-guided injection into a caudal articular process joint (C6–C7). The needle is visualized on the left-hand side of the image and is being directed into the joint space. The fluid is visualized being injected into the joint space.

http://bit.ly/1mv09t2

(This will take you directly to the video on Wiley Blackwell's companion website)

Video 52 Sacroiliac region: cranial aspect

Ultrasound-guided injection into the cranial aspect of the sacroiliac region. The needle is directed in from the right-hand side of the image, deep to the iliac wing. The distal end of the needle can not be visualized close to the sacroiliac joint due to the artifact that is created by the overlying iliac wing. The back-flow of the fluid medication being injected can also sometimes be seen, as in this case.

http://bit.ly/1fiQHTY

(This will take you directly to the video on Wiley Blackwell's companion website)

Video 53 Lumbar facet joint

Ultrasound-guided injection into a lumbar facet joint (L3–L4). The needle is directed towards the joint from the left-hand side of the image.

http://bit.ly/1e9o7jm

(This will take you directly to the video on Wiley Blackwell's companion website)

SECTION 2

REPRODUCTION

Section 2a: Ultrasonography of the Stallion Reproductive Tract

CHAPTER ELEVEN

Ultrasonography of the Internal Reproductive Tract

Malgorzata A. Pozor

College of Veterinary Medicine, University of Florida, Gainesville, FL, USA

The internal reproductive tract in a normal stallion consists of the pelvic urethra, the two vasa deferentia with their glandular portions (ampullae), the paired vesicular glands (seminal vesicles), the bilobed prostate, and the paired bulbourethral glands (Figure 11.1).

Normal Anatomy

The vasa deferentia run from the epididymal tails, through the inguinal canals, and turn backwards towards the pelvic cavity, where their diameter increases to form the glandular portions of the vasa deferentia, called ampullae. The ampullae run over the dorsal surface of the urinary bladder, dive under the isthmus of the prostate, where they come very close together, often holding the uterus masculinus between them [1]. The vasa deferentia narrow down again, and continue their course within the urethral wall, beyond the prostatic isthmus, to join the excretory ducts of the vesicular glands, and to form the short ejaculatory ducts [2]. The ejaculatory ducts open on the colliculus seminalis, a summit of the urethral mucosa, as the ejaculatory orifices. In approximately 15% of individuals the vasa deferentia do not fuse with the excretory ducts of the vesicular glands, and open separately [1].

A rudimentary remnant of the uterus masculinus and the urogenital sinus, called utriculus masculinus, is often present within the colliculus seminalis and has its opening in the middle of this structure, between the ejaculatory orifices [3,4]. If the utriculus masculinus has a blind ending, it has a tendency to form cysts,

which can enlarge with age, and may affect the ejaculatory process [5].

The vesicular glands have a shape of pyriform sacs, which lie on both sides of the bladder, and are partially enclosed in the urogenital fold. Each gland consists of the fundus, the body, and the neck or the excretory duct, which runs under the prostate before it unites with the ipsilateral vas deferens [6]. The mucous membrane of the vesicular glands has a columnar epithelium and forms a network of numerous folds [1].

The prostate gland lies on the neck of the bladder and the beginning of the urethra, and has two lobes, connected by the isthmus. The lobes have prismatic shapes, while the isthmus is a thin transverse band lying on the junction of the bladder neck and the urethra. The prostatic isthmus covers terminal parts of the ampullae, the necks of the vesicular glands, and the distal portion of the uterus masculinus. The prostate is completely enclosed in the musculo-glandular capsule, and has numerous spheroid or ovoid lobules separated by trabeculae [1]. The secretion is collected in central spaces of the lobules, called tubular diverticula, and is excreted via prostatic ducts to the urethra on both sides of the colliculus seminalis [1].

Just behind the prostate the lumen of the pelvic urethra dilates, and it then narrows again at the level of the ischial arch, between the bulbourethral glands. The caudal part of the prostate and the pelvic urethra are covered by the urethralis muscle, which consists of dorsal and ventral layers of transverse fibers, forming an elliptical sphincter around the urethra [1].

The bulbourethral glands are ovoid in shape, and are located on the both sides of the pelvic urethra [1].

Atlas of Equine Ultrasonography, First Edition. Edited by Jessica A. Kidd, Kristina G. Lu, and Michele L. Frazer.
© 2014 John Wiley & Sons, Ltd. Published 2014 by John Wiley & Sons, Ltd.
Companion Website: www.wiley.com/go/kidd/equine-ultrasonography

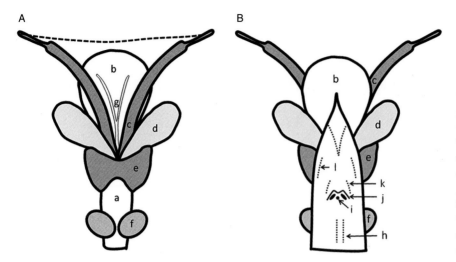

Figure 11.1 Diagram of the internal genitalia in a stallion: (A) dorsal view; (B) ventral view (urethra cut open). a: urethra; b: urinary bladder; c: ampulla of vas deferens; d: vesicular gland; e: prostate gland; f: bulbourethral gland; g: uterus masculinus; h: openings of bulbourethral ducts; i: opening to utriculus masculinus; j: colliculus seminalis; k: openings of prostatic ducts; l: openings of urethral glands.

These glands have a similar structure to the prostate and have numerous excretory ducts. The excretory ducts open to the urethra in two parallel rows of small papillae, just behind the prostatic ducts. Each bulbourethral gland is covered by the bulboglandularis muscle, which forms a capsule around the gland [6].

The blood supply to the stallion internal genitalia is derived mainly from the prostatic artery, which gives off the numerous branches to all accessory sex glands and the terminal portion of the vasa deferentia [7].

PALPATION *PER RECTUM*

Transrectal ultrasonography (TRUS) is the method of choice for evaluating the internal genitalia in stallions [8], but palpation *per rectum* is always done first. The pelvic urethra is most prominent and easy to find. It lies directly on the midline, and is detectable just before it curves around the ischial arch as a firm tube. Since the entire length of the pelvic urethra in a mature stallion is only 10–13 cm (4–5 inches) [1], the examiner does not need to introduce his/her hand deeper than up to the wrist in order to detect this structure. Palpation of the prostate gland *per rectum* is unrewarding in the horse [9]: the capsule is thick and its surface is flat, making detection of this gland difficult.

The next structures of interest are the ampullae of the vasa deferentia. Both ampullae are palpable on the neck of the bladder, just before they dive under the isthmus of the prostate. They are rigid small tubes, often lying very close together, and are easily palpable using fingertips. If the urinary bladder is large, the ampullae are more spread apart, and are found on the lateral aspects of the bladder.

Narrow parts of the vasa deferentia are too small to palpate. However, the internal vaginal rings should be located during palpation *per rectum*. In order to find one of these rings, the examiner's hand moves over the pelvic brim, turns laterally and sweeps the caudoventral aspect of the body wall on each side. The internal vaginal ring can be recognized as an elliptical slit, easily accommodating one to two fingertips. Palpation of the vas deferens or testicular vessels passing through the ring is difficult, but detection of a retained testis or herniating intestines is possible.

Palpation of the vesicular glands is often challenging in the stallion. They are detectable only when filled with secretion as fluctuant sacs lateral to the ampullae, or more cranially, occasionally hanging over the pelvic brim. The bulbourethral glands are not palpable, due to the thick muscular capsules that completely cover these glands.

ULTRASONOGRAPHY OF THE NORMAL INTERNAL REPRODUCTIVE TRACT

Transrectal ultrasound evaluation (TRUS) of the internal genitalia is performed immediately after palpation *per rectum*. A linear transducer with a high frequency (7.5–10 MHz), and high resolution is needed to detect the fine structure of the internal genitalia. Small, microconvex, transverse transducers are also very useful in evaluating the area of the colliculus seminalis. The easiest structure to detect is the pelvic urethra with its urethralis muscle (Figures 11.1, 11.2). The dorsal and ventral layers of this muscle appear as thick hypoe-

A

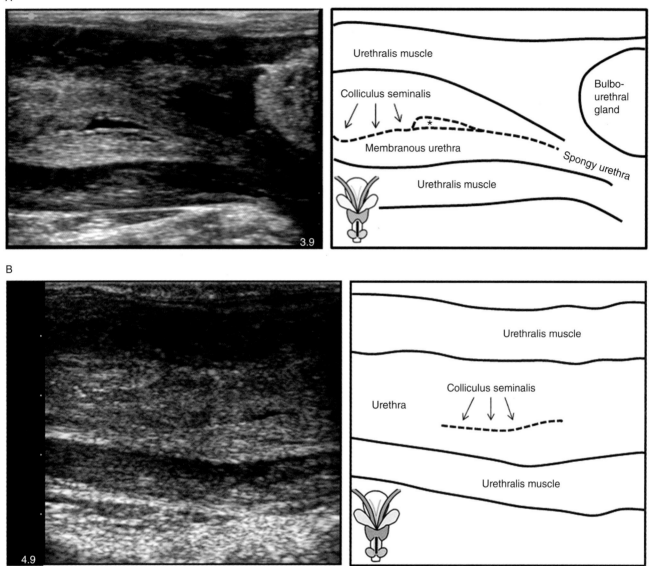

B

Figure 11.2   Pelvic urethra. (A) Ultrasound image of the distal part of the pelvic urethra (membranous urethra), and the proximal part of the spongy urethra. A small amount of anechoic semen, prostatic secretion, or urine is present in the urethral lumen, just behind the colliculus seminalis (*). (B) Ultrasound image of the membranous part of the pelvic urethra in a stallion. Urethralis muscle appears as two hypoechoic, thick lines, parallel to each other. Urethra is uniformly echogenic. This area often serves as a landmark during transrectal ultrasound examination of the internal genitalia of a stallion. (C) Ultrasound image of the membranous part of the pelvic urethra in a stallion. Colliculus seminalis is less echogenic than the urethra, and has a hyperechoic contour. (D) Ultrasound image of the membranous part of the pelvic urethra in an aged stallion. Terminal portions of the vasa deferentia (a) and the excretory ducts of the vesicular glands (b) contain hyperechoic concretions.

choic lines, when the linear transducer is positioned on the midline, parallel to the long axis of the animal. The urethra itself is an echogenic tube, but contains a few structures with varied echogenicity. The colliculus seminalis can be visualized in the most caudal aspect of the pelvic urethra (Figures 11.2A,C, 11.3, 11.4 (focus on 11.4J)). It appears as a roundish, echogenic or hypoechoic protrusion from the dorsal wall of the urethra, often with an anechoic outline due to the small accumulation of urine, prostatic secretion, or semen in this area. Single or multiple anechoic cysts of the colliculus seminalis may be also found (Figure 11.3). Most often, these cysts have an oval or tear shape, but can also be spindle shaped or rectangular. Occasionally, echogenic or hyperechoic contents may be observed within a cyst.

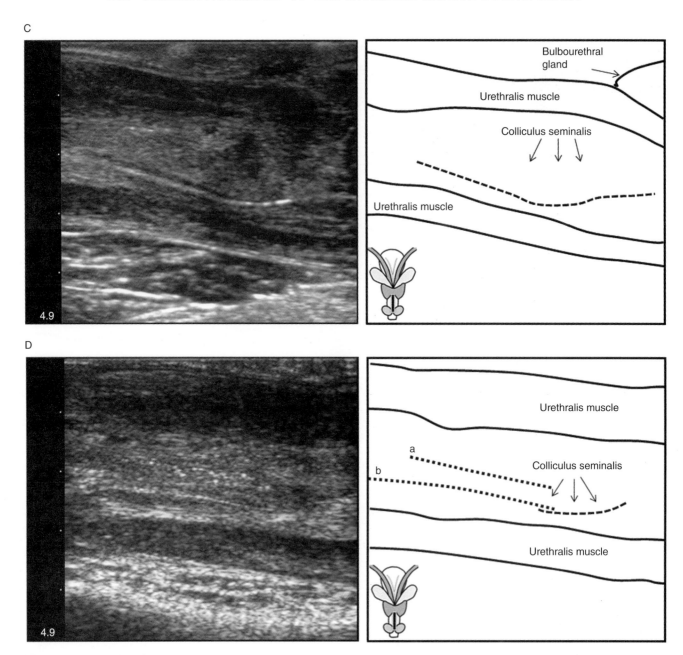

Figure 11.2 *Continued*

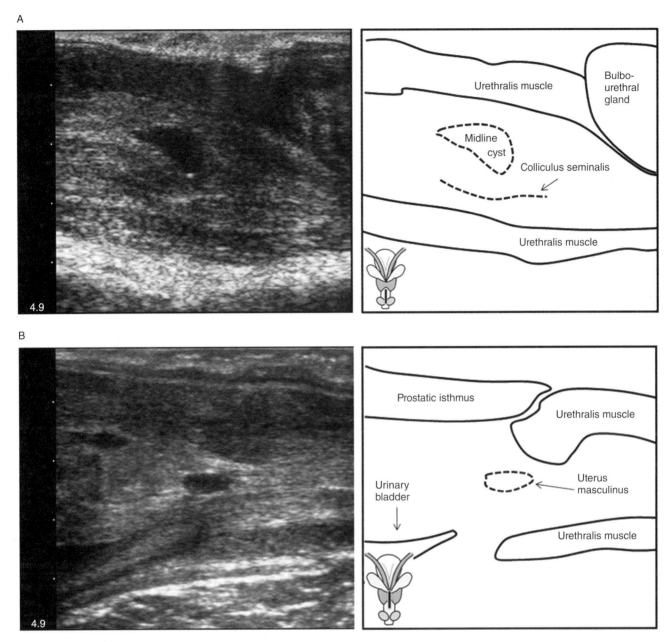

Figure 11.3 (A) Ultrasound image of a midline cyst of the colliculus seminalis in a stallion with ejaculatory problems. The cyst is anechoic and has a tear shape. (B) Ultrasound image of a small cyst of the uterus masculinus, which was found between the terminal parts of the ampullae of the vasa deferentia. This was an incidental finding; the stallion did not have any problems with ejaculation. (C) Ultrasound image of a spindle-shaped cyst of the uterus masculinus, which was found in the urogenital fold of a stallion. This stallion was experiencing ejaculatory problems. (D) Ultrasound image of a cyst near the terminal part of the ampulla of the vas deferens. A hyperechoic plug is present in the ampullary lumen.

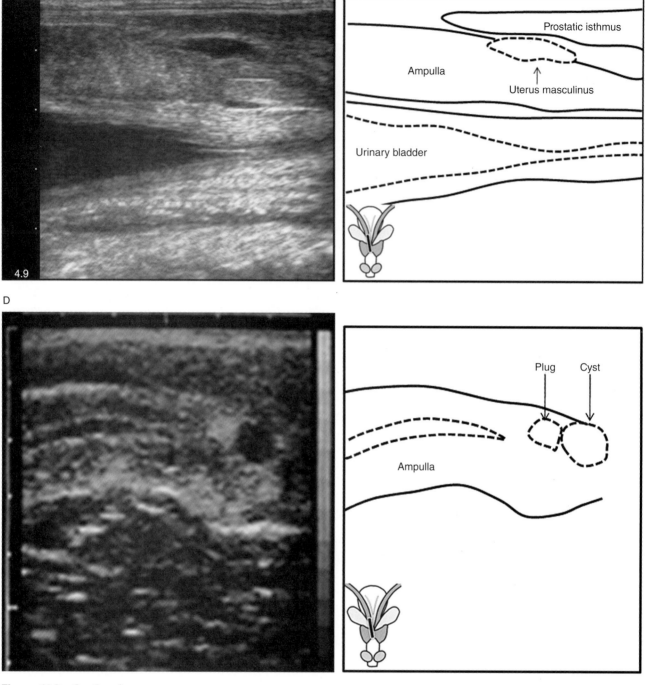

C

Prostatic isthmus

Ampulla

Uterus masculinus

Urinary bladder

4.9

D

Plug   Cyst

Ampulla

Figure 11.3 *Continued*

Figure 11.4 (A) Ultrasound image of the cross-sections of the ampullae of the vasa deferentia and the urinary bladder. (B) Ultrasound image of the cross-sections of the ampullae of vasa deferentia and the urinary bladder – close view. (C) Ultrasound image of the cross-sections of the ampullae of the vasa deferentia, the vesicular glands, and the urinary bladder. (D) Ultrasound image of the cross-sections of the ampullae of the vasa deferentia, and the prostatic isthmus in a sexually aroused stallion. (E) Ultrasound image of the cross-sections of the ampullae of the vasa deferentia, the excretory ducts of the vesicular glands, and the prostate. (F) Ultrasound image of the cross-sections of the ampullae of the vasa deferentia, the excretory ducts of the vesicular glands, and the prostate in a sexually aroused stallion. (G) Ultrasound image of the cross-sections of the very terminal portions of the ampullae of the vasa deferentia, the excretory ducts of the vesicular glands, and the prostatic ducts. (H) Ultrasound image of the cross-sections of the terminal portions of the vasa deferentia, excretory ducts of the vesicular glands, and the cyst of the uterus masculinus in a normal stallion. (I) Ultrasound image of the cross-sections of the terminal portions of the vasa deferentia, excretory ducts of the vesicular glands, and the utriculus masculinus in a normal stallion. (J) Ultrasound image of the cross-sections of the colliculus seminalis in a normal stallion.

A

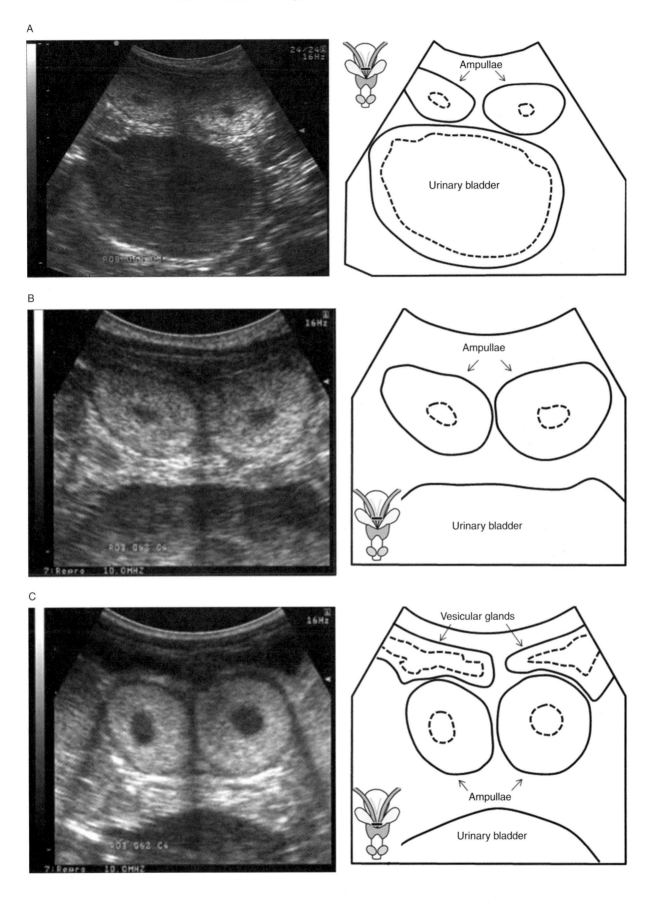

Ampullae

Urinary bladder

B

Ampullae

Urinary bladder

C

Vesicular glands

Ampullae

Urinary bladder

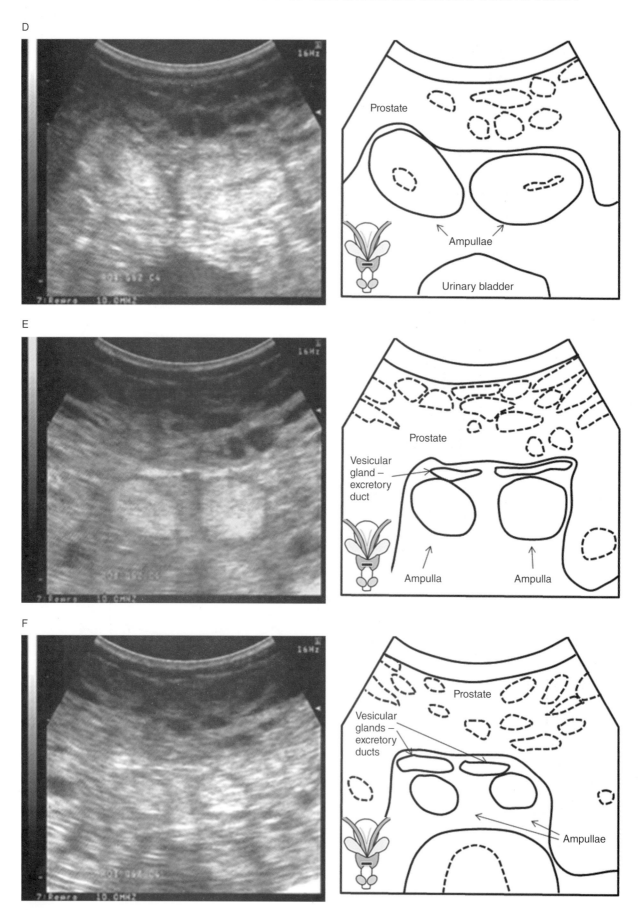

Figure 11.4 *Continued*

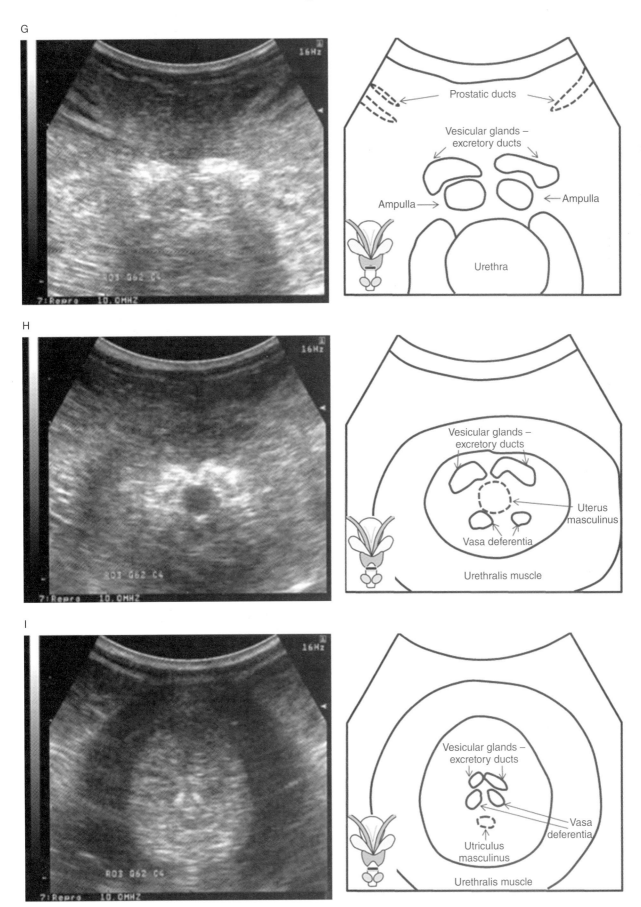

Figure 11.4 *Continued*

J

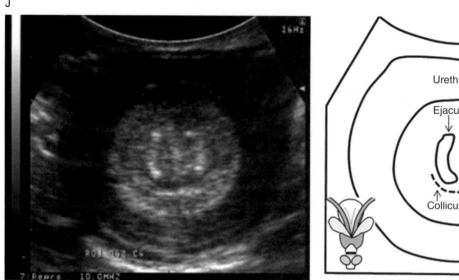
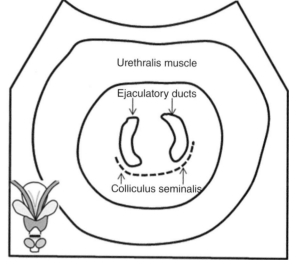

Figure 11.4 *Continued*

After localizing the colliculus seminalis, the examiner moves the transducer cranially, making an attempt to trace the ejaculatory ducts, the most terminal and narrow parts of the vasa deferentia, and the excretory ducts of the vesicular glands (Figures 11.4 (focus on 11.4G,H,I), 11.5). All these ducts travel through the urethral wall, and can be seen as hyperechoic lines, running parallel to each other. The vasa deferentia gradually thicken, and look like tips of sharpened pencils in a transition to the ampullae, which initially run under the isthmus of the prostate, and continue their path on the laterodorsal aspect of the urinary bladder (Figure 11.5, focus on 11.5B,C). Each ampulla of the vas deferens appears as a thick, echogenic tube, which is separated from the surrounding structures by the hyperechoic layer of connective tissue. This tube often has a small, anechoic lumen. Secretion of numerous tubulo-alveolar glands, which are present in the mucous membrane of the ampulla, can be visualized as hypoechoic spaces within the ampullary wall. Occasionally, hyperechoic, inspissated sperm appear in the lumen and in the glandular alveoli. Each ampulla can be traced individually, using the linear transducer, until it loses its glandular component and becomes a thin-walled vas deferens again (Figures 11.5, 11.6, 11.7, 11.8). Tracing the narrow part of the vas deferens is difficult, and requires good quality equipment and an experienced operator. The skill of tracing the vasa deferentia in a stallion can be quite helpful in localizing a cryptorchid testis (Figure 11.9).

The ultrasound appearance of the vesicular glands is very variable, and depends on the amount of secretion. Most often, the fundus of each gland can be found either cranially to the bladder and laterally to the ipsilateral ampulla, or on the level of the bladder, dorsal to the ipsilateral ampulla. The normal vesicular gland has a thin, echogenic wall, and hypoechoic or echolucent content in the lumen. However, if the secretion of the vesicular gland is very viscous and thick, it may have a highly echogenic or hyperechoic appearance. This is often observed in stallions that have been exposed to mares for a prolonged period of time, and have not had an opportunity to ejaculate. The shape of the most distal pole of the vesicular gland is usually roundish, like a fluid-filled sac, but it can be also triangular if the gland is compressed between the intestines and the bladder. The body of the gland can be traced caudally until it dives under the prostatic isthmus and becomes the excretory duct. The excretory ducts often have a hyperechoic appearance and penetrate through the urethral wall under a small angle. Occasionally, there is a small amount of anechoic or echogenic secretion in the body, or in the excretory ducts of the vesicular glands. Identifying empty vesicular glands may be difficult. In such cases, it may be easier to detect this gland tracing it from the midline of the urethra rather than trying to find it blindly (Figures 11.4 (focus on 11.4C,E,F,G,H,I) 11.6 (focus on 11.6B,C), 11.10, 11.11, 11.12, 11.13).

The lobes of the prostate gland are easily visualized using ultrasonography. They are found on the both sides of the neck of the urethra, with the linear transducer held parallel to the long axis of the animal. The

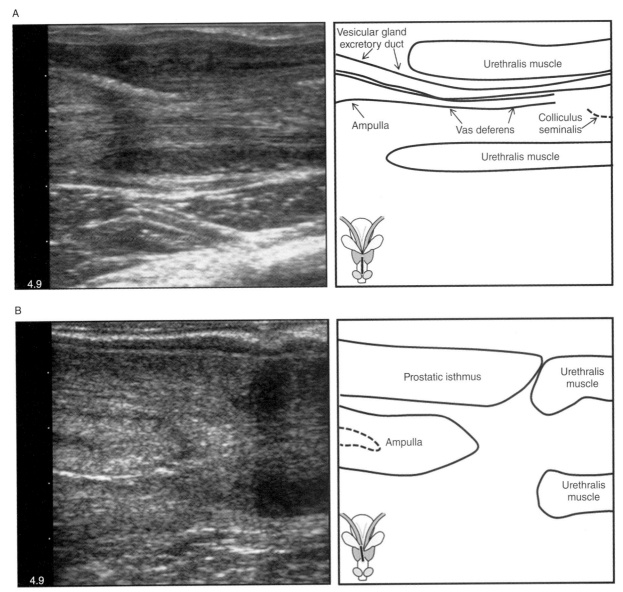

Figure 11.5 (A) Ultrasound image of the terminal portion of the vas deferens and the excretory duct of the vesicular gland. The vas deferens narrows down significantly before joining the excretory duct of the vesicular gland to form the ejaculatory duct. (B) Ultrasound image of the distal part of the prostatic part of the pelvic urethra. The ampulla of the vas deferens appears as an uniformly echogenic tube with a hypoechoic lumen. (C) Ultrasound image of the proximal part of the ampulla of the vas deferens. The ampulla is "diving" under the prostatic isthmus. (D) Color Doppler ultrasound image of the vas deferens branch of the prostatic artery. (E) Ultrasound image of the prostatic isthmus in a sexually aroused stallion. The prostatic acini are filled with anechoic secretion.

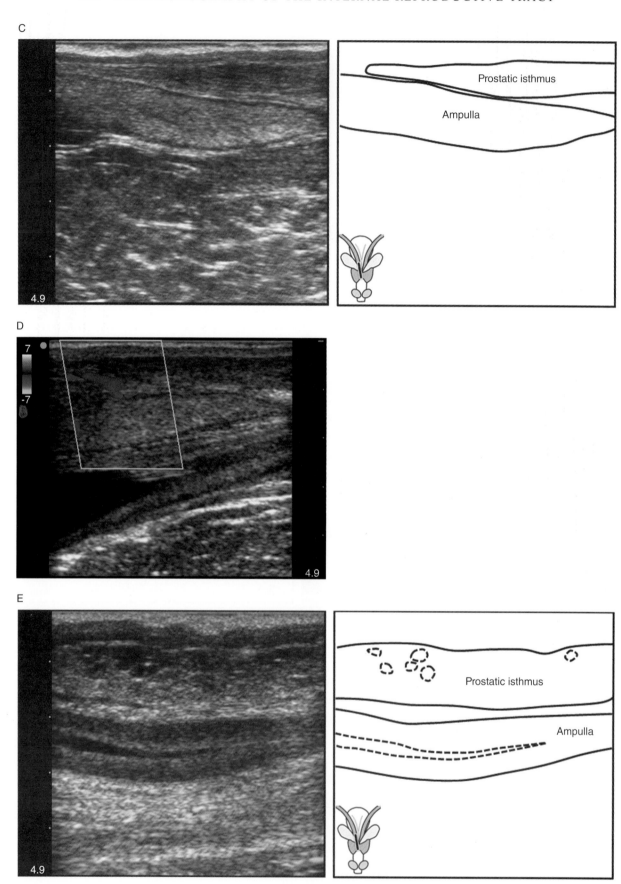

Figure 11.5   *Continued*

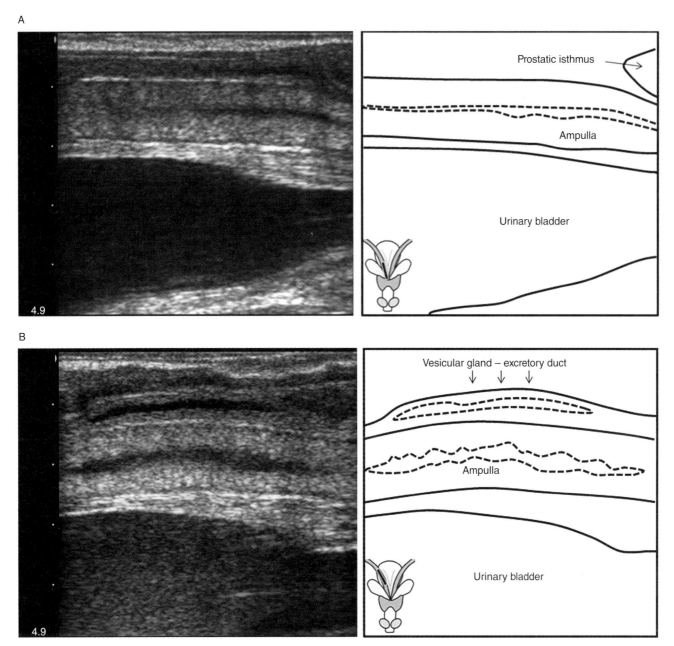

Figure 11.6   (A) Ultrasound image of the ampulla of the vas deferens – longitudinal section. The course of the entire ampulla is followed until it narrows down before entering the vaginal ring. (B) Ultrasound image of the ampulla of the vas deferens, as well as the excretory duct of the ipsilateral vesicular gland. (C) Ultrasound image of the distal part of the ampulla, which bends ventrally towards the ipsilateral vaginal ring. The fundus of the vesicular gland is lying on the top of the ampulla. (D) Ultrasound image of the narrow part of the vas deferens and its glandular part – the ampulla.

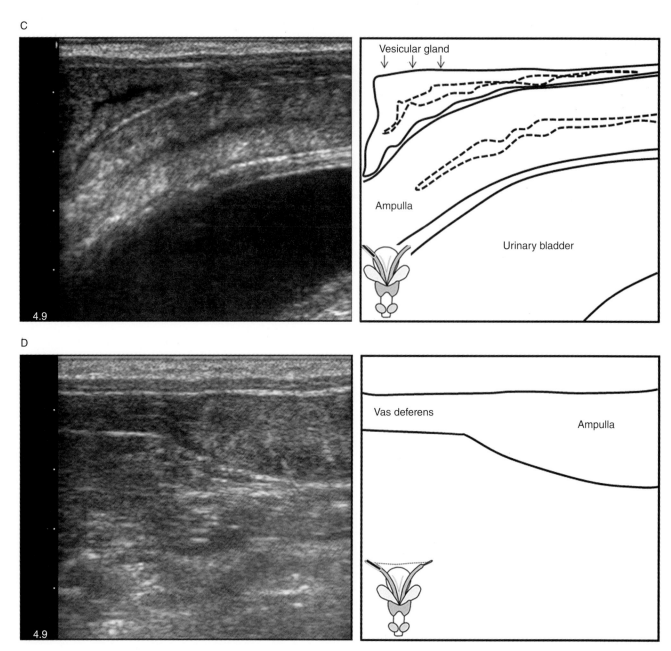

Figure 11.6 *Continued*

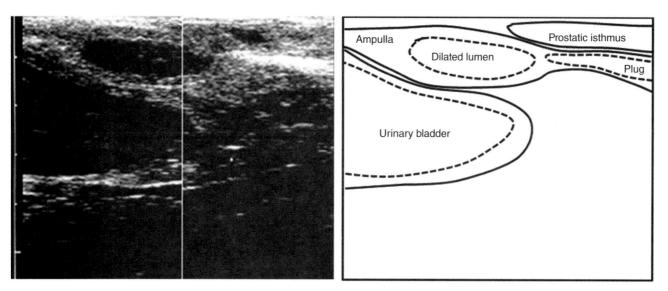

Figure 11.7 Ultrasound image of the occluded ampulla of the vas deferens. The ampullar lumen is significantly dilated. A long hyperechoic plug is present in the lumen of the vas deferens, just distal to the ampulla.

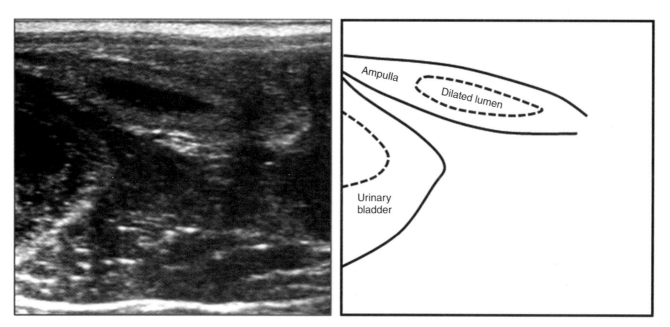

Figure 11.8 Ultrasound image of the dilated ampulla of the vas deferens.

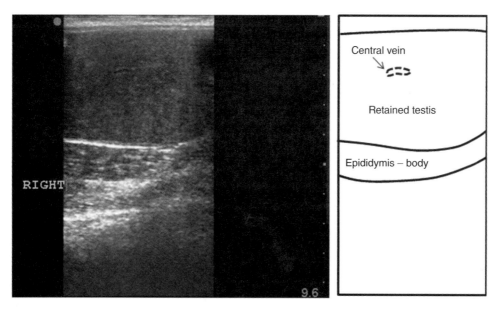

Figure 11.9 Ultrasound image of the abdominal testis of a cryptorchid. Typical features of testis are present: uniform echogenicity, hyperechoic capsule, anechoic central vein.

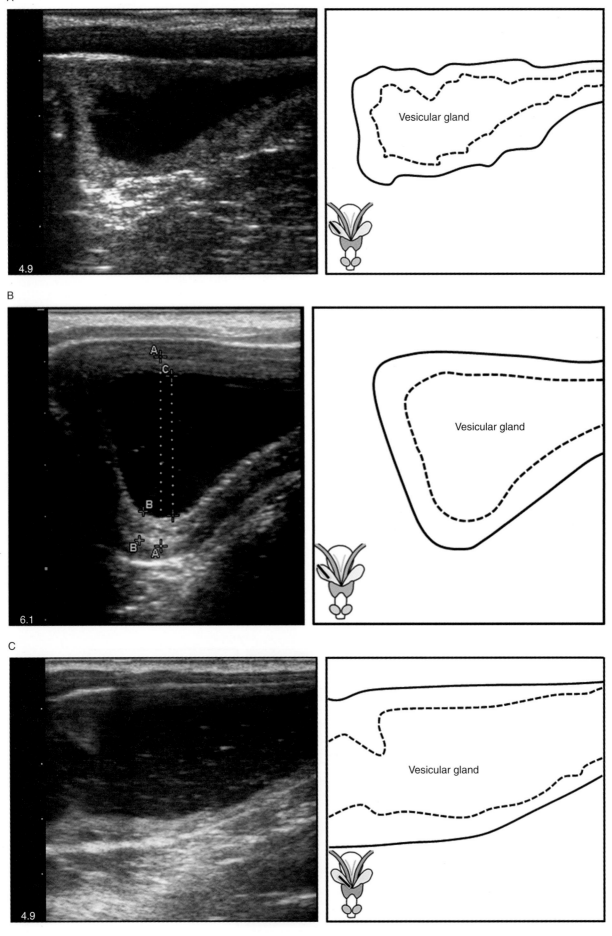

A

4.9

Vesicular gland

B

6.1

Vesicular gland

C

4.9

Vesicular gland

Figure 11.10 (A) Ultrasound image of the fundus of the vesicular gland. The gland contains anechoic secretion. (B) Ultrasound image of the fundus of the vesicular gland. Measurements of the total diameter of the gland, thickness of the glandular wall, as well as diameter of the glandular lumen are taken using the ultrasonographic caliper. (C) Ultrasound image of the vesicular gland in a stallion. The gland contains mildly echogenic secretion with hyperechoic concretions. This stallion was exposed to mares but did not have a chance to ejaculate for a prolonged period of time, which led to the formation of the viscous secretion. (D) Ultrasound image of the fundus of the vesicular gland. The gland contains hyperchoic secretion due to a high viscosity of the glandular secretion. (E) Ultrasound image of the vesicular gland in a teaser stallion.

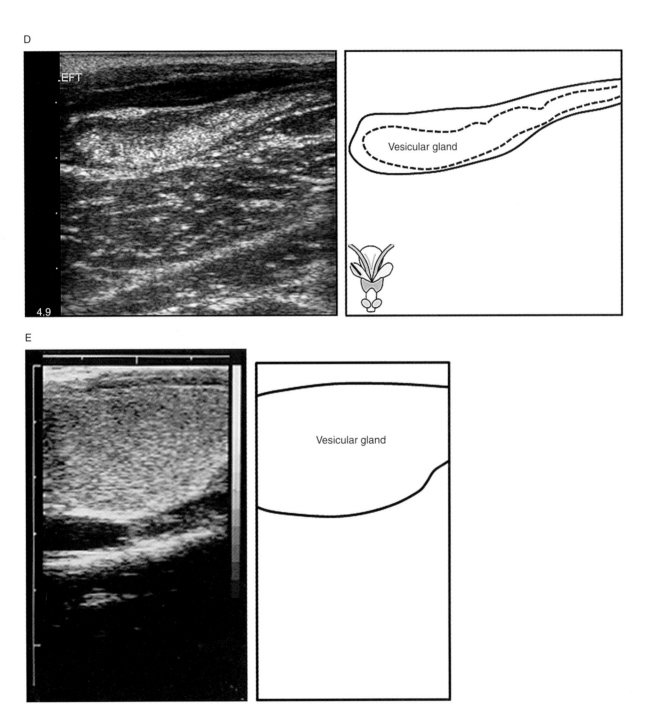

Figure 11.10 *Continued*

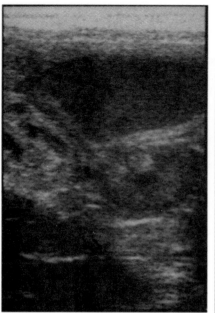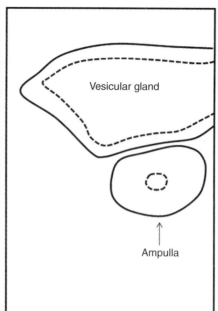

Figure 11.11 Ultrasound image of the vesicular gland and ampulla of the vas deferens (cross-section) in a stallion with seminal vesiculitis.

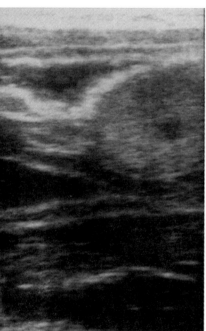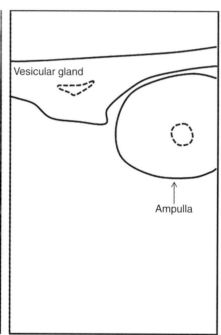

Figure 11.12 Ultrasound image of the vesicular gland and ampulla of the vas deferens (cross-section) in a stallion with seminal vesiculitis. The wall of the vesicular gland was thickened and had abnormally increased echogenicity.

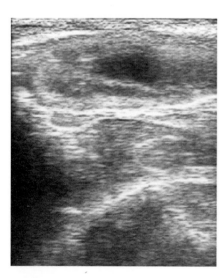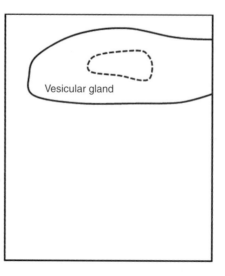

Figure 11.13 Ultrasound image of the vesicular gland in a stallion with seminal vesiculitis. The wall of the vesicular gland was significantly thickened.

ultrasound appearance of the prostate is often described as "Swiss-cheese like", due to the multiple acini filled with anechoic secretion. The sizes of the acini vary, depending on the level of sexual stimulation of a stallion. Stallions exposed to mares prior to examination have large amounts of prostatic secretion stored in the acini and the tubular diverticula, which are easy to visualize. Stallions not exposed to mares may have only a few, small, anechoic spaces in their prostates.

The rest of the prostatic lobe is uniformly echogenic with a hyperechoic capsule. The isthmus of the prostate is quite thin, but it may also contain spaces filled with secretion. The isthmus can be visualized dorsally to the distal portions of the ampullae (Figures 11.4 (focus on 11.4D,E,F,G), 11.5 (focus on 11.5B,C,D), 11.14, 11.15, 11.16).

The bulbourethral glands are usually examined at the end of the ultrasound examination of the internal

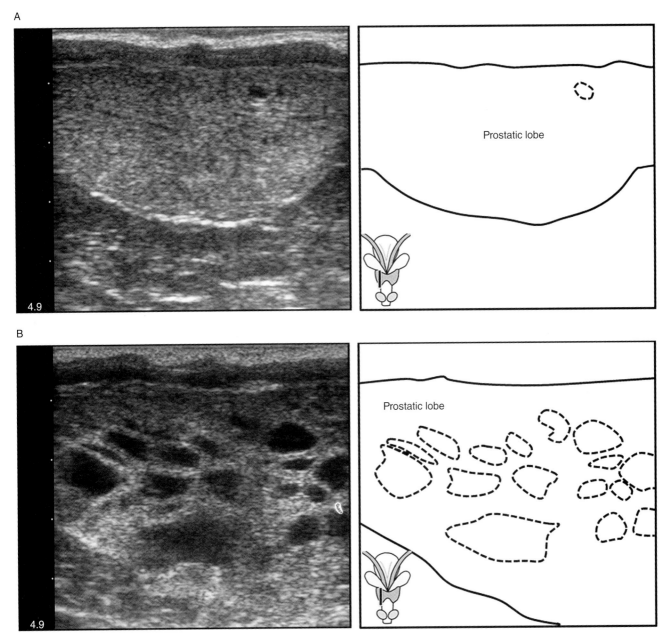

Figure 11.14 (A) Ultrasound image of the prostatic lobe of a stallion at sexual rest. (B) Ultrasound image of the prostatic lobe of a sexually aroused stallion. The prostatic acini are filled with anechoic secretion. (C) Ultrasound image of the prostatic lobe of a sexually aroused stallion – oblique section. The prostatic ducts are dilated by anechoic secretion. (D) Color Doppler ultrasound image of the prostatic vein. (E) Color Doppler ultrasound image of the prostatic vein and artery.

C

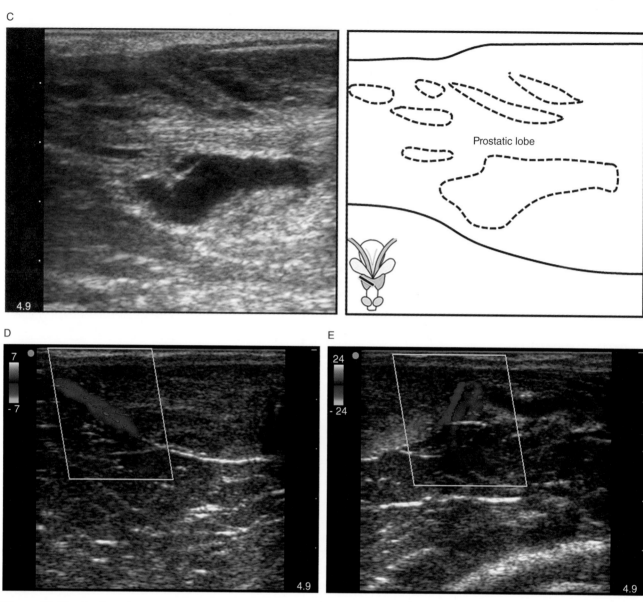

Prostatic lobe

D

E

Figure 11.14 *Continued*

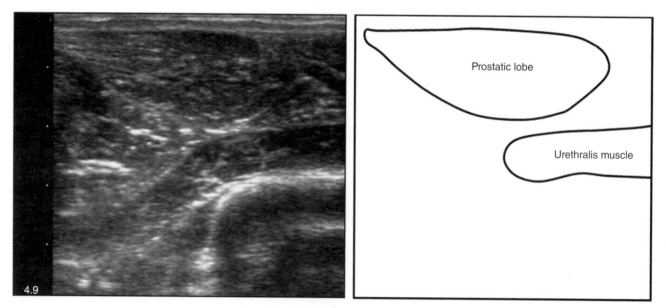

Prostatic lobe

Urethralis muscle

Figure 11.15 Ultrasound image of the prostatic lobe in a gelding. All accessory sex glands are significantly smaller in long-term geldings than in intact stallions [9].

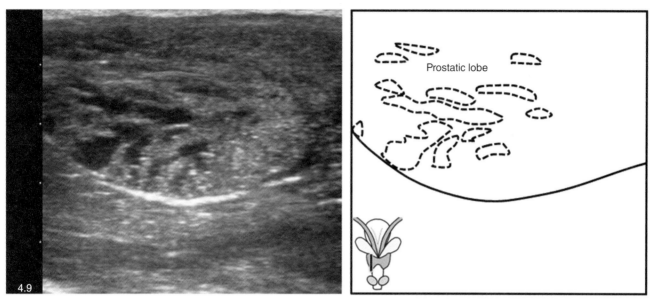

Figure 11.16 Ultrasound image of the prostatic lobe of the sexually aroused unilateral abdominal cryptorchid. This prostate has a size comparable with a prostate of an intact stallion, and contains a moderate amount of prostatic secretion.

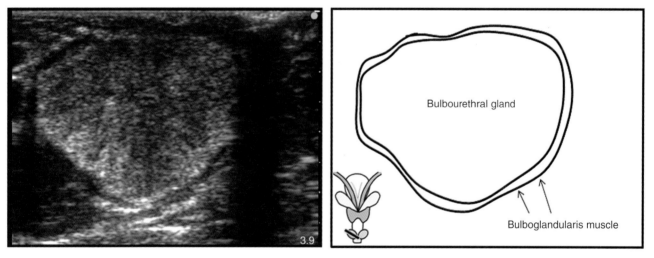

Figure 11.17 Ultrasound image of the bulbourethral gland in a sexually rested stallion. The gland is surrounded by the hypoechoic bulboglandularis muscle.

genitalia of a stallion. They are found on both sides of the most caudal portion of the pelvic urethra, at the level of the ischial arch where the urethra narrows. With the hand of the examiner partially out of the rectum, a transducer is moved slightly laterally and angled slightly caudolaterally to image the longitudinal section of the bulbourethral gland. The muscular capsule is hypoechoic and gives a nice outline of this ovoid gland. The appearance of the parenchyma of this gland is similar to that of the pros-

tate lobe. The number and size of anechoic spaces with glandular secretions visualized during the examination depends on the sexual stimulation of the stallion (Figures 11.17, 11.18, 11.19, 11.20).

The internal genitalia of the stallion can be also evaluated using small, micro-convex transducers, which are available as either "I" or "T" shaped finger-grip probes. These transducers are particularly helpful in visualizing cross-sections of the urethra, colliculus seminalis, ejaculatory ducts, vasa deferentia with

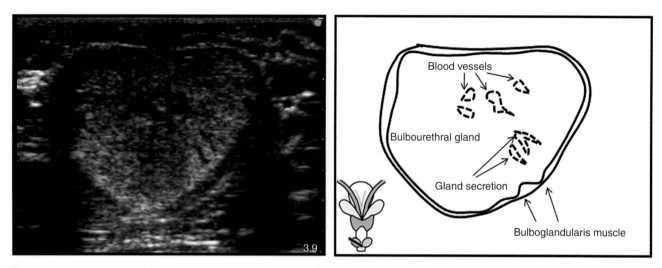

Figure 11.18 Ultrasound image of the bulbourethral gland. Blood vessels appear as hypoechoic spaces in the center of the gland.

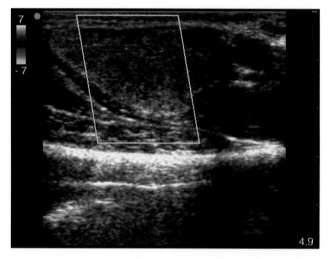

Figure 11.19 Color Doppler ultrasound image of the bulbourethral gland. Blood vessels appear as red and blue lines in the center of the gland.

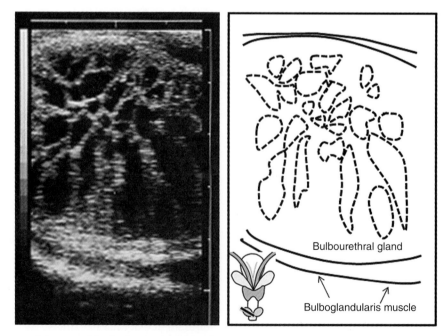

Figure 11.20 Ultrasound image of the bulbourethral gland in a teaser stallion after a long exposure to mares. The sacs and tubules are dilated with anechoic secretion.

ampullae, as well as the excretory ducts of the vesicular glands and the prostatic isthmus. Cysts of the colliculus masculinus and their effects on the ejaculatory ducts can be accurately identified using these transducers (Figure 11.4).

Blood vessels can be visualized using color Doppler ultrasonography. Prostatic arteries and their branches are located on the lateral and dorsal aspects of the accessory sex glands [7].

PATHOLOGIES OF THE INTERNAL GENITALIA

The most common pathologic condition affecting the internal genitalia of stallions is ampullary occlusion. This problem occurs periodically in some individuals after prolonged periods of time of sexual abstinence and lack of ejaculation. The inspissated sperm accumulates in the terminal portions of the vasa deferentia causing partial or complete occlusion [10, 11]. The back flow of semen causes significant distention of the ampullary lumen (Figure 11.7). Large cysts of the uterus masculinus in the area of the prostatic isthmus, or cysts of the utriculus masculinus in the colliculus seminalis, may compress the vasa deferentia or ejaculatory ducts and affect the ejaculatory process (Figures 11.21, 11.22, 11.23). Furthermore, this may lead to the accumulation of sperm and bacteria, which form firm concretions causing occlusion. The clinical signs of this condition are oligospermia, azoospermia, a low percentage of morphologically normal sperm, a high percentage of tail-less sperm heads, and a palpable enlargement of the distal ampullae. Ultrasound evaluation reveals the distended lumen of the ampullae, with either hypoechoic or echogenic contents. Hyperechoic concretions are also often found in the terminal, narrow parts of the vas deferens of the affected stallions (Figures 11.3 (focus on 11.3D), 11.7, 11.8). All stallions with typical symptoms of ampullary occlusion have to be carefully examined for presence of the cystic uterus masculinus and the cystic utriculus masculinus prior to any treatment. Stallions accumulating sperm due to sexual abstinence respond well to manual massage of the ampullae, and/or administration of oxytocin (20I.U., IV) 5–10 minutes before ejaculation. Large numbers of immotile spermatozoa are usually expelled. Small concretions of inspissated sperm can also be found in the first ejaculate. Multiple collections of semen are recommended in order to remove sperm stored in the excretory system. The quality of semen usually improves significantly after several semen collections. In contrast to so-called "sperm accumulators", stallions with ampullary occlusion due to the physical compression of the vas deferens do not respond to manual massage of the ampullae *per rectum*. Furthermore, low frequency of ejaculations is recommended for these individuals, since a high pressure of semen in the ampullae seems to be necessary to force its contents through the compressed ducts into the

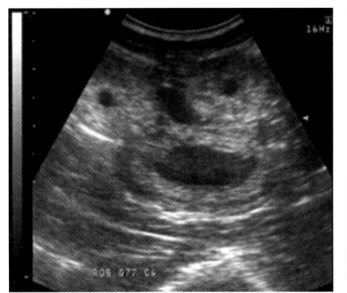
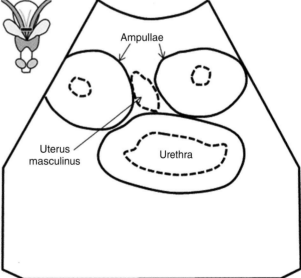

Figure 11.21 Ultrasound image of the cross-sections of the ampullae of the vasa deferentia and the urinary bladder. A large cyst of the uterus masculinus is also present between the ampullae. This stallion was experiencing ejaculatory problems.

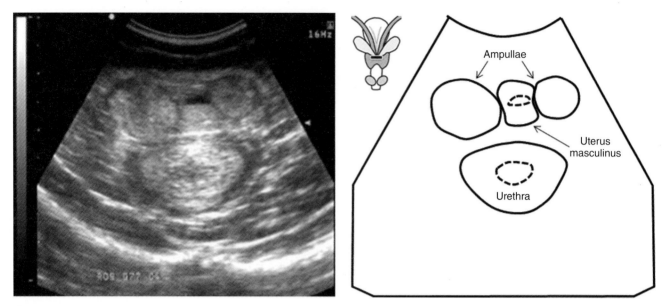

Figure 11.22 Ultrasound image of the cross-sections of the ampullae of the vasa deferentia and the urinary bladder in a stallion with ejaculatory problems. The multicystic uterus masculinus has anechoic, watery content, as well as echogenic, highly viscous content.

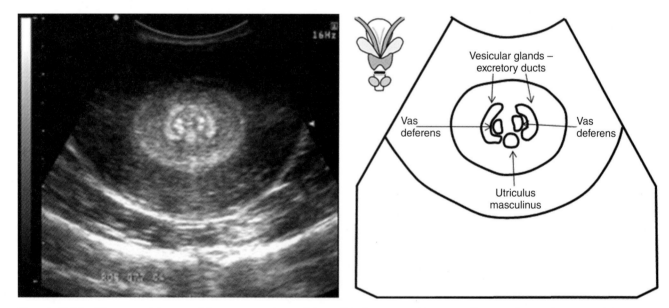

Figure 11.23 Ultrasound image of the cross-sections of the colliculus seminalis in a stallion with ejaculatory problems. The terminal portions of the vasa deferentia contain numerous hyperechoic concretions.

urethra, and to trigger the ejaculatory process [5]. Administration of oxytocin prior to semen collection seems to also be helpful in these cases. Ultrasound evaluation performed after successful ejaculation confirms that the diameter and contents of the ampullary lumen are appreciably decreased.

Seminal vesiculitis is a less common pathologic condition in stallions (Figures 11.11, 11.12, 11.13). Usually,

it is due to bacterial infection, but the exact pathogenesis of this condition is not well known yet. Perhaps a reflux of urine and semen during ejaculation can contribute to this infection, or an ascending or descending infection comes from other sites of the reproductive tract. Clinical signs include a presence of inflammatory cells and/or blood in the ejaculate, positive bacterial culture from semen, and/or enlarged or painful vesicular glands [12]. Typically, as seen in the ultrasound evaluation, inflamed vesicular glands have thickened walls and cloudy luminal contents (Figures 11.11, 11.12, 11.13) [13]. However, echogenic luminal contents within seminal vesicles are not always indicative of seminal vesiculitis, as this appearance may also be seen in normal stallions [14]. Therefore, presumptive diagnosis is made from semen evaluation rather than based on the ultrasound examination alone. Seminal vesiculitis can be treated using antibiotics delivered directly into the lumen of the vesicular glands using a flexible endoscope. However, there are reports of a limited success with treatment of seminal vesiculitis using systemic antibiotics, such as enrofloxacin.

A Powerpoint file showing the recommended order of scanning for the stallion internal reproductive tract is available on the companion website: www.wiley.com/go/kidd/equine-ultrasonography.

REFERENCES

[1] Sisson, S. (1910) *A Textbook of Veterinary Anatomy*. W.B. Saunders, Philadelphia.

[2] McFadyean, J. (1884) *The Anatomy of the Horse. A Dissection Guide*. W&AK Johnson, Edinburgh and London.

[3] Swoboda, A. (1929) Beitrag zur Kenntnis des Utriculus Masculinus der Haustiere. *Zeitschrift für Anatomie und Entwicklungsgeschichte*, 89, 494–512.

[4] Guyon, L. (1939) Recherches sur Litricule Prostatique chez le Cheval Entier ou Castre. *Comptes Rendus des Séances de la Société de Biologie et de ses Filiales*, 131, 1167–1169.

[5] Pozor, M., Macpherson, M.L., Troedsson, M.H., *et al.* (2011) Midline cysts of colliculus seminalis causing ejaculatory problems in stallions. *Journal of Equine Veterinary Science*, 31, 722–731.

[6] Little, V.L. & Holyoak, G.R. (1992) Reproductive anatomy and physiology of the stallion. *Veterinary Clinics of North America: Equine Practice*, 8, 1–29.

[7] Ginther, O.J. (2007) *Ultrasonic Imaging and Animal Reproduction: Color-Doppler Ultrasonography. Book 4*. Equiservices, Cross Plains, WI.

[8] Little, T.V. & Woods, G.L. (1987) Ultrasonography of accessory sex glands in the stallion. *Journala of Reproduction and Fertility*, 35(Suppl), 87–94.

[9] Nickel, R., Schummer, A., & Seiferle, E. (1979) *The Viscera of the Domestic Mammals*. Springer-Verlag, Hamburg.

[10] Love, C.C., Riera, F.L., Oristaglio, R.M., *et al.* (1992) Sperm occluded (plugged) ampullae in the stallion. *Proceedings of the Society for Theriogenology*, 117–125.

[11] Klewitz, J., Probst, J., Baackmann, C., *et al.* (2012) Obstruktion der Samenleiterampullen ["plugged ampullae"] als Ursache einer Azoospermie bei einem Hengst. *Pferdeheilkunde*, 28, 14–17.

[12] Varner, D.D., Blanchard, T.L., Brinsko, S.P., *et al.* (2000) Techniques for evaluating selected reproductive disorders of stallions. *Animal Reproduction Science*, 60–61, 493–509.

[13] Malmlgren, L. (1992) Ultrasonography: a new diagnostic tool in stallions with genital tract infection? *Acta Veterinaria Scandinavica*, 88(Suppl), 91–94.

[14] Pozor, M. & McDonnell, S.M. (2002) Ultrasonographic measurements of accessory sex glands, ampullae, and urethra of normal stallions of various size types. *Theriogenology*, 58, 1425–1433.

CHAPTER TWELVE

ULTRASONOGRAPHY OF THE PENIS

Malgorzata A. Pozor

College of Veterinary Medicine, University of Florida, Gainesville, FL, USA

ANATOMY

The stallion penis consists of three parts: the root, the body or the shaft, and the glans. The root has two crura, which are attached to the tubera ischii via the ischiocavernous muscles on each side. Suspensory ligaments deliver further support and stabilization to this attachment [1]. The crura fuse below the ischial arch and form the laterally compressed corpus cavernosum. The urethra is surrounded by the corpus spongiosum, which starts at the bulb of the penis and continues all the way to the urethral process. The urethra lies in the urethral groove, on the ventral side of the penile body [1]. The bulbospongiosus muscle runs along the ventral aspect of the penis and encloses the corpus spongiosum of the urethra (Figure 12.1). The corpus cavernosum is enclosed by a thick fibrous sheet termed the tunica albuginea (Figure 12.1), the elastic properties of which allow limited expansion of the penis during erection [2]. Further anteriorly, the corpus cavernosum divides into three processes – one central process and two lateral processes. The central process is the longest and runs all the way into the glans penis. The glans penis is the most distal part of the penis and has two distinct parts – neck and corona glandis. The erectile body of the glans is called the corpus spongiosum glandis (Figure 12.2). The corpus spongiosum glandis has a dorsal process, which covers the dorsal and lateral sides of the corpus cavernosum penis for approximately 10–15 cm (4–6 inches) [3]. The glans can expand significantly during erection due to a profound elasticity of the surrounding tissues. The most distal part of the glans penis has a deep depression, the fossa glandis, which hosts the terminal portion of the urethra, the urethral process. Furthermore, the fossa glandis has a bilocular diverticulum, called the urethral sinus [3]. Smegma may accumulate in the urethral sinus and form thick "beans", which are often manually removed prior to semen collection (Figure 12.2).

The main source of blood supply to the stallion penis is the internal pudendal artery, as well as the obturator artery [4]. The internal pudendal artery gives off the artery of the bulb, the deep artery of the penis, and the dorsal artery of the penis. The obturator artery gives off the middle artery of the penis, which anastomoses with the dorsal artery of the penis and with the cranial artery of the penis [5]. The latter comes from the external pudendal artery.

ULTRASOUND EVALUATION OF THE STALLION PENIS

Ultrasound evaluation of the stallion penis is not performed routinely. However, this technique is helpful in detecting penile pathologies, mostly associated with paraphimosis, priapism, and penile trauma. Prior to the ultrasound examination of the penis in a normal stallion, sedatives are given to induce the penis to drop from the preputial cavity. Phenothiazine derivatives should be avoided as they can cause paraphimosis. High-frequency (7.5–10 MHz) linear or micro-convex transducers are recommended. Prior to the examination, the penis should be washed with warm water in order to remove smegma, which could interfere with penetration of the ultrasound waves. A copious amount of warm ultrasound gel is then applied to the penis. Once the examination is completed, the remaining gel is washed off with warm water and a cotton towel.

The ultrasound architecture of the corpora cavernosa, the corpus spongiosum of the urethra, and the

Atlas of Equine Ultrasonography, First Edition. Edited by Jessica A. Kidd, Kristina G. Lu, and Michele L. Frazer.
Companion Website: www.wiley.com/go/kidd/equine-ultrasonography

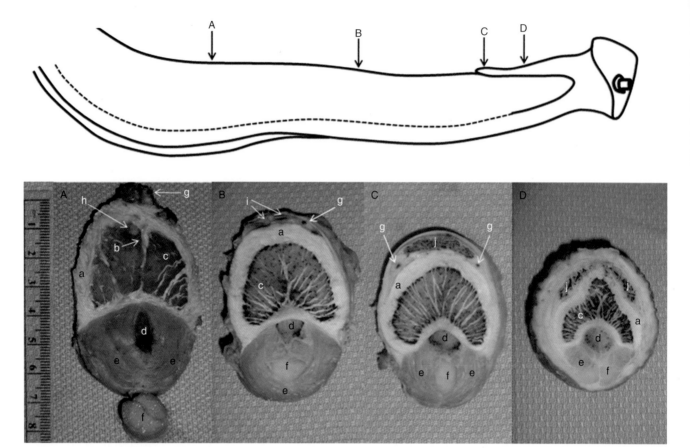

Figure 12.1 Diagram of stallion penis and cross-sections through a specimen: A – proximal part of the penile body; B – middle part of the penile body; C – free part of the penile body; D – distal part of the penile body. a: tunica albuginea; b: incomplete septum; c: corpus cavernosum; d: corpus spongiosum and urethra; e: bulbospongiosus muscle; f: retractor penis muscle; g: dorsal artery; h: deep artery; i: dorsal vein; j: corpus spongiosum glandis – dorsal process.

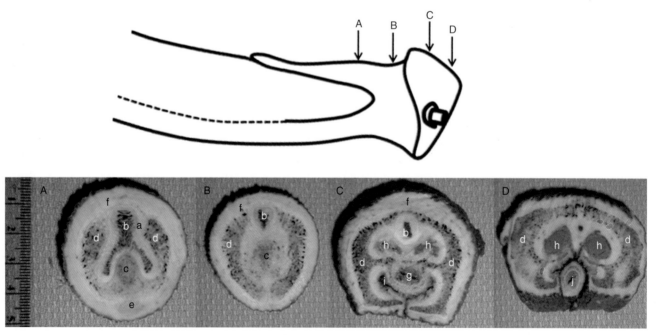

Figure 12.2 Diagram of a distal part of stallion penis and cross-sections through a specimen: (A) distal penis; (B) collum glandis; (C) corona glandis; (D) distal part of the glans penis. a: tunica albuginea; b: corpus cavernosum; c: corpus spongiosum and urethra; d: corpus spongiosum glandis; e: retractor penis muscle; f: connective tissue and penile fascias; g: urethra; h: diverticula of urethral sinus; i: fossa glandis; j: urethral process.

corpus spongiosum of the glans are visualized on the longitudinal and cross-sections of the organ (Figures 12.3, 12.4, 12.5, 12.6, 12.7, 12.8, 12.9, 12.10, 12.11, 12.12, 12.13, 12.14). The integrity of all these structures is carefully assessed. Color and power Doppler ultrasonography may be helpful in visualizing the vascularization of the penis (Figures 12.3, 12.6, 12.7). Ultrasound evaluation of the erect penis is difficult in stallions. Some stallions may tolerate ultrasound evaluation after they have been exposed to estrous mare urine, which usually causes them to develop a penile erection. However, the operator has to be very cautious in order to avoid injury.

Spectral Doppler ultrasound assessment of the penile blood flow is often performed in men with erectile dysfunction after pharmacological induction of erection [6]. Prostaglandin E1 is injected into the corpora cavernosa in a "stepwise" fashion and any changes in the diameter of the cavernosal arteries, as well as in the peak systolic velocity (PSV) in these blood vessels are determined. Similar tests may be introduced to veterinary medicine.

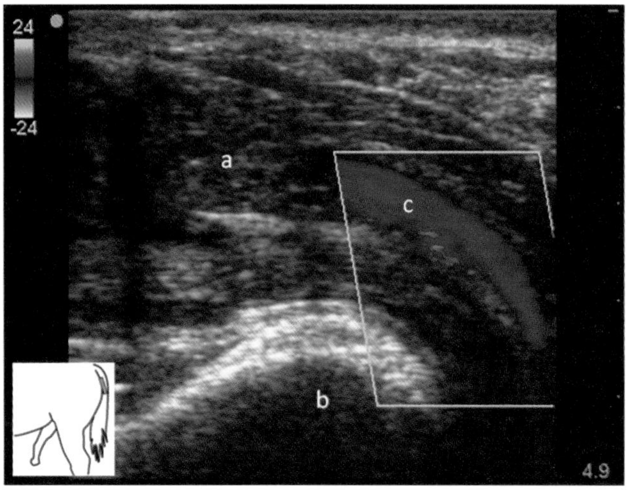

PENILE PATHOLOGIES

The most common penile pathology in a stallion is paraphimosis (inability to retract the penis back into the prepuce). Paraphimosis affects normal blood and lymphatic circulation in the penis leading to gravitational edema, especially in the preputial ring (Figures 12.15, 12.16, 12.17). The corpus spongiosum of the glans is thickened and contains dilated vessels and trabeculae (Figure 12.18). Blood flow is slow and blood clots are often formed in the corpus cavernosum, which can be visualized using ultrasonography (Figure 12.19). Priapism (persistent erection) occurs rarely in stallions, but can be devastating to the reproductive career.

Hyperechoic contents in the trabeculae of the corpus cavernosum and the corpus spongiosum of the glans

Figure 12.3   Color Doppler ultrasound image of the dorsal artery of the penis at the level of the ischial arch. a: penile bulb; b: ischial arch; c: dorsal artery of the penis.

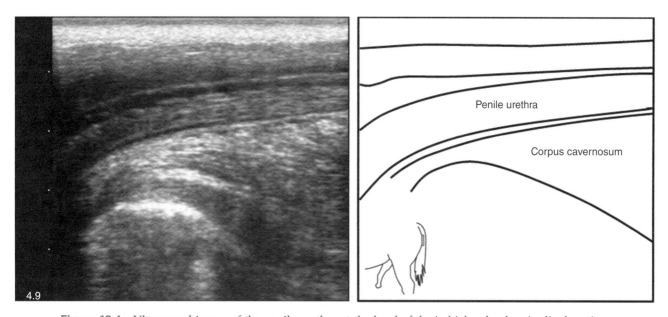

Figure 12.4   Ultrasound image of the penile urethra at the level of the ischial arch – longitudinal section.

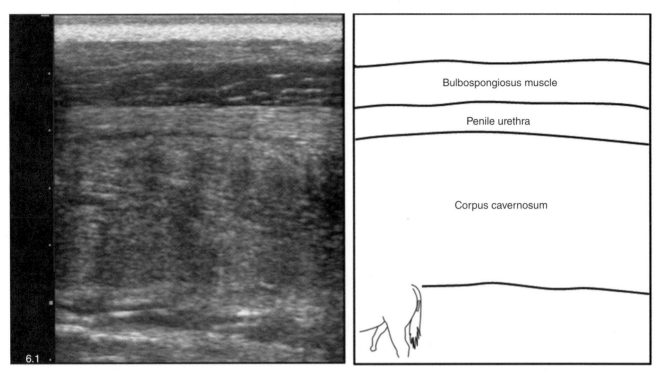

Figure 12.5 Ultrasound image of the proximal part of the penile body – longitudinal section.

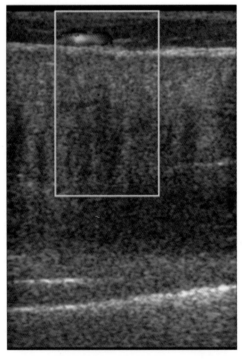

Figure 12.6 Power Doppler ultrasound image of the erect penis – longitudinal section. The dorsal artery of the penis is visualized on the dorsal surface of the penis (orange color).

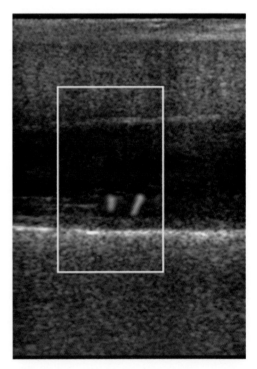

Figure 12.7 Power Doppler ultrasound image of the erect penis – longitudinal section. The helicine arteries appear as short, straight lines. These vessels assume a coiled disposition again when the penis becomes flaccid.

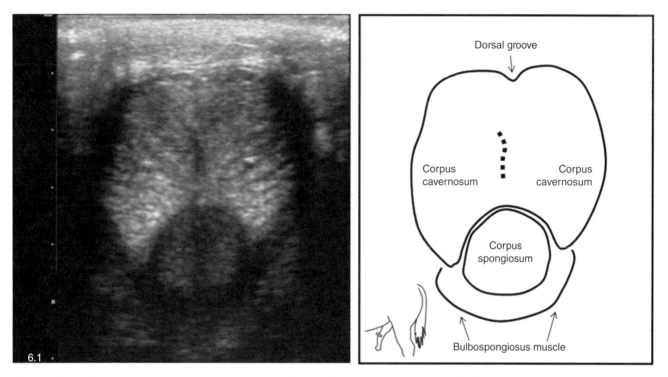

Figure 12.8   Ultrasound image of the free part of the penile body – cross-section. Trabeculae of the corpus cavernosum appear as hypoechoic spots. The incomplete septum (septum pectiniforme) and the dorsal groove are visible.

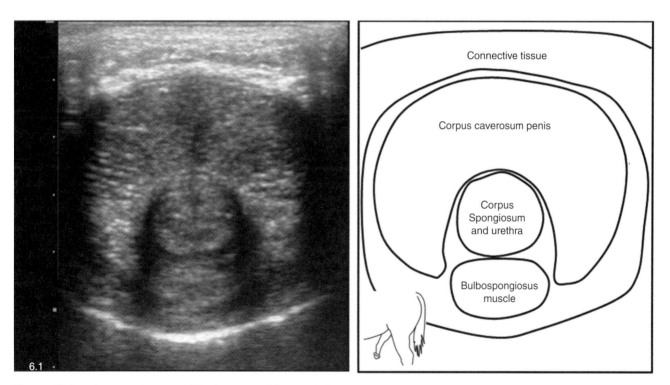

Figure 12.9   Ultrasound image of the free part of the penile body. The cross-section of the more distal part of the penile body becomes round.

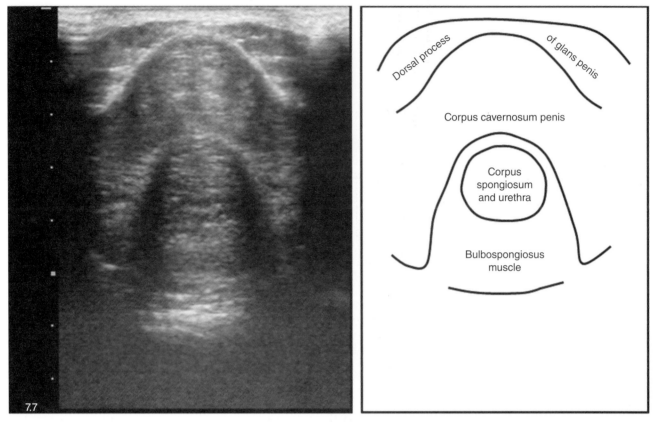

Figure 12.10 Ultrasound image of the penile body. The dorsal process of glans penis covers the dorsal aspect of the corpus cavernosum.

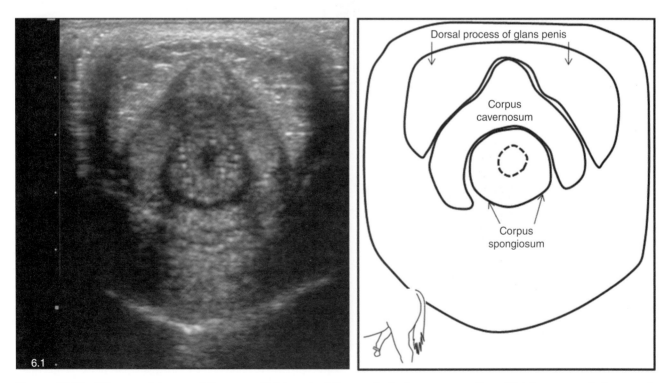

Figure 12.11 Ultrasound image of the more distal part of the penile body – cross-section. Distal process of glans penis becomes larger, while the corpus cavernosum becomes smaller.

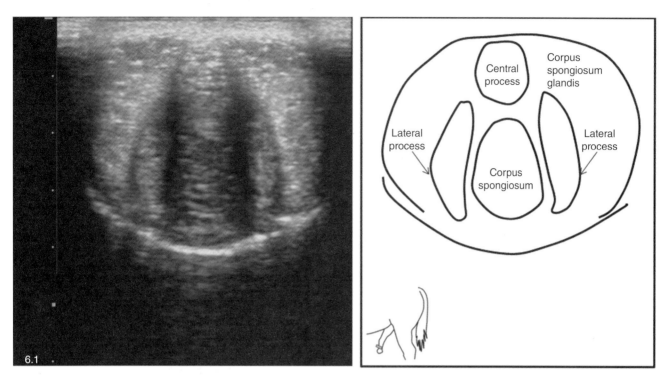

Figure 12.12 Ultrasound image of the distal part of the penile body – cross-section. Corpus cavernosum divides into three processes: long central, and two blunt, short lateral processes.

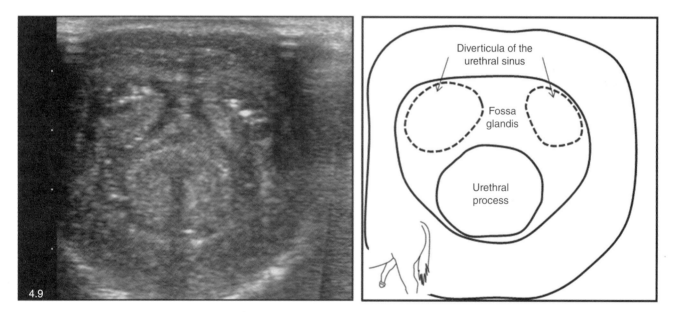

Figure 12.13 Ultrasound image of the glands penis. Hyperechoic smegma is accumulated in the urethral sinus.

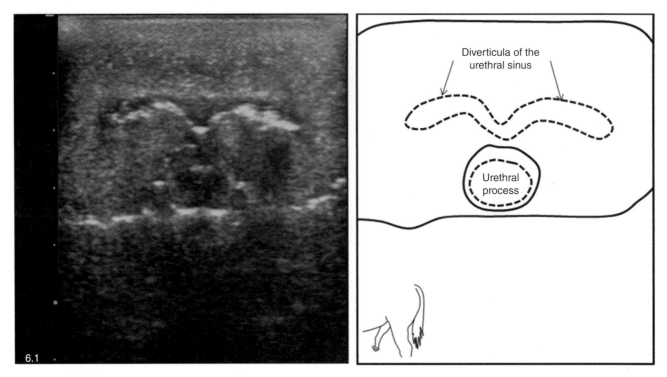

Figure 12.14 Ultrasound image of the urethral process and the urethral sinus with accumulated smegma.

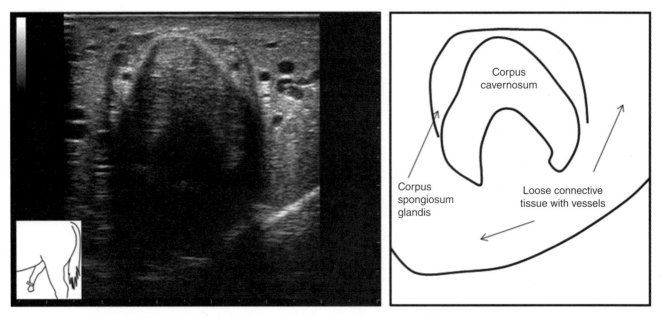

Figure 12.15 Ultrasound image of the distal part of the penile body in a stallion with chronic paraphimosis. Massive edema of the prepuce and the corona glandis are present. Vessels are engorged.

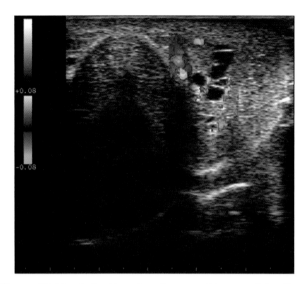

Figure 12.16   Color Doppler ultrasound image of the distal part of the penile body in a stallion with chronic paraphimosis. The preputial vessels are dilated.

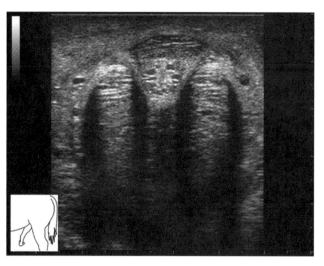

Figure 12.18   Ultrasound image of the distal part of the penile body in a stallion with chronic paraphimosis (ventral aspect). Trabeculae in the corpus spongiosum and the corpus cavernosum are engorged.

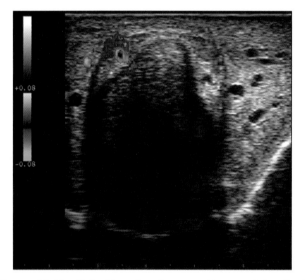

Figure 12.17   Color Doppler ultrasound image of the distal part of the penile body in a stallion with chronic paraphimosis. The vessels in the corpus spongiosum glandis are visualized and color coded.

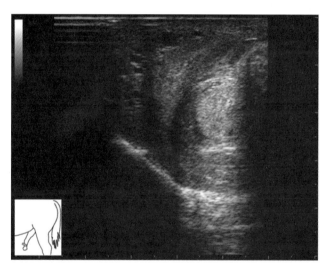

Figure 12.19   Ultrasound image of the distal part of the penile body in a stallion with chronic paraphimosis. Hyperechoic blood clot is present in the lateral process of the corpus cavernosum.

suggest blood clotting (Figures 12.20, 12.21), which needs to be immediately addressed by an aggressive flushing with heparinized saline. Ultrasonography is also helpful in assessing the degree of damage caused by penile trauma (Figure 12.22). The integrity of the tunica albuginea is essential for penile function, and it therefore needs to be carefully examined. Rupture of the tunica albuginea has to be repaired surgically, while penile hematomas or mild contusions can be managed medically, supplemented with physiotherapy.

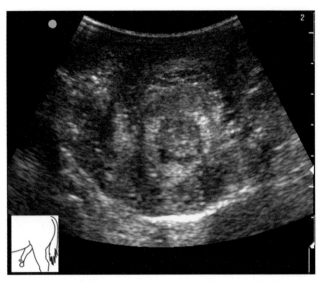

Figure 12.20 Ultrasound image of the distal part of the penile body in a stallion with priapism. Hyperechoic contents of the trabeculae of the corpus cavernosum and the corpus spongiosum suggest blood clotting. This was later confirmed during surgery.

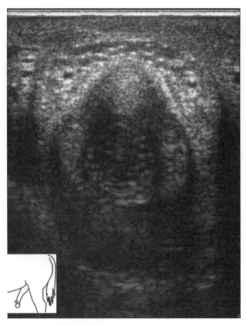

Figure 12.21 Ultrasound image of the distal part of the penile body in the stallion with priapism.

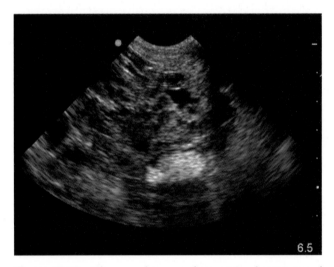

Figure 12.22 Ultrasound image of organizing hematoma of the penis in a stallion, due to a breeding accident.

REFERENCES

[1] Sisson, S. (1910) *A Textbook of Veterinary Anatomy*. W.B. Saunders, Philadelphia.

[2] Nickel, R., Schummer, A., & Seiferle, E. (1979) *The Viscera of the Domestic Mammals*. Springer-Verlag, Hamburg.

[3] Little, V.L. & Holyoak, G.R. (1992) Reproductive anatomy and physiology of the stallion. *Veterinary Clinics of North America: Equine Practice*, 8, 1–29.

[4] Budras, K., Sack, W.O., & Röck, S. (2009) *Anatomy of the Horse*, 5th edn. Schlütersche VerlagsgesellschaftmbH & Co.KG., Hannover.

[5] Nickel, R., Schummer, A., & Seiferle, E. (1981) *The Anatomy of the Domestic Animals*, Volume 3. Verlag Paul Parey,Berlin, Hamburg.

[6] Wilkins, C.J., Sriprasad, S., & Sidhu, P.S. (2003) Colour Doppler ultrasound of the penis. *Clinical Radiology*, 58, 514–523.

CHAPTER THIRTEEN

ULTRASONOGRAPHY OF THE TESTES

Charles Love

Texas A&M University College of Veterinary Medicine, College Station, TX, USA

Ultrasonographic evaluation of the scrotal contents in the stallion includes the spermatic cord (the spermatic artery, ductus deferens, and spermatic venous network (pampiniform plexus), cremaster muscle, nerves, lymphatics), the epididymis (head, body and tail), the testis, vaginal cavity, and scrotum (skin, dermis). The clinician should be able to identify position, location, and the normal echoic pattern of these structures. The examination of the scrotal contents, in addition to determining normalcy, should also include measurement of the length, width, and height of each testis. These measures are then used to calculate testis volume and determine the efficiency of sperm production.

STALLION POSITION AND LOCATION

The clinician is required to perform the examination in the vicinity of the flank area of the stallion. For obvious reasons this is a risky position for the clinician. If semen collection is performed in conjunction with the evaluation, stallions tend to be more tractable following semen collection. Regardless, it is recommended to sedate the stallion to facilitate a thorough and complete evaluation. The ultrasound evaluation of the scrotal contents should be considered a stand-alone primary procedure and therefore sufficient time and patience should be allotted to allow for a thorough examination of the scrotal contents as well as an accurate measurement of the testes dimensions. An inadequate examination can result in erroneous testis measurements leading to an incorrect clinical interpretation.

The stallion can be evaluated from the left flank, either confined in a stock or free-standing in the stall following sedation.

PROBE TYPE

The location of the scrotum is in a relatively restricted area between the hind legs of the stallion, which can limit manipulation and probe placement. The linear array probe commonly used for *per rectum* examination is satisfactory, but its size (i.e. length) can limit examination of discrete structures such as the epididymis. Sector probes can also be used, particularly the "finger" type probe, that is small (surface area ~2.5 cm) and allows easier access to specific areas of interest. The T-type linear probe allows ease of handling and placement in the scrotal area. See Figure 13.1.

EXAMINATION

Ultrasound evaluation should be preceded by a thorough manual evaluation of the scrotum and its contents to detect any specific areas that require scrutiny. Ultrasound gel or a similar lubricant can be applied to the probe. Since the scrotum in the stallion has very little hair there is no need to clip the scrotum. However, since sweat glands are present, artifactual changes due to lather and bubble formation require gel removal and gel reapplication to maximize image resolution.

Testis Measures

Measurement of the testis dimensions (width, height, and length) can be performed first.

Height

The height is measured by placing the probe ventrally and directing the beam dorsally so that the central vein

Atlas of Equine Ultrasonography, First Edition. Edited by Jessica A. Kidd, Kristina G. Lu, and Michele L. Frazer.

is approximately two thirds of the distance from the surface and the spermatic artery can be visualized dorsally. There is no need grasp or manipulate the testis for this measure (Figures 13.2, 13.3).

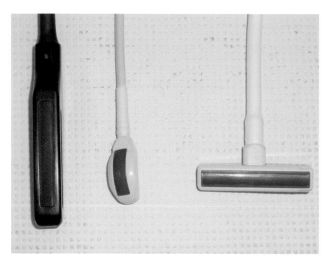

Figure 13.1 Ultrasound probes used for scrotal content evaluation. Left: standard linear array; middle: "finger" sector scanner; right: T-type linear array.

Length

The length is usually measured from the caudal aspect of the scrotum in the vicinity of the tail of the epididymis, directing the beam cranially. The ultrasound probe should be rotated slightly in a horizontal direction so that the maximum length is visualized. The maximum distance can be determined by visualizing the hyperechoic cranial edge of the tunica albuginea of the testis. Similar to the height measurement, the length should be measured *in situ* (Figure 13.4).

Width

The left testis is measured by placing the probe on the left lateral surface of the scrotum and directing the beam horizontally and medially (Figure 13.5). At the same time the right testis should be pushed dorsally so that the shape of measured testis is not distorted. For the measurement of the right testis, the left testis is pushed dorsally to allow measurement. Grabbing of the scrotal neck, similar to the technique used to measure ruminant testes, should be avoided for several reasons. First, it is easier to perform the examination using only one hand to manipulate the probe on the

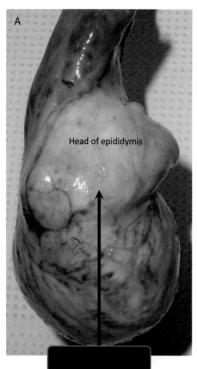
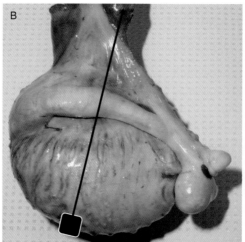
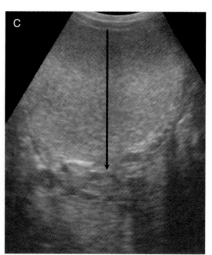

Figure 13.2 (A) Cranial–caudal view of the left testis. (B) Lateral view of the left testis. The height of the testis is measured by placing the ultrasound probe ventrally with the beam directed dorsally. (C) The line denotes the orientation of the arrow in B. Notice the hyperechoic line at the tip of the arrow identifying the tunica albuginea on the dorsal surface of the testis. Below the arrow (dorsal) is the caudal edge of the spermatic cord.

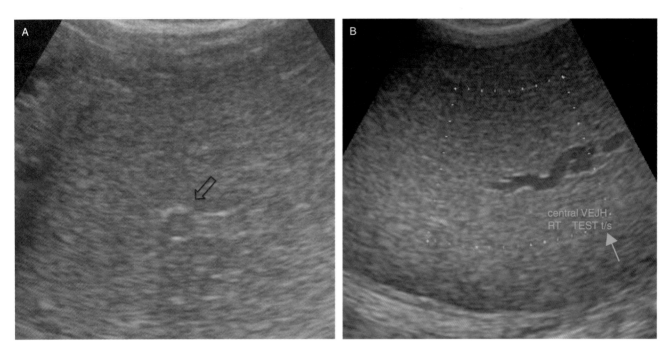

Figure 13.3 (A) Central vein in cross-section and (B) longitudinally.

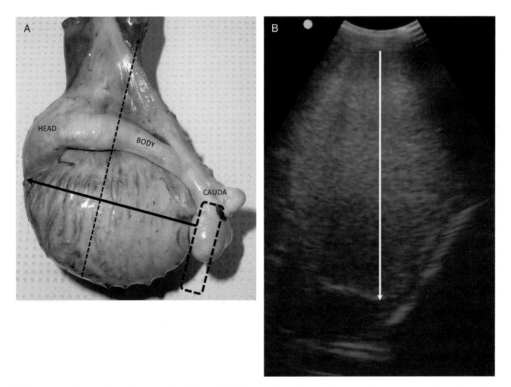

Figure 13.4 (A) Lateral view of the left testis. The solid black line shows the length measure that should extend from the cranial to the caudal edge of the testis, making sure to not include the cauda epididymis. The ultrasound probe is located caudally on the scrotum. Notice the long axis of the testis is not located horizontally, but rather is angled in a dorsocranial direction. (B) Ultrasound picture of the long axis of the testis. The white line corresponds to the black line in A. Notice the hyperechoic line at the tip of the arrow denoting the cranial edge of the testis.

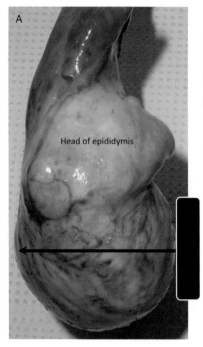

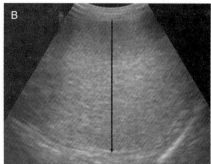

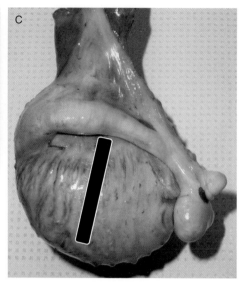

Head of epididymis

Figure 13.5 (A) Cranial–caudal view of the left testis. The width of the testis is measured by placing the ultrasound probe laterally at the widest point of the testis with the beam directed medially. (B) Line denotes the orientation of the beam in A. Notice the hyperechoic line at the end of the arrow identifying the tunica albuginea on the medial side of the testis. (C) The location of the probe on the lateral surface of the testis at the widest point of the testis.

testis, while the testis hangs freely. Even if the testis is in an inguinal position, the testis can be accurately measured without the need to manually draw the testis into the scrotum. Second, it tends to cause strong contraction of the cremaster muscle, which may elicit a similarly strong response from the stallion (i.e. kick).

Qualitative Evaluation of the Scrotal Contents

The echotexture of the scrotal contents can be evaluated following testes measurement. A routine should be followed to ensure a thorough evaluation is completed. The routine followed by the author starts at the neck of the scrotum and visualizes the spermatic cord above the testis.

Spermatic Cord

The primary structure visualized is the tortuous spermatic artery as it winds to the testis (Figure 13.6). Pathology of the spermatic cord includes spermatic cord torsion, which commonly occurs 1–3 cm dorsal to the testis (Figures 13.7, 13.8, 13.9). Varicocele (Figure 13.10), dilation of the pampiniform plexus, while

uncommon, may also be detected here. In addition, generalized edema resulting from inflammation, such as orchitis or epididymitis, may present as hyperechoic inconsistencies in the spermatic cord (Figure 13.11).

Testis

Following the examination of the spermatic cord the ultrasound probe is passed laterally on the testis to examine the parenchyma, which should be homogeneous in echotexture, devoid of hyper- or hypoechoic foci, commonly associated with neoplasia (Figures 13.12, 13.13) or benign structures (Figure 13.14). In cross-section the testis shape may be round to oblong.

Epididymis

The epididymis includes head, body, and tail regions that are located craniolaterally, dorsolaterally and caudally respectively, on the horizontally oriented testis. The epididymal tail (Figure 13.15) should be evaluated for location and size. Spermatic cord rotation of 180° occurs where the epididymal tail is located dorsocranially. In addition, the size and ultrasonographic appearance of the tail can vary from small, in the case of

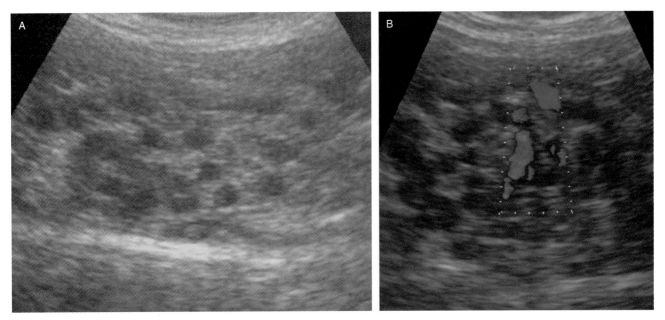

Figure 13.6   (A) Cross-section of the spermatic cord showing the spermatic artery and (B) confirming blood flow with Doppler ultrasound.

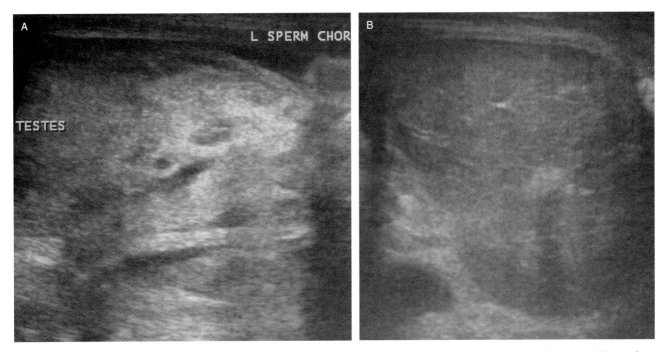

Figure 13.7   Spermatic cord torsion. (A) Spermatic cord dorsal to the testis in a case of spermatic cord torsion. Notice loss of the "Swiss cheese" appearance of the spermatic artery and the increase in the hyperechoic appearance of the cord due to loss of circulation, blood stagnation, and edema. (B) Testis associated with the cord lesion. Notice the hyperechoic areas, probably a result of venous congestion.

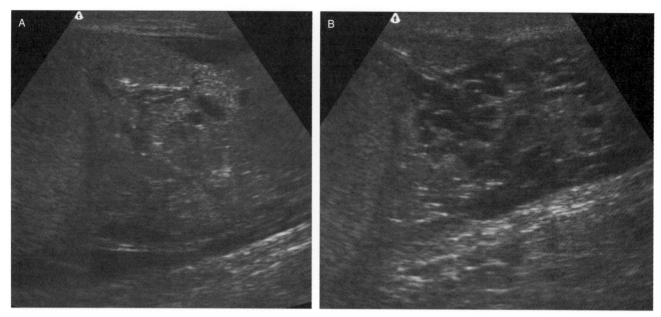

Figure 13.8 (A) Ultrasonographic appearance of a spermatic cord following torsion of the spermatic cord compared to (B) normal contralateral spermatic cord. Notice the lack of circulation in A compared to the hypoechoic areas of circulation in the normal cord.

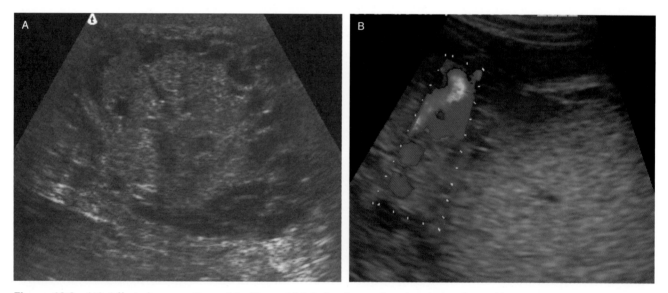

Figure 13.9 (A) Affected spermatic cord in Figure 13.8 1 day later, after the torsion has self-corrected. (B) The spermatic artery is patent (Doppler flow), but there is residual edema in the center of the cord.

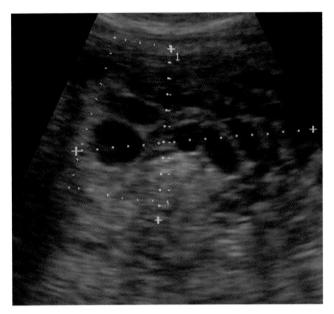

Figure 13.10 Distended venous supply (varicocele) dorsal to the testis.

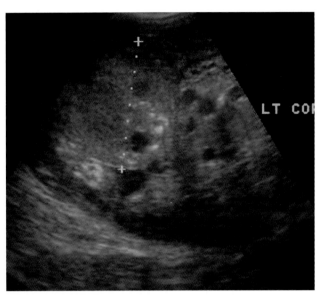

Figure 13.11 Generalized edema resulting from inflammation such as orchitis or epididymitis may present as hyperechoic inconsistencies in the spermatic cord.

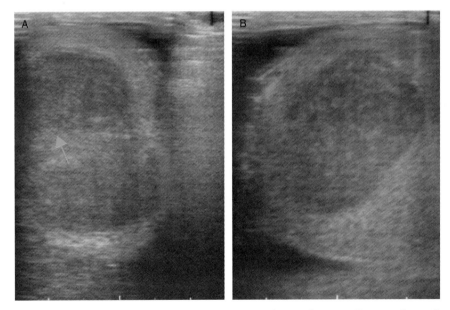

Figure 13.12 (A,B) Heterogeneous mass within the testis parenchyma that was diagnosed as a Sertoli cell tumor.

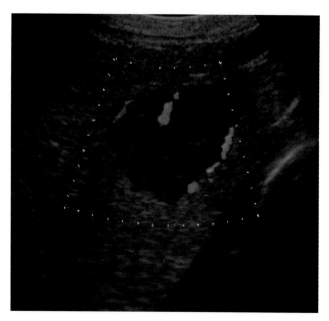

Figure 13.13 Heterogeneous mass within the testis parenchyma that was diagnosed as a seminoma. Notice the prominent vascular channels at the periphery and within the body of the mass.

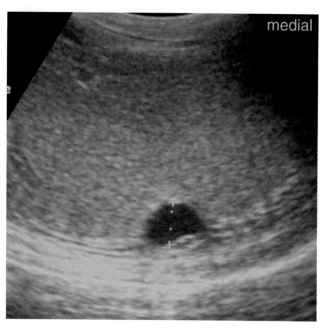

Figure 13.14 Discrete hypoechoic lesion beneath the tunica albuginea of the testis. These lesions tend to be benign, but should be monitored for growth and vascularity.

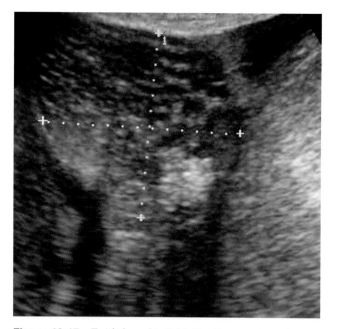

Figure 13.15 Epididymal tail. Notice the prominent lumen in cross-section.

hypoplasia, to prominent, when the tail is distended with sperm or due to inflammation. A tail distended by sperm only, may be common in stallions at sexual rest or in cases of sperm accumulation when sperm accumulates from the ampulla all the way back to the ductus deferens and epididymis (Figures 13.16, 13.17).

Vaginal Cavity

The vaginal cavity is a potential space that communicates with the peritoneal cavity through the inguinal canal and therefore, peritoneal contents such as fluid and intestines have the potential to pass through the canal and occupy the vaginal cavity. In addition, circulatory (artery, vein, lymphatic) compromise to the spermatic cord can result in free fluid accumulation (hydrocele). This fluid tends to accumulate around the epididymal tail (Figure 13.18).

MEASUREMENT AND INTERPRETATION OF TESTES VOLUME

Measurement of testes size is an important part of the stallion breeding soundness evaluation since testes size is associated with sperm production. The number of sperm produced by the stallion may impact fertility and, thus, the number of mares that a stallion can breed. Historically, testes size was determined using the linear measure, total scrotal width, in which calipers were used to measure the combined width of the testes, the mediastinum testes, and the scrotum. This technique, however, does not determine the three-dimensional shape (i.e. volume) of each testis. While

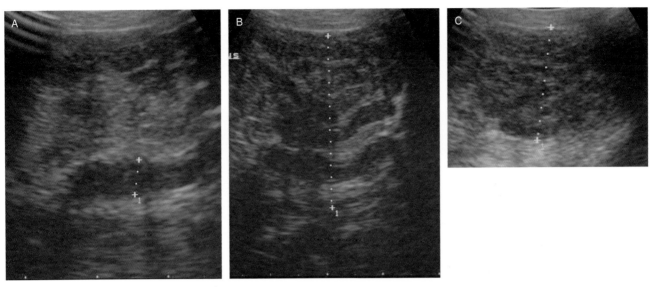

Figure 13.16   (A) Dilated (~0.5 cm) ductus deferens associated with (B) distended (~3.0 cm) cauda epididymal tail. (C) Contralateral epididymal tail that measures 1.7 cm.

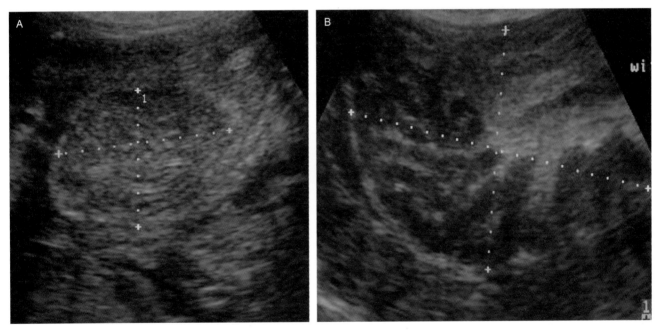

Figure 13.17   Comparison of the size and distension level of the (A) left (1.6 × 2.1 cm) and (B) right epididymal tails (2.5 × 4.0 cm) from the same stallion. Lack of a prominent lumen (A) may result from recent ejaculation or indicate reduced sperm production from that testis. A prominent lumen is usually due to sperm. It may be associated with plugged ampullae (accumulation) or may occur in a stallion at sexual rest.

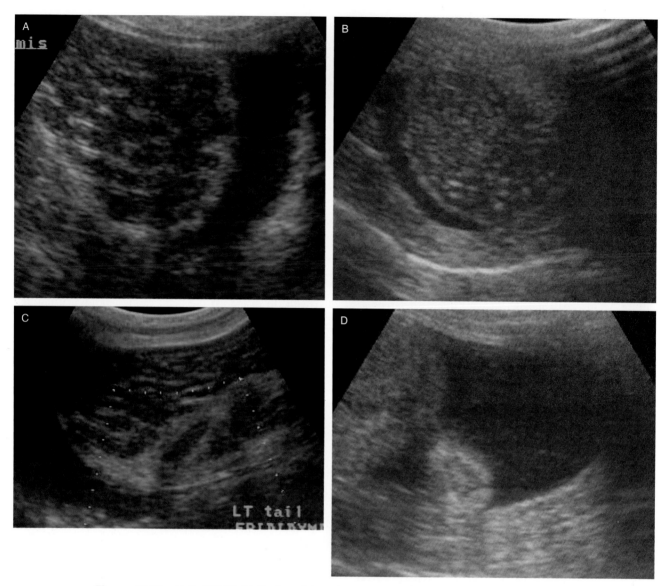

Figure 13.18 (A,B,C,D) Fluid (hydrocele) in the vaginal cavity around the epididymal tail.

the relationship of length, width, and height tends to be proportional, there are instances where they are not, and the determination of each dimension will more accurately determine volume.

Subsequently, ultrasonography has been introduced as a technique to measure and evaluate the testes. This technique has the advantage of being specific and accurate since the clinician can visualize the testis parenchyma and identify landmarks that assure measurement of the length, width, and height.

Measurements (length, width, and height) from each testis are performed as described in the preceding section. The measures from each testis are then inserted in a formula that approximates the volume of an ellipsoid [1]:

Testis volume in cm^3

$$= \frac{4\pi}{3}\left(\frac{length\ in\ cm}{2}\right)\left(\frac{width\ in\ cm}{2}\right)\left(\frac{height\ in\ cm}{2}\right)$$

$$= 0.5238(length\ in\ cm)(width\ in\ cm)(height\ in\ cm)$$

The volumes from each testis are combined to give the total testicular volume (TTV).

The TTV is then inserted into the regression formula to calculate the expected daily sperm output (DSO). Formulae are based on the author's previous two publications in which semen was collected once daily for 7 consecutive days from reproductively normal stallions [2,3]. The total sperm number (in billions) was averaged from days 5–7 and this was considered to be daily sperm output. The TTV was then calculated after measuring the length, width, and height of each testis. The following regression formulae were created from that data:

$$\text{Predicted DSO (billions)} = 0.024\,(TTV) - 1.26\ [2]$$
$$= 0.024\,(TTV) - 0.76\ [3]$$

These formulae differ because there were more stallions included in the second study than the first. The only mathematical difference between the two formulae is the constant (i.e. 0.76 vs. 1.26). When calculating the expected DSO the author uses both formulae to give an expected range.

Example:

	Left testis	Right testis
Length (cm)	8.1	8.3
Width (cm)	4.2	5.0
Height (cm)	5.2	5.6
Volume (cm³)	93	122
Total testes volume	215 cm³	

The TTV of this stallion is 215 cm³. This value would then be inserted in the two formulae to give a range of expected DSO from 3.9–4.4 billion sperm.

Interpretation

The intent of measuring the TTV is as follows:

1. Determine the *absolute* volume measure. The average total testes volume for the population of stallions measured in the two studies was approximately 250 cm³. Based on this TTV the *average* stallion should produce approximately 4.7–5.2 billion sperm when at DSO. This translates to a spermatogenic efficiency of approximately 18 million sperm/cm³ testis parenchyma/day. The absolute value becomes particularly important when measuring sexually immature stallions retired to stud following performance careers. The clinician is often asked to render an opinion on a stallion's testes size in relation to his potential as a breeding stallion. Recognizing that a 2–4-year-old stallion has a TTV similar to the average sexually mature stallion is useful when rendering an opinion. The clinician must also recognize that TTV alone does not "qualify" a stallion as fertile, but a "normal" testes size does reduce the risk of "subfertility."

2. Compare the *expected* DSO value to the *actual* number of sperm collected from the stallion (Figure 13.19). Ideally the clinician would like to collect a stallion once daily for 5–7 days to determine DSO.

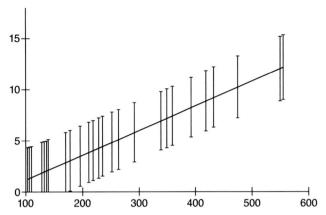

Figure 13.19 The relationship between total testes volume (TTV, cm³) on the x-axis and predicted daily sperm output (billions) on the y-axis. Regression coefficient (y = 0.024 (TTV) − 1.26). Error bars represent ±2 standard deviations. (Source: Love et al, 1991 [2]. Reproduced with permission of Bioscientifica.)

Oftentimes this is impractical due to time and monetary constraints and a lesser collection frequency is more practical. Stich *et al.* reported that testes volume will affect the number of days required to reach DSO with a smaller TTV (148–245 ml; ml = cm³) reaching DSO sooner (day 5) than medium (253–274 ml; day 6) or large testes (292–466 ml; day 6–7) [4]. In lieu of collecting from a stallion for 5–7 days, collecting two ejaculates 1 hour apart and using the second ejaculate as an approximation of DSO, is a useful compromise. In most cases, the clinician is not interested in whether the stallion is producing *too much* sperm, but rather whether he is producing *too little* when compared to the expected DSO value.

References

[1] Oberg, E.V. (1984) *Machinery's Handbook: A Reference for the Mechanical Engineer*, 22nd edn. Industrial Press, New York, 54.

[2] Love, C.C., Garcia, M.C., Riera, F.R., & Kenney, R.M. (1991) Evaluation of measures taken by ultrasonography and caliper to estimate testicular volume and predict daily sperm output in the stallion. *Journal of Reproduction and Fertility*, 44, 99–105.

[3] Love, C.C., Garcia, M.C., Riera, F.R., & Kenney, R.M. (1990) Use of testicular volume to predict daily sperm output in the stallion. *Proceedings of the American Association of Equine Practitioners*, 36, 15–21.

[4] Stich, K., Brinsko, S., Thompson, J., *et al.* (2002) Stabilization of extragonadal sperm reserves in stallions: application for determination of daily sperm output. *Theriogenology*, 58, 397–400.

Section 2b: Ultrasonography of the Mare Reproductive Tract

CHAPTER FOURTEEN

USE OF ULTRASONOGRAPHY IN THE EVALUATION OF THE NON-PREGNANT MARE

Walter Zent

Hagyard Equine Medical Institute, Lexington, KY, USA

In preparation for the ultrasonographic evaluation of the non-pregnant mare, a manual transrectal examination of the reproductive tract should be performed. This palpation allows the examiner to arrange the mare's reproductive tract so as to make the ultrasonographic examination easier. The tract should be arranged so that it is free of any intestine and the ovaries should be positioned so that they are not behind the broad ligament. The operator should be able to follow the tract from one ovary to the other without any obstruction. This will allow the examination to be done without the interference of abdominal structures that can make the examination difficult and in some instances cause confusion in interpretation. More importantly, this examination allows the operator to become aware of possible abnormalities that will need closer visualization when the ultrasonographic examination is being performed.

In order to properly perform an ultrasonographic examination of the reproductive tract it is very important that the mare be properly restrained. The amount of restraint that is required will differ greatly depending on the temperament of the mare and the quality of the available help. Older mares that have been examined multiple times often need very little restraint, while younger, more fractious individuals may need considerable restraint. It is very important that the animal is handled so that the safety of the animal, help and veterinarian is maintained. Remember that the veterinarian is often times the only professional involved and therefore the person responsible for the proper execution of the procedure. If stocks are not available the mare is frequently positioned with the

hindquarters in a stall door, in order to prevent too much lateral movement and give some protection to the operator and equipment. If the mare is not accustomed to being palpated some form of minor sedation can be helpful. The author would rather not use acepromazine for sedation as it will cause a profound loss of uterine tone and thus make examination difficult. Xylazine (0.5–1.1 mg/kg) will cause much less uterine relaxation and will provide ample sedation in most instances. Detomidine (0.02–0.04 mg/kg IV) is also a good choice. If the mare resists transrectal examination by persistent straining or if the operator must do extensive manipulation of the reproductive tract, a small dose of N-butylscopolammonium bromide (Buscopan, 20–40 mg IV) can be given to relax the rectum and make examination easier on the operator and the patient.

When scanning is being performed it is important for the operator to hold the probe in a manner that will allow the head of the probe to have full contact with the ovaries and uterus. The author believes that this can best be done by grasping the probe in a way that the index finger is placed along the dorsal surface of the probe, with the thumb on one side and the remaining fingers on the other, being careful not to cover the crystals on the bottom. The middle finger can be used as a guide to move the probe along the anterior edge of the uterus so that the probe will be easily centered over the uterus while the examination of the horns is being performed (Figure 14.1).

The examination should always be done in the same manner so that all of the structures are examined thoroughly and the operator will be able to cover the entire tract. The author palpates left handed so it is easiest

Atlas of Equine Ultrasonography, First Edition. Edited by Jessica A. Kidd, Kristina G. Lu, and Michele L. Frazer.
© 2014 John Wiley & Sons, Ltd. Published 2014 by John Wiley & Sons, Ltd.
Companion Website: www.wiley.com/go/kidd/equine-ultrasonography

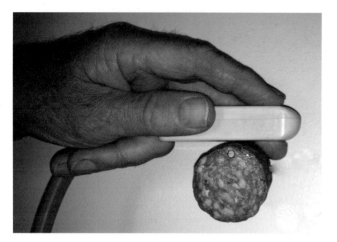

Figure 14.1 Proper method of gripping probe for good visualization of the uterus.

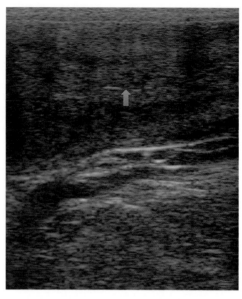

Figure 14.3 Longitudinal section of uterine body during diestrus; there is no edema and no fluid in the lumen of the uterus. The lumen is often visualized by a hyperechoic horizontal line (arrow).

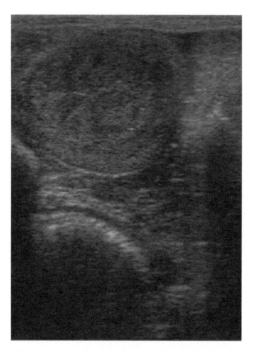

Figure 14.2 Cross-section of uterine horn.

for him to start at the right ovary, and then examine the right horn, left horn, left ovary, body and cervix, ending with the vagina. It is very important that the operator makes sure that the entire uterus is examined. If the probe is held correctly the horns of the uterus will appear as a cross-section of a piece of sausage on the screen and can easily be followed from one ovary to the other (Figure 14.2). The body of the uterus will be seen longitudinally (Figure 14.3). When scanning the body of the uterus, sometimes the body is wider than the width of the probe and parts of the lateral

areas can be missed. In order to make sure that the operator has covered the entire uterus the probe is moved from left to right. This is particularly important when mares are being examined for very early pregnancies.

The ultrasound examination of the non-pregnant mare's reproductive tract can be done as a single examination, for reasons such as breeding soundness examination or purchase, or as one of a series of examinations, such as when the mare is being examined over several days for mating. Whatever the reason it is important to remember that the ultrasonographic examination is only one part of the evaluation of the mare's reproductive tract and must be coupled with the history, the mare's mental condition (in behavioral estrus or not), a speculum examination to evaluate the condition of the vagina and cervix, and palpation of her reproductive tract. Only when all of this information is put together can a proper interpretation of the examination be made. The normal mare should go together like a puzzle and if she does not, then, in the author's view, she has deviated from normal.

It is important to be aware of the mare's position in her reproductive cycle so that you know what you are expecting the normal mare's reproductive tract to look like. During the period of anestrus that mares pass through during the winter, most mares, on palpation, will have no follicular development, their uterus will be relaxed, and the cervix toneless. She will be non-responsive to the teaser and on speculum examination the vagina and cervix will be pale and dry. The cervix will have very little tone. The ultrasound examination will find ovaries that are very small and may have small, less than 10 mm follicles present on them and a uterus with no edema (Figure 14.4) and no fluid in the lumen.

The mare that is entering and passing through the transitional period will have a reproductive tract that shows many different degrees of development. This can be the most difficult period for a veterinarian to interpret. The ovaries may have no follicles or clusters of small follicles (Figure 14.5) and the mare may be showing strong estrous behavior or no estrous behavior at all. Often the most confusing times for owner and veterinarian are when the mare is showing strong estrus and has no follicles, which may be a normal finding during transition. The uterus usually has very little tone and no edema or fluid, and the cervix will be pale and relaxed. Ginther [1] has described in great detail the changes that occur during this period of a mare's reproductive life.

As the mare moves into the cycling period, the first signs of estrus will be the beginning of uterine edema, follicular development, and the development of cervical edema, relaxation, and pinker color (Figure 14.6).

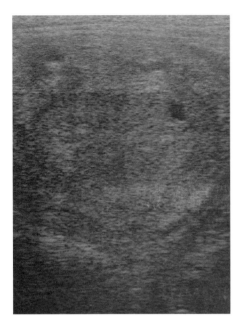

Figure 14.4 Cross-section of uterine body during transition from anestrus to cyclicity. There is no edema in the uterine wall or fluid in the lumen of the uterus.

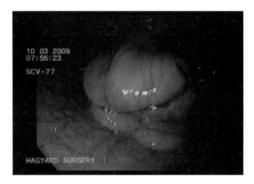

Figure 14.6 Cervix during early estrus with some edema; cervix is beginning to relax.

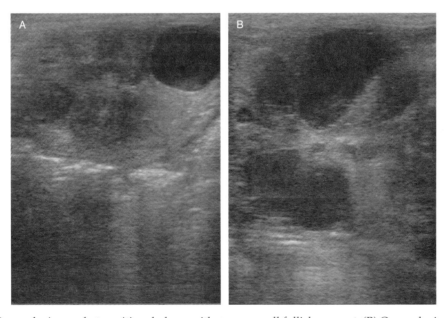

Figure 14.5 (A) Ovary during early transitional phase with a very small follicle present. (B) Ovary during transitional phase with several small follicles (cluster).

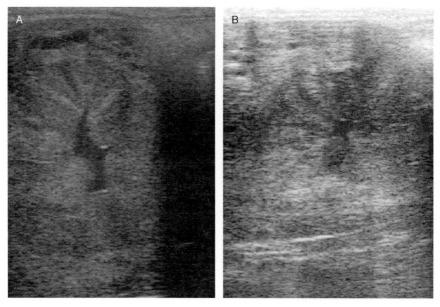

Figure 14.7 (A,B) Cross-section of uterus with edema and normal fluid that is often present during early estrus.

As estrus progresses, uterine edema will increase and a small amount of fluid may normally be present in the mare's uterus (Figure 14.7), follicular activity will become greater with the development of a dominant follicle (Figure 14.8), and behavioral signs of estrus will increase. The approach of ovulation will be signaled by the reduction of uterine edema (Figure 14.9), further relaxation of the cervix (Figure 14.10) and vulva, and stronger behavioral signs of estrus. The follicle will lose its spherical shape and begin to migrate towards the ovulation fossa (Figure 14.11).

When ovulation occurs the mare will begin to be less receptive to the teaser, the follicle will collapse and a corpus hemorrhagicum (Figure 14.12) will begin to form. The uterine edema will resolve and there should be no fluid in the mare's uterus. The mare's cervix will appear paler and begin to close (Figure 14.13). A much more detailed description of follicular growth and development can be found [2].

As the mare enters diestrus she will become non-receptive to the stallion, the vulva will be less relaxed, and the cervix (Figure 14.14) will be closed, pale, and dry. The uterus will have some tone on palpation. The ovaries may or may not have palpable follicles and a corpus luteum will usually be palpable at the site of ovulation. Ultrasound examination of the uterus and ovaries should find a significant reduction in edema, no fluid in the lumen of the uterus (Figure 14.15), and the ovaries may or may not have significant follicular development but should have a visible corpus luteum (Figure 14.16) present at the site of ovulation.

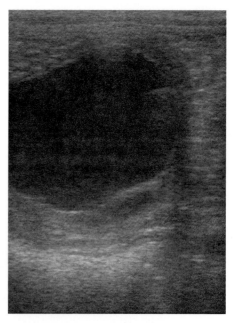

Figure 14.8 Dominant follicle developing during the middle of the estrus period.

It is important to remember that mares can be very much individuals and not always progress through their estrous cycle in a prescribed path. The examining veterinarians must use their clinical skills to properly interpret the mare's position in her estrous cycle so that she can be properly managed.

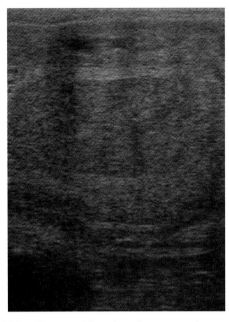

Figure 14.9 Uterus with reduced estrous edema as ovulation approaches.

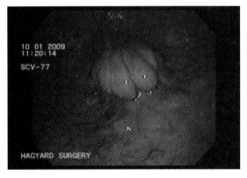

Figure 14.10 Cervix is relaxed and edematous as ovulation approaches.

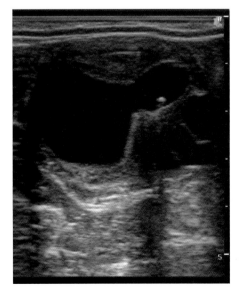

Figure 14.11 Preovulatory follicle has thickening of the follicular wall and is losing its spherical shape.

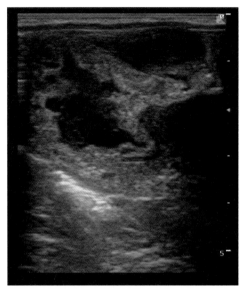

Figure 14.12 Corpus hemorrhagicum and secondary follicle.

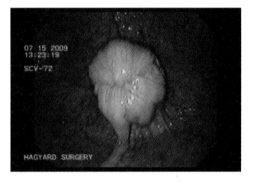

Figure 14.13 Cervix after ovulation.

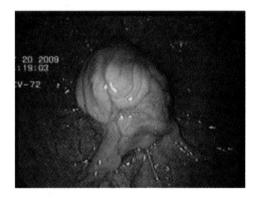

Figure 14.14 The cervix during diestrus is pale and closed.

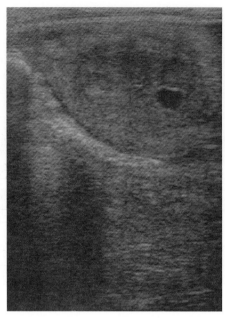

Figure 14.15 Diestrus uterus has lost its edema.

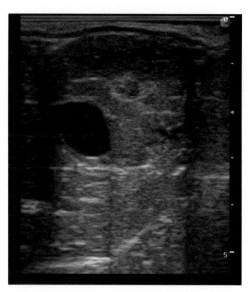

Figure 14.16 Ovary with a visible corpus luteum.

REFERENCES

[1] Ginther, O.J. (1992) *Reproductive Biology of the Mare: Basic and Applied Aspects,* 2nd edn. Equiservices, Cross Plains, 135–172.

[2] Gastal, E.L. (2011) Ovulation: Part 2. Ultrasonographic Morphology of the Preovulatory Follicle. In: *Equine Reproduction,* 2nd edn (eds A.O. McKinnon, E.L. Squires, W.E. Vaala & D.D. Varner). Wiley Blackwell, Oxford, 2032–2054.

CHAPTER FIFTEEN

USE OF ULTRASONOGRAPHY IN THE MANAGEMENT OF THE ABNORMAL BROODMARE

Jonathan F. Pycock

Equine Reproductive Services, Ryton, UK

INTRODUCTION

To carry out ultrasound examinations safely, mares should be suitably restrained. Ideally, one should have a set of stocks approximately 75 cm (30 inches) wide and just longer than an average mare. This is adequate for most animals and will even accommodate large draft mares. In a few cases, a twitch may be required to provide additional restraint. Foals should be restrained in front of, or to the side of the mare. Tying the tail to one side keeps it out of the way, and prevents hairs entering the rectum.

Precautions necessary for transrectal examinations also apply to ultrasound examinations and transrectal examination should always precede ultrasound examination. An initial rectal and transrectal examination ensures removal of all fecal material, facilitates rapid location of the tract during scanning and provides information on texture of structures.

The scanner should be as close to eye level as practicable and the control panel of the machine within easy reach of the operator. The scanner can be placed on either side of the mare. Where the operator's left hand holds the transducer, the scanner is placed obliquely to the right side of the mare's hindquarters allowing the right hand to make any notes or adjustments to the controls. To facilitate correct orientation of the transducer, a groove for the finger of the operator is usually located on the transducer, on the opposite side to the transducer face. The fingers should always be in front of the transducer as it is being introduced and later manipulated rather than pushing the transducer on ahead. For reasons of hygiene, it may be

desirable to have the transducer in a plastic sleeve. Coupling gel should be used to exclude air from between the transducer and its protective cover. Using copious amounts of lubricant, which also acts as a coupling medium to ensure good contact and prevent air interference, the transducer and hand are gently inserted into the rectum. Should the mare strain, the examination should be stopped and one should wait for the rectum to relax. However, straining is usually not a significant problem.

It is best to examine the reproductive tract systematically and to scan the entire uterus and both ovaries at least twice. The transducer is usually held within the rectum in the longitudinal plane. Since the uterus of the mare is T-shaped, the uterine body appears as a rectangular image in the longitudinal plane. When scanning the uterine body, it is important to move the transducer forwards and backwards and from side to side so that no feature is missed. It is important to move the transducer slowly at all times. To image the uterine horns and ovaries the transducer should be rotated slowly to the right and then the left side. Therefore, the uterine horns appear as circular images in cross-section. If difficulties are encountered with finding a structure, the transducer can be withdrawn a short distance and the structure located by palpation. Ultrasound examination can then be resumed.

Both the ovaries and the uterus need to be examined thoroughly at every examination of an abnormal mare.

Ovarian features to note are:

- ovarian size, shape, and ultrasound appearance;
- follicle size, softness, and shape;

Atlas of Equine Ultrasonography, First Edition. Edited by Jessica A. Kidd, Kristina G. Lu, and Michele L. Frazer.
© 2014 John Wiley & Sons, Ltd. Published 2014 by John Wiley & Sons, Ltd.
Companion Website: www.wiley.com/go/kidd/equine-ultrasonography

- echogenicity and thickness of the granulosa layer;
- presence of small echogenic particles within the follicular fluid.

ABNORMAL FOLLICLES

In the 48 hours, but more obviously in the 24-hour period before ovulation, the wall of the follicle (granulosa layer) becomes increasingly echogenic [1]. As ovulation approaches, the follicle wall often becomes intensely hyperechoic and irregular in outline. Small echogenic particles may appear in the follicular fluid close to ovulation. These particles are thought to be the result of preovulatory hemorrhage (Figure 15.1). If the particles continue to increase in density and become widespread these follicles rarely ovulate and are termed hemorrhagic anovulatory follicles (HAFs).

Ultrasonographic collapse of the follicle may be rapid, within several seconds, or more prolonged over several minutes with eventual complete or almost complete evacuation of the follicular antrum. The length of time does not appear to impact fertility. Ovulation failure occurs in almost 10% of estrous cycles according to a study by McCue and Squires (2002) [2]. These authors report that the majority of anovulatory follicles luteinize (85.7%) but some remain as persistent follicular structures (14.3%). More recently it has been suggested that the incidence is between 5% and 20% of estrous cycles [3]. All types of anovulatory follicles are infertile since follicular collapse and oocyte release (ovulation) has not occurred. It is difficult to predict if a dominant follicle will fail to ovulate [4]. The best indicator is the "snow storm" appearance of echogenic particles in the follicular fluid and an increase in follicular size. The follicles continue to grow and may occasionally reach diameters of 125 mm. The particles are likely to be the result of hemorrhage into the follicle. In some situations, hemorrhage into the follicular antrum is minimal and the "snow storm" appearance disperses and the follicle returns to normal appearance (Figures 15.2, 15.3).

The hemorrhage in anovulatory follicles may organize to form a cobweb-like network of narrow hyperechoic fibrin strands (Figures 15.4, 15.5). Alternatively a more solid structure may form from organization of the fibrin (Figures 15.6, 15.7). These structures can be confused with a granulosa theca cell tumor.

Luteinized anovulatory follicles invariably have some echogenic material present, allowing differentiation from non-luteinized anovulatory follicles. Differentiation can be confirmed by measurement of blood progesterone values, as luteinized follicles will be associated with elevated progesterone values, unlike non-luteinized follicles. These luteinized anovulatory follicles usually respond to an injection of prostaglandin $F_{2\alpha}$ (PGF$_{2\alpha}$) and as low a dose as possible should

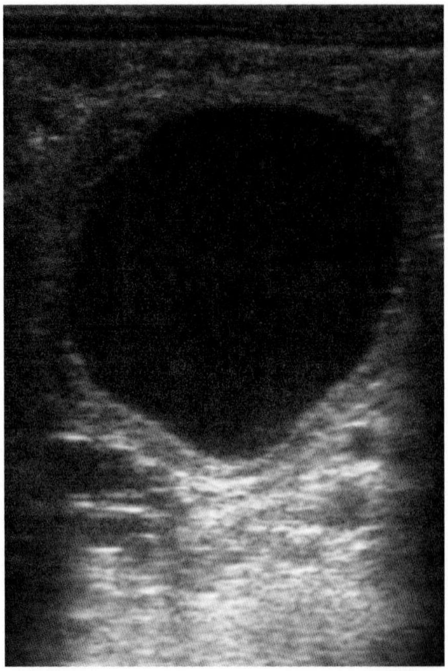

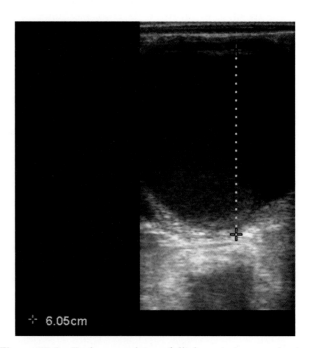

Figure 15.1 Small, indistinct echogenic particles only just visible at the ventral margin of the follicular fluid are normal in the 48-hour period preceding ovulation.

Figure 15.2 Early anovulatory follicle: note increase in size of follicle with some echoic particles.

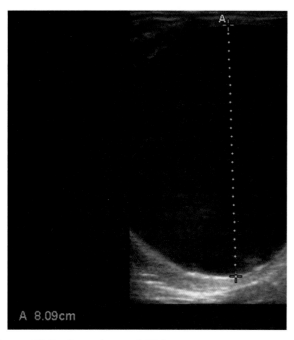

A 8.09cm

Figure 15.3 Anovulatory follicle continuing to grow and develop more echogenic particles.

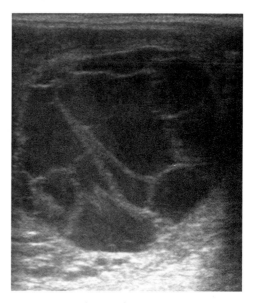

Figure 15.5 Anovulatory follicle with increasing fibrin strands.

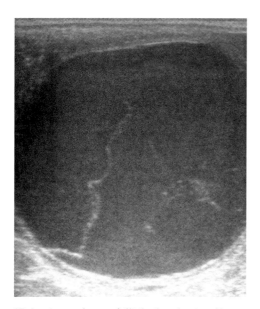

Figure 15.4 Anovulatory follicle developing fibrin strands.

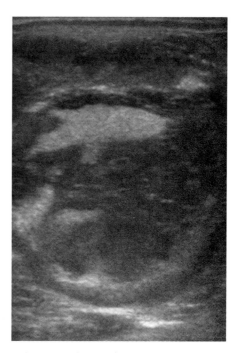

Figure 15.6 Anovulatory follicle with fibrin organizing into solid masses.

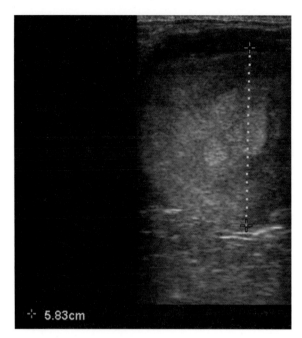

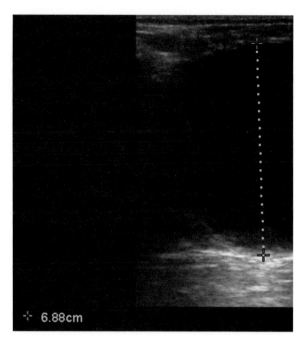

Figure 15.7 Anovulatory follicle with solid appearance. Anovulatory follicles with this appearance can be difficult to differentiate from normal corpora lutea. Anovulatory follicles are usually larger than normal corpora lutea and there is no collapsed stage detected. Of course, it may just be that the examination interval frequency meant that a collapsed stage was not detected. This is the reason the author believes it is not always possible with certainty to differentiate anovulatory follicles from normal corpora lutea.

Figure 15.8 Non-luteinized anovulatory follicle.

be used. The naturally occurring PGF$_{2\alpha}$, dinoprost, or the synthetic prostaglandin analog, cloprostenol, are equally effective. The recommended dose for a 500 kg mare is 5 mg of dinoprost or 250 μg of cloprostenol. However, since it is reported that higher doses of PGF$_{2\alpha}$ represent an increased risk for formation of anovulatory follicles [5], a low dose of dinoprost (1.5 mg) or cloprostenol (50 μg) should be used in mares prone to formation of anovulatory follicles.

Non-luteinized anovulatory follicles are more difficult to treat, as they do not respond to prostaglandin. If the mare ovulates normally from another follicle, treatment may not be necessary, but occasionally treatment is needed either due to the physical size of the structure or its suppression of any other follicular development. Attempts to induce their disappearance with human chorionic gonadotrophin or deslorelin are usually unsuccessful. Sometimes a 12-day course of altrenogest (0.044 mg/kg PO SID) followed by an ovulation induction agent may be successful. Fortunately, they usually spontaneously regress although this can take as long as 4 weeks (Figure 15.8). Rarely, they

persist beyond this period and transvaginal puncture may be useful in these rare cases.

The most challenging aspect of these anovulatory follicles is their recognition. As stated earlier, some echogenic particles appear in normal follicles in the 48-hour period preceding ovulation. These particles may be transient and are gone when the follicle is evaluated 24 hours later. In addition, a second follicle may be developing normally elsewhere on the same ovary or on the opposite ovary. This follicle may go on to ovulate normally. It is, therefore, important when examining mares in which the development of a hemorrhagic anovulatory follicle is suspected, to look very carefully for a normal preovulatory follicle developing. For these reasons, if the mare has been bred, the author does not administer prostaglandin, but makes a note in the mare's record that an anovulatory hemorrhagic follicle was suspected. Certain mares seem prone to development of anovulatory follicles and there is often a history of repeated prostaglandin administration and/or endometritis in these mares. Exogenous prostaglandin is best avoided in mares prone to development of hemorrhagic follicles. This topic has recently been described in detail and there is evidence that the incidence of hemorrhagic follicles is greater in mares treated with ovulation induction agents compared with those with spontaneous cycles [5].

It is debatable whether the condition ovarian hematoma exists as a separate entity from anovulatory

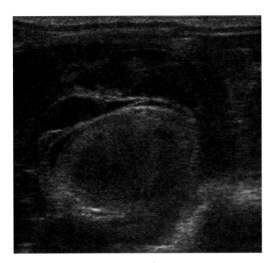

Figure 15.9   Ovarian hematoma.

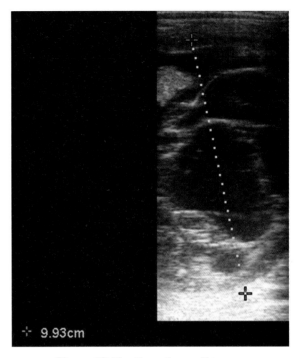

9.93cm

Figure 15.10   Granulosa cell tumor.

hemorrhagic follicles (AHFs). Structures previously reported as ovarian hematomas (Figure 15.9) might be examples of AHFs where the hemorrhage forms a particularly solid-appearing mass.

GRANULOSA CELL TUMORS

The most common ovarian tumor in the mare is the granulosa cell tumor. The ultrasonographic appearance is highly variable, from a multicystic, honeycomb-like appearance (Figure 15.10), to a solid mass with just the occasional cyst (Figure 15.11). On palpation the affected ovary is typically enlarged with no ovulation fossa being palpable. The contralateral ovary is usually small, firm and inactive. The variable ultrasonographic appearance of granulosa cell tumors confuses differentiation from normal ovaries as well as anovulatory follicles and endocrine assays are typically required to confirm the diagnosis. Until recently, measurement of inhibin was the most reliable means, but recently anti-Mullerian hormone has proved to be a reliable marker for granulosa cell tumors [6].

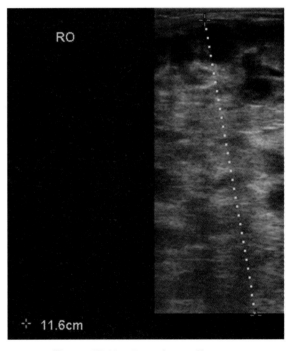

RO

11.6cm

Figure 15.11   Granulosa cell tumor.

PERSISTENT ENDOMETRIAL CUPS

Persistent endometrial cups are relatively rare in the mare, but are a consideration when a mare demonstrates irregular ovarian activity in the form of repeated formation of anovulatory follicles [7]. They are not easy to identify ultrasonographically and are more easily seen once they become mineralized. Figure 15.12 is of persistent endometrial cups visible as 2–8 mm hyperechoic areas at the base of the right horn. They can resemble air in the uterus (Figure 15.13, 15.14) or fetal remnants (see Figure 15.27).

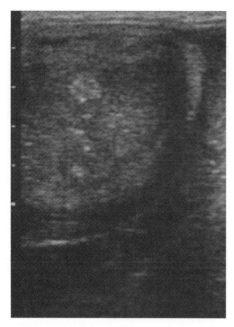

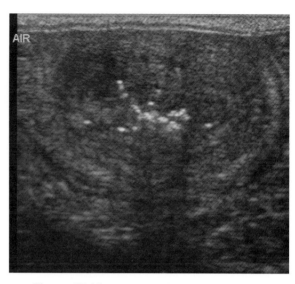

Figure 15.14   Air in the horn of the uterus.

Figure 15.12   Persistent endometrial cups at the base of the right horn of the uterus of a mare.

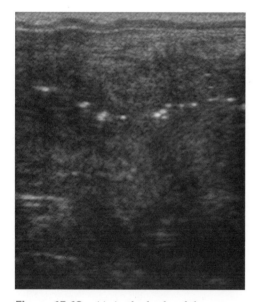

Figure 15.13   Air in the body of the uterus.

Air in the Uterus (Pneumometra)

The integrity of the vulvar lips and its anatomic relation with the perineal area and anus are essential components of a mare's fertility because they provide the first barrier to contamination between the external environment and the uterus. Absence (natural or acquired) of a normal perineal conformation can facilitate the entry of air (pneumovagina, also called "wind-sucking"), feces, and potential pathogens into the reproductive tract, which jeopardizes the mare's fertility. The initial vaginitis may lead to cervicitis and acute endometritis resulting in subfertility. In a mare with an incompetent vulval seal, ultrasonographic examination of the uterus of such a mare may reveal the presence of air as hyperechoic foci in the body (Figure 15.13) or one of the horns of the uterus (Figure 15.14).

Endometrial Cysts

Endometrial cysts are often cited as a cause of infertility, however, a cause and effect relationship has not been clearly established. Rather than being viewed as a cause of infertility, endometrial cysts should be considered as an indication of underlying pathologic changes in the uterus. Endometrial cysts are of lymphatic origin, and their occurrence may be associated with a disruption of lymphatic function. The incidence of endometrial cysts increases with mare age. Endometrial cysts are best diagnosed with ultrasonography. Cysts can be identified as hypoechoic, immovable structures with a clear border, as opposed to intraluminal fluid, which is movable and has a less distinct shape or border. Endometrial cysts can complicate early pregnancy diagnosis. Oftentimes an endometrial cyst can be similar in size and appearance to an early conceptus (Figure 15.15). See also Figures 15.16 and 15.17.

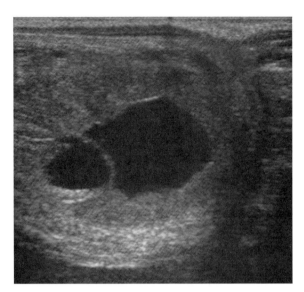

Figure 15.15 20-day pregnancy and cyst. In this image an embryo is not yet detectable in the 20-day pregnancy (right), the cyst can be seen to the bottom left of the image. Note the relatively thick, hyperchoic wall of the cyst.

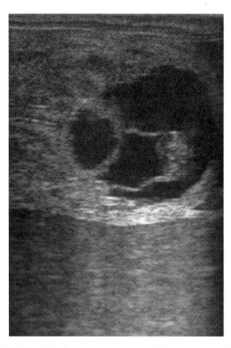

Figure 15.17 29-day pregnancy with embryo visible to right of image and cyst to left of image.

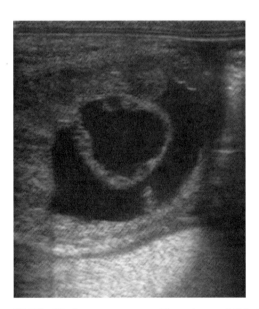

Figure 15.16 22-day pregnancy with embryo visible in six o'clock position and cyst in dorsal aspect of pregnancy.

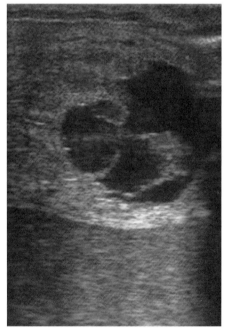

Figure 15.18 This is the same mare as imaged in Figure 15.17, but the ultrasound transducer has been reoriented changing the appearance of the cyst.

To evaluate cysts thoroughly, it is important to reorient the ultrasound transducer in several positions as this can allow more thorough evaluation of any structure suspected of being a cyst (Figure 15.18). If a cyst is spherical, it can be very difficult to distinguish from an early pregnancy (Figure 15.19).

UTERINE FLUID

Fluid accumulation in the uterus is the most common cause of reproductive failure in mares, particularly older mares and mares being bred for the first time in their teenage years. This subfertility is due to an

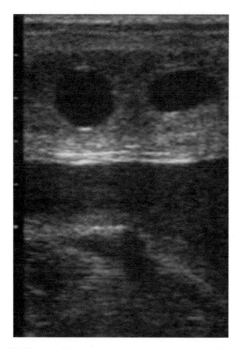

Figure 15.19 In this image the pregnancy is on the left and the cyst on the right.

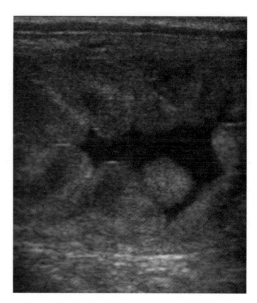

Figure 15.21 Ultrasonographic image of grade 1 uterine fluid: anechoic.

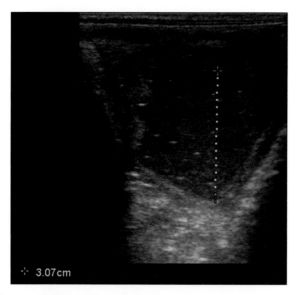

3.07cm

Figure 15.20 Ultrasonographic image of the uterus of a mare with fluid accumulation.

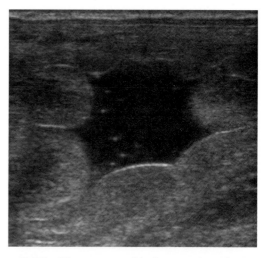

Figure 15.22 Ultrasonographic image of grade 2 uterine fluid: hypoechoic with hyperechoic particles.

unsuitable environment within the uterus for the developing conceptus, and in some instances the ensuing endometritis persists and causes early regression of the corpus luteum. In addition, uterine fluid may damage the ability of spermatozoa to survive in the uterus or oviduct, or even fertilize once in the oviduct.

Ultrasonographic examination to detect uterine luminal fluid (Figure 15.20) has proved useful to iden-

tify mares that accumulate fluid and is the most useful technique in practice.

Intraluminal uterine fluid can be graded according to the degree of echogenicity; for example the author uses grades 1 to 4, where grade 1 is anechoic and grade 4 is hyperechoic (Figures 15.21, 15.22, 15.23, 15.24). The more echogenic the fluid, the more likely the fluid contains debris, including white blood cells. However, cellular fluid can appear relatively anechoic, so care is needed in interpretation. Inspissated pus can be so echogenic that it is overlooked. The actual appearance of the fluid and the ultrasonographic appearance

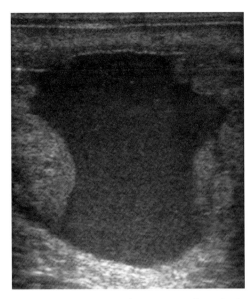

Figure 15.23 Ultrasonographic image of grade 3 uterine fluid: moderately echogenic.

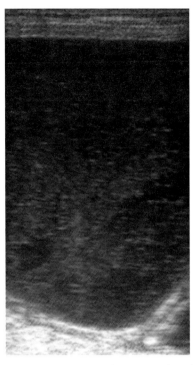

Figure 15.25 Ultrasonographic image of a full urinary bladder.

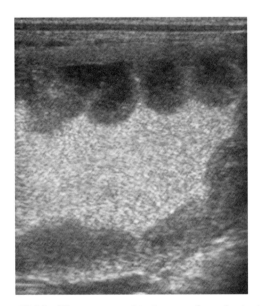

Figure 15.24 Ultrasonographic image of grade 4 uterine fluid: hyperechogenic fluid in the uterus of a mare with bacterial endometritis.

might not be as closely linked as was once thought. Ultrasonographic appearance may be proportional to the size and concentration of particulate matter within the fluid, rather than the viscosity of the fluid; for example, purulent exudates can appear more hypoechoic than expected. Air appears as hyperechoic foci, and fluid with air bubbles can appear as fluid with cellular debris. Urine in the bladder can appear echo-

genic, despite being a watery liquid (Figure 15.25). Ultrasonographic appearance of urine varies according to diet. Diets high in protein (lucerne and clover) produce echogenic urine from secretions. Grass diets produce relatively anechoic urine.

FOREIGN BODIES IN THE UTERUS

Using ultrasound, various foreign bodies can be imaged in the uterus. These include glass marbles placed as an intrauterine device to suspend cyclicity and suppress estrous behavior in some mares (Figure 15.26). Occasionally mineralized fetal parts may be imaged following fetal mummification (Figure 15.27).

Certain intrauterine medications may appear hyperechoic on ultrasonographic examination; an example is procaine penicillin suspension in the uterus (Figure 15.28).

VAGINAL HEMATOMA

Vaginal trauma can result in hematoma formation and ultrasonography provides a useful diagnostic tool as

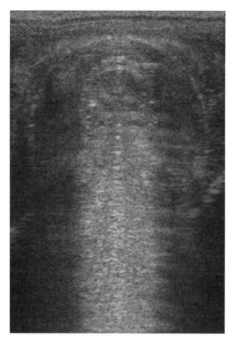

Figure 15.26 Ultrasonographic image of a 35 mm marble in the uterus of a mare.

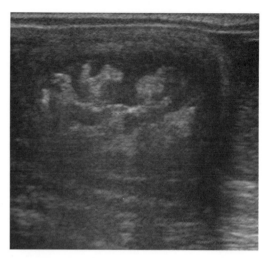

Figure 15.28 Ultrasonographic image of intrauterine antibiotic suspension.

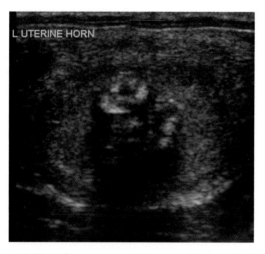

Figure 15.27 Ultrasonographic image of hyperechoic fetal remnants following mummification.

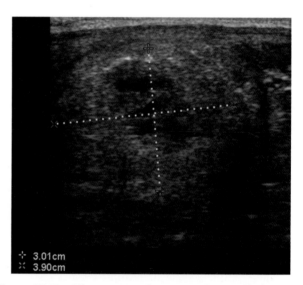

Figure 15.29 Ultrasonographic image of vaginal hematoma.

well as allowing monitoring of the regression of the hematoma (Figure 15.29).

VAGINAL POLYP

Vaginal polyps occur rarely in mares and ultrasound can be useful to image their extent (Figure 15.30).

OVARIAN CYSTS

Cysts lying within the ovarian stroma near the ovulation fossa of the ovary arise from the surface epithelium and are often seen in older mares during examination of the ovary (Figure 15.31). They are known as "retention", "inclusion", or "fossa" cysts and generally have no adverse effect on fertility. Para-ovarian cysts are remnants of the mesonephric ducts which can vary in size from a few mm to 2 cm. If large, they may be confused with the ovary on rectal palpation or ultrasound evaluation. They are of no consequence to fertility unless they impinge on the oviduct.

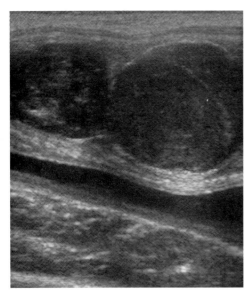

Figure 15.30   A large bilobed vaginal polyp.

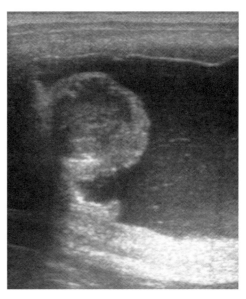

Figure 15.32   Ultrasonographic image of a uterine leiomyoma (with surrounding intrauterine fluid).

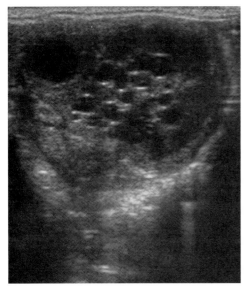

Figure 15.31   Ultrasonographic image of an 18-year-old mare with inclusion cysts in the ovary.

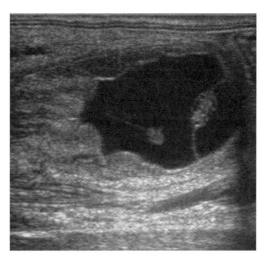

Figure 15.33   Ultrasound image of an unknown structure during a scan of a 28-day pregnancy.

UTERINE NEOPLASIA

Leiomyomas are the most frequently diagnosed equine uterine tumors. They may not directly affect fertility and are usually small and benign. In Figure 15.32, the typical pedunculated appearance of a leiomyoma can be seen.

UNKNOWN

Very occasionally a structure is imaged which is not an artifact, but of unknown origin. In Figure 15.33, an image of a day-28 pregnancy, a structure resembling a second embryo can be seen on the left-hand side. However, careful evaluation failed to reveal any heartbeat present. The mare went on to develop a normal single pregnancy and the structure was not visible at a subsequent ultrasound examination 10 days later. The mare foaled normally. Suggestions as to what the structure is would be welcomed by the author!

REFERENCES

[1] Gastal, E.L., Gastal, M.O., & Ginther, O.J. (1998) The suitability of echotexture characteristics of the follicular wall for identifying the optimal breeding day in mares. *Theriogenology*, 50, 1025–1038.

[2] McCue, P.M. & Squires, E.L. (2002) Persistent anovulatory follicles in the mare. *Theriogenology*, 58, 541–543.

[3] Ginther, O.J., Gastal, E.L., Gastal, M.O., Jacob, J.C., & Beg, M.A. (2008) Induction of hemorrhagic anovulatory follicles in mares. *Reproduction in Domestic Animals*, 20, 947–954.

[4] McCue, P.M. (2007) Ovulation Failure. In: *Current Therapy in Equine Reproduction* (eds J.C. Samper, J.F. Pycock, & A.O. McKinnon). Saunders Elsevier, St. Louis, 83–86.

[5] Cuervo-Arango, J. & Newcombe, J.R. (2009) The effect of hormone treatments (hCG and cloprostenol) and season on the incidence of haemorrhagic anovulatory follicles in the mare: a field study. *Theriogenology*, 72, 1262–1267.

[6] Ball, B.A., Almeida, J., & Conley, A.J. (2013) Detection of serum anti-Mullerian hormone concentrations for the diagnosis of granulosa-cell tumors in mares. *Equine Veterinary Journal*, 45, 199–203.

[7] Crabtree, J.R., Chang, Y., & de Mestre, A.M. (2012) Clinical presentation, treatment and possible causes of persistent endometrial cups illustrated by two cases. *Equine Veterinary Education*, 24, 251–259.

Transrectal Ultrasonography of Early Equine Gestation – the First 60 Days

Christine Schweizer

Early Winter Equine PLLC, Lansing, NY, USA

Introduction

Direct examination of the mare's reproductive tract for the purposes of pregnancy detection and evaluation during the first 60 days of gestation is best accomplished via transrectal palpation and ultrasonography. Effective and efficient breeding management of the mare is facilitated by early and accurate detection of pregnancy [1]. Prompt detection of mares who fail to become pregnant on a given bred cycle, or whose pregnancies fail to thrive prior to 35 days of gestation, presents the opportunity for follow-up diagnostics and rebreeding attempts within the confines of a limited breeding season [2]. Early detection of multiple embryos (see Chapter 17) provides the opportunity for effective reduction management prior to endometrial cup formation. For the purposes of this discussion gestational age will be measured as days from ovulation, where the date of ovulation is identified as day 0.

Transrectal Technique

Safety

Transrectal examination of the reproductive tract of the mare is a standard part of any reproductive practitioner's repertoire of technical skills. Appropriate restraint of the mare is indicated for both the mare's and the clinician's safety [3]. The risk of damage to the rectal mucosa and the possibility of producing a fatal rectal tear during the course of any transrectal examination should be foremost in the examiner's mind and govern the movement and manipulation within the rectum so that it is gentle and careful. The ample use of rectal lubricant facilitates the safe removal of fecal material from the mare's rectum and the safe movement of the examiner's hand and arm against the rectal mucosa, as well as providing effective contact between the ultrasound probe and rectal wall [3,4]. In the case of pregnancy diagnosis and evaluation it is important that practitioners be gentle in their manipulation in order to thoroughly ultrasound the mare's tract without damaging a developing embryo.

Palpation

Once all fecal material has been safely evacuated, the practitioner first performs a gentle palpation of the mare's uterus, cervix, and ovaries. This helps orient the position of the structures in the "mind's eye" and provides for an assessment of uterine and cervical tone. Visualizing an accurate mental picture of the reproductive anatomy of the mare's ovaries, uterus, and cervix during the course of both the palpation and ultrasound examinations of the tract will help accurately guide the examiner's hand and facilitate interpretation of what is being felt and visualized.

Uterine tone in the normal pregnant mare will be consistent with diestrus and becomes more prominent,

Atlas of Equine Ultrasonography, First Edition. Edited by Jessica A. Kidd, Kristina G. Lu, and Michele L. Frazer.
© 2014 John Wiley & Sons, Ltd. Published 2014 by John Wiley & Sons, Ltd.
Companion Website: www.wiley.com/go/kidd/equine-ultrasonography

with a distinct "two-humped" feeling to the base of each uterine horn (uterine bifurcation between them), beginning around 1–15 days of gestation. Uterine tone goes on to become especially pronounced and tubular between 18 and 30 days. With the development of pronounced uterine tone in the pregnant mare the uterine horns may become "kinked" especially at the base, sometimes turning back along the uterine body. Palpation can help identify this when it is present, and allows for gentle manual repositioning facilitating a complete examination. Starting at around 30 days of gestation (especially in maiden mares) the development of a palpable ventral bulge in the base of one uterine horn will aid in the identification of pregnancy. The cervix in the normal pregnant mare will be tubular and firm. Once palpation is completed the ultrasound probe can be introduced into the mare's rectum.

Imaging Technique

In most instances it is standard practice from 0–60 days of gestation to use a 5–10 MHz linear probe to perform the ultrasonographic pregnancy examination in real time [4]. Care should be taken to choose a probe that has smooth sides and rounded edges to protect the rectal wall during the course of the exam. The ample use of lubricant will help produce good contact between the probe surface and rectal wall with minimal pressure. The goal is a clear image without distorting the shape of, or possibly even damaging, the structures being examined (Figure 16.1). The early spherical

equine embryo is mobile within the mare's uterus for approximately the first 16 days of gestation until it becomes "fixed" within the uterine lumen. Therefore, detection of an equine pregnancy prior to fixation requires the practitioner to be able to scan the entire uterine lumen during the course of the ultrasound examination before the presence of an embryo or embryos can accurately be determined.

The uterine body is imaged from cervix to apex in a longitudinal plane and the horns are imaged from base to tip in cross-section [3] (Figure 16.2). As the tip of each horn is visualized to its conclusion, each ovary should then be imaged with careful note being made of the presence or absence and number of corpora lutea (CLs) present. The practitioner should develop a routine whereby they systematically and completely scan the uterus (Figure 16.3a). When imaging the cross-section of the horns it is important to center the round cross-sectional image on the ultrasound screen noting the direction orientation of the probe and the image. This helps the practitioner to stay on the uterus and notice if the probe skips over a section of the uterine horns (especially at the bifurcation). Likewise, when scanning longitudinally along the uterine body, gently rotating the probe along the long axis so that the image of the uterine body appears as "thick" as possible dorsal to ventral, helps image the lumen of the body completely (Figure 16.3b). Lastly, carefully scanning the cervix and vagina and noting the bladder and urethra as the probe is withdrawn from the rectum completes the exam and helps check for the presence of uro- or pneumovagina.

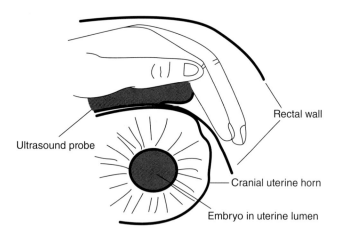

Figure 16.1 Probe cupped within the examiner's hand so that it is under control at all times. Tips of the examiner's closed fingers "lead" the probe so that they are free to gauge the tightness of the rectal wall and simultaneously "hook" the free cranial edge of the uterine horns to facilitate the complete imaging of the uterine lumen.

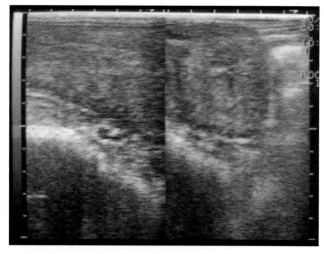

Figure 16.2 Left: longitudinal view of uterine body. Right: cross-section of uterine horn.

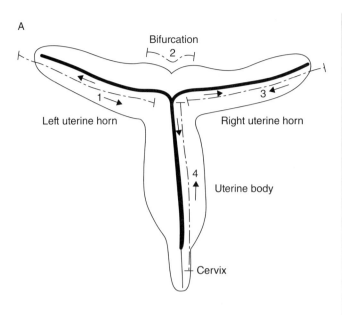

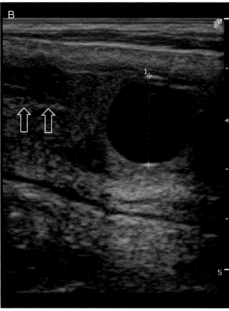

Figure 16.3 (A) Technique for completely evaluating the uterus, starting 1) at the base of one horn out to its tip, back down to its base, 2) carefully through the bifurcation from the base of one horn to the other, 3) from the base of that opposite horn out to its tip and back down again to its base and bifurcation, and finally 4) from the bifurcation to the connected apex of the uterine body and caudally through the uterine body back to the cervix. (B) Longitudinal ultrasonography of the uterine body. The hyperechoic line (arrows) indicates the uterine lumen. A 17-mm vesicle is present in the cranial uterine body.

IMAGE MILESTONES IN EMBRYONIC, PLACENTAL, AND FETAL DEVELOPMENT

The normal equine pregnancy develops in a predictable sequence in regards to size and development of visible structures through the embryonic stage (days 0–39) and through the fetal period covered in this chapter (days 40–60) [5,6]. While being careful to be gentle and non-disruptive to the developing pregnancy it is good technique to carefully scan through the entire pregnancy vesicle and piece together a three-dimensional image in the mind's eye of what is being presented on the screen.

Days 9–16

Prior to day 9 post-ovulation, it is not possible via ultrasound to identify the developing blastocyst after it arrives within the uterine lumen from the oviducts on or about day 6 post-ovulation [5,6,7]. The image of the pregnant mare's uterus at this stage will be consistent with a normal, non-pregnant diestrus mare. Uterine and cervical tone should be palpably increased relative to that of an estrus mare, and there should be no endometrial edema or free uterine fluid visible. One or more ovulatory CLs should be readily identifiable on one or both ovaries, and follicle sizes will depend on the point of follicular wave development at the time of the examination. In some cases (pristine uterus, excellent image quality, and sharp-eyed examiner) the developing embryo can be identified via ultrasound as early as day 9–11 when it is only <3–5 mm in diameter [5,6], but this is unreliable in most mares under field conditions and will necessitate re-examination regardless.

In the author's experience the normally developing embryo (Figure 16.4) can typically be first reliably identified starting at day 12 post-ovulation when it appears as an approximately less than or equal to 1-cm diameter, anechoic (fluid-filled), circular (spherical) structure located within the uterine lumen. After day 12, ultrasound imaging detects the anechoic, fluid-filled yolk sac [5,6] within the uterine lumen in contrast to surrounding uterine soft tissue echogenicity. There is often a characteristic, definable specular reflection, visible as lines of bright echogenicity dorsally and ventrally, on the tangent of the circumference of the embryo that is parallel to the probe (Figure 16.5) [5,6].

The embryo maintains its general anatomy, but increases in size in a linear fashion through day 16 (Figure 16.6). The embryo remains mobile within the uterine lumen until its increasing size and increasing uterine tone at approximately day 16 causes it to become "fixed", typically at the base of a uterine horn

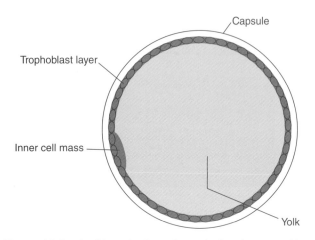

Figure 16.4 At this point in embryonic development (day 12) the embryonic vesicle is composed of a spherical layer of trophoblast cells (ectoderm) and endoderm [4] (by day 14 a mesodermal layer is added [4]) with a specialized embryonic disc region that is contained by and expanded against a glycoprotein capsule [8]. The capsule protects the embryo and helps the developing vesicle maintain a spherical shape around its yolk sac [5,6].

[5,6]. This embryonic migration is most pronounced around 14 days gestation when successful maternal recognition of pregnancy in the mare requires that the embryo make contact with the entire endometrial surface in order to block prostaglandin release by the uterus [5,6,8]. During the mobile period it is possible to visualize the contractions of the myometrium moving the embryo back and forth in real time if the examiner carefully stills the probe over the embryo and watches for them [5,6, and personal observation].

Days 17–28

Between days 17 and 26 dorsal–ventral diameter expansion of the embryonic vesicle plateaus [5,6], but between approximately days 18 and 20 the embryo loses its spherical structure, allowing the trophoblast cells (which form the chorionic surface of the placenta [5,6,9]) to conform to the irregular surface of the surrounding endometrium. In so doing the fluid-filled embryo acquires an irregular contour (Figure 16.7). As the embryo becomes "fixed" at day 16, normal vesicles become oriented so that the embryonic disc comes to rest against the ventral surface of the uterine lumen [5,6]. It is the cells of the embryonic disc that subsequently develop into the "embryo proper" which is the actual developing foal (Figures 16.8, 16.9) [4,5,6]. On or about day 23, the developing allantoic cavity first

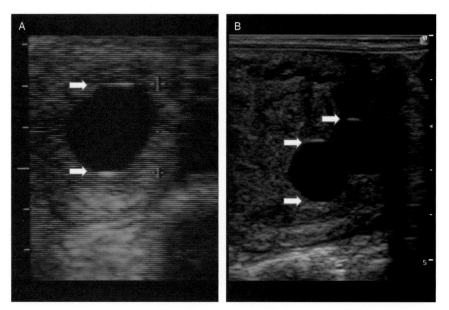

Figure 16.5 (A,B) The yolk sac is anechoic surrounded by the gray soft tissue density of the uterine wall. The uterine lumen "expands" immediately around the embryo accommodating its size, but otherwise the uterine wall remains in "tight" visual apposition immediately in front of and behind the embryo(s). Characteristically there is often a definable specular reflection, visible as lines of bright echogenicity dorsally and ventrally on the circumference of the embryo (white arrows).

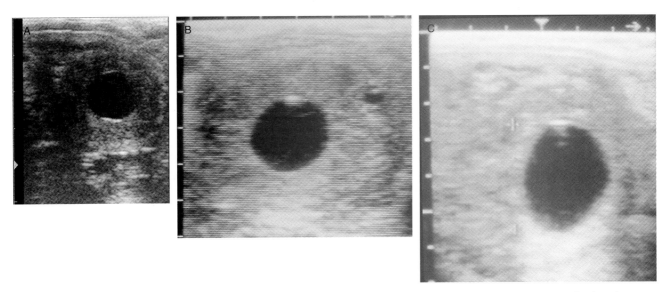

Figure 16.6 (A) 1.5-cm 14-day vesicle. (B) 2.0-cm 15-day vesicle. (C) 3-cm 17-day vesicle. Markers to the left of each image are in 1-cm increments.

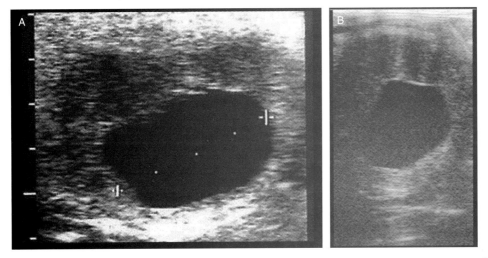

Figure 16.7 (A,B) 18-day vesicle. The fluid-filled embryo takes on an irregular contour after losing its capsule. It also begins to expand longitudinally in small but detectable amounts [5,6] and this can be appreciated as the practitioner scans through the vesicle distally along the horn from the base.

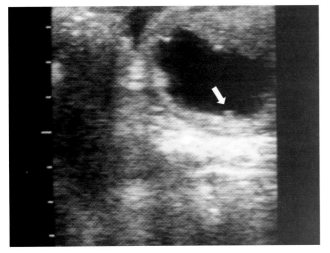

Figure 16.8 20–21-day embryo. The embryo proper first becomes visible as a small, ventral, echogenic projection (arrow) into the fluid-filled embryonic vesicle, typically by day 21.

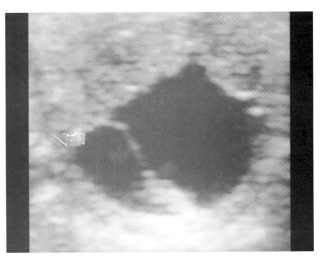

Figure 16.9 29-day embryo. At this time the shape of the entire embryonic vesicle sometimes takes on a "guitar pick" shape [1,5,6] but still retains the irregular contours of the surrounding endometrial folds.

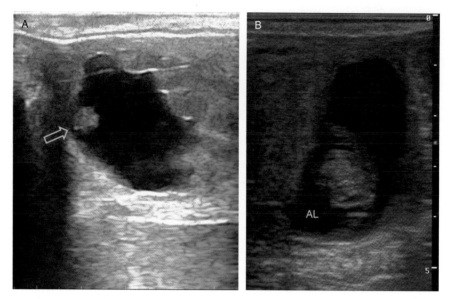

Figure 16.10 (A) 24-day embryo with anechoic, small developing allantoic cavity (arrow). The heartbeat should be easily detected at this stage. (B) 26-day embryo with developing allantoic cavity (AL). The heartbeat was also detected. (Source: Part A – Image courtesy of Dr Christy Cable DVM, DACVS.)

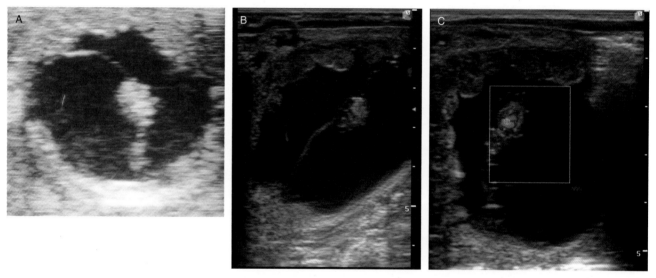

Figure 16.11 (A,B,C) 28-day embryos. The embryo proper appears suspended on an echogenic line that represents the apposition of the membranes of the yolk sac and allantois and divides the fluid-filled space into two cavities with the yolk sac dorsal and the allantoic space ventral. By 28–30 days this dorsal migration of the embryo proper has brought the developing embryo to a characteristic equatorial position within the vesicle. The heartbeat should be detectable.

becomes visible as it emerges from the hindgut of the embryo proper [4,5,6], and appears as a fluid-filled cavity ventral to the embryo proper (Figure 16.10). Over the course of the next 8 days the allantoic cavity enlarges and moves the embryo proper progressively dorsally through the embryonic vesicle (Figure 16.11) [5,6]. Also during this period the embryo proper has increased in size and a detectable heartbeat has devel-

oped. These features make this gestational age a common landmark for monitoring the development and viability of the embryo. In the author's experience the heartbeat can sometimes first be imaged by about 23 days, detectable as a rapid flicker centralized within the embryo proper. The heartbeat becomes more pronounced and more readily detectable as the embryo proper increases in size.

Days 30–40

From day 30 through day 35 the embryo proper continues its dorsal migration through the embryonic vesicle until it is almost resting against the dorsal wall, with a small yolk sac still visible dorsally (Figure 16.12). True implantation of the embryo does not begin to occur until very late in equine gestation, day 34–38 [8]. The epitheliochorial placentation of the equine is minimally to non-invasive, and true interdigitation of the chorionic and endometrial surfaces takes a while to develop. (Interdigitation is first recognizable at approximately day 45, but is not complete until after day 80 [9].) However, beginning on about day 35, trophoblast cells migrate from the chorionic girdle region of the embryonic vesicle [5,6,8,9] (visible on ultrasound where the line of apposition between the membranes of the yolk sac and the developing allantoic cavity meet the circumference of the vesicle [5,6]) to invade the endometrium and form the endometrial cups [8,9]. Once the endometrial cups form they will remain functional through what would be their normal lifespan (day 35–120+) whether or not the developing embryo/fetus remains viable [8,9]. The cups themselves are not normally discernible within the endometrium on routine ultrasound examination, although mineralized structures in non-pregnant mares with retained endometrial cups may be visible at the base of a previously pregnant horn in rare instances of abnormal cup retention [5,6, and author's observation]. Production of equine chorionic gonadotropin (eCG) by the formed endometrial cups stimulates the development of secondary CLs on both ovaries (Figure 16.13) [8,9].

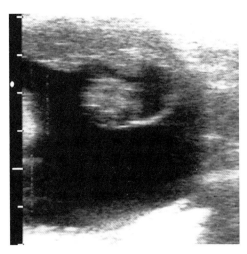

Figure 16.12 37-day embryo. The embryo proper has moved dorsally with the expansion of the allantois.

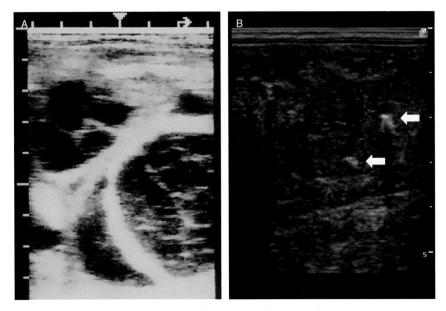

Figure 16.13 (A) Accessory corpora lutea on the ovary. Production of equine chorionic gonadotropin (eCG; pregnant mare serum gonadotrophin (PMSG)) by the endometrial cups stimulates the development of secondary/accessory CLs on both ovaries. In the author's experience, secondary CL development can be appreciated by the appearance of hemorrhagic-looking follicles and corpora hemorrhagicum-looking structures on one or both ovaries in addition to the original primary/ovulatory CL(s) (good records help identify) by day 40 to before day 60. (B) Mineralized, retained endometrial cups (arrows) in a non-pregnant mare.

Days 40–60

By day 40 the fetus is dorsal within the allantoic cavity and the umbilical cord has formed by the circumferential enclosure of the yolk sac by the allantoic membranes (Figure 16.14) [4,5,6]. Between days 45 and 50 the umbilical cord lengthens and the fetus begins a ventral descent through the allantoic cavity, suspended by the umbilical cord (Figure 16.15) [4,5,6]. By day 60 of gestation, the fetus has come to rest once again against the ventral surface of the uterine lumen, now readily identifiable as a foal with discernible anatomy (Figure 16.16) [8].

Spontaneous fetal movement, in addition to an identifiable heart beat, confirms fetal viability at the time of examination. Fetal movements likewise develop on a characteristic time line and have been previously described as the development of a head nod by day 40, whole body motion by day 45, limb motion after day 45, body raises by day 50, and fetal mobility by day 55 [5,6]. As the fetus ages the frequency and duration of spontaneous fetal movement also increases [4,5,6].

The chorioallantoic membrane begins to expand beginning day 40, and extends into the entire luminal space by day 65 [4,5,6] (day 80–85 [8]). The pregnancy is typically contained to the base of the pregnant (cord horn) through day 50 with the rest of the uterine lumen remaining "tightly collapsed" such that the non-pregnant horn, uterine body, and distal pregnant horn remain free of discernible fluid during the course of most routine examinations (Figure 16.17). By day 60, fluid expansion is more readily apparent through the bifurcation to the base of the non-pregnant horn and into the apex of the uterine body, with the fetus itself sometimes visible extending into the spaces from its anchoring cord horn.

Understanding the normal timeline of embryonic, fetal, and placental development makes it possible to

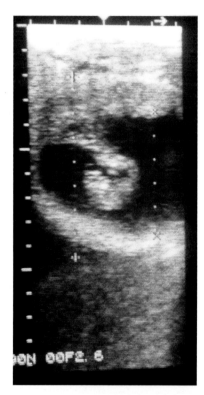

Figure 16.14   42-day fetus.

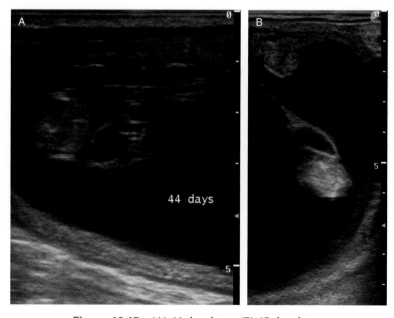

Figure 16.15   (A) 44-day fetus. (B) 45-day fetus.

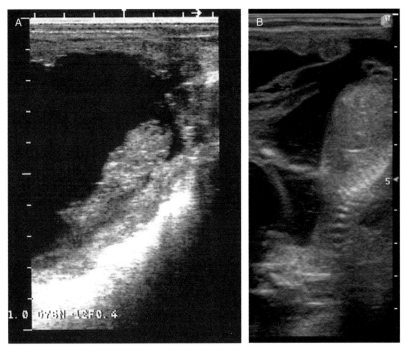

Figure 16.16 (A) 55-day fetus. (B) 62-day fetus.

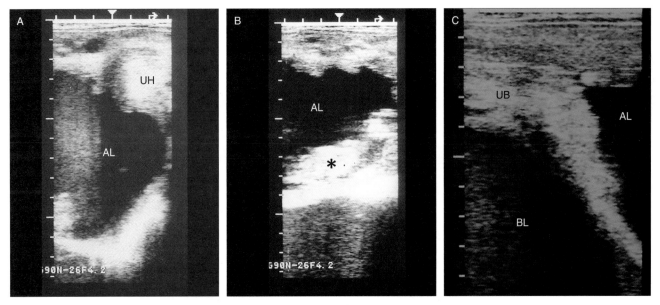

Figure 16.17 (A) 56-day pregnancy with allantoic fluid (AL) visible in the base of uterine horn but distal uterine horn (UH) appears contracted and fluid free. Ultrasonographic artifact makes the caudal portion of the allantoic fluid appear echogenic. (B) 56-day fetus (*) in base of uterine horn. Amniotic sac not always easily identifiable. Majority of fluid (AL) is allantoic. (C) Uterine body in a 56-day pregnancy. Note the caudal uterine body (UB) lumen appears to be fluid free and the fluid-filled allantoic cavity (AL) appears to only be present in the apex of the body. Urine in the bladder (BL) can have similar echogenicity to fetal fluids.

evaluate appropriate development relative to a known ovulation date, or to estimate gestational age of a pregnancy when an ovulation date is unknown. In the majority of successful pregnancies the landmarks of development are reliable, constant, and a key feature of interpreting the ultrasound images produced by the examination.

PREGNANCY FAILURE

In the author's practice, five routine pregnancy exams of otherwise normal mares and their pregnancies during the first 60 days of gestation are scheduled for day 14–15, day 16–17, day 28–30 (heart beat check), day 35–45, and day 60–70. At each examination the uterus is thoroughly imaged and an assessment of pregnancy development and rechecking for possible multiple pregnancies is performed. The schedule is set up so that there is a decreased likelihood that twins will be missed if they are present. It is also set up so that if a mare fails to successfully conceive or a pregnancy is lost after initial diagnosis but prior to day 35 the occurrence is readily identified so that the mare can be quickly prepared for rebreeding if indicated. Periodic examinations beyond day 35 help to identify mares that fail to maintain a viable pregnancy in spite of development of endometrial cups, and may offer insight into the reasons for pregnancy failure at these later dates (Figure 16.18). Multiple, accurate checks take on even more importance for those mares that are being supplemented with altrenogest or exogenous progesterone, so that these therapies can be discontinued and the mare allowed to return to estrus, either for rebreeding or to facilitate the resorption/expulsion of any non-viable fetal tissues (>day 40).

Pregnancy loss prior to day 40 has been reported to occur in 5–30% of pregnancies [2,7,10]. In infertile mares this loss may occur most often prior to day 6 when the embryo is still in the oviduct and ultrasound confirmation of conception is not possible [7]. Older mares (>18 years of age especially) experience embryonic loss at the upper end of the percentile, as compared to young fertile mares that experience a lower overall incidence of loss [2,7,10]. Note, however, that the incidence of pregnancy loss across all classes of mares is never zero, and for this reason it is recommended that all pregnancies be monitored at least through the embryonic and early fetal stages so that detectable losses are identified.

Ultrasound findings indicative of possible impending embryonic loss include an embryo that is small for its gestational age, an embryo that fails to increase in size or progress in development, failure of an embryonic vesicle to develop a visible embryo proper, an embryo in improper alignment relative to the ventral surface of the vesicle, failure of an embryo to develop a heartbeat at the expected time, or loss of a previously detected heartbeat [Personal observation, 2,7,10]. Embryos that "fix" in locations other than the base of a uterine horn (especially caudal uterine body pregnancies [2]) may also represent an increased risk of loss and bear monitoring. In the author's experience it is not unusual to detect a limited, mild amount of

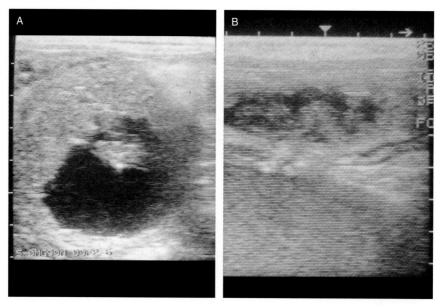

Figure 16.18 (A) Day 34 seemingly normal viable pregnancy. (B) Same pregnancy as (A) no longer viable at day 63.

endometrial edema around an otherwise healthy embryo between days 14 and 18 [4,5,6], but widespread or exaggerated endometrial edema or the presence of free uterine fluid are indicative of a pregnancy that is in jeopardy (Figures 16.19 and 16.20) [10].

Not every pregnancy between days 0–60 that varies in its development from the expected progression is doomed to fail, and it is sometimes important to watch and be patient. Many pregnancies that start out small for gestational age or behind in their expected devel-

opment, "catch up" in their development and go on to successfully produce normal, viable foals at term (Figure 16.21). Examinations that fail to identify an embryo at day 14–15 can be followed by examinations even as late as day 18 that reveal a mare that has failed to return to estrus and now has an identifiable embryo, albeit small for gestational age. Likewise an embryo that has a heart beat but with an otherwise small vesicular size sometimes rallies (Figure 16.22). It is therefore prudent in many instances to perform serial examinations [10] over the course of several days to be sure that an embryo is truly absent or is truly non-viable before reaching for the prostaglandin to terminate a "retained" CL (Figure 16.23).

DISTINGUISHING ENDOMETRIAL CYSTS FROM DEVELOPING EMBRYOS

The presence of endometrial cysts in a mare's uterus can complicate accurate pregnancy detection [7,11]. While glandular endometrial cysts are typically microscopic [7], lymphatic cysts can range in size from ≤10 mm in diameter to several centimeters [11]. Like the early equine embryo, endometrial cysts appear as fluid-filled structures within the lumen of the endometrium. In general, cysts do not appear as perfectly round structures and are usually "off center" relative to the uterine lumen, extending partially if not fully into the wall of the endometrium on the ultrasound image (Figure 16.24). Likewise, cysts do not

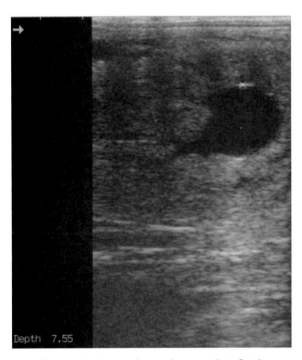

Figure 16.19   14-day embryo within fluid.

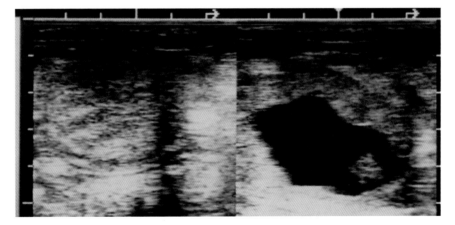

Figure 16.20   Widespread abnormal endometrial edema (left) accompanying an ultimately non-viable 27-day embryo (right). The finding of abnormal endometrial edema may represent inflammation and/or failure of luteal function with return to estrus imminent. In some instances, when these warning signs are detected while the embryo is still viable, it may be possible to intervene with supportive therapy and the pregnancy successfully continues [2,7]. Other times the pregnancy is lost and there is nothing to do but re-evaluate the mare for any possible underlying addressable reasons and try again.

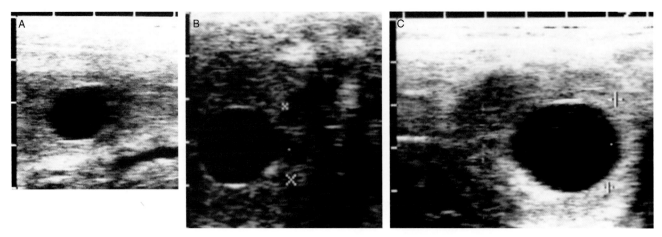

Figure 16.21   (A) Small for gestational age embryo that was only 12 mm at 14 days post ovulation. (B) Same embryo as A; still small for gestational age but growing. (C) Same embryo as A and B; small for gestational age, growing, and developed successfully to term.

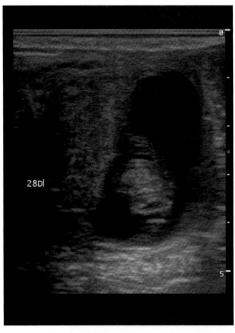

Figure 16.22   Small vesicle at 28 days but contains embryo with heartbeat that ultimately carried to term.

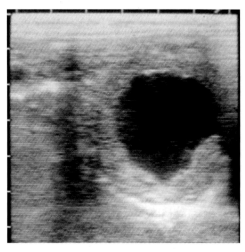

Figure 16.23   20-day embryo that fixed in the distal uterine horn rather than the base; the pregnancy was found to be viable at 60 days and the mare went on to foal successfully.

usually appear to increase in diameter over the course of several days, although sometimes cysts do prove to be somewhat dynamic and increase in size relative to estrus and diestrus, and "shrink" in some post-foaling mares between their foal heats and 30-day heats [author's observation]. Lastly, cysts do not move (Figure 16.25).

Many times, however, a practitioner is presented with a mare for pregnancy examination that he or she did not manage through the breeding, and may or may not have breeding dates for. If the presented mare also has unfamiliar and/or undocumented endometrial cysts this can make accurate diagnosis of the presence of an early embryo (<21 days gestation), and especially the presence of possible multiple embryos, challenging. In such instances it may become necessary and prudent to follow the mare over the course of multiple examinations beginning before 16 days of gestation to detect growth, location change of any embryo-like structure prior to 16 days of gestation (i.e. before fixation), or the eventual development of a visible embryo proper within the possible vesicle if more than 16 days of gestation (Figure 16.26). Patience and multiple examinations are required if a final correct assessment of the pregnancy is to be made, and the possibility of two embryos of differing gestational ages is to be accurately determined.

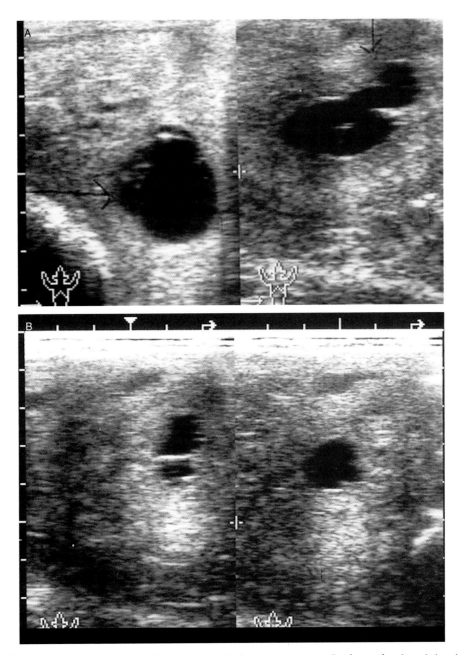

Figure 16.24 (A,B) Recording images of multiple endometrial cysts in a mare. In the author's opinion it is good breeding management to make careful note of the size and position of any cysts present within a mare's uterus during the course of breeding exams and carefully record that information in the record for future reference. Recording ultrasound images may also be useful. As a matter of routine, a well managed mare is monitored with ultrasonography in order to detect day of ovulation, multiple ovulations, and any possible post-breeding inflammation/fluid. Once examination has confirmed ovulation, this is an opportune moment to fully "map" the mare's endometrial cysts so the information is readily available for referral and comparison during the course of the upcoming pregnancy examinations [11].

CONCLUSION

As in all effective reproductive management, accurate and thorough record keeping will greatly aid the practitioner in identifying and interpreting the images that appear on the ultrasound screen during the course of pregnancy examinations during the first 60 days of gestation. Thorough and gentle examination techniques provide for efficient examinations that can be accomplished in a minimal amount of time with little

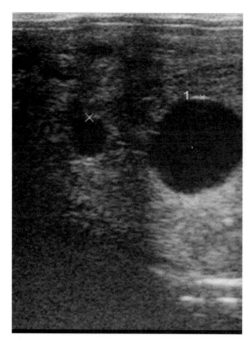

Figure 16.25 Mare with a 2-cm round, centered cyst adjacent to a smaller, slightly irregular cyst in the apical uterine body. Mapping cysts is especially useful when a mare has an endometrial cyst that strongly resembles an early embryo [4,11] that might be easily confused for a pregnancy or a twin.

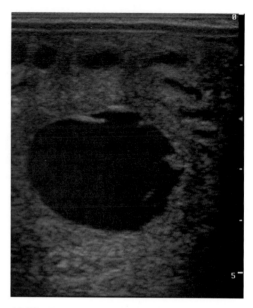

Figure 16.26 In some mares, the presence of numerous or multiloculated cystic structures, even when known and thoroughly documented, may make it impossible to be sure of the presence of an embryo or embryos until a heart beat can be definitively detected. This is especially worrisome if two CLs are detected on the mare's ovaries during the pregnancy exam and/or when it is definitively known that the mare experienced an asynchronous double ovulation.

discomfort to the mare and little risk to the developing pregnancy.

ACKNOWLEDGMENTS

The author would like to thank Dr Christy Cable DVM, DACVS, and Dr Kirsty Gallagher BVMS, DACT, for contributing images to this chapter.

REFERENCES

[1] Sertich, P.L. (1998) Ultrasonography of the Genital Tract of the Mare. In: *Equine Diagnostic Ultrasound* (ed. V.B. Reef). W.B. Saunders Company, Philadelphia, 405–424.

[2] Vanderwall, D.K. (2011) Early Embryonic Loss. In: *Equine Reproduction*, 2nd edn (eds A.O. McKinnon, E.L. Squires, W.E. Vaala, & D.D. Varner). Wiley Blackwell, Oxford, 2118–2122.

[3] Pycock, J.F. (2011) Ultrasonography. In: *Equine Reproduction*, 2nd edn (eds A.O. McKinnon, E.L. Squires, W.E. Vaala, & D.D. Varner). Wiley Blackwell, Oxford, 1914–1921.

[4] Bergfelt, D.R, Adams, G.P. (2011) Pregnancy. In: *Equine Reproduction*, 2nd edn (eds A.O. McKinnon, E.L. Squires, W.E. Vaala, & D.D. Varner). Wiley Blackwell, Oxford, 2065–2079.

[5] Ginther, O.J. (1998) Equine pregnancy: physical interactions between the uterus and conceptus. *Proceedings of the 44th Annual Convention of the American Association of Equine Practitioners*, 44, 73–104.

[6] Ginther, O.J. (1999) *Equine Pregnancy: Eleven Months of Intrauterine Activity* (Video). Equiservices Publishing, Cross Plains, Wisconsin.

[7] Ball, B.A. (2011) Embryonic Loss. In: *Equine Reproduction*, 2nd edn (eds A.O. McKinnon, E.L. Squires, W.E. Vaala, & D.D. Varner). Wiley Blackwell, Oxford, 2325–2338.

[8] Allen, W.R., Gower, S., & Wilsher, S. (2011) Fetal Membrane Differentiation, Implantation and Early Placentation. In: *Equine Reproduction*, 2nd edn (eds A.O. McKinnon, E.L. Squires, W.E. Vaala, & D.D. Varner). Wiley Blackwell, Oxford, 2187–2199.

[9] deMestre, A.M., Antczak, D.F., & Allen, W.R. Equine Chorionic Gonadotropin (eCG). In: *Equine Reproduction*, 2nd edn (eds A.O. McKinnon, E.L. Squires, W.E. Vaala, & D.D. Varner). Wiley Blackwell, Oxford, 1648–1664.

[10] McKinnon, A.O. & Pycock, J.F. (2011) Maintenance of Pregnancy. In: *Equine Reproduction*, 2nd edn (eds A.O. McKinnon, E.L. Squires, W.E. Vaala, & D.D. Varner). Wiley Blackwell, Oxford, 2455–2478.

[11] Stanton, M.E. (2011) Uterine Cysts. In: *Equine Reproduction*, 2nd edn (eds A.O. McKinnon, E.L. Squires, W.E. Vaala, & D.D. Varner). Wiley Blackwell, Oxford, 2665–2668.

CHAPTER SEVENTEEN
USE OF ULTRASONOGRAPHY IN TWIN MANAGEMENT

Richard Holder
Hagyard Equine Medical Institute, Lexington, KY, USA

Is it better to attempt to try to avoid twinning or to manage it once it occurs?

The development of twin-management techniques with the use of ultrasound has saved millions of dollars for horse owners and turned the incidence of abortions due to twinning from commonplace to a rare occurrence.

Avoidance of twinning can be attempted in a couple of different ways. Careful examination of the ovaries to detect multiple follicles to try to breed between the ovulations, or not breeding at all with multiple follicles would lessen the incidence of twinning. Avoidance of ovulation induction products (e.g. deslorelin, hCG), which encourage multiple follicles to ovulate, would reduce the incidence of twinning. The presence of multiple follicles and multiple ovulations increase the chance of the mare becoming pregnant; consequently, in the author's opinion it is better to increase the chance of becoming pregnant and deal with the occurrence of twins should they occur, rather than have a barren mare.

There are many useful questions that should be considered when deciding to manually reduce a twin vesicle during early gestation (~14–16 days of gestation).

- Are there definitely multiple vesicles or is it a cyst and a singleton?
- Is the vesicle that I am leaving definitely a pregnancy?
- Will the vesicle move?
- Has the vesicle grown from the day before?
- Is the vesicle large enough to be easily pinched or is it so small it may be difficult to express?
- If I have difficulty, cannot express the twin and have to try again later, will I know which vesicle I manipulated?

- Should I let the vesicles grow a day? What day of pregnancy is it?
- Should I come back in a few hours or try to separate the unilateral twins now?
- Is there a good chance the twin will reduce on its own? Approximately 75% unilateral twins at 17 days reduce on their own (personal experience).
- Is there a large size discrepancy between the vesicles? Is the size discrepancy related to ovulation dates?

All of these questions should be answered before manually reducing a twin.

Examination for pregnancy at the proper stage of gestation is mandatory to detect twins and have the opportunity to successfully express the selected twin vesicle. Some practitioners like to check 15–16 days from breeding to be sure they are still in the mobility phase. Some like to check 14–15 days from ovulation. It is sometimes difficult to tell when ovulation exactly occurs and accuracy of ovulation date is dependent upon when the mare is checked post breeding. If the mare is examined 2 days after breeding for ovulation then ovulation could have occurred anytime from when she was last checked before breeding to 2 days after breeding. This could be a 3-day span. Personal preference dictates when the examinations are done but it is important not to wait longer than 16 days from conception. After that time, if the twins are unilateral, they could be very difficult to separate. The author uses 15–16 days from breeding because the pregnancy cannot be any older than 15 or 16 days.

At 14–15 days from conception the vesicles are in their mobility phase and can be found anywhere in the uterus. A thorough examination of the mare's uterus is mandatory, regardless of the number ovulations thought to have occurred. It is important to examine

Atlas of Equine Ultrasonography, First Edition. Edited by Jessica A. Kidd, Kristina G. Lu, and Michele L. Frazer.
© 2014 John Wiley & Sons, Ltd. Published 2014 by John Wiley & Sons, Ltd.
Companion Website: www.wiley.com/go/kidd/equine-ultrasonography

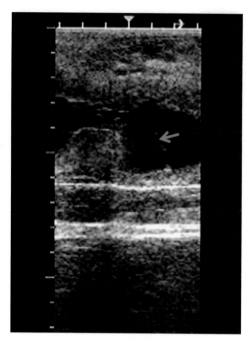

Figure 17.1   Twin vesicles. Careful evaluation may be necessary to observe the line of demarcation (arrow) between closely apposed twins.

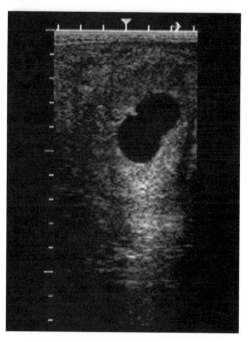

Figure 17.2   Twin vesicles. When twins are in close apposition and less than 16 days of gestation, re-evaluation at a later time may reveal them to have separated.

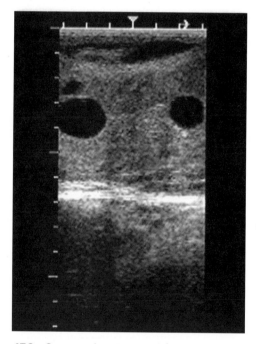

Figure 17.3   Separated twin vesicles in the uterine body. The size difference may be due to different gestational ages or delayed growth of the smaller vesicle.

the most distal tip of each horn and near the cervix. If the examination occurs after 16 days from conception and the twins are unilateral, it is often difficult to separate the vesicles due to increased tone of the uterus from the progesterone influence from the corpus luteum. Thus, the examination is best done during the mobility phase, before 17–18 days post conception.

During the mobility phase the twins can be separated, even if they are unilateral and in close proximity. Sometimes two yolk sac membranes will come together forming a very faint line indicating twins. (Figure 17.1) This can be difficult to see. If the twins are touching closely it is sometimes best to leave and return in 4–5 hours (Figure 17.2). If they are in the mobility phase they frequently will separate on their own when given time to move (Figure 17.3). If they continue to be in close proximity or re-examination is not possible, 10 mg IV of acepromazine maleate (Vedco, Inc., Saint Joseph, MO, USA) relaxes the increased tone of the uterus resulting from the elevated blood progesterone level. Allow about 5 minutes after acepromazine administration before attempting to separate unilateral twins transrectally. The twins can then be separated manually much more easily with less risk of unintentionally injuring either vesicle. The trick is to only injure the vesicle you are trying to rupture and not both. If the mare is straining or resisting your examination, it is important to use a rectal spasmolytic such as N-butylscopolammonium bromide (Buscopan

Injectable Solution, 60 mg IV, Boehringer Ingelheim Vetmedica, Saint Joseph, MO, USA) or propantheline (30 mg IV), to allow ease in handling the uterus. It is difficult to use delicate manipulation when the mare is straining against you. Sometimes gentle nudging of

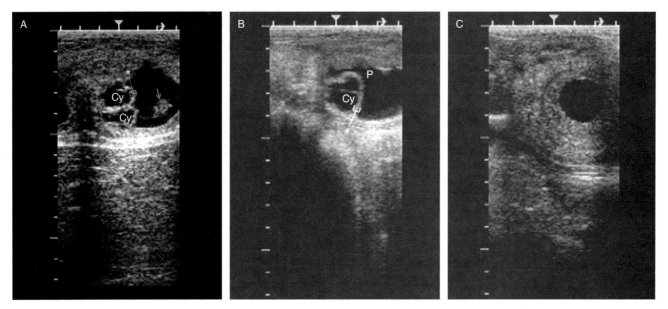

Figure 17.4 (A) 29-day pregnancy adjacent to two cysts (Cy). Identifying a heartbeat within the embryo (blue arrow) differentiates pregnancy from cysts. Note the hyperechoic, thick walls (*) of these cysts. (B) Endometrial cyst (Cy) with hyperechoic wall (*) protruding into a pregnancy (P). (C) Endometrial cyst that appears similar to a pregnancy.

both the vesicles will slightly separate them enough to allow placement of the ultrasound transducer between them to gently spread them apart. Slow and gentle pushing of the transducer into the area between the vesicles causes the vesicles to separate. For good results it is best to manipulate the uterus and vesicles as little as possible. With proper technique the percentage of normal single pregnancies at 60 days from twins that have been pinched at ~15 days is equal to a group of mares pregnant with a single pregnancy at ~15 days (personal experience).

If there are cysts present in the uterus, it is critical to be certain that the vesicle being left is a true pregnancy. A cyst can often be identified by having a visible wall that can be readily seen (Figure 17.4A,B). Cysts usually have an irregular shape and thickened wall, while the yolk sac of a 15-day pregnancy should be spherical or slightly oval in shape with a wall that is difficult to visualize (Figures 17.5, 17.6). Occasionally cysts appear just like a pregnancy (Figure 17.4C). Pregnancies at 18+ days can be slightly irregular in shape (Figure 17.7). A cyst cannot move much in comparison to a vesicle that can move from one end of the uterus to the other before 17 days. A cyst does not grow in size when examined the next day, while a pregnancy grows very noticeably at the 14–15-day stage. The size of the vesicle should be the proper size for the number of days of the pregnancy.

When encountering two vesicles of different sizes it is a good idea to try to reduce the smaller twin if pos-

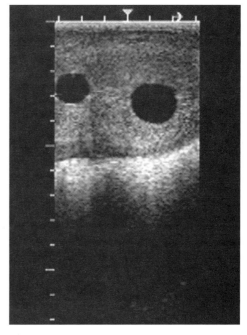

Figure 17.5 Twin vesicles of different diameters, either from ovulations that occurred on different days or due to growth rate differences.

sible (Figure 17.5). Sometimes a vesicle is smaller than expected because it is from a later ovulation, but it is possible that it is smaller because it is defective for some reason. If a vesicle is smaller than 15 mm, it is frequently evasive and difficult to express (Figure

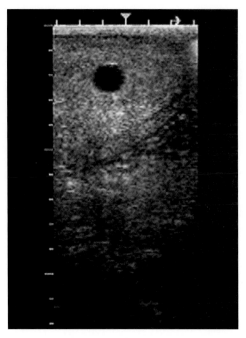

Figure 17.6 Unexpectedly small vesicle for a 15-gestational-day pregnancy evaluation (markers beside image are 10 mm apart).

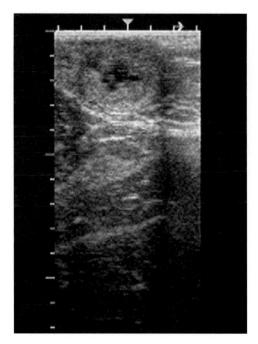

Figure 17.8 Vesicle after pinch.

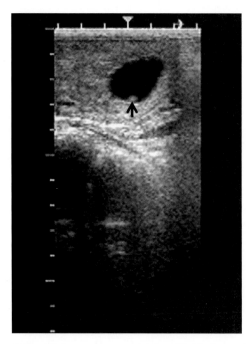

Figure 17.7 21-day pregnancy. After 17–18 days of gestation, vesicles can have an irregular shape that can make distinguishing them from an endometrial cyst difficult. Embryo proper indicated with arrow.

17.6). It is preferable to let a vesicle grow 1 day to become larger than 15 mm to facilitate expressing it and to avoid extensive manipulation of the uterus. Letting the vesicle grow 1 day is another good way to differentiate a cyst from a pregnancy; the pregnancy

should increase noticeably in size daily while the cyst will remain the same size. Monitoring the vesicles with measurements and saved ultrasonographic images is useful to determine size changes.

When a vesicle is reduced it can be pinched between the thumb and forefingers or it can be expressed by pressure between the transducer and the pelvis. There should be a very slight fremitus (vibration) felt as the vesicle ruptures and a small amount of free fluid is visible in the uterus at the spot of the rupture (Figure 17.8). Frequently the fluid from the ruptured vesicle migrates toward, and can be seen around, the pregnancy that is still present (Figure 17.9). If a twin is near the cervix, it can be expressed by forming cup with the four fingers of the hand around the vesicle and dragging the hand posteriorly, toward the cervix, pressing down on the floor of the pelvis until the vesicle ruptures. If you are expressing a twin in the horns of the uterus while one twin is in the body or near the cervix, be careful that the forearm does not put pressure on or accidentally rupture a twin near the cervix. If the twin is in the horn of the uterus it usually can be pushed to the tip of the horn where it can be easily trapped and expressed.

After the vesicle is reduced, in the author's opinion, it worthwhile to treat the mare with flunixin meglumine (1.1 mg/kg IV) once daily for 3 days. This has an antiprostaglandin effect in case there is a prostaglandin release from the manipulation of the uterus or in response to fluid from the vesicle. Some clinicians

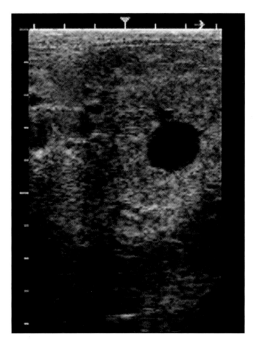

Figure 17.9 Trace anechoic fluid from pinched vesicle surrounding remaining vesicle.

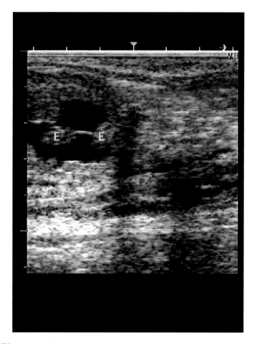

Figure 17.10 28-day adjacent twins (E: embryo).

recommend altrenogest (0.044 mg/kg PO SID, Regu-Mate, Intervet) in case there is compromise of the corpus luteal tissue supporting the pregnancy.

It is possible when examining a mare during the mobility phase at 15 days post ovulation that the mare could have a 14–15-day pregnancy and a 9–10-day pregnancy. Missing the 9–10-day pregnancy would be easy to do because it is so small. A transrectal scan 4–5 days later at 19–20 days from breeding should alleviate that problem because the 9–10-day pregnancy would have grown and be easy to see at that time.

The next exam should be at 28–30 days of gestation, again looking for twins that could have been missed. If twins are found at this stage and are bilateral they can be expressed with about a 50–60% success rate (personal experience). If the twins found at this examination are unilateral, it is very difficult to express one without injuring the other (Figure 17.10). It is best to follow the twins until about 33–34 days of gestation to see if they reduce to a singleton on their own. Finding two viable heartbeats is the best indicator of twins persisting. At ~35 days, the endometrial cups are forming, which may prevent the mare from returning to estrus if pregnancy loss were to occur. The endometrial cups produce pregnant mare serum gonadotropin (PMSG; equine chorionic gonadotrophin), causing secondary corpora lutea development for maintenance of the pregnancy. Prior to endometrial cup formation, and taking into consideration if there is time to rebreed

in the breeding season, the mare can be given prostaglandin to bring her back in heat and rebred. Most mares do well becoming pregnant again from this or subsequent breedings. If it is too late in the breeding season to rebreed the mare, it is best to see if the twin reduces on its own. The author has had poor results from manually expressing twins past 40 days, transvaginal twin aspiration and transabdominal twin injection.

If twins persist beyond 40 days, the author recommends a procedure associated with about a 60% success rate [1]: manual cranio-cervical dislocation of the fetal head to terminate one fetus in attempt to preserve the other. This can be performed transrectally after 60–70 days up to about 110 days of gestation. This involves grasping the head of the fetus and breaking down the tissue at the base of the posterior skull to sever it from the spinal cord. This does not immediately result in death of the twin but it will usually die in a few weeks. The untouched twin will be born normal about 50–60% of the time, while 40–50% of mares will abort both fetuses. This technique can be very difficult to perform transrectally, consequently a sterile surgical procedure was developed via a flank incision and grasping the head of the fetus through the uterine wall and dislocating it. The head is dislocated by manual manipulation at the base of the fetal skull with the thumb. The uterine wall stays intact. An advantage of this procedure is that a fetal

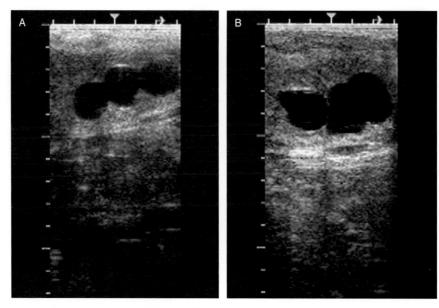

Figure 17.11   (A,B) Triplets.

sex determination can be performed and when there is a filly and a colt, the owner can select which sex to keep. A fetal sex determination is performed with transrectal ultrasonography during the surgery by another practitioner (Video 54), and the proper fetus is identified for elimination to the surgeon going in through the flank.

Video 54 Ultrasound of 58-day twins with views to allow fetal sexing

http://bit.ly/1fB0AJi

(This will take you directly to the video on Wiley Blackwell's companion website.)

Occasionally more than two pregnancies are present (Figure 17.11). The procedure is the same as for twin reduction. Some clinicians like to reduce one vesicle and come back the next day to reduce one more. This prevents a large amount of fluid from the rupture of two vesicles being released into the uterus at one time.

A twin vesicle is more easily expressed in a maiden mare than in a post-foaling mare with a larger uterus because the wall of the maiden mare's uterus is thinner. The ability to express a vesicle is difficult at first but becomes much easier with experience. The procedure is well worth the time and effort spent to become adept at manual reduction of twin vesicles and it is a very worthwhile service to offer to mare owners.

RECOMMENDED READING

Ginther, O.J. (1992) *Reproductive Biology of the Mare: Basic and Applied Aspects*, 2nd edn. Equiservices, Cross Plains.
Sheerin, P.C. (2010) Manual reduction of twins in the mare: effect of operator, mare age, and treatment. *Proceedings of the American Association of Equine Practitioners*, 56, 322.

REFERENCE

[1] Wolfsdorf, K.E., Rodgerson, D., & Holder, R. (2005) How to manually reduce twins between 60 and 120 days gestation using cranio-cervical dislocation. *Proceedings of the American Association of Equine Practitioners*, 51, 284–287.

CHAPTER EIGHTEEN

USE OF ULTRASONOGRAPHY IN EQUINE FETAL SEX DETERMINATION BETWEEN 55 AND 200 DAYS OF GESTATION

Richard Holder

Hagyard Equine Medical Institute, Lexington, KY, USA

Fetal sex determination between 55 days and 200 days of gestation is a worthwhile service to provide for clients. The procedure is difficult to learn and will require approximately 300–400 attempts at diagnosis to become accurate and confident of your diagnosis. Once it is learned it is not forgotten and will become easier and quicker with each subsequent examination.

STAGES OF GESTATION

There are primarily three different stages of gestation during which the determinations can be made: 1) between 55 and 90 days gestation, 2) between 90 and 150 days gestation, and 3) beyond 150 days gestation.

Fetal Development at Different Stages

55–60 days. The fetus is very accessible but it is small. The genital tubercle is difficult to see, and the tubercle may or may not have fully migrated.

60–70 days. This is the *ideal time* for the examination. The tubercle is distinct, fully migrated, and the fetus is easily accessible for viewing.

70–80 days. The fetus is slightly more difficult to reach and the tubercle is slightly less distinct.

80–90 days. It is more difficult to view the fetus, the tubercle is less distinct, the genitalia development is just beginning, and the fetus is frequently out of reach. Maiden mares often can be done at this time.

90–110 days. The fetus is usually accessible and the genitalia are gradually becoming more evident.

110–120 days. This is the *ideal time* for examination at the mid-gestation stage. The fetus is very accessible and the genitalia are very well developed.

120–140 days. The genitalia are well developed, but the posterior of the fetus may be difficult to access.

140–150 days. The fetus is large with the posterior difficult to access.

150+ days. The fetus is large with an anterior presentation and the posterior is usually out of reach transrectally. The transabdominal approach is best after 150 days of gestation.

Fetal Sexing 55–90 Days of Gestation

This stage involves finding the genital tubercle, a small, ~2 mm, hyperechoic bilobed structure, resembling an equal sign. It is the precursor to the penis in the male and the clitoris in the female. The genital tubercle must be identified and located in relation to other fetal anatomic structures. The tubercle can be seen as early as 52 or 53 days of gestation located between the hind legs on the ventral midline. As the fetus ages the tubercle appears to migrate toward the umbilical cord in the male and toward the tail in the female. Around day 55 from conception the tubercle has usually migrated enough to make a determination. At this time the fetus is easily accessible by transrectal palpation and an accurate determination (99%+ accuracy) can be made a very high percentage

Atlas of Equine Ultrasonography, First Edition. Edited by Jessica A. Kidd, Kristina G. Lu, and Michele L. Frazer.
© 2014 John Wiley & Sons, Ltd. Published 2014 by John Wiley & Sons, Ltd.
Companion Website: www.wiley.com/go/kidd/equine-ultrasonography

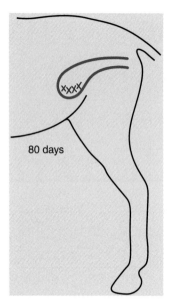

Figure 18.1 Schematic of the uterus and fetal location within the abdomen at 80 days of gestation.

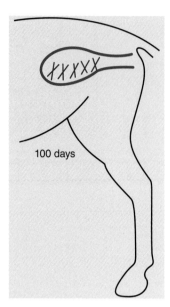

Figure 18.2 Schematic of the uterus and fetal location within the abdomen at 100 days of gestation.

(~98%) of the time with one examination. This examination of the fetus takes 10 seconds to 2–3 minutes depending on the experience of the examiner. The fetus is easily accessible until around 75 days of gestation. At this time, in some mares, the fetus can be difficult to access. Usually, it can be done until about day 80.

At about 80 days of gestation, the fluid of the pregnancy pulls the uterus over the rim of the pelvis. The fetus is small and falls to the most ventral part of the uterus in the allantoic fluid. However, after ~90 days, the uterus does not continue to move more ventrally into the abdomen. It actually elevates in the abdominal cavity as it becomes larger and the fetus is usually visible again at about 90–95 days of gestation. As the fetus grows it often extends back into the pelvic cavity and is readily visible after around 100 days. At this time the external genitalia are used to make a sex determination (Figures 18.1, 18.2).

Fetal Sexing 90–150 Days of Gestation

At 90 days the fetus comes back into view, as the uterus seems to elevate dorsally in the abdominal cavity and is easily accessible. The genital tubercle is less prominent now but the external genitalia (penis, prepuce, glans penis, and the gonads in the male, and the mammary gland, teats, clitoris, and the gonads in the female) are just beginning to be evident. Determinations are somewhat more subjective at this stage because of the need to evaluate the tissue densities

between prepuce and muscle or mammary gland and muscle. Other fetal tissues frequently obscure the genitalia. The optimum time for determination at this stage is between 110 and 125 days. It is usually not as clear as the genital tubercle evaluations, and it may take anywhere from 30 seconds to 5–10 minutes. A sex determination can be made 90% of the time at this stage, with 98+% accuracy, with one examination.

Fetal Sexing after 150 Days of Gestation

If the posterior part of the fetus cannot be accessed transrectally, it is worthwhile to attempt transabdominal ultrasonography using a 2.5–3.5 MHz sector scanner. With the proper equipment good visualization of the posterior area of the fetus can frequently be achieved. The transducer should be placed on the midline of the mare's abdomen slightly anterior to the udder and moved anteriorly until the fetus is located. Locate the heart of the fetus for orientation and locate the umbilical entrance to the abdomen. Follow the ventral midline of the fetus posteriorly from the umbilical entrance to the abdomen until the base of the tail is reached. In the male, the prepuce and hyperechoic area of the glans penis will be seen just posterior to the entrance of the umbilical cord. The mammary gland and teats of a female fetus will also be seen in this area. Moving posteriorly it is possible to see a clitoris on the fetal midline before the base of the tail is reached.

The external genitalia on a transabdominal scan appear the same as the 100+ day transrectal views but they are not quite as clear. When attempting transabdominal fetal sexing, the heart and the umbilical entrance into the abdomen are the most useful markers. Adjusting the ultrasound to a deep penetration reduces the visual size of the fetus and allows for better visualization of a larger area of the fetus. This is helpful in relating the location of certain structures to other fetal anatomic structures. The genitalia can be seen on the ventral midline, between the umbilical entrance to the abdomen and the base of the tail. These include the prepuce, glans penis, and penis in a colt and the mammary gland, teats, and clitoris in a filly. These structures are difficult to visualize but can be seen with much practice.

ULTRASONOGRAPHIC PLANES

- Plane I (primarily useful for colts) (Figure 18.3)
- Plane II female (ideal view for filly diagnosis) (Figure 18.4)
- Plane II male (similar to female view but slightly more anterior for colts) (Figure 18.5)
- Plane III (primarily useful for colt diagnosis) (Figure 18.6, focus on 18.6A)

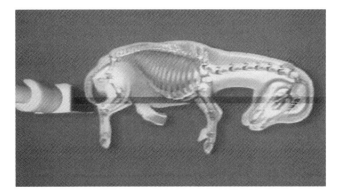

Figure 18.3 Plane I, primarily useful for colt diagnosis.

Take Home Hints

1. If the image is not clear, push down gently on the uterus with the probe to bring the fetus closer to the probe. This changes the focal point for various areas of the fetus and creates movement of the allantoic fluid, causing the fetus to change position slightly.
2. If the view of fetus is not productive, turn the transducer 90° to the left. If the view is still not productive, turn the transducer 180° to the right. Somewhere in this 180° span is the proper scanning plane for viewing the tubercle.
3. If the mare is straining, do not hesitate to use propantheline (30 mg IV) or butylscopolamine bromide (Buscopan, Boehringer Ingelheim GmbH) (40 mg IV) to lessen straining. This enables one to move the probe to various positions to get different angles of view of the fetus.
4. Darkened ambient light makes the details of the genital tubercle easier to recognize.
5. It may be necessary to place the probe in front of the hand to reach older fetuses. This is difficult to do without a stiff probe cord.
6. Evacuate fecal material as far anteriorly as possible.
7. View a cross-section of the fetal abdominal cavity to identify ribs. This will give you dorsoventral orientation (the dorsoventral orientation is very critical in differentiating the hyperechoic tailhead and tibias). Proceed posteriorly until you have moved off the fetus. The bright spot on the dorsal area of the posterior fetus as you move back on the fetus will be the tailhead. The two bright spots on the ventral area of the posterior fetus will be the tibias.

PROCEDURE AT 55–90 DAYS

Place proper restraint on the mare and evacuate feces thoroughly. If the mare is straining, a smooth muscle relaxant may need to be given (propantheline 30 mg or Buscopan 30–40 mg IV). First, determine the anterior–posterior positioning of the fetus. Find the skull (good anterior marker), the heart (good ventral marker), and

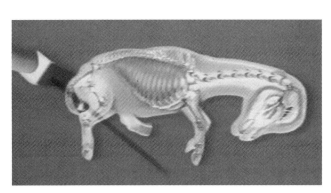

Figure 18.4 Plane II female. Ideal view for filly diagnosis.

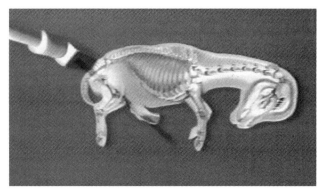

Figure 18.5 Plane II male. Ideal view for colt diagnosis.

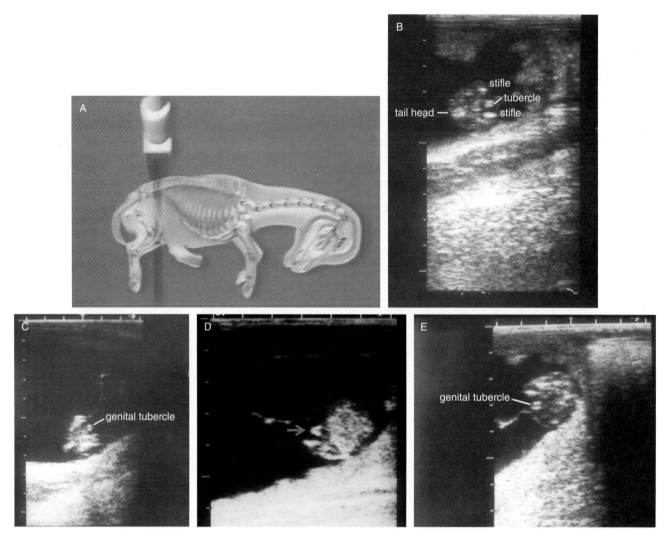

Figure 18.6 (A) Plane III, primarily useful for colt diagnosis. (B) Colt. (C) Colt. (D) Colt, with a prominent hyperechoic bilobed genital tubercle (arrow). (E) Colt.

the umbilical entrance to the abdomen (good ventral marker), which appears as a 3–4-mm dark hole on the posterior abdominal midline (Figure 18.7, focus on 18.7B). The ribs coming off the vertebrae (Figures 18.8, 19.9) and the tail are good dorsal and posterior markers, respectively (Figures 18.10, 18.11, 18.12 (focus on 18.12A), 18.13 (focus on 18.13A)). Using these markers for orientation, scan the area to see if an obvious genital tubercle is present.

Next, try to get a transverse view of the abdomen where the plane of the ultrasound beam transects the fetus perpendicular to the axis of the fetal spine (plane III) (Figures 18.6, 18.8, 19.9, 18.14). It is necessary to look for markers (ribs) that identify dorsal and ventral orientation of the fetus. The spinal column exhibits as a hyperechoic equal sign and is a good dorsal marker (this looks slightly like a genital tubercle but is on the

dorsal side rather than the ventral side) (Figure 18.9). Ribs coming off of the vertebrae are often the most useful dorsal marker (Figure 18.8, 19.9). The umbilical cord entering the abdominal cavity is a very good ventral marker (Figure 18.15). These markers give an idea of where you should be looking for the genital tubercle.

The genital tubercle for the male will be on the ventral midline just posterior to the umbilical entrance into the abdominal cavity (Figures 18.7A,B,C). The genital tubercle for the female will be on the fetal ventral midline just under the tail head. (Figure 18.12). If you have a transverse ultrasound plane (perpendicular to the axis of the spine), continue with this plane until you leave the posterior part of the fetus. After there is no fetus in view, keeping this same plane, ease back toward the fetus. The first hyperechoic area

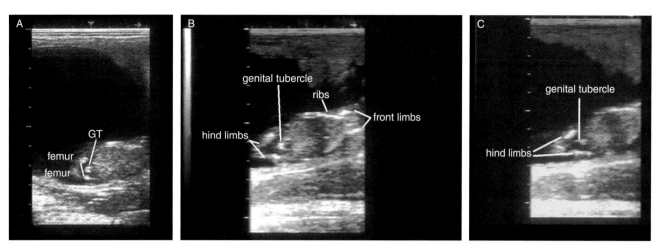

Figure 18.7 (A) Colt, viewed in plane I. GT: genital tubercle. (B) Colt, viewed in plane I; note the anechoic umbilical entrance to the abdominal cavity just cranial to the genital tubercle. (C) Colt, viewed in Plane I.

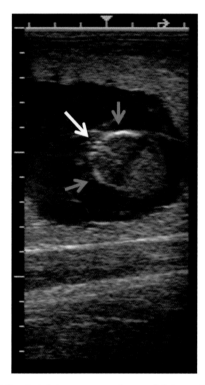

Figure 18.8 Axial transverse plane of fetus with hyperechoic ribs (blue arrows) and vertebrae (white arrow). Ribs are an easily viewed dorsal reference.

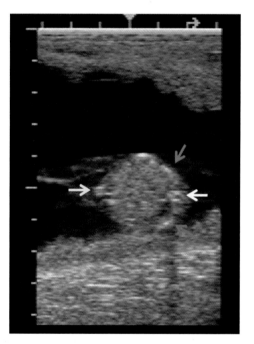

Figure 18.9 Colt, 65 days of gestation, viewed with Plane III technique. Ribs (blue arrows) and vertebrae (white arrow) provide dorsal reference. Genital tubercle indicated with yellow arrow.

that you see on the dorsal side will be the tailhead. The next hyperechoic areas will be the genital tubercle just under the tail (in a female) and two hyperechoic areas (tibias), with no muscle mass around them, about 1–2 cm from the tail, depending on the age of the fetus (Figures 18.12, 18.13A). There now should be thee or four hyperechoic areas in view. If it is a colt there will be three hyperechoic areas forming a tailhead–tibia triangle with no hyperechoic area within this triangle (Figure 18.11). If it is a filly, a bilobed hyperechoic equal sign will appear within the tailhead–tibia triangle slightly closer to the tailhead (Figures 18.12, 18.13A). This view is a requirement for identifying a filly. A colt tubercle can be visualized from many different angles

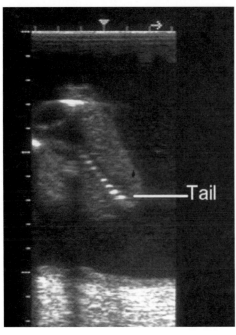

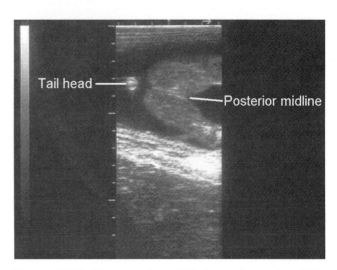

Figure 18.11 Posterior fetus, 113 days of gestation. Tailhead is dorsal reference. Posterior midline discernable with absence of clitoris suggesting a colt.

Figure 18.10 Posterior fetus viewing the tail. Line points to the most dorsal aspect of tail.

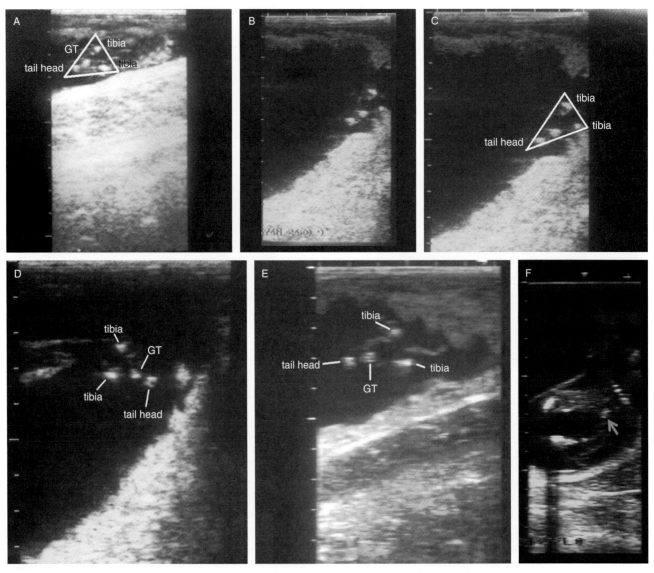

Figure 18.12 (A) Filly, 63 days of gestation. Tailhead provides dorsal reference. GT: genital tubercle in the middle of triangle created by tailhead and tibias. (B) Filly. (C) Filly. (D) Filly; GT: genital tubercle. (E) Filly. (F) Filly, 78 days of gestation. Tailhead and tail to right, tibias to the left, with clitoris (arrow) within the triangle formed by the tailhead and tibias.

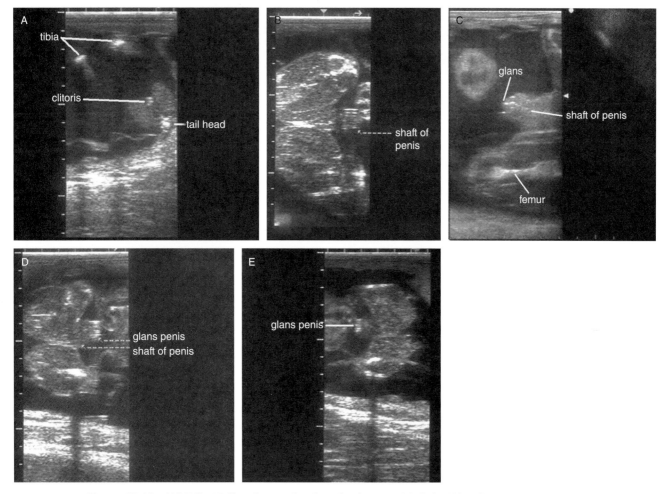

Figure 18.13 (A) Filly. Tailhead provides dorsal reference. (B) Colt. (C) Colt. (D) Colt. (E) Colt.

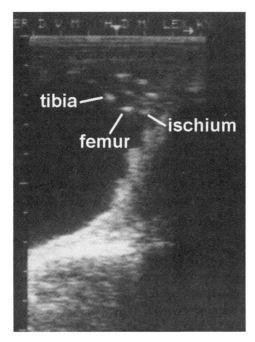

Figure 18.14 Pelvic bones, visualized while orienting for plane II or plane III views.

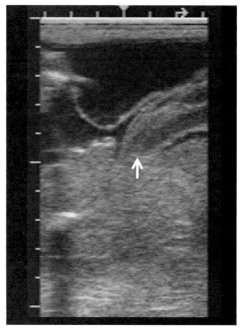

Figure 18.15 Colt, 115 days of gestation. Oblique sagittal view of penis caudal (left) to umbilical cord insertion (indicated with arrow). The umbilical cord attachment to the fetus is a good ventral reference.

including a frontal plane (plane I, Figure 18.7A,B) that exhibits the front legs, ventral abdomen, and hind legs. The tubercle will appear on the ventral midline slightly anterior to a line drawn between the stifles and slightly posterior to the umbilical entrance into the abdominal cavity (Figure 18.7A,B,C).

If there is a negative filly view (nothing within the triangle) then advance the plane of the scan anteriorly on the fetus. The male tubercle will appear just at the ventral edge of the abdominal wall as a hyperechoic bilobed equal sign (Figure 18.6D). Moving the ultrasound plane toward plane I you will see the umbilical entrance to the abdominal cavity (appears as a small black hole, Figure 18.7B). If you move the transducer to plane II you will see a tubercle between the hind legs (Figure 18.6B,C,E). The tubercle should be anterior to a line drawn between the stifles to make sure it is a colt. Remember that at 52–53 days the tubercle is between the hind limbs in both male and female. We

have to wait at least until 55 days of gestation to determine which direction the tubercle appears to be moving. If the tubercle is anterior to a line drawn between the stifles it will be a colt. If the tubercle is posterior to a line between the stifles it will be a filly. If it is difficult to decide, wait 3 or 4 days and look again.

PROCEDURE 90–150 DAYS

This procedure involves finding the external genitalia of the fetus. After 90 days the fetus begins to come back into transrectal view with the ultrasound. It is best to scan the entire fetus to get oriented anteriorly, posteriorly, dorsally, and ventrally. It is good to get a cross-sectional view of the posterior abdomen (Figure 18.16, focus on 18.16F) and keeping that plane move off the fetus posteriorly. As one comes back on to the fetus it

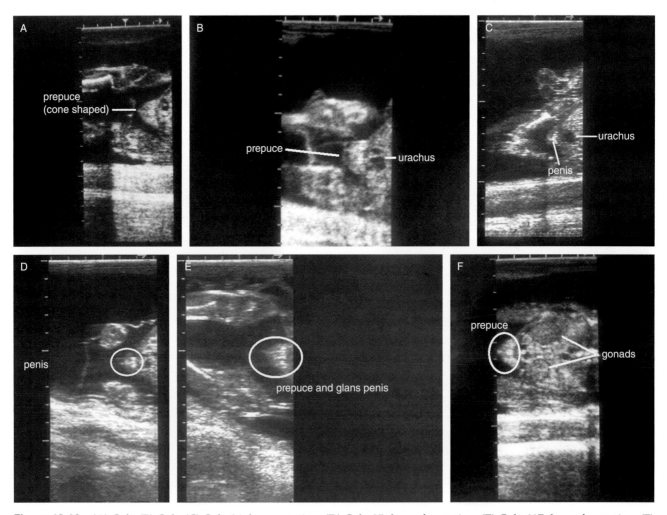

Figure 18.16   (A) Colt. (B) Colt. (C) Colt, 94 days gestation. (D) Colt, 95 days of gestation. (E) Colt, 117 days of gestation. (F) Colt, with prepuce and gonads in view.

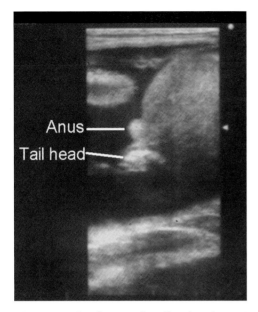

Figure 18.17   122 day fetus with tailhead and anus in view.

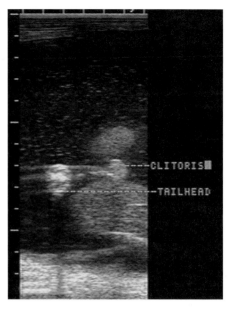

Figure 18.19   Filly, 110 days of gestation.

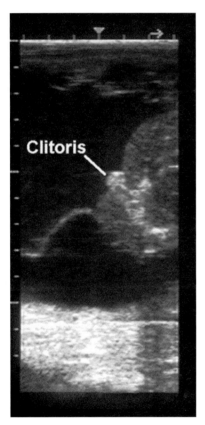

Figure 18.18   Filly.

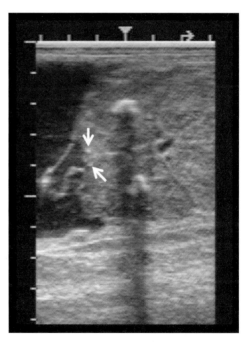

Figure 18.20   Filly, 105 days of gestation. Clitoris indicated by arrows.

is possible to get the same tailhead–tibia triangle with the clitoris showing up just under the tailhead within the triangle (Figure 18.12F, 18.13A). If the structure on the midline is too close to the tail it could be the anus (Figure 18.17). If nothing is under the tailhead, notice the prominent ventral midline (appears as a white line) (Figure 18.12). In a filly, following the prominent ventral midline posteriorly to the tailhead will lead to the clitoris (small round hyperechoic mass (Figure 18.12F, 18.13A, 18.18, 18.19)), that may appear as two hyperechoic dots lying on each side of the ventral midline (Figure 18.20). Following the ventral midline anteriorly from the tailhead leads to the mammary gland (Figure 18.21). The mammary gland consists of

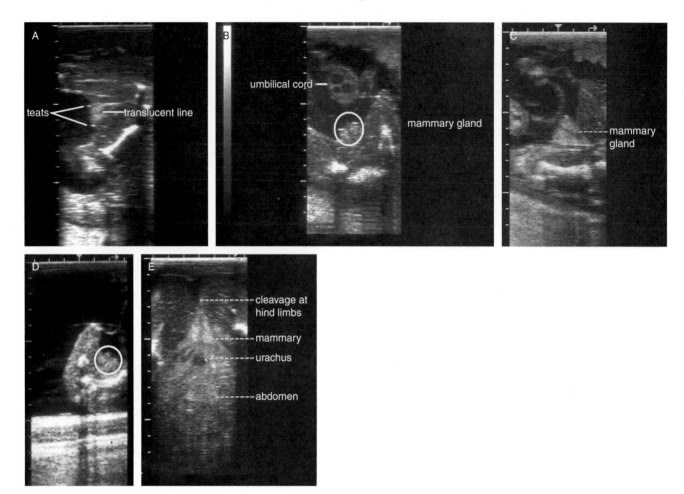

Figure 18.21   (A) Filly, 124 days of gestation. (B) Filly, mammary gland within white circle. (C) Filly, 129 days of gestation. (D) Filly, mammary gland within white circle. (E) Filly, 134 days gestation, Plane I view.

three distinct parts: the bright small hyperechoic teats, on each lateral side of the gland (Figure 18.21A,B,C), and two dense halves of the mammary gland separated by a hypoechoic line between the two halves (Figure 18.21). Preputial tissue is not as dense as a mammary gland and does not have a hypoechoic line separating the halves, and obviously has no hyperechoic teats.

In a male, following the ventral midline posteriorly using plane II, nothing is encountered before reaching the tailhead (Figure 18.11). Following the ventral midline anteriorly from the tailhead will lead to the prepuce (a cone-shaped structure that comes to a point (Figure 18.16A,B)). The penis can often readily be seen as a shaft-like structure with a bright hyperechoic mass on the end (Figure 18.13B,C,D,E). This bright hyperechoic tip is the glans penis. Figure 18.22 is a sagittal view through the flank of a shaft of a penis with a hyperechoic tip. Using a plane III view (a cross-section of the posterior abdomen) the prepuce will be seen as a cone-shaped structure off the ventral abdomen. Fre-

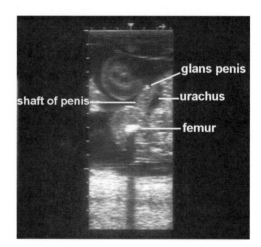

Figure 18.22   Sagittal view of colt, 109 days of gestation.

quently the hyperechoic mass of the glans penis will be seen within the prepuce (Figure 18.16). It is possible to get a plane III view of the glans penis without any of the prepuce in view (the glans penis frequently protrudes out the front of the prepuce). This will appear

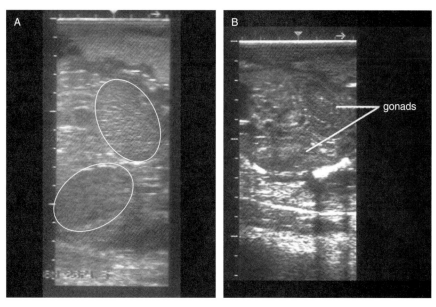

Figure 18.23 (A) Colt, 130 days of gestation. Gonads (circled) have homogeneous appearance. (B) Filly, 119 days of gestation. Female gonads have a central dense area surrounded by a more translucent peripheral oval ring.

as a hyperechoic mass off the ventral abdominal wall just posterior to the umbilical entrance into the abdominal cavity (Figure 18.16C). The main marker to be utilized is the prominent ventral midline (Figure 18.11).

The gonads can readily be seen but should be used to support a diagnosis and not to make a diagnosis. The male gonads usually appear very homogeneous (Figure 18.23A) whereas the female gonads have a central dense area surrounded by a more translucent peripheral oval ring (Figure 18.23B). These can be difficult determinations and are not reliable for a diagnosis by themselves.

PROCEDURE FOR TRANSABDOMINAL SCAN POST 150+ DAYS

Mares usually do not object to transabdominal ultrasonography. Generally no restraint is used on the mare, but if a mare will not stand quietly she can be sedated or tranquilized. Alcohol is applied liberally over the ventral midline of the mare's abdomen. Lubricant can be used to enhance coupling. It is good to have a stool to sit on during the examination.

Scan the entire ventral midline until the fetus is located. When the fetus is located, locate the beating heart then proceed posteriorly on the fetus. Locate the umbilical entrance to the abdominal wall (Figure

18.15). The transducer must be manipulated in many different directions to expose recognizable anatomic structures. Moving very slowly, look for a hyperechoic mass (glans) just posterior the umbilicus. If nothing is seen, slowly proceed posteriorly until the area of the posterior abdominal midline and the hind legs converge. A prepuce, glans, and penis in the male (Figure 18.13D) or the triangular mammary gland and teats in the female will be in this area (Figure 18.21A). If nothing is definitely identifiable proceed along the fetal ventral midline between the hind legs to the tailhead. The clitoris can be seen on the midline in a female before the tailhead is reached. At this stage of gestation the external genitalia are large and can be seen but it is often difficult to distinguish between a mammary gland and a prepuce. The prepuce will have varying degrees of a hyperechoic glans and penis (Figure 18.13B,C,D,E), whereas a triangular mammary gland will have no definite hyperechoic area except for two small hyperechoic teats (Figure 18.21A). The triangular mammary gland will be more dense and echoic than the surrounding tissue. These scans are difficult at first and may take considerable time. Trying different sides of the mare sometimes gives better exposure if the posterior fetus is not on the midline. This also allows switching and resting of the arms handling the transducer.

Post 150 days is not the preferred time to do fetal sexing. However clients sometimes decide at a later date that it needs to be done. Days 60–70 is still the optimum time to do the sexing: it is quicker and easier for the mare and the practitioner and cheaper for the client!

RECOMMENDED READING

Ginther, O.J. (1985) *Ultrasonic Imaging and Animal Reproduction. Horses*. Equiservices, Cross Plains.

Ginther, O.J., Curran, S., & Ginther, M. (1995) *Fetal Gender Determination in Cattle and Horses* (video). Equiservices, Cross Plains, WI. (Instructional video available from Equiservices, 4343 Garfoot Road, Crossplains, WI 53528 (telephone 608-798-4910))

Holder, R.D. (2011) Chapter 218. In: *Equine Reproduction*, 2nd edn (eds A.O. McKinnon, E.L. Squires, W.E. Vaala, & D.D. Varner). Wiley Blackwell, Oxford, 2080–2093.

Holder, R.D. (2001) Sex determination in the mare between 55–150 days gestation. *Proceedings of the 46th Annual Convention of the American Association of Equine Practitioners*, 46, 321–324.

Holder, R.D. (1997) *A Guide to Equine Fetal Sexing 55–150 days*. Instructional video available from Hagyard Equine Medical Institute, 4250 Iron Works Pike, Lexington KY, 40505 (telephone 859-255-8741).

Holder, R.D. (2007) Chapter 53. Fetal sex determination. In: *Current Therapy in Equine Reproduction* (eds J.C. Samper, J. Pycock, A.O. McKinnon). Saunders Elsevier, St. Louis, MO, 343–356.

Holder, R.D. (2003) Chapter 5.22. Determination of fetal gender. In: *Current Therapy in Equine Medicine*, 5th edn (ed. N.E. Robinson). Saunders, Philadelphia, 288–294.

CHAPTER NINETEEN

USE OF ULTRASONOGRAPHY IN FETAL DEVELOPMENT AND MONITORING

Stefania Bucca

Qatar Racing and Equestrian Club, Doha, Qatar

INTRODUCTION

Ultrasonography offers safe and continuous viewing of fetal life in the mare, from completion of fetal organogenesis (day 40) to term. The combination of transrectal and transabdominal scanning techniques provides extensive investigation of fetal growth and development and monitoring of the fetal environment [1,2,3,4,5,6,7,8,9]. Doppler technology represents an additional tool to assess fetal viability, by characterizing blood flow through maternal, fetal, and placental circulations. Clinical applications of Doppler technology to the pregnant mare are currently limited by the necessity of specific equipment, the difficult visualization of some vascular structures in advanced gestation (i.e. the umbilical cord), and the lack of reference values for physiologic and pathologic conditions of equine gestation.

APPLICATIONS

Applications of ultrasonography in early gestation (40–120 days) generally include identification and management of multiple fetuses [10,11] and fetal sexing [12,13,14]. In addition, elective feto-placental evaluations are carried out from 4 months of gestation to term in mares with histories of previous complicated pregnancies and potentially at risk of an unfavorable gestational outcome. Emergency feto-placental evaluations are performed when gestational complications or maternal disease are recognized and fetal distress or compromise may be anticipated [4,5]. Repeated examinations are usually required to assess fetal viability and response to treatment. Finally, routine scanning of term mares is carried out on some breeding farms to assess presentation and identify other factors that may complicate birth, suggesting the need for assistance to the mare at delivery or to the neonate shortly after birth.

EQUIPMENT AND TECHNIQUE

Linear, convex and sector ultrasound technologies can all be successfully used to image the equine pregnancy. Complete ultrasonographic feto-placental assessment is based on the acquisition of a series of biophysical parameters that requires both transrectal and transabdominal imaging. Transrectal ultrasound scanning provides access to the caudal aspects of the gravid uterus and should always be performed at any stage of gestation. Ultrasound scanning per rectum usually employs linear technology with frequencies ranging from 5–10 MHz. Convex and sector transducers better adapt to the curvilinear contour of the mare's abdomen and are preferred for percutaneous ultrasonography of the gravid uterus. The equine fetus becomes visible by this route from day 100 of gestation on. A wide range of frequencies, spanning from 2–8 MHz, is needed by this route to reach scanning depths of up to 30 cm and visualize the growing fetus from mid-gestation to term. Optimal skin preparation greatly enhances image quality, as per standard percutaneous ultrasonography.

Atlas of Equine Ultrasonography, First Edition. Edited by Jessica A. Kidd, Kristina G. Lu, and Michele L. Frazer.
© 2014 John Wiley & Sons, Ltd. Published 2014 by John Wiley & Sons, Ltd.
Companion Website: www.wiley.com/go/kidd/equine-ultrasonography

ULTRASONOGRAPHIC DATABASE

The *sonographic* profile of the feto-placental unit requires the establishment of a minimum database to ensure adequate fetal growth and development for the stage of gestation and to demonstrate appropriate levels of activity and responsiveness within an adequate environment.

FETAL GROWTH AND DEVELOPMENT

Several parameters can be measured to estimate fetal size in order to identify growth trends. Orbital diameters/eye volume [9,15,16] (Figure 19.1), aortic diameter (Figure 19.2), bi-parietal diameter (Figure 19.3), and, to a lesser extent, fetal chest and femur length [7] have all been reported as useful indicators of fetal growth. The aortic diameter correlates to fetal size more efficiently than any other anatomic structure and measurement should be taken in systole, on a longitudinal scan of the fetal left hemithorax, in close proximity to the spinal cord [9] (Figure 19.4). Ultrasonography provides excellent anatomic detail of the fetus in mid to late gestation (up to 9 months) (Figures 19.5, 19.6, 19.7, 19.8), when fetal sexing diagnosis can be easily accomplished (Figure 19.9, 19.10, 19.11, 19.12, 19.13) and congenital abnormalities identified. Developmental abnormalities commonly detected during late gestational scans include microphthalmus (Figure 19.14), hydrocephalus, small and large intestinal segmental atresia (Figure 19.15), and renal abnormalities (Figure 19.16). After 9 months of gestation, the quality of the image may decline due to fetal size and positioning within the mare's abdomen. Ossified remnants of the vitelline sac can be visualized from early to late gestation with no need for concern (Figure 19.17).

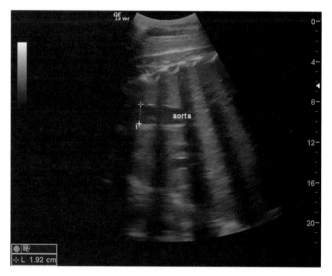

Figure 19.2 Transabdominal convex sonogram of a 250-day-old fetus showing the cranial chest and aorta; cranial aspect of fetus oriented to the left.

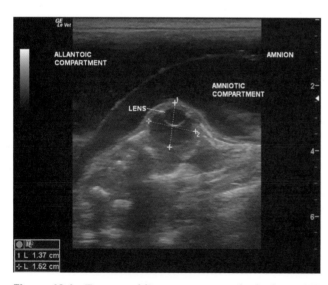

Figure 19.1 Transrectal linear sonogram of a fetal eye, 105 days gestation; measurements of the orbital diameters taken from a still image, when the lens was visualized.

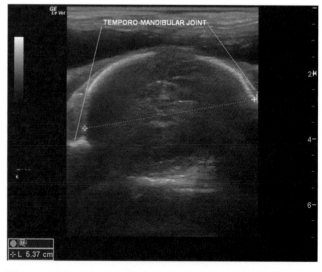

Figure 19.3 Transrectal linear sonogram showing a fetal skull, 133 days of gestation: the bi-parietal diameter is measured at its widest point, between the two temporomandibular joints.

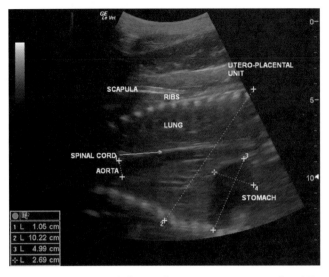

Figure 19.4 Transabdominal convex sonogram of a 161-day-old fetus, displaying the chest and cranial abdomen; measurements of the aortic diameter are taken as the aorta emerges from the cardiac area, in close proximity to the spinal cord, within the left hemithorax.

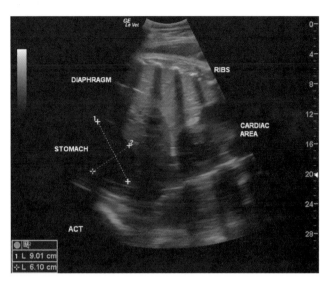

Figure 19.6 Transabdominal convex sonogram of a 272-day-old fetus, showing an incomplete view of thoracic and abdominal organs, on a frontal plane.

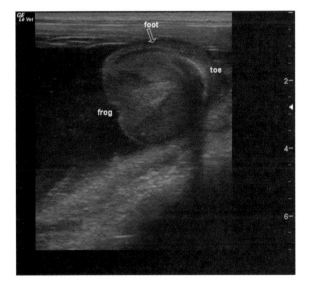

Figure 19.5 Transrectal linear sonogram of a 205-day-old fetus, showing detailed imaging of the foot; it is interesting to note the absence of the eponychium, which develops at a later stage of gestation.

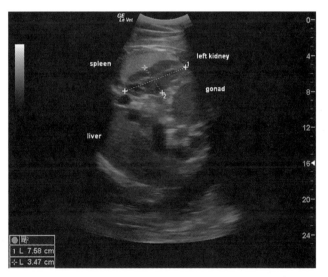

Figure 19.7 Transabdominal convex sonogram of a 225-day-old fetus, showing a cross-sectional oblique view of the left kidney and gonad.

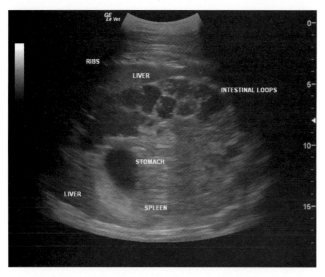

Figure 19.8 Transabdominal convex sonogram of a 204-day-old fetus, showing a frontal view of the abdomen; cranial aspect of fetus oriented to the left.

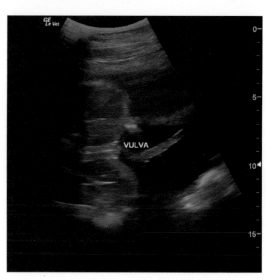

Figure 19.11 Transabdominal convex sonogram of a 192-day-old filly fetus; cross-sectional oblique view of the perineum, showing the vulvar rim and clitoris.

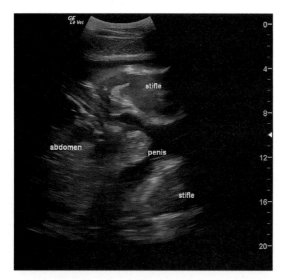

Figure 19.9 Transabdominal convex scan of a 209-day-old colt fetus; cross-sectional imaging of the ventral pelvis shows the penis encased within the prepuce.

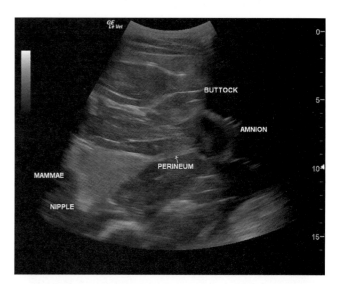

Figure 19.12 Transabdominal convex sonogram of a 214-day-old filly fetus; frontal view showing mammary gland, nipples, and perineum.

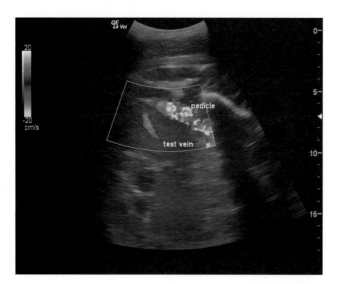

Figure 19.10 Transabdominal sonogram of a 204-day-old fetus; color Doppler ultrasonography of the male gonad in a frontal view, showing the vascular pedicle and the course of the testicular vein.

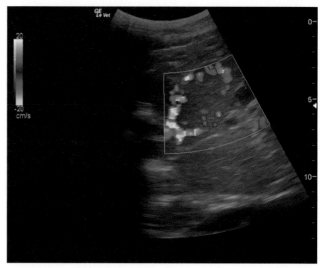

Figure 19.13 Transabdominal sonogram of a 164-day-old filly fetus; color Doppler of the female gonad in a frontal view, showing different vascular patterns between cortex and medulla.

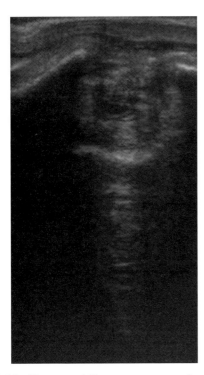

Figure 19.14 Transrectal linear sonogram of a term fetus, showing disruption of ocular anatomic architecture (compared to normal fetal eye, Figure 19.1). Bilateral microphthalmus was confirmed at birth.

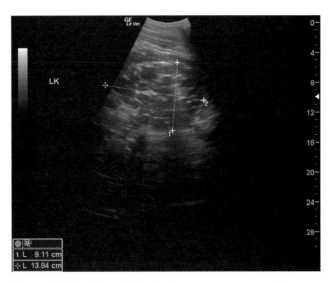

Figure 19.16 Transabdominal convex sonogram of a term fetus; cross-sectional view of a polycystic left kidney.

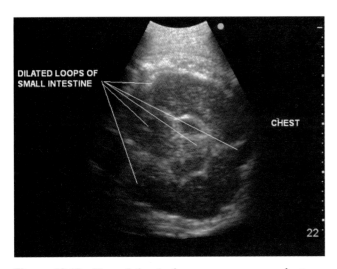

Figure 19.15 Transabdominal convex sonogram of a term fetus with congenital segmental atresia of the small intestine, showing marked dilation of intestinal loops.

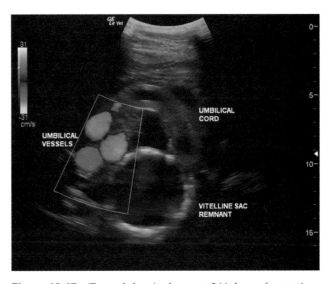

Figure 19.17 Transabdominal scan at 264 days of gestation, displaying views of the umbilical cord with attached remnant of the yolk sac in its allantoic portion.

FETAL ACTIVITY AND RESPONSIVE PATTERNS

Fetal activity and tone reflect central nervous system (CNS) function and development, with decreased activity and declining muscular strength resulting from depressed CNS function. Activity is required to ensure satisfactory muscular development and skeletal joint function, to promote successful postnatal adaptation. Dormant (inactive) phases are observed at all stages of pregnancy, but are more common and prolonged in late gestation, where they can last up to 60 minutes or longer on occasion. Lack of fetal movements and sudden bouts of excessive activity followed by abrupt cessation have both been associated with a negative outcome [5]. Rhythmic breathing movements may be observed in all fetuses in advanced gestation (from 7 months), when the diaphragm is visualized

(Figure 19.6). Nevertheless, fetal breathing is intermittent in nature and cannot be consistently evaluated.

FETAL HEART RATE

Fetal heart rate (FHR) and FHR reactivity represent the most sensitive indicators of fetal well-being. Cardiac frequency is obtained by M-mode echocardiography and automatically calculated by the cardiac calculation software, in-built in the ultrasound unit (Figure 19.18). FHR frequencies of around 100–130 beats per minute (bpm) are commonly recorded in mid-gestation depending on the level of fetal activity. A gradual decline occurs towards term, with values ranging around 55–65 bpm at rest and 80–100 bpm post-activity in healthy pregnancies [9]. Sustained tachycardia [4,5,17,18] or a large range of FHRs may indicate fetal distress, but could be brought on by painful maternal systemic problems. Sustained bradycardia [4,5,17,18], inappropriate FHR for gestational age, or lack of heart rate reactivity suggest CNS depression, probably attributable to hypoxia and may indicate impending fetal demise. Fetal cardiac rhythm is usually regular, and cardiac arrhythmias [19] are commonly associated with a negative outcome.

ADEQUATE ENVIRONMENT

Evaluation of fetal environment includes assessment of fetal orientation, volume and quality of fetal fluids, combined thickness and contiguity of the uteroplacental unit, cervical relaxation, and, of course, should confirm the presence of a single fetus.

FETAL ORIENTATION: PRESENTATION

Abnormal presentation causes dystocia and early detection may prevent a serious perinatal crisis, by implementation of specific strategies at delivery. Under normal circumstances, fetal mobility gradually decreases as gestation advances. After 9 months, rotation along the short axis, allowing changes in presentation, is restricted by fetal body size and the encasing of the fetal hind limbs within the gravid uterine horn [20,21]. Detection of an abnormal presentation after 9 months of gestation should raise concern and be investigated as term approaches to enable formulation of an appropriate plan of action.

VOLUME AND QUALITY OF FETAL FLUIDS

The equine pregnancy includes an allantoic and an amniotic compartment. The distribution of allantoic fluid is directly related to fetal dynamics and uterine tone, with no preferential area of maximal fluid depth detectable. Amniotic fluid tends to collect more frequently around the cranio-ventral half of the fetus (Figure 19.19). Minimal and maximal allantoic and amniotic fluid depth values are reported in the literature [2,4,6,8].

Free-floating particles (vernix) are commonly observed swirling within the fetal fluids and become

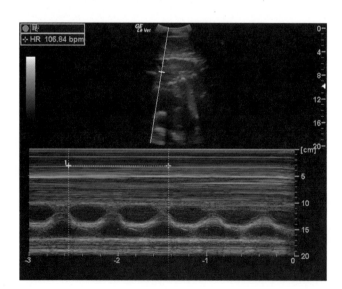

Figure 19.18 Transabdominal convex sonogram, showing an M-mode tracing of cardiac activity taken from a 244-day-old fetus, at rest.

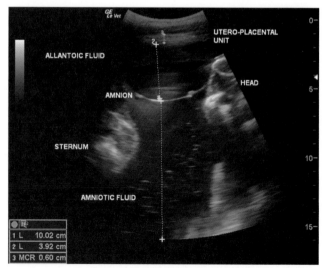

Figure 19.19 Transabdominal convex sonogram at 164 days gestation, showing a pocket of amniotic fluid collecting ventral to the neck of the fetus; note the typical hyperechogenicity of amniotic fluid.

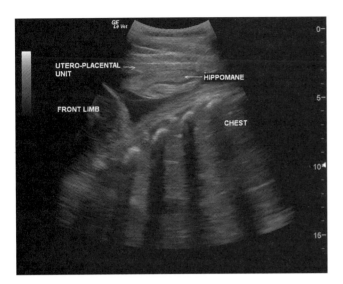

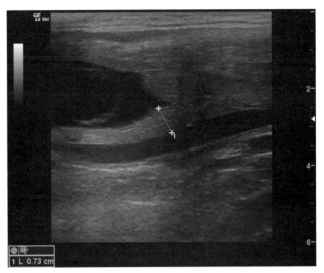

Figure 19.20 Transabdominal convex sonogram in late gestation, showing the hippomane within the allantoic compartment, compressed between the fetus and the mare's ventral abdominal wall.

Figure 19.21 Transrectal linear sonogram of the caudal gravid uterus at 8 months of gestation, showing measurement of the combined thickness of the uteroplacental unit, using the ventral uterine vasculature as landmark; caudal aspect of mare oriented to the right.

more visible during episodes of fetal activity, particularly in the amniotic sac (Figure 19.19). The hippomane is defined as an allantoic calculus and can often be visualized floating within the allantoic fluid, with its typical oval shape and onion-like, concentric structure (Figure 19.20). Sudden release of meconium (fetal diarrhea) in the amniotic compartment may sometimes be observed in highly distressed fetuses just prior to birth, stillbirth, or abortion. Pathologic increases in fetal fluids have been reported (*hydramnion* and *hydroallantois*) [22,23,24,25,26,27]. Markedly reduced volumes of amniotic fluid (*oligohydroallantois*) may be observed in mares with severe systemic illness. An association of the condition with a poor fetal outcome has been reported. Objective assessment of fetal fluid depth requires extensive scanning of the mare's abdomen and is best carried out during phases of fetal quiescence.

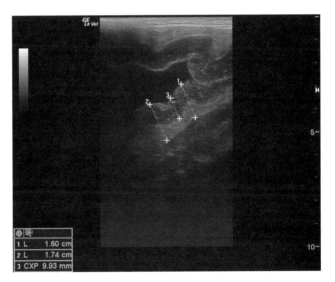

Figure 19.22 Transrectal linear sonogram of the caudal gravid uterus at term, showing diffuse sonolucency of the fetal membranes; caudal aspect of mare oriented to the right.

COMBINED THICKNESS AND CONTINUITY OF THE UTEROPLACENTAL UNIT

The literature reports reference values for the combined measurement of the uteroplacental unit at different stages of gestation [3,4,8,28,29,30,31] (Figure 19.21). Both uterus and placenta should present with similar echotexture up until term, when diffuse sono-

lucency of the inner layers of the placenta may be observed (Figure 19.22). Adequate uteroplacental contact should also be maintained throughout gestation. However, small areas of separation of the placental membranes and uterus are commonly observed in normal pregnancies without any apparent effect on the health of the fetus. An average combined thickness of the uteroplacental unit of 1.26 ± 0.33 cm has been

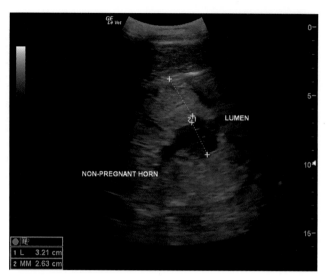

Figure 19.23 Transabdominal convex sonogram at day 266 of gestation showing a cross-section of the non-pregnant uterine horn.

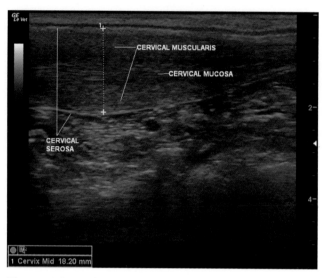

Figure 19.24 Transrectal linear sonogram of the caudal end of a pregnant cervix at 7 months of gestation, showing a tight, compact mucosal layer and wider muscularis.

reported in mares with normal term pregnancies. Measurements should be taken avoiding areas of compression of the uteroplacental thickness by the fetus.

The thickness of the uteroplacental unit is affected by numerous factors, which may reduce the efficiency of placental function. Such conditions include placentitis/degenerative changes of fetal membranes, placental edema, and premature placental separation. Large and/or progressively enlarging areas of placental separation may lead to inefficient exchanges, adversely affecting fetal growth and well-being, and resulting in red bag delivery at parturition and decreased neonatal viability. The non-pregnant horn presents with a folded, thickened appearance and, although normal, could be mistakenly interpreted as uteroplacental thickening (Figure 19.23). The lumen of the non-pregnant horn is relatively small, but may suddenly increase to accommodate larger volumes of fetal fluids in response to uterine dynamics and fetal shifting; a marked reduction in the combined thickness of the uterus and the placenta of the non-pregnant horn can be observed under these circumstances (author personal observations).

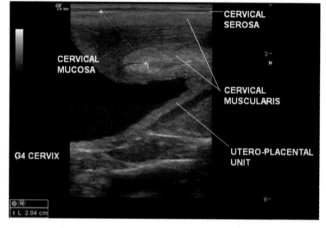

Figure 19.25 Transrectal linear sonogram of the cranial end of a term pregnant cervix, displaying mucosal widening, indicating cervical relaxation.

sonographic appearance was also demonstrated (Figures 19.24, 19.25).

CERVICAL PARAMETERS

Recent data on cervical size and echotexture in the pregnant mare suggest a high degree of cervical tone maintained up to 9 months of gestation, followed by progressive cervical relaxation until delivery [32]. A high degree of correlation between cervical size and

REFERENCES

[1] Pipers, F.S. & Adams-Brendemuehl, C.S. (1984) Techniques and application of transabdominal ultrasonography in the pregnant mare. *Journal of the American Veterinary Medical Association*, 185, 766–771.

[2] Adams-Brendemuehl, C.S. & Pipers, F.S. (1987) Antepartum evaluation of the equine foetus. *Journal of Reproduction and Fertility*, 35(Suppl), 565–573.

[3] Reef, V.B., Vaala, W.E., Worth, L.T., Spencer, P.L., & Hammett, B. (1995) Ultrasonographic evaluation of the foetus and intrauterine environment in healthy mares during late gestation. *Veterinary Radiology & Ultrasound*, 36, 533–541.

[4] Reef, V.B., Vaala, W.E., Worth, L.T., Sertich, P.A., & Spencer, P.L. (1996) Ultrasonographic assessment of fetal well-being during late gestation: development of a biophysical profile. *Equine Veterinary Journal*, 28, 200–208.

[5] Reimer, J.M. (1997) Use of transcutaneous ultrasonography in complicated latter-middle to late gestation on pregnancies in the mare: 122 cases. *Proceedings of the 43rd Annual Convention of the American Association of Equine Practitioners*, 259–261.

[6] Renaudin, C.D., Gillis, C.L., Tarantal, A.F., & Coleman, D.A. (1998) Ultrasonographic evaluation of equine fetal growth from 100 days gestation to parturition. *Proceedings of the 7th International Symposium on Equine Reproduction*, 71–72.

[7] Pantaleon, L.G., Bain, F.T., Zent, W., & Powell, D.G. (2003) Equine fetal growth and development. *Compendium on Continuing Education for the Practicing Veterinarian*, 25, 470–476.

[8] Bucca, S., Fogarty, U., Collins, A., & Small, V. (2005) Assessment of foeto-placental well-being in the mare from mid-gestation to term: transrectal and transabdominal ultrasonographic features. *Theriogenology*, 64, 542–557.

[9] Bucca, S. (2011) Ultrasonographic monitoring of the fetus. In: *Equine Reproduction*, 2nd edn (eds A.O. McKinnon, E.L. Squires, W.E. Vaala, & D.D. Varner). Wiley Blackwell, Oxford, 39–54.

[10] Rantanen, N.W. & Kincaid, B. (1998) Ultrasound guided fetal cardiac puncture: a method of twin reduction in the mare. *Proceedings of the 34th Annual Convention of the American Association of Equine Practitioners*, 173–179.

[11] Wolfsdorf, K.E., Rodgerson, D., & Holder, R. (2005) How to manually reduce twins between 60 and 120 days gestation using cranio-cervical dislocation. *Proceedings of the 51st Annual Convention of the American Association of Equine Practitioners*, 284–287.

[12] Curran, S. & Ginther, O.J. (1993) Ultrasonic fetal gender diagnosis during months 5 to 11 in mares. *Theriogenology*, 40, 1127–1135.

[13] Holder, R.D. (2001) Fetal sex determination in the mare between 55 and 150 days gestation. *Proceedings of the 47th Annual Convention of the American Association of Equine Practitioners*, 321–324.

[14] Bucca, S. (2011) Fetal gender determination from mid gestation to term. In: *Equine Reproduction*, 2nd edn (eds A.O. McKinnon, E.L. Squires, W.E. Vaala, & D.D. Varner). Wiley Blackwell, Oxford, 2094–2098.

[15] McKinnon, A.O., Voss, J.L., Squires, E.L., & Carnevale, E.M. (1993) Diagnostic Ultrasonography. In: *Equine Reproduction*, 1st edn (eds A.O McKinnon & J.L. Voss). Lea & Febiger, Philadelphia, 266–302.

[16] Turner, R.M., McDonnell, S.M., Feit, E.M., Grogan, E.H., & Foglia, R. (2006) Real-time ultrasound measure of the fetal eye (vitreous body) for prediction of parturition date in small ponies. *Theriogenology*, 66, 331–337.

[17] Smith, L.J. & Schott, H. (1990) Abstract. Xylazine-induced foetal bradycardia. In: *Proceedings of the Second International Conference on Veterinary Perinatology* (ed. P.D. Rossdale), 36.

[18] Colles, C.M., Parkes, R.D., & May, C.J. (1978) Foetal electrocardiography in the mare. *Equine Veterinary Journal*, 10, 32–37.

[19] Yamamoto, K., Yasuda, J., & Too, K. (1992) Arrhythmias in the newborn thoroughbred foals. *Equine Veterinary Journal*, 24, 169–173.

[20] Ginther, O.J. & Griffin, P.G. (1993) Equine fetal kinetics; presentation and location. *Theriogenology*, 40, 1–11.

[21] Ginther, O.J. (1998) Equine pregnancy: physical interactions between the uterus and conceptus. *Proceedings of the 44rd Annual Convention of the American Association of Equine Practitioners*, 73–103.

[22] Wintour, A.M., Barnes, A., Brown, A.J., *et al.* (1977) The role of deglutition in the production of hydramnios. *Theriogenology*, 8, 160.

[23] Bucca, S. & Romano, G. (2000) Un caso di idramnios in una fattrice in gestazione avanzata. *Ippologia*,11, 35–38.

[24] Allen, W.E. (1986) Two cases of abnormal equine pregnancy associated with excess foetal fluid. *Equine Veterinary Journal*, 18, 220–222.

[25] Sertich, P.L., Reef, V.B., Oristaglio-Turner, R.M., Habecker, P.L. & Maxson, A.D. (1994) Hydrops amnii in a mare. *Journal of the American Veterinary Medical Association*, 204, 1481–1482.

[26] Vandeplassche, M., Bouters, R., Spincemaille, M. & Bonte, P. (1976) Dropsy of the foetal sacs in mares: induced and spontaneous abortions. *Veterinary Record*, 99, 67–69.

[27] Oppen, T.V. & Bartmann, C.P. (2001) Two cases of hydroallantois in the mare. *Pferdeheilkunde*, 17(6), 593–596.

[28] Renaudin, C.D., Troedsson, M.H.T., Gillis, C.L., King, V.L., & Bodena, A. (1997) Ultrasonographic evaluation of the equine placenta by transrectal and transabdominal approach in the normal pregnant mare. *Theriogenology*, 47, 559–573.

[29] Troedsson, M.H.T., Renaudin, C.D., Zent, W.W., & Steiner, J.V. (1997) Transrectal ultrasonography of the placenta in normal mares and mares with pending abortion: a field study. *Proceedings of the 43rd Annual Convention of the American Association of Equine Practitioners*, 256–258.

[30] Colon, J.L. (2008) Trans-rectal ultrasonographic appearance of abnormal combined utero-placental thickness in late-term gestation and its incidence during routine survey in a population of Thoroughbred mares. *Proceedings of: 54th Anual American Association of Equine Practitioners Convention*, 279–285.

[31] Sheerin, P.C., Morris, S., & Kellerman, A. (2003) Diagnostic efficiency of transrectal ultrasonography and plasma progestins profiles in identifying mares at risk of premature delivery. *Proceedings of the Focus on Equine Reproduction Meeting*, 22–23.

[32] Bucca, S. & Fogarty, U. (2011) Ultrasonographic cervical parameters throughout gestation in the mare. *Proceedings of the 57th Annual Convention of the American Association of Equine Practitioners*, 235–241.

CHAPTER TWENTY

ULTRASONOGRAPHY OF THE POST-FOALING MARE

Peter R. Morresey
Rood and Riddle Equine Hospital, Lexington, KY, USA

INTRODUCTION

Abdominal discomfort in the post-foaling mare may result from normal uterine contractions or be indicative of visceral compromise. The uterus and associated structures may be affected or non-reproductive viscera may be involved. Transabdominal ultrasonography is valuable because it is a non-invasive technique that allows assessment of peritoneal fluid quantity and quality, evaluation of visceral disposition, and estimation of visceral integrity. Transrectal ultrasonography, when appropriate, improves identification of structures distinguished by palpation *per rectum*.

TECHNIQUE

A lower-frequency transducer (3.5 MHz) is preferred in larger horses as penetration of the ultrasound beam is enhanced, however smaller horses and foals can be adequately imaged with higher-frequency probes. Clipping of the abdomen and the use of ultrasound coupling gel may give the best image, but, in practical settings, wetting with alcohol and slicking down hair in the direction of growth to expel air is sufficient. The probe is then held perpendicular to the abdominal wall which is systematically covered in a dorsal–ventral direction and, when along the midline, in a cranial–caudal direction. The more cranial aspects of the abdominal cavity are located within the thoracic rib cage and imaging of this area uses a similar technique to that detailed for thoracic ultrasonography.

NORMAL ANATOMY

On the left side of the horse, the liver is adjacent to the diaphragm medially and lung fields ventrally between approximately the seventh and ninth intercostal spaces (ICS) [1]. The liver is lateral to the spleen in this region, with the stomach visualized deep to this interface; however, the stomach may have variable contact with the body wall depending on degree of fill. The spleen is imaged over the majority of the left side of the abdominal cavity, extending medial to the body wall from the paralumbar fossa to the eighth ICS and, further cranially, medial to the liver as noted above. The spleen extends ventrally to the midline and may extend to the right ventral abdomen. Spleen size is variable. The left kidney lies medial to the spleen and is found from the sixteenth ICS through the paralumbar fossa. Gas-filled viscera may obstruct complete visualization of the left kidney.

On the right side of the abdominal cavity, the liver is from approximately the sixth to fifteenth ICS medially and from the lung to diaphragm ventrally [1]. The right kidney is located dorsally and superficially in the same region, adjacent to the caudal-most aspects of the liver in the fourteenth to the seventeenth ICS region.

The intestinal tract is imaged via the caudal and ventral abdomen. Small intestine is variable in location, and may be visualized on the left or right side and is often seen on both. Ventral colon is adjacent to the ventral abdominal wall and identified by sacculations (haustra). Liver is not imaged from the ventral

Atlas of Equine Ultrasonography, First Edition. Edited by Jessica A. Kidd, Kristina G. Lu, and Michele L. Frazer.
© 2014 John Wiley & Sons, Ltd. Published 2014 by John Wiley & Sons, Ltd.
Companion Website: www.wiley.com/go/kidd/equine-ultrasonography

abdomen in the normal horse [1]. The right dorsal colon can be visualized medial to the liver on the right side. The cecum is visualized in the right paralumbar fossa traversing caudally and ventrally before the tip trends cranially.

The bladder is located on the ventral midline of the caudal abdomen and visualization improves when it is urine filled. The non-pregnant uterus is not typically discernible with transabdominal ultrasound. Varying stages of pregnancy and uterine pathology can be noted depending on uterine size and disposition.

Portions of the intestinal tract may be visualized lateral to the spleen on the left side, with some appearing dorsal and lateral to the dorsal most aspect of the spleen. In the absence of content in the nephrosplenic space, this does not appear to cause problems.

Limitations of Transabdominal Ultrasonography

The limitations of transabdominal ultrasonography are a result of the size of the abdominal cavity relative to the penetrating ability of the ultrasound transducer, which depends on the nominal frequency.

Pathology, Abdominal Cavity

Ruptured Body Wall, Rectus Abdominis, and Prepubic Tendon

Ruptured body wall, ruptured *rectus abdominis*, and ruptured prepubic tendon cause abrupt changes in

shape of the body wall. Subcutaneous edema, fluid, hemorrhage, and muscle fiber disruption are visible with ultrasonography (Figures 20.1, 20.2). Diagnosis of the specific tissue involved can be difficult [2]. Prepubic tendon rupture results in ventral abdominal wall deviation, regional edema, and pain [2]. Herniation of the abdominal wall has the potential to incarcerate gut [2].

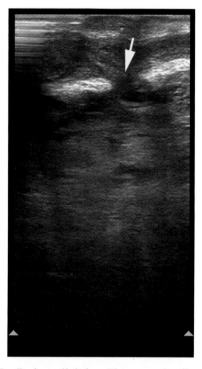

Figure 20.2 Body wall defect. This mare developed a defect in her body wall (arrow) 5 days after a Cesarean section. This sonogram was obtained from the ventral abdomen with a linear probe operating at 7.5 MHz at a depth of 6 cm.

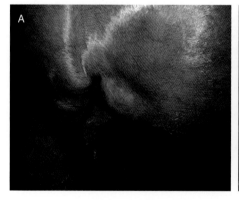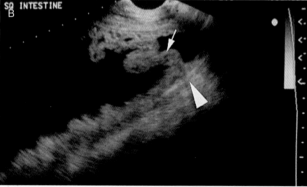

Figure 20.1 Body wall defect. (A) This picture is of a post-foaling mare with acute swelling of her lateral body wall. (B) This image shows body wall (arrowhead) with cecum (arrow) through a defect and into the subcutaneous tissue. This sonogram was obtained from the right abdominal wall using a curvilinear probe operating at 3.5 MHz at a depth of 10 cm.

Diaphragmatic Hernia

Diaphragmatic hernia is a rare parturient complication [3] and prognosis is considered guarded. One review involving various horse signalments reported a 23% survival rate in diagnosed cases and 46% survival rate following surgical correction [4]. Viscera reported involved include small intestine, large intestine, stomach, spleen, and liver [4,5]. With ultrasonography, strangulation of gut may be visible as thickened intestinal wall and increased peritoneal fluid. Intrathoracic intestine may be noted cranial to the diaphragm shadowing the lung due to gaseous content, and pleural fluid may be increased (Figure 20.3). An intraluminal air–fluid interface may be present [6].

Retroperitoneal Hemorrhage and Pelvicitis

With retroperitoneal hemorrhage into the pelvic cavity and pelvicitis, transrectal ultrasonography may detect fluid or fibrin caudal to the peritoneal reflection. Caudal vaginal or rectal trauma during parturition may be sufficient to cause hemorrhage, tissue necrosis, sepsis, or perforation. This may not be reflected in grossly observable changes in the adjacent peritoneal cavity.

PATHOLOGY, PERITONEAL CAVITY

Changes in the peritoneal fluid reflect the altered integrity of the viscera within the peritoneal cavity. These include ultrasonographically detectable changes in peritoneal fluid volume, echogenicity, and, sometimes, disposition. Increase in value of two or more fluid variables, including total protein, nucleated cell count, and percentage neutrophils, is considered significant [7].

Hemoperitoneum

Periparturient hemorrhage (Figures 20.4, 20.5, 20.6) can develop in mares of any age or parity, however, it is more common in older mares [8,9,10]. It was the second most common reason for emergency presentation of post-partum mares in one review [9]. Ultrasonographic appearance will vary with rate of bleeding, volume of hemorrhage, and duration of time since cessation of bleeding. Hemoperitoneum has a characteristic ultrasonographic appearance in the initial stages, being cellular and swirling (smoke-like) in response to diaphragmatic and visceral movements.

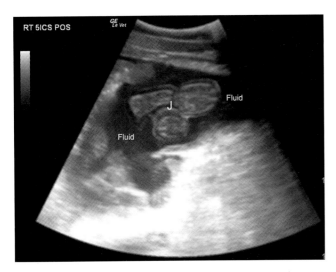

Figure 20.3 Diaphragmatic tear with intestine in thoracic cavity. Jejunum (J) is visible in the pleural space adjacent to the pulmonary parenchyma. Hypoechoic fluid surrounds the intestine in the thoracic cavity. Fibrin deposits on the lung and diaphragm suggest the lesion is chronic. Diaphragmatic hernia should be considered a differential diagnosis for colic in the post-partum mare, particularly if she had a dystocia. This sonogram was obtained from the right fifth ICS using a curvilinear probe operating at 4.0 MHz at a depth of 12 cm.

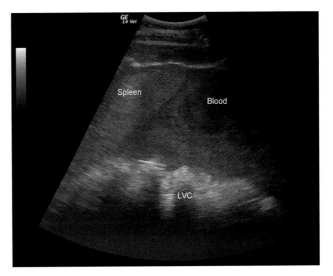

Figure 20.4 Acute hemoperitoneum in a post-foaling mare. In this post-partum mare with intra-abdominal hemorrhage, the peritoneal fluid (blood) is heterogeneous and diffusely echogenic. Swirling is present within the fluid due to erythrocyte rouleaux formation as well as diaphragmatic and visceral movement. Continued blood loss into the abdominal cavity may also contribute to the swirling or "smokey" appearance of the fluid. Spleen and left ventral colon (LVC) are visible. This sonogram was obtained from the left inguinal region using a curvilinear probe operating at 4.0 MHz at a depth of 18 cm.

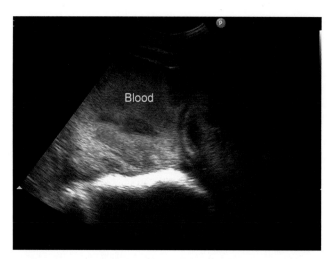

Figure 20.5   Acute hemoperitoneum in post foaling mare. This image is from a mare with acute colic 18 hours after foaling. This image shows swirling fluid (blood) in the abdominal cavity consistent with ongoing intra-abdominal hemorrhage. This sonogram was obtained from the ventral abdomen using a curvilinear probe operating at 3.0 MHz at a depth of 16 cm.

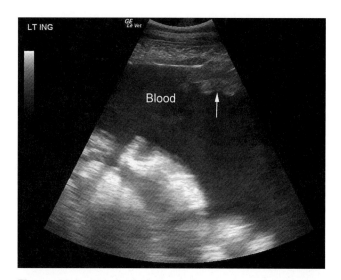

Figure 20.6   Resolving hemoperitoneum in a post-foaling mare. Several days after intra-abdominal hemorrhage, peritoneal blood becomes less echogenic. Clot formation (arrow) is apparent as ventrally located irregular hyperechoic foci. This sonogram was obtained from the left inguinal area using a curvilinear probe operating at 4.0 MHz at a depth of 18 cm.

Within a few days, this progresses to clot formation ventrally with relatively anechoic fluid remaining dorsally. Hemorrhage may be acute and overwhelming, or may persist at a lower level over a number of days. While the genital tract is the most likely source in the periparturient mare, examination of the liver, spleen,

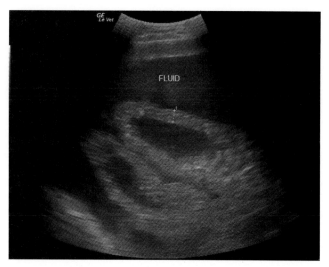

Figure 20.7   Peritonitis in a post-foaling mare. Diffusely heterogeneously echogenic fluid is present in the abdomen. Fibrin tags may be located on the peritoneal surfaces. Thickened, inflamed gastrointestinal tract (cursors) is present. Causes for peritonitis in the post-foaling mare include rupture of the gastrointestinal tract, uterus, an abdominal abscess, or bladder. This sonogram was obtained from the right inguinal region using a curvilinear probe operating at 4.0 MHz at a depth of 15 cm.

and kidneys is prudent if a readily identifiable source is not present. Mesenteric disruption can also lead to hemoperitoneum.

Peritonitis

Peritonitis (Figure 20.7) may result when intestinal bruising, strangulation, and ischemia progress to mural necrosis and rupture of the affected segment. The condition may progress over a number of days, with apparent abdominal discomfort and fever preceding overt signs of sepsis as bacterial translocation increases across devitalized gut wall. Spillage of gastrointestinal content precipitates a rapid onset of systemic deterioration. Peritonitis has also been reported secondary to bladder wall necrosis [11]. Peritoneal fluid appears echogenic (cellular, flocculent, or turbid) and may, in advanced cases, contain fibrin strands, either free or attached to regional visceral and parietal peritoneal surfaces. Gas echoes or highly echogenic particles are consistent with a ruptured viscus. Abscess formation within the mesentery (Figure 20.8) may occur.

Uroperitoneum and Bladder Rupture

Normal, urine filled bladder (Figure 20.9) is visualized in the inguinal region transabdominally or transrec-

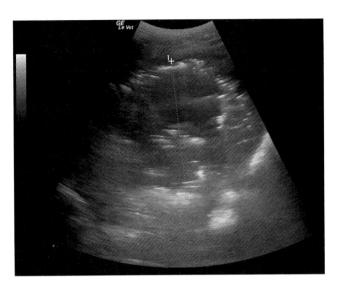

Figure 20.8 Mesenteric abscess in a post-partum mare. This image shows a heterogeneous mass (cursors) with diffuse, hypoechoic foci. The mass is a mesenteric abscess. The mare had been diagnosed with hemoperitoneum post partum 1 month previously. This sonogram was obtained from the ventral abdomen using a curvilinear probe operating at 4.0 MHz at a depth of 15 cm.

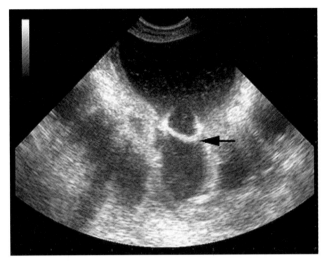

Figure 20.10 Ruptured bladder. This image shows a defect in the bladder (arrow). Ruptured bladder should be considered as a differential diagnosis for a mare with increased abdominal fluid either prior to or after foaling. This sonogram was obtained from the caudal aspect of ventral midline using a curvilinear probe operating at 3.5 MHz at a depth of 25 cm. (Source: Image courtesy of Dr. Fairfield Bain, University of Queensland Veterinary Medical Centre, Queensland, Australia.)

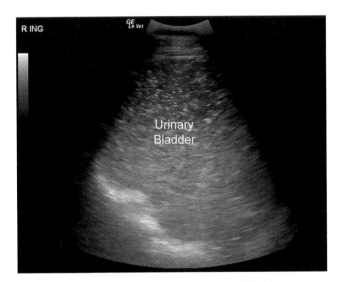

Figure 20.9 Normal bladder. The urinary bladder appears as a rounded structure high in the inguinal region. Content is heterogeneous with diffuse hyperechogenic foci. The urine-filled bladder can be confused with uterine hematomas depending on appearance. The bladder will appear near the midline and similar from both sides, however. This sonogram was obtained from the right inguinal region using a curvilinear probe operating at 4.0 MHz at a depth of 20 cm.

tally. Uroperitoneum and bladder rupture (Figure 20.10) may occur if the bladder wall becomes traumatized and devitalized by compression against the pelvic brim during parturition [12]. This is reported to be a rare occurrence [13]. Uroperitoneum may result [14], with anechoic peritoneal fluid containing increased creatinine and calcium carbonate crystals [3]. The bladder may be seen as folded or collapsed, however, the lesion is unlikely to be visualized.

PATHOLOGY, ABDOMINAL VISCERA

Uterus and Associated Structures

The arterial supply to the uterus is within the broad ligament. The majority consists of the uterine artery (from the external iliac artery), with a cranial branch supplying the proximal uterine horn and a caudal branch supplying the distal uterine horn and body. This is anastomosed cranially by a uterine branch of the ovarian artery, and caudally by a uterine branch of the vaginal artery [15]. Rupture of these vessels leads to hematoma formation between the layers of the broad ligament. Rupture occurs most commonly

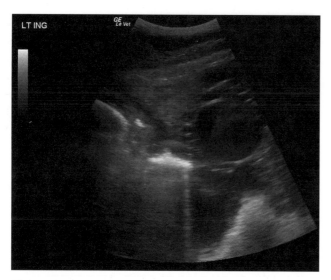

Figure 20.11 Acute, broad ligament hematoma in a post-partum mare. Note the linear separation occurring within the encapsulated blood. This sonogram was obtained from the left inguinal region using a curvilinear probe operating at 4.0 MHz at a depth of 12 cm.

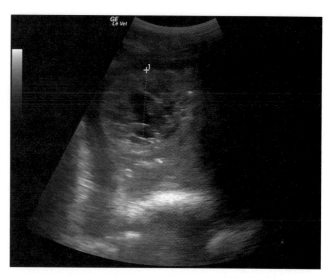

Figure 20.13 Organized, broad ligament hematoma (cursors) in a post-partum mare. The mass has a relatively smooth surface with echodense content and occasional fluid pockets. This sonogram was taken from the left inguinal area using a curvilinear probe operating at 4.0 MHz at a depth of 13 cm.

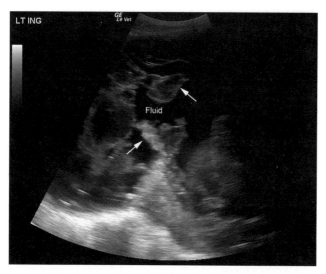

Figure 20.12 Organizing, broad ligament hematoma in a post-partum mare. Separation of the fibrinous material (arrows) and fluid components of the blood has occurred. This sonogram was obtained from the left inguinal area using a curvilinear probe operating at 4.0 MHz at a depth of 17 cm.

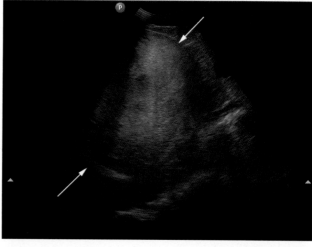

Figure 20.14 Chronic broad ligament hematoma. This image shows a hematoma (arrows) in the broad ligament several days after foaling. The hematoma has smooth margins and organized, echodense material in it. This sonogram was taken from the right inguinal area using a curvilinear probe operating at 3.5 MHz at a depth of 25 cm.

during parturition, but has been reported to occur both before and after parturition [10]. The hematoma initially appears uniformly hyperechoic. With time, a heterogeneous appearance develops, and blood separates into areas of anechoic fluid and areas of hyperechoic organizing hematoma (Figures 20.11, 20.12, 20.13,

20.14). Tearing of the broad ligament in the acute to subacute phase will allow leakage of blood into the peritoneal cavity and this may precipitate profound life-threatening hypovolemia. No reported predilection for side of rupture exists [10], however, most tears occur in the proximal uterine artery [16].

Mural Hematoma

Mural hematomas may occur when trauma to the uterine wall causes hemorrhage within or between any or all of the endometrium, myometrium, and serosal layers. Initially appearing as a hyperechoic mass, this subsequently progresses to anechoic fluid adjacent to heterogeneous organizing tissue (Figures 20.15, 20.16).

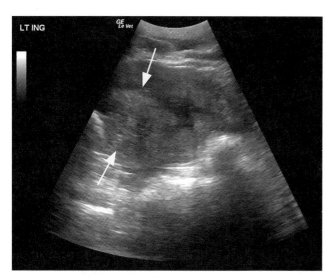

Figure 20.15 Acute, mural hematoma. Hemorrhage occurred within the uterine lumen and a hematoma (arrows) formed in the uterine wall. This sonogram was obtained from the left inguinal area using a curvilinear probe operating at 4.0 MHz at a depth of 17 cm.

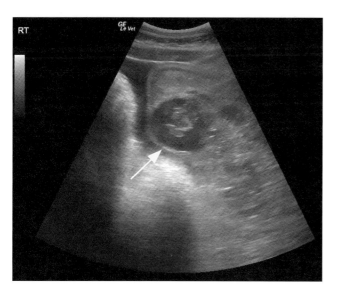

Figure 20.16 Organized, mural hematoma. A hematoma (arrow) in the uterine wall has become round and taken on typical characteristics of an organizing blood clot. This sonogram was taken from the right inguinal area using a curvilinear probe operating at 4.0 MHz at a depth of 17 cm.

Over time, abscessation may develop or the hematoma may dissect into the uterine lumen or peritoneal cavity. A full-thickness uterine defect may result with potential for peritonitis or pneumoperitoneum.

Intrauterine Fluid

The presence of a small amount of fluid within the uterine lumen and endometrial edema is common in the initial post-partum period (Figure 20.17). However, uterine involution (Figure 20.18) progresses rapidly and persistence of a high volume indicates failure of uterine clearance (Figure 20.19). Post-partum lochia is predominantly hypoechoic in nature. Septic fluid appears flocculent. Gas echoes within the fluid indicate anaerobic infection, sepsis of placental remnants, or failure of the perineal, vestibular or cervical seals allowing aerophagia (Figure 20.20). Intraluminal hemorrhage appears diffusely uniformly echogenic in nature, consistent with the appearance of peritoneal hemorrhage (Figure 20.21).

Mural Laceration, Necrosis, and Perforation

The peritoneal cavity may display characteristics of hemorrhage, peritonitis, or both depending on the degree of integrity loss and the duration of time since formation. Acute full-thickness laceration of the uterine

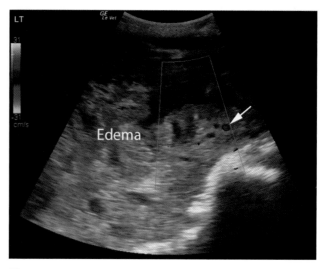

Figure 20.17 Normal uterine edema in post-partum mare. Uterine edema is a normal finding in a post-partum mare. This image was taken 12 hours post foaling. Loose folding of the uterine wall and prominent endometrial edema is a common finding. Color Doppler identifies a vessel (arrow) in the uterine wall. This sonogram was obtained from the left inguinal region using a curvilinear probe operating at 4.0 MHz at a depth of 12 cm.

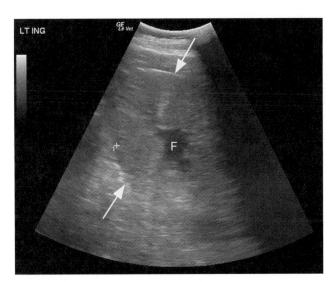

Figure 20.18 Normal uterine involution. This image shows the uterus (arrows) 2 days post partum. The uterus has decreased considerably from prepartum size. Normal intraluminal lochia (F) appears hypoechoic. The relatively thick uterine wall (cursors) is a normal finding caused by increased muscular tone during involution. This sonogram was obtained from the left inguinal area using a curvilinear probe operating at 4.0 MHz at a depth of 15 cm.

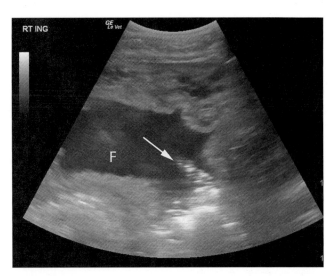

Figure 20.20 Gas in intraluminal uterine fluid. This image shows hyperechoic foci (arrow) within the intraluminal fluid (F). These foci are gas pockets and suggest either aerophagia or uterine infection with a gas-producing organism. This sonogram was obtained from the right inguinal area using a curvilinear probe operating at 4.0 MHz at a depth of 12 cm.

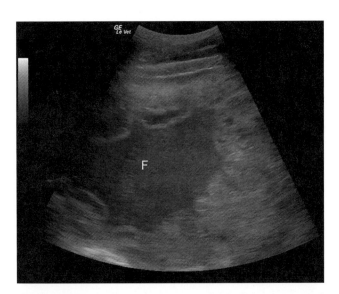

Figure 20.19 Intraluminal uterine fluid. The uterine wall has poor mural tone and the lumen is enlarged and contains heterogeneous content (F). The uterine fluid was septic. This sonogram was obtained using a curvilinear probe operating at 4.0 MHz at a depth of 15 cm.

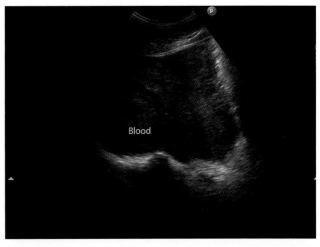

Figure 20.21 Hemorrhage into uterus. This image shows acute hemorrhage (blood) into the uterus several hours after foaling. Note the swirling appearance to the intrauterine fluid. This sonogram was obtained from the right inguinal area using a curvilinear probe operating at 3.5 MHz at a depth of 17 cm.

wall may appear initially as hemoperitoneum before progressing to septic peritonitis (see Figure 20.7). Mural necrosis followed by perforation may initially present with signs of peritoneal inflammation before rupture occurs and fulminant bacterial peritonitis ensues. Expulsion of intraluminal uterine fluid will exacerbate peritonitis, especially if endometritis is present post partum. Sudden onset of colic signs after uterine lavage, with concurrent appearance of a large volume of relatively anechoic peritoneal fluid, is highly

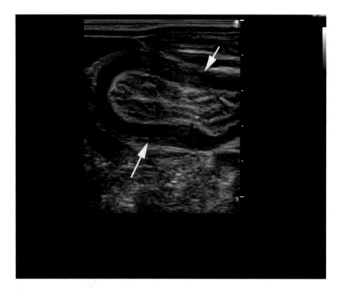

Figure 20.22 Inverted uterine horn. This image shows a uterine horn (arrows) that has inverted in a post-partum mare. Note the multilayered appearance and edematous outer layer of the uterine wall. This sonogram was obtained transrectally using a linear probe operating at 7.5 MHz at a depth of 5 cm.

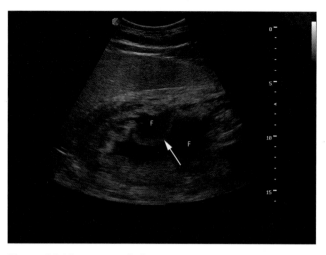

Figure 20.23 Retained placenta. Note the irregular contour of the retained placental tissue relative to the uterine wall. Fluid (F) of identical echogenicity is present on both sides of the free placental membrane (arrow). This sonogram was obtained from the left inguinal area using a curvilinear probe operating at 4.0 MHz at a depth of 15 cm.

suggestive of a pre-existing uterine perforation. Tears are more likely to occur in the uterine body [17]. Medical and surgical treatment have both been reviewed [17,18].

Inverted Uterine Horn

Inverted uterine horn tip may occur following uncoordinated uterine contraction or uterine fatigue post foaling, or overzealous traction in cases of placental retention. The characteristic target sign appearance may be difficult to obtain with transabdominal ultrasonography (Figure 20.22).

Retained Placenta

Retained placenta should not be confused with the ultrasonographically prominent definition of the endometrium and myometrium resulting from edema in the wall of the post-partum uterus. The presence of an extra tissue layer with variable or discontinuous attachment to the endometrium is highly suggestive of placental retention (Figure 20.23) Gas echoes may be present due to bacterial decomposition (Figure 20.24). Small fragments retained in the more proximal regions of the uterine horns may be difficult to image transabdominally. When this is suspected, secondary indicators such as the presence of increased or turbid

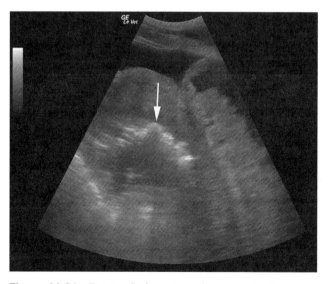

Figure 20.24 Retained placenta with gas production. Placental tissue is firmly adhered to the uterine wall. The hyperechoic line (arrow) is gas production from septic decomposition of the placental tissue. This sonogram was obtained from the left inguinal area using a curvilinear probe operating at 4.0 MHz at a depth of 20 cm.

intraluminal fluid warrant investigation ultrasonographically *per rectum* or manually *per vaginam*.

Pneumometra

Pneumometra, accumulation of air in the uterus, has been reported as a cause of postpartum colic [19]. This

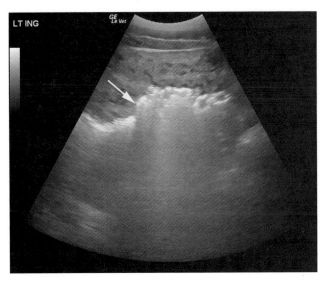

Figure 20.25 Pneumometra. Aspiration of air secondary to an incompetent vulval or vestibulovaginal seal causes a hyperechogenic interface (arrow) and loss of all ventral tissue detail. This sonogram was obtained from the left inguinal area using a curvilinear probe operating at 4.0 MHz at a depth of 18 cm.

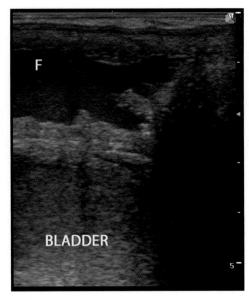

Figure 20.26 Vaginal fluid. Fluid is visualized in the vaginal vault. The cervix is visible "floating" in the fluid. In this image, caudal is on the left and cranial is on the right. This sonogram was obtained transrectally using a linear probe operating at 5.0 MHz at a depth of 5 cm.

appears as hyperechogenic particles within the uterine lumen or as a hyperechoic gas interface adjacent to and within the uterine wall, obscuring ventral structures (Figure 20.25). Poor perineal conformation leading to aspiration of air or endometrial infection with a gas-producing organism is the typical cause.

Vaginal Fluid

Fluid may accumulate in the vaginal vault (Figure 20.26) in the post-foaling mare from urine pooling, hemorrhage, trauma, or infection.

Gastrointestinal Tract

The entirety of the intestinal tract cannot be imaged; therefore, the only indication of intestinal compromise or rupture may be the onset of fulminant peritonitis and clinical signs of endotoxemia. Ultrasonographic findings are not pathognomonic for any particular lesion; however, deviation from normal viscera location or size warrants further investigation.

Large Colon

Edematous colon in the post-parturient mare may occur from colitis, peritonitis, or colon torsion (Figures 20.27, 20.28, 20.29). The large colon is at increased risk of torsion in the post-partum mare [20]. In one review,

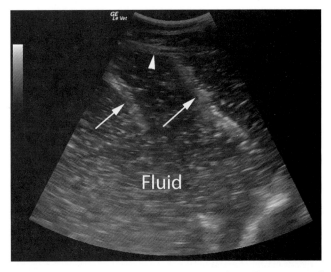

Figure 20.27 Colitis in right ventral colon. This image of the right ventral colon shows increased luminal fluid and prominent outlining of the haustra (arrow). Note the loss of sacculations along the colon wall (arrowhead). This sonogram was obtained from the right ventral abdomen with a curvilinear probe operating at 4.0 MHz at a depth of 15 cm.

this was the most common diagnosis of emergency presentations of post-partum mares at a referral center [9]. More chronic cases may have vague presenting clinical signs including inappetence and depression [21]. Ultrasonographic changes include increased wall

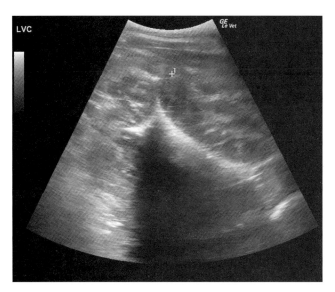

Figure 20.28 Thickened wall of left ventral colon. This post-partum mare developed severe, necrotizing typhlocolitis. Note the thickened wall (cursor) of the left ventral colon. This sonogram was taken from the left ventral abdomen with a curvilinear probe operating at 4.0 MHz at a depth of 12 cm.

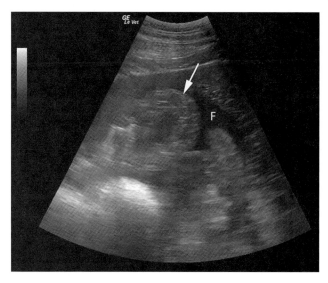

Figure 20.30 Thickened wall of jejunum. This image shows an amotile loop of jejunum with thickened walls (arrow). Flocculent peritoneal fluid (F) indicates intestinal devitalization with ensuing peritonitis. This sonogram was taken from the right inguinal region using a curvilinear probe operating at 4.0 MHz at a depth of 18 cm.

Small Colon Injury

The small colon may suffer bruising from compression during foaling or avascular necrosis from disruption of the mesenteric attachments. Segmental necrosis and entrapment may result from rents in the mesocolon [25]. Lesser trauma may result in impaction and colic. The small colon cannot be directly visualized transabdominally, and increased peritoneal fluid with inflammatory changes (see Figure 20.7), in conjunction with signs of endotoxemia, may be the first indication of devitalization.

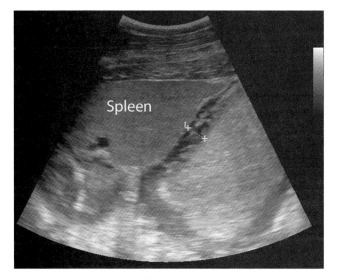

Figure 20.29 Colon wall edema. Adjacent to the spleen, the left dorsal colon wall (cursors) is grossly thickened and edematous. Causes for edematous colon wall include colitis, peritonitis, and colon torsion. This sonogram was obtained from the left abdomen using a curvilinear probe operating at 4.0 MHz at a depth of 13 cm.

Cecum

The most likely site of post-partum rupture is the tip of the cecum [3]. In parturient mares, fetal hoof on tympanic cecal wall is thought to lead to pressure necrosis [26]. Ultrasonographic findings are indicative of peritonitis (see Figure 20.7).

Jejunum

Ultrasonography has been reported to be 100% sensitive and 100% specific for small intestinal strangulation when distension, mural thickening (Figure 20.30), and loss of motility are noted [27]. Dilated small intestine with motility was associated with large colon lesions, and wall thickening with motility was present in peritonitis [27].

thickness, gaseous distension, and loss of sacculations due to profound distension [22]. The cecal and colonic mesenteric vessels are usually visualized in the right paralumbar fossa coursing ventrally. With colonic displacement or torsion, these vessels may become engorged and tortuous [23,24].

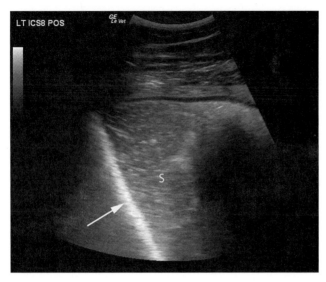

Figure 20.31 Dilated stomach. The stomach was dilated in this post-partum mare secondary to enteritis. The stomach (S) has increased contact with the body wall. The hyperechoic line (arrow) is a prominent air–fluid interface in the stomach. This sonogram was taken from the left eighth ICS using a curvilinear probe operating at 4.0 MHz at a depth of 15 cm.

Jejunum, or even small colon, may become incarcerated through a tear or rent in the mesentery [28]. Alternatively, disruption of the blood supply to the intestine may cause mural necrosis to ensue. This is especially important for the small colon due to its relatively short mesocolon, which can tear with passage of the fetus [2,25].

Stomach

Gastric distention (Figure 20.31), stasis, and rupture have also been reported secondary to other complications post partum, including small intestinal ileus [29]. In these cases, the characteristic shape and location of the stomach is altered from normal, with the arc of the stomach wall becoming irregular from loss of appropriate tension and displaced from close proximity to the liver and spleen.

SUMMARY

Ultrasonography provides a rapid and non-invasive method of assessing the viscera and genital tract of the post-foaling mare. In conjunction with consideration of the amount and characteristics of the peritoneal fluid, decisions regarding the health of the mare can be made.

REFERENCES

[1] Reef, V.B., Whittier, M., & Allam, L.G. (2004) Sonographic evaluation of the adult abdomen. *Clinical Techniques in Equine Practice*, 3(3), 294–307.
[2] Hanson, R.R. & Todhunter, R.J. (1986) Herniation of the abdominal wall in pregnant mares. *Journal of the American Veterinary Medical Association*, 189(7), 790–793.
[3] Frazer, G.S. (2003) Post partum complications in the mare. Part 2: Fetal membrane retention and conditions of the gastrointestinal tract, bladder and vagina. *Equine Veterinary Education*, 15(2), 91–100.
[4] Romero, A.E. & Rodgerson, D.H. (2010) Diaphragmatic herniation in the horse: 31 cases from 2001–2006. *Canadian Veterinary Journal*, 51(11), 1247–1250.
[5] Moll, H.D., Wallace, M.A., Sysel, A., *et al.* (1999) Large colon strangulation due to a diaphragmatic hernia in a mare: A case report. *Journal of Equine Veterinary Science*, 19(1), 58–59.
[6] Hartzband, L.E., Kerr, D.V., & Morris, E.A. (1990) Ultrasonographic diagnosis of diaphragmatic rupture in a horse. *Veterinary Radiology*, 31(1), 42–44.
[7] Frazer, G., Burba, D., Paccamonti, D., *et al.* (1997) The effects of parturition and peripartum complications on the peritoneal fluid composition of mares. *Theriogenology*, 48(6), 919–931.
[8] Arnold, C.E., Payne, M., Thompson, J.A., *et al.* (2008) Periparturient hemorrhage in mares: 73 cases (1998–2005). *Journal of the American Veterinary Medical Association*, 232(9), 1345–1351.
[9] Dolente, B.A., Sullivan, E.K., Boston, R., *et al.* (2005) Mares admitted to a referral hospital for postpartum emergencies: 163 cases (1992–2002). *Journal of Veterinary Emergency and Critical Care*, 15(3), 193–200.
[10] Williams, N.M. & Bryant, U.K. (2012) Periparturient arterial rupture in mares: a postmortem study. *Journal of Equine Veterinary Science*, 32(5), 281–284.
[11] Snalune, K.L. & Mair, T.S. (2006) Peritonitis secondary to necrosis of the apex of the urinary bladder in a post parturient mare. *Equine Veterinary Education*, 18(1), 20–26.
[12] Nyrop, K., DeBowes, R., Cox, J., *et al.* (1984) Rupture of the urinary bladder in two postparturient mares. *The Compendium on Continuing Education for the Practicing Veterinarian*, 6(9), S510–S513.
[13] Higuchi, T., Nanao, Y., & Senba, H. (2002) Repair of urinary bladder rupture through a urethrotomy and urethral sphincterotomy in four postpartum mares. *Veterinary Surgery*, 31(4), 344–348.
[14] Jones, P.A., Sertich, P.S., & Johnston, J.K. (1996) Uroperitoneum associated with ruptured urinary bladder in a postpartum mare. *Australian Veterinary Journal*, 5, 354–358.
[15] Lofstedt, R. (1994) Haemorrhage associated with pregnancy and parturition. *Equine Veterinary Education*, 6(3), 138–141.

[16] Ueno, T., Nambo, Y., Tajima, Y., *et al.* (2010) Pathology of lethal peripartum broad ligament haematoma in 31 Thoroughbred mares. *Equine Veterinary Journal*, 42(6), 529–533.

[17] Javsicas, L.H., Giguere, S., Freeman, D.E., *et al.* (2010) Comparison of surgical and medical treatment of 49 postpartum mares with presumptive or confirmed uterine tears. *Veterinary Surgery*, 39(2), 254–260.

[18] Brooks, D.E., McCoy, D.J., & Martin, G.S. (1985) Uterine rupture as a postpartum complication in two mares. *Journal of the American Veterinary Medical Association*, 187(12), 1377–1379.

[19] Livesey, L.C., Carson, R.L., & Stanton, M.B. (2008) Postpartum colic in a mare caused by pneumouterus. *Veterinary Record*, 162(19), 626–627.

[20] Hance, S.R. & Embertson, R.M. (1992) Colopexy in broodmares: 44 cases (1986–1990). *Journal of the American Veterinary Medical Association*, 201(5), 782–787.

[21] Doyle, A.J., Freeman, D.E., Sauberli, D.S., *et al.* (2002) Clinical signs and treatment of chronic uterine torsion in two mares. *Journal of the American Veterinary Medical Association*, 220(3), 349–353.

[22] Abutarbush, S.M. (2006) Use of ultrasonography to diagnose large colon volvulus in horses. *Journal of the American Veterinary Medical Association*, 228(3), 409–413.

[23] Grenager, N.S. & Durham, M.G. (2011) Ultrasonographic evidence of colonic mesenteric vessels as an indicator of right dorsal displacement of the large colon in 13 horses. *Equine Veterinary Journal*, 43, 153–155.

[24] Ness, S.A.L., Bain, F.T., Zantingh, A.J., *et al.* (2012) Ultrasonographic visualization of colonic mesenteric vasculature as an indicator of large colon right dorsal displacement or 180° volvulus (or both) in horses. *Canadian Veterinary Journal*, 53(4), 378–382.

[25] Dart, A.J., Pascoe, J.R., & Snyder, J.R. (1991) Mesenteric tears of the descending (small) colon as a postpartum complication in two mares. *Journal of the American Veterinary Medical Association*, 199(11), 1612–1615.

[26] Platt, H. (1983) Caecal rupture in parturient mares. *Journal of Comparative Pathology*, 93(2), 343–346.

[27] Klohnen, A., Vachon, A.M., & Fischer, A.T. (1996) Use of diagnostic ultrasonography in horses with signs of acute abdominal pain. *Journal of the American Veterinary Medical Association*, 209(9), 1597–1601.

[28] Gayle, J.M., Blikslager, A.T., & Bowman, K.F. (2000) Mesenteric rents as a source of small intestinal strangulation in horses: 15 cases (1990–1997). *Journal of the American Veterinary Medical Association*, 216(9), 1446–1449.

[29] Hillyer, M.H., Smith, M.R.W., & Milligan, P.J.P. (2008) Gastric and small intestinal ileus as a cause of acute colic in the post parturient mare. *Equine Veterinary Journal*, 40(4), 368–372.

SECTION 3

INTERNAL MEDICINE

Section 3a: Ultrasonography of the Thoracic Cavity

CHAPTER TWENTY-ONE

ULTRASONOGRAPHY OF THE PLEURAL CAVITY, LUNG, AND DIAPHRAGM

Peter R. Morresey

Rood and Riddle Equine Hospital, Lexington, KY, USA

THORACIC ULTRASONOGRAPHY

Ultrasonography has largely replaced radiography in the diagnosis of pulmonary disease since it can be performed stall-side relatively quickly without the need for transport to a referral center. The pleural surfaces, the pleural space, and the surface of the lung can be rapidly evaluated for mild to severe pathological changes. In some cases of thoracic disease, the extent of involvement of the pleural space and lung may be subtle and unable to be detected by auscultation, radiography, or percussion; but these changes may be readily detected by ultrasonography. Severity of pulmonary consolidation is better assessed with ultrasonography, and consolidation can be readily identified in horses with pleural effusion. The musculature of the thoracic wall, bony and cartilaginous continuity of the ribs, and the integrity of the diaphragm can also be evaluated.

Technique

The entire thorax should be examined in a dorsal to ventral direction from the third to seventeenth intercostal space (ICS). While clipping this area provides the best image, removal of hair is best reserved for discrete areas of pathology, if at all necessary, to maintain cosmesis. Acceptable acoustic contact can be achieved by thoroughly wetting the hair with isopropyl alcohol before slicking down the hair to remove trapped air.

The probe is placed in the ICS parallel to the ribs to maximize the acoustic window, beginning at the most dorsal aspect of the visualized lung and traversing down the ICS to past the level of the diaphragm to ensure the entire lung field and pleural space are imaged. The probe is generally placed perpendicular to the thoracic wall; however, the areas shielded by the ribs can be assessed during horizontal oscillations applied to the probe to sweep the ultrasound beam along this plane. Assessment of the cranial thorax (cranial to the third ICS) presents some difficulty as the triceps musculature covers this area. The probe may be applied to the triceps muscle with depth adjusted to allow pleural and pulmonary evaluation. Alternatively, the probe can be placed under the right triceps musculature with this limb protracted cranially, and the probe angled appropriately to image the cranial mediastinum.

NORMAL ANATOMY

The cranial thorax encompasses the heart which is deep to the triceps musculature [1]. The cardiac notch of the lung allows visualization of the heart, extending from the third rib to the fourth ICS on the right side, and the third to sixth ribs on the left side [1]. The diaphragm (Figure 21.1) extends cranially to contact the heart, with the most ventral aspect reflecting caudally. Always identify the hyperechoic diaphragmatic musculature as it reflects on to the thoracic wall to provide visual separation between the lung fields and the abdominal viscera. This will ensure the correct location is ascribed to any fluid seen, and determines whether

Atlas of Equine Ultrasonography, First Edition. Edited by Jessica A. Kidd, Kristina G. Lu, and Michele L. Frazer.
© 2014 John Wiley & Sons, Ltd. Published 2014 by John Wiley & Sons, Ltd.
Companion Website: www.wiley.com/go/kidd/equine-ultrasonography

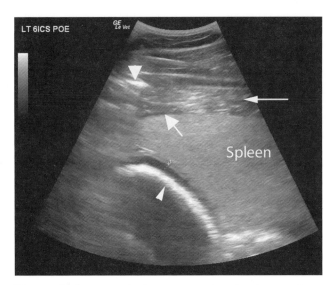

Figure 21.1 Normal diaphragm. The diaphragm (long arrow) provides a muscular layer of separation between the thoracic and abdominal cavities. It inserts on the thoracic wall at approximately the eighth to ninth costal cartilage and curves caudodorsally to the eighteenth rib. It then reflects craniomedially and ends at the seventeenth ICS. Also visible in this image is spleen, the curvilinear surface of the stomach (small arrowhead), liver (short arrow), and tip of lung (large arrowhead). This sonogram was obtained from the left sixth ICS with a curvilinear probe operating at 4.0 MHz at a depth of 16 cm.

contact is occurring between the viscera and the lungs resulting from discontinuity of the diaphragm.

Examination of the left hemithorax caudal to the heart finds the left liver lobe deep to the diaphragm. Traversing caudally, the spleen will come into view, adjacent and medial to the left lobe of the liver. The stomach may be noted in cross-section deep to this interface alongside the splenic vein. The spleen is visible between the seventh and seventeenth ICS [2].

Examination of the right hemithorax ventrally, caudal to the heart, reveals the diaphragm and right lobe of the liver extending from the ninth to sixteenth ICS, with the large colon medial to the liver or in apposition with the diaphragm [2]. Dorsally, as on the left side, the lung fields are easily visualized moving across the screen in time with inspiration and expiration during breathing. Mid-thorax, deep to the diaphragm, the liver and right dorsal colon may be seen in close apposition. Caudally, between ICS sixteen and seventeen, the cranial aspect of the right kidney is visible [2].

The apposition of the parietal and visceral pleura may be noted as a hyperechoic interface with evenly spaced reverberation artifacts indicating a highly reflective interface (Figures 21.2, 21.3, 21.4). Motion of the pulmonary parenchyma can be seen synchronously with thoracic excursions during respiration.

An anechoic space from a small amount of fluid (up to 3.5 cm reported) [1] is present in the majority of horses over the right cranioventral lung field. This fluid creates separation of the parietal and visceral

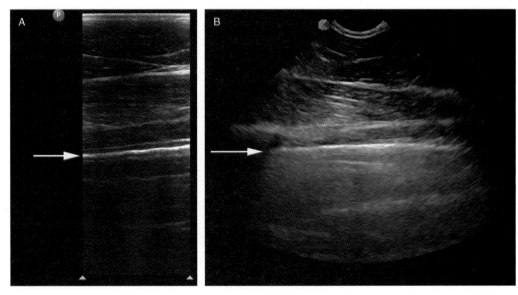

Figure 21.2 Normal lung. Ultrasound is used to image the superficial areas of lung contacting the thoracic body wall. This lung field is triangular in shape and extends caudally to the sixteenth ICS. In these images, the hyperechoic line (arrow) is the pleural surface of normal lung. (A) This sonogram was obtained from the left eighth ICS using a linear probe operating at 5.0 MHz at a depth of 8 cm. (B) This sonogram was obtained from the left eighth ICS using a micro-convex probe operating at 6.6 MHz at a depth of 6 cm.

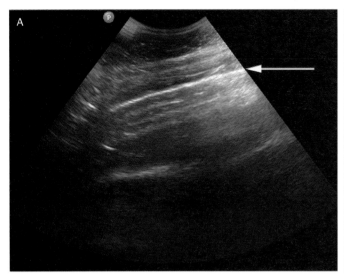
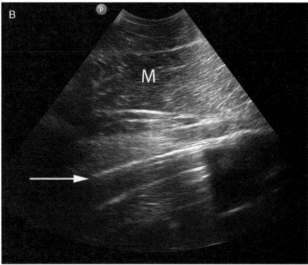

Figure 21.3 Normal lung. The most cranial aspect of the lung field is located under the triceps musculature. (A) To scan this portion of lung, the forelimb must be pulled forward and the ultrasound probe moved under the triceps muscle. The hyperechoic line (arrow) is the normal lung surface. This sonogram was obtained from the fourth ICS using a curvilinear probe operating at 3.5 MHz at a depth of 15 cm. (B) Also, the cranial lung can be imaged by increasing the display depth and scanning through the triceps muscle (M). The hyperechoic line (arrow) is the pleural surface of normal lung. This sonogram was obtained by imaging through the triceps musculature over the shoulder using a curvilinear probe operating at 3.5 MHz at a depth of 18 cm.

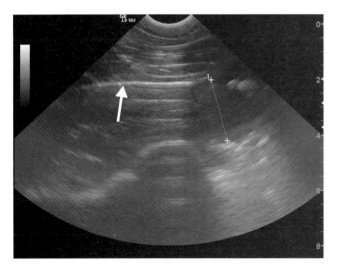
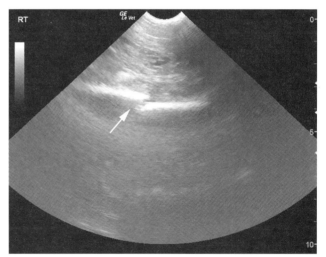

Figure 21.4 Pleural echogenicity, normal (arrow) with adjacent abscess. Note the hyperechogenic interface between the thoracic wall and lung parenchyma corresponding to an abrupt change in echodensity in the unaffected area. This prominent interface is lost with pulmonary parenchymal disease (in this case an abscess indicated by the calipers) due to enhanced transmission of the ultrasound beam through the non-aerated tissue. This sonogram was obtained from the right eighth ICS using a micro-convex probe operating at 8.0 MHz at a depth of 6 cm.

Figure 21.5 Fractured rib. This image shows a rib fracture (arrow) in a neonatal foal. The distal segment has minimal displacement, so diagnosis of the fracture by palpation alone may have been difficult. This sonogram was obtained from right thorax using a micro-convex probe operating at 6.0 MHz at a depth of 8 cm.

PATHOLOGY

Thoracic Wall

pleura. This may also be present in a lesser amount on the left side in these horses. This is not an indicator of a disease state, rather this is thought necessary for lubrication of the pleural surfaces.

Rib fractures (Figures 21.5, 21.6, 21.7, 21.8) are more readily detected by ultrasonography than radiography

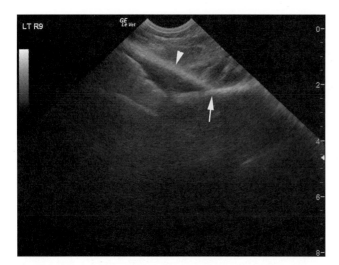

Figure 21.6 Fractured rib with displacement. This image shows an acute fractured rib in a neonatal foal. The fracture has overriding of the proximal (arrowhead) and distal fragments (arrow) with associated pleural hemorrhage. This sonogram was taken from the left thorax, ninth rib using a micro-convex probe operating at 8.0 MHz at a depth of 8 cm.

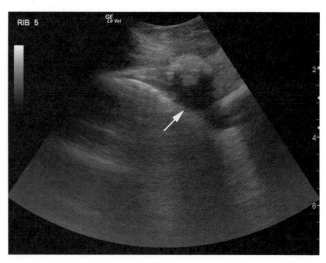

Figure 21.8 Fractured rib with hematoma. This image shows a fractured rib with an organizing hematoma (arrow). This is the first stage of fracture stabilization prior to callus formation. This sonogram of the right fifth rib was obtained with a probe operating at 8.0 MHz at a depth of 8 cm.

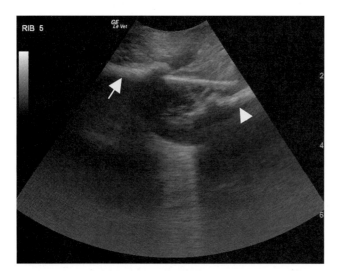

Figure 21.7 Fractured rib with lung trauma. In this rib fracture, the proximal rib fragment (arrow) is overriding the distal portion (arrowhead), and a free rib fragment is present. Pulmonary contusion can be inferred from the increased echodensity of the adjacent lung. This sonogram was taken from the left thorax, ninth rib using a micro-convex probe operating at 8.0 MHz at a depth of 6 cm.

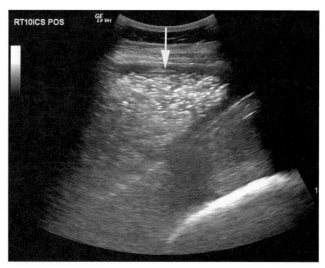

Figure 21.9 Pleural abscess. This image shows a pleural abscess (arrow) in an adult horse. Note the encapsulated heterogeneous mass at the diaphragmatic reflection. This sonogram was obtained from the right tenth ICS using a curvilinear probe operating at 4.0 MHz at a depth of 12 cm.

in neonatal foals [3]. Changes in continuity of the hyperechoic border of the ribs, as well as size and location of rib fragments, are visualized. Associated subcutaneous and intramural hematomas can also be detected and their extent assessed.

Pleural Abscess

Abscesses may form on the pleural surface (Figures 21.4, 21.9) and image as hypo- or hyperechoic, encapsulated structures.

Pleuritis

Uniformly aerated lung adjacent to the parietal pleura creates a hyperechoic gas echo and is responsible for the smooth appearance of healthy lung sliding rhyth- mically past the thoracic wall. With pleuritis (Figures 21.10, 21.11, 21.12, 21.13, 21.14), comet tail artifacts result from discrete small amounts of fluid in the pleural space or cellular infiltrate in the pulmonary periphery. This leads to transmission of the ultrasound

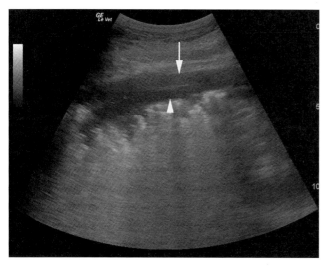

Figure 21.10 Pleuritis. This image shows demarcation between thickened pulmonary (arrowhead) and thoracic (arrow) pleura. This sonogram was obtained from the right ninth ICS using a curvilinear probe operating at 4.0 MHz at a depth of 14 cm.

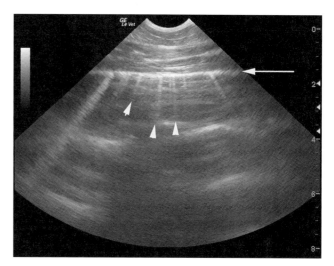

Figure 21.11 Comet tail artifact. This image shows comet- tail artifact (arrowheads) on the surface of the lung (arrow). Irregularities on the pulmonary surface cause diffraction of the ultrasound beam and shadowing. This sonogram was taken from the right seventh ICS using a micro-convex probe operating at 8.0 MHz at a depth of 8 cm.

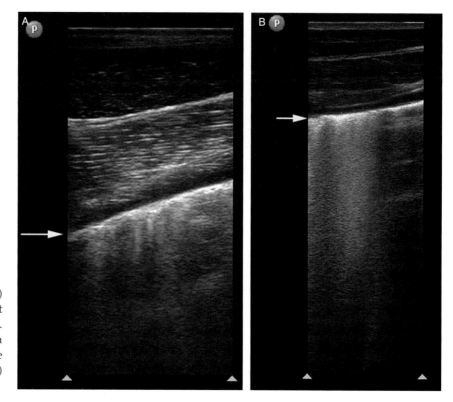

Figure 21.12 Comet tail artifact. (A,B) These images show comet tail artifact on the surface of the lung (arrow). These sonograms were obtained from the left ninth ICS with a linear probe operating at 5.0 MHz at a depth of (A) 7 cm and (B) 10 cm.

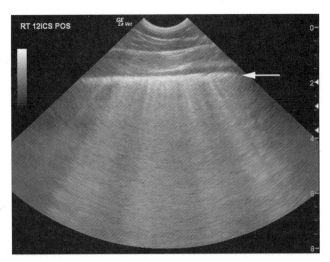

Figure 21.13 Comet tail artifact. This image shows more severe comet tail artifacts on the surface of the lungs (arrow) than those in Figures 20.11 and 20.12. More severe inflammatory changes cause coalescing of adjacent ultrasound shadowing. This sonogram was obtained from the right twelfth ICS using a micro-convex probe operating at 8.0 MHz at a depth of 8 cm.

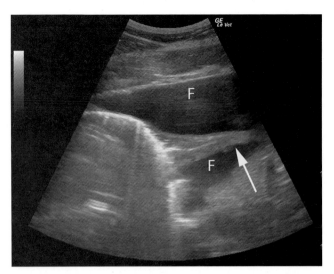

Figure 21.15 Pleuropneumonia. This image shows pleural effusion (F) surrounding atelectic (collapsed) lung (arrow). This sonogram was obtained with a curvilinear probe operating at 4.0 MHz at a depth of 13 cm.

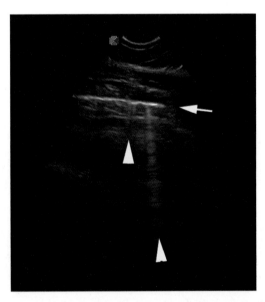

Figure 21.14 Caudodorsal lung changes. This image shows comet tail artifact (arrowhead) from the surface of the lung (arrow) in the caudodorsal lung field. Changes in this area of the lungs have been associated with exercise-induced pulmonary hemorrhage. This image was obtained from the left sixteenth ICS using a curvilinear probe operating at 4.0 MHz at a depth of 10 cm.

beam and then reflection at an air interface, resulting in the classic hyperechoic shadowing appearance. This hyperechoic shadow is a non-specific indicator of pulmonary pathology and may result from inflammatory conditions, pulmonary edema, metastatic infiltrative conditions, granulomatous diseases, fibrosis, and acute infectious causes of disease [4,5]. Resolved areas of pleural or pulmonary inflammation also retain this appearance.

Pleural Effusions

Pleural effusions (Figures 21.15, 21.16, 21.17, 21.18, 21.19, 21.20, 21.21) are typically a transudate or modified transudate and are, therefore, anechoic in appearance. As cell count and protein content increase, ultrasonographic character changes from hypoechogenic to echogenic. Fibrin strands appear filamentous and echogenic in relation to the fluid around them. They may coalesce to form fluid pockets in a web-like structure joining the lungs, parietal pleura, and diaphragm, or consolidate to a relatively echogenic mass. Small, hyperechogenic foci within the pleural fluid suggest the presence of gas (Figure 21.17), indicating anaerobic infection or bronchopleural fistula formation. Gas echoes within pleural fluid are a reliable indicator of anaerobic infection. Do not confuse the pericardial diaphragmatic ligament (Figure 21.18), especially when floating in increased pleural fluid, with pathological fibrin deposition. The pericardial diaphragmatic ligament is visualized as an undulating uniform solitary hyperechoic strand, in contrast to fibrin which is more filamentous and composed of multiple strands.

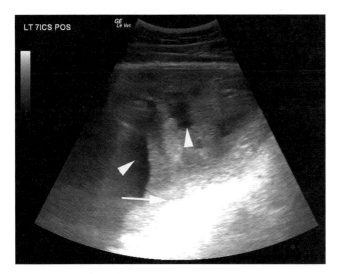

Figure 21.16 Fibrinous pleuritis. This image shows pleural effusion with fibrin coalescing in the pleural space. Pocketing of fluid is present (arrowheads). Enhanced transmission of the ultrasound beam through the fluid and fibrin has caused an enhancement of the reflection at the tissue interface (arrow). This sonogram was obtained from the left seventh ICS with a curvilinear probe operating at 4.0 MHz at a depth of 15 cm.

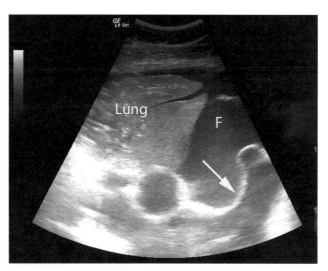

Figure 21.18 Pericardial diaphragmatic ligament. This image shows the pericardial diaphragmatic ligament (arrow) surrounded by pleural fluid (F). This structure is not visualized in the normal thorax, but is apparent when bathed in fluid. Do not confuse the ligament with fibrin strands. Atelectic lung is also visible. This image was obtained from the left seventh ICS using a curvilinear probe operating at 4.0 MHz at a depth of 17 cm.

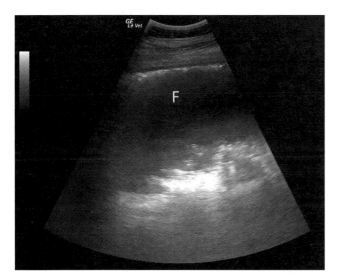

Figure 21.17 Pleural space gas. In this image of pleural effusion, hyperechoic foci are present within the pleural fluid (F) indicating the presence of gas. This image was obtained from the left seventh ICS with a curvilinear probe operating at 4.0 MHz at a depth of 20 cm.

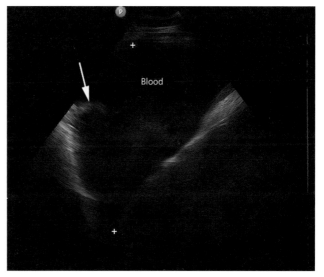

Figure 21.19 Acute hemothorax. This image shows hemorrhage into the pleural cavity. Note the swirling appearance to the fluid suggesting ongoing hemorrhage. The atelectic lung tip (arrow) is visible. This sonogram was obtained from the left sixth ICS with a curvilinear probe operating at 3.5 MHz at a depth of 30 cm.

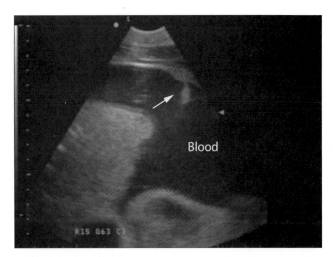

Figure 21.20   Acute hemothorax. This image shows recent hemorrhage into the pleural cavity. The blood swirls with respiratory movements. Fibrin deposits (arrow) are seen on the thoracic pleura. This sonogram was obtained from the right sixth ICS with a curvilinear probe operating at 4.0 MHz at a depth of 14 cm.

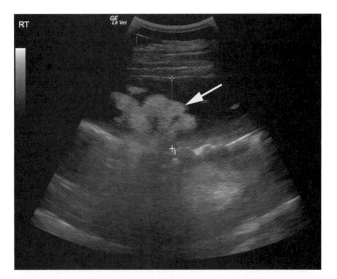

Figure 21.21   Organizing hemothorax. This image shows hemorrhage into the pleural cavity after clotting has started. Echodense masses (arrow) are present within relatively hypoechogenic fluid. This sonogram was taken from the right seventh ICS using a curvilinear probe operating at 4.0 MHz at a depth of 16 cm.

Hemothorax

Hemothorax (Figures 21.19, 21.20, 21.21) images as a large, relatively anechoic effusion in the pleural space. With respiratory movements, swirling is noted which is likely the result of erythrocyte rouleaux formation. Swirling of the blood may also indicate continued blood loss to the thoracic cavity.

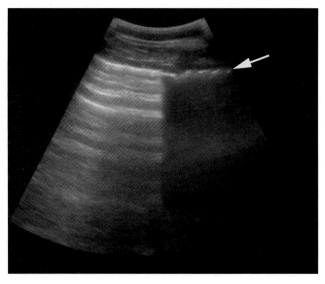

Figure 21.22   Pneumothorax and pleuritis. The lung parenchyma is no longer in contact with the thoracic wall because of air in the pleural cavity. The reverberating, hyperechoic line (arrow) shadows more medial structures and confirms the diagnosis of pneumothorax. This sonogram was obtained from the left fifteenth ICS using a curvilinear probe operating at 4.0 MHz at a depth of 19 cm.

Pneumothorax

Pneumothorax (Figure 21.22), or the presence of gas within the pleural space, results in loss of the normal pulmonary architecture. A hyperechoic reverberating line is present in place of the parietal pleural reflection. Scanning the ICS from dorsal to ventral will ascertain the interface between air accumulation and normal lung parenchyma movement. As pneumothorax may be the sole pathology and located dorsally, examination of the entire thoracic cavity is important to detect this condition.

Pulmonary Disease

Diffuse inflammation of the lung parenchyma can result in interstitial pneumonia (Figure 21.23). Interstitial pneumonia images as diffuse shadowing or a "ground glass" appearance. Causes of interstitial pneumonia include bacteria, viral, or fungal infection, environmental factors, and acute respiratory distress syndrome (ARDS).

Consolidated lung (Figures 21.24, 21.25, 21.26, 21.27) appears as hypoechoic areas within the lung. Consolidated areas may be of varying shape, ranging from irregular to spherical. The overall shape of the lung is preserved. Accumulation of fluid and cellular infiltration alters the echogenicity of the lung as these areas

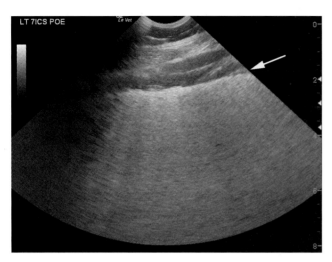

Figure 21.23 Interstitial pneumonia. This image shows diffuse shadowing of the lung. The arrow identifies lung surface. Generalized inflammation of the pulmonary parenchyma, such as in this case of interstitial pneumonia, can cause loss of all detail in the deeper lung parenchyma. This sonogram was obtained from the left seventh ICS using a micro-convex probe operating at 8.0 MHz at a depth of 8 cm.

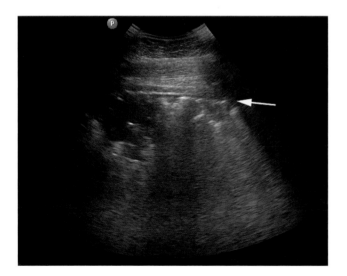

Figure 21.24 Aspiration pneumonia. This image shows aspiration pneumonia secondary to chronic esophageal obstruction in an adult horse. The arrow identifies the surface of the lung. This sonogram was obtained from the left seventh ICS with a curvilinear probe operating at 3.5 MHz at a depth of 15 cm.

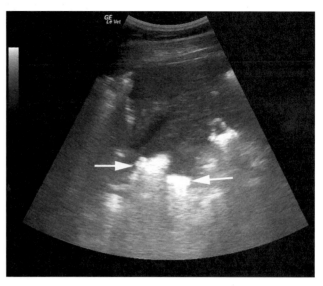

Figure 21.25 Pulmonary consolidation. Enhanced transmission of ultrasound is possible through more echodense pulmonary parenchyma. Blood vessels and airways are apparent. Hyperechoic areas with shadowing indicate areas of gas/air trapping (arrows). This sonogram was obtained from the left ninth ICS using a curvilinear probe operating at 4.0 MHz at a depth of 16 cm.

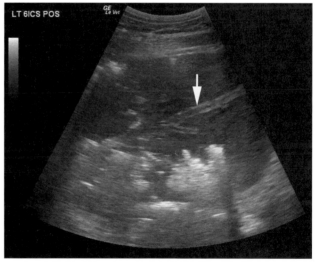

Figure 21.26 Pulmonary consolidation. An airway (arrow) is clearly delineated within an area of consolidated lung. This sonogram was obtained from the left sixth ICS using a curvilinear probe operating at 4.0 MHz at a depth of 16 cm.

are poorly aerated and hence not acoustically reflective. The pulmonary vascular and bronchial tree may still be evident, however if tissue degeneration ensues, these structures will be lost and the area becomes more hypoechoic. Diffuse small hypoechoic areas throughout the lung fields may be indicative of a multifocal disease process, such as neoplasia or granulomatous lung disease (Figure 21.28).

Pulmonary Atelectasis

Pulmonary atelectasis is collapse or compression of lung parenchyma and appears relatively hypoechoic. It may result from pleural effusion or pneumothorax. When associated with pleural effusion, the cranioventral lung tip is affected and appears bathed within

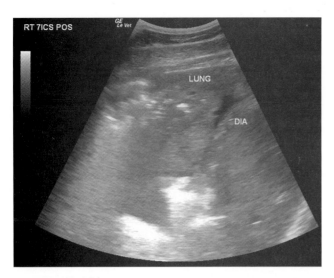

Figure 21.27 Pulmonary consolidation. This image shows consolidated lung with gas trapping within the consolidated area. This gas leads to shadowing of more medial structures. Diaphragm (DIA) is visible. This sonogram was obtained from the right seventh ICS with a curvilinear probe operating at 4.0 MHz at a depth of 16 cm.

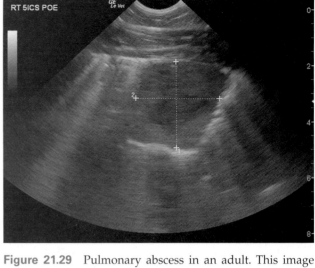

Figure 21.29 Pulmonary abscess in an adult. This image shows an abscess (cursors) on the surface of the lung in an adult horse. The heterogeneous fluid content of the abscess leads to less shadowing of more medial structures than the abscess in Figure 21.30. This image was obtained from the right fifth ICS with a micro-convex probe operating at 8.0 MHz at a depth of 8 cm.

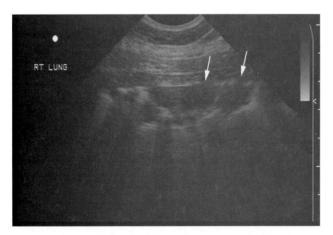

Figure 21.28 Granulomatous lung disease. Multiple, coalescing, relatively hypoechogenic structures (arrows) are present on the lung surface. Normally aerated lung located medially has obscured deeper lesions. At necropsy, the lung was uniformly populated with granulomatous foci. Hyperechoic streaks present at the bottom of the image are artifact from damaged crystals in the probe. This sonogram was obtained from the right tenth ICS using a curvilinear probe operating at 4.0 MHz at a depth of 7 cm.

Pulmonary Abscessation

Pulmonary abscesses (Figures 21.29, 21.30, 21.31) that contact the surface of the lung can be imaged with ultrasonography. They may also be seen within consolidated lung, but cannot be imaged if aerated lung is present between the abscess and the ultrasound transducer. They may appear as a heterogeneous hypoechoic region with hyperechoic margins. Gas may also be present leading to a mixture of hyperechoic and hypoechoic reflections within the cavitation. There is a significant association between the presence of hyperechoic gas echoes and the presence of anaerobic infection [6].

Increased Pulmonary Volume

Increased pulmonary volume may occur with recurrent airway obstruction (RAO). As seen with ultrasound, lung fields in horses with RAO may extend more caudally than normal, suggesting expansion of the lung field from pulmonary hyperinflation or emphysema [7]. Variation in the caudal extent of the lung fields is noted between horses, however the seventeenth ICS consistently does not contain lung in the normal horse [8].

pleural fluid (see Figure 21.15). Pneumothorax leads to compression of the more dorsal aspect of the lung resulting in a hypoechoic region of lung at the junction of normal parenchyma and the pleural space air.

Diaphragmatic Disruption

Herniation of abdominal content into the thoracic cavity (Figure 21.32) may be suspected if curved, hyperechoic interfaces attenuate the ultrasound beam and cause reverberation cranial and dorsal to the dia-

phragmatic line [9]. Peristaltic waves may also be noted when intestine has herniated into the thoracic cavity. Anechoic fluid may be noted ventrally in the thorax consistent with concurrent pleural effusion. The muscular borders of the diaphragmatic tear may appear thickened as they retract through loss of

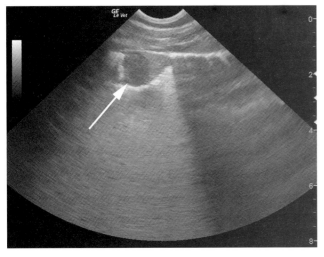

Figure 21.30 Pulmonary abscess in a foal. This image shows an abscess (arrow) on the surface of the lung in a foal. The more fluid content of this abscess (compared to Figure 21.29) enhances transmission of the ultrasound beam and creates a more pronounced reflection at the fluid–tissue interface. The result is a more hyperechoic interface with increased shadowing of medial structures. This sonogram was obtained from the right eighth ICS with a micro-convex probe operating at 8.0 MHz at a depth of 7 cm.

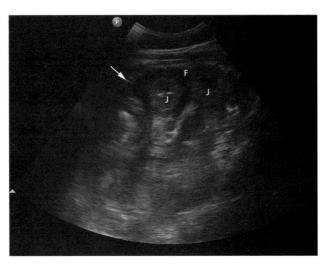

Figure 21.32 Diaphragmatic hernia. This image shows herniation of small intestine into the pleural cavity. The loops of jejunum (J) are in direct apposition with the lung parenchyma (arrow). Diaphragm is not visible between the intestine and lung. This sonogram was obtained from the right fifth ICS with a curvilinear probe operating at 3.5 MHz at a depth of 15 cm. (Source: Image courtesy of Dr. Nathan Slovis, Hagyard Equine Medical Institute, Lexington, KY, USA.)

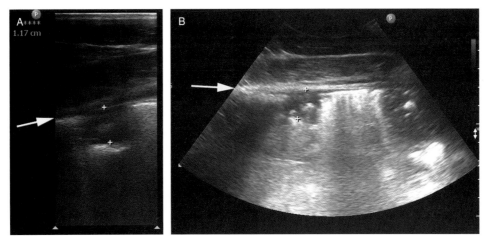

Figure 21.31 Pulmonary abscess in foal. These images show abscesses (cursors) on the surface of the lungs (arrow) in two foals diagnosed with *Rhodococcus equi* infection. (A) This image was obtained from the right sixth ICS with a linear probe operating at 5.0 MHz at a depth of 7 cm. (B) This sonogram was obtained from the right seventh ICS with a curvilinear probe operating at 5.0 MHz at a depth of 10 cm.

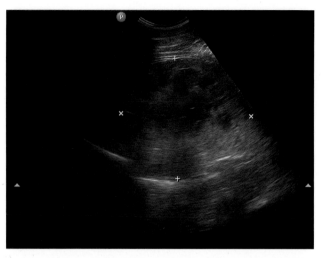

Figure 21.33 Diaphragmatic mass. This image shows a mass (cursors) in the thoracic cavity. Histopathology of a biopsy sample confirmed a diagnosis of hemangiosarcoma. This image was obtained from the left tenth ICS with a curvilinear probe operating at 3.5 MHz at a depth of 20 cm. (Source: Image courtesy of Dr. Nathan Slovis, Hagyard Equine Medical Institute, Lexington, KY, USA.)

tension. Herniation through the central tendon may be difficult to detect as the defect is not visible and viscera may not be adjacent to the thoracic wall.

Neoplastic disease, including lymphosarcoma or hemangiosarcoma, may manifest as nodular lesions in the diaphragm (Figure 21.33).

LIMITATIONS OF THORACIC ULTRASONOGRAPHY

With respect to intrapulmonary disease, radiography remains a superior diagnostic modality. Ultrasound is unable to penetrate air-filled lung, raising the specter of significant pathology being shielded from view by normal aerated lung parenchyma. In these cases, when used in conjunction with ultrasonography, radiography allows the most thorough imaging of the thoracic content to be achieved.

SUMMARY

Thoracic ultrasonography allows rapid assessment of pleural and pulmonary health. However, ultrasonography should not be considered a substitute for a thorough physical examination of the patient and careful thoracic auscultation. Rather, the information it provides the clinician is complementary and confirmatory in nature, adding weight to clinical suspicions already raised from the horse's history and physical examination.

REFERENCES

[1] Rantanen, N.W. (1986) Diseases of the thorax. *Veterinary Clinics of North America: Equine Practice*, 2(1), 49–66.

[2] Rantanen, N. (1981) Ultrasound appearance of normal lung borders and adjacent viscera in the horse. *Veterinary Radiology*, 22(5), 217–219.

[3] Jean, D., Picandet, V., Macieira, S., et al. (2007) Detection of rib trauma in newborn foals in an equine critical care unit: a comparison of ultrasonography, radiography and physical examination. *Equine Veterinary Journal*, 39(2), 158–163.

[4] Gross, D.K., Morley, P.S., Hinchcliff, K.W., et al. (2004) Pulmonary ultrasonographic abnormalities associated with naturally occurring equine influenza virus infection in standardbred racehorses. *Journal of Veterinary Internal Medicine*, 18(5), 718–727.

[5] Marr, C.M. (1993) Thoracic ultrasonography. *Equine Veterinary Education*, 5(1), 41–46.

[6] Reimer, J.M., Reef, V.B., Spencer, P.A. (1989) Ultrasonography as a diagnostic aid in horses with anaerobic bacterial pleuropneumonia and/or pulmonary abscessation: 27 cases (1984–1986). *Journal of the American Veterinary Medical Association*, 194(2), 278–282.

[7] Bakos, Z., Voros, K., Kellokoski, H., et al. (2003) Comparison of the caudal lung borders determined by percussion and ultrasonography in horses with recurrent airway obstruction. *Acta Veterinaria Hungarica*, 51(3), 249–258.

[8] Bakos, Z. (2011) Ultrasonographic description of the caudal and ventral lung borders in normal Warmblood horses. *Equine Veterinary Education*, 23(8), 416–421.

[9] Hartzband, L.E., Kerr, D.V., & Morris, E.A. (1990) Ultasonographic diagnosis of diaphragmmatic rupture in a horse. *Veterinary Radiology*, 31(1), 42–44.

CHAPTER TWENTY-TWO

ULTRASONOGRAPHY OF THE HEART

Colin C. Schwarzwald

University of Zurich, Zurich, Switzerland

Over the last three decades, echocardiography has become a standard diagnostic tool in equine cardiology. Development of M-mode and two-dimensional (2D) real-time echocardiography and introduction of various Doppler modalities, including continuous wave (CW) Doppler, pulsed-wave (PW) Doppler, and color flow Doppler, provided the basis for comprehensive evaluation of internal cardiac structures, chamber dimensions, blood flow characteristics, and mechanical function of the equine heart [1,2,3]. Newer echocardiographic modalities, including tissue Doppler imaging (TDI) and 2D speckle tracking (2DST), might become valuable tools for assessment of cardiac function in horses in the near future [4,5,6,7,8]. Nonetheless, accurate and reliable assessment of chamber dimensions and mechanical function of the heart will remain challenging and is limited by a variety of technical, anatomic, and physiologic issues that must be considered when performing echocardiographic examinations [3,9,10]. Knowledge of the technical principles of ultrasonography, strict adherence to a routine protocol in order to obtain high-quality standard sonographic images, and comprehensive knowledge of normal cardiac anatomy and abnormal findings in horses with heart disease are prerequisites to the successful use of echocardiography. Also, despite the availability of quantitative echocardiographic methods, subjective assessment of recordings will remain a cornerstone of echocardiography and must not be neglected. Finally, independent of the methods used, the findings obtained during echocardiography should be critically assessed in the light of medical history and clinical findings.

TECHNICAL CONSIDERATIONS

The ultrasonographic equipment should include a phased-array sector transducer working at frequencies between 1.5 and 3.5 MHz. Tissue harmonic imaging often improves the image quality, particularly in the far field and in large horses, by providing a higher signal-to-noise ratio, better contrast, and higher spatial resolution. Frame rates of at least 15 Hz (15 images/second) are required for real-time 2D imaging of the moving structures of the heart, but frame rates of 25 Hz or higher are preferable. Newer applications, such as anatomical M-mode [11] or 2D speckle tracking [6,7,8] demand a frame rate between 40 and 90 Hz to achieve sufficient temporal resolution. The depth of penetration should reach at least 25–30 cm to scan the heart of an adult horse. Simultaneous recording of a surface electrocardiogram (ECG) is required and allows exact timing of flow events and echocardiographic measurements. Modern echocardiography systems offer digital raw data storage of still frames and cine loop recordings. This is extremely useful since it reduces the contact time with the patient and allows post processing and off-line analysis of the stored data.

ULTRASONOGRAPHIC EXAMINATION OF THE NORMAL EQUINE HEART

The echocardiographic examination should take place in a location where the horse can be safely restrained. If possible, the patient should not be sedated prior to

Atlas of Equine Ultrasonography, First Edition. Edited by Jessica A. Kidd, Kristina G. Lu, and Michele L. Frazer.
© 2014 John Wiley & Sons, Ltd. Published 2014 by John Wiley & Sons, Ltd.
Companion Website: www.wiley.com/go/kidd/equine-ultrasonography

the examination, since cardiac dimensions, indices of cardiac function, and color Doppler signals of regurgitant flow or shunt flow might be altered because of drug effects on preload, afterload, contractility, heart rate, and rhythm [12,13,14,15]. However, some horses do not tolerate the echocardiographic procedure and require sedation to allow safe examination with sufficient quality and at normal heart rates.

A systematic approach using standardized image planes is important for comparison of studies over time and for comparison of studies obtained by different examiners (Figures 22.1, 22.2, 22.3, 22.4, 22.5). By

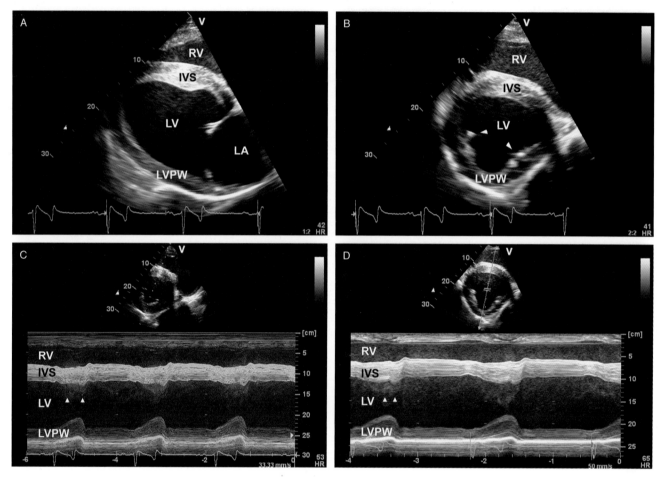

Figure 22.1 Standard echocardiographic views for assessment of left ventricular size and function. (A) Right-parasternal long-axis four-chamber view centered on the left ventricle (LV). The transducer is positioned in the right fourth intercostal space at a level slightly above the olecranon, angled caudally, and rotated clockwise to the 1 o'clock position. Slight changes in transducer placement may be necessary to optimize the image plane. This view is best suited to assess the structures, dimensions, and mechanical function of the LV. Since this image is centered on the LV, the left atrium (LA) may not be imaged in its entirety throughout the cardiac cycle. Assessment of the right heart is limited due to its anatomic position, its complex geometry, and its visualization in the narrow near field of the imaging sector. (B) Right-parasternal short-axis view of the LV at the level of the chordae tendineae (arrowheads). This view is obtained by rotating the transducer 90° clockwise from a four-chamber view. It is commonly used for measurement of the diameter and the area, respectively, of the LV, and evaluation of LV systolic function. (C) Right-parasternal short-axis view (top) and corresponding M-mode recording (bottom) of the LV at the chordal level. The motion of the interventricular septum (IVS) and the left ventricular peripheral wall (LVPW) are displayed over time. The right ventricle (RV) and the right ventricular free wall are displayed in the near field. A small amount of spontaneous echo contrast is frequently seen in the ventricular lumen (arrowheads). Measurement of LV wall thickness and internal dimensions, evaluation of septal motion, and calculation of LV fractional shortening allow assessment of LV size and systolic function. (D) Anatomic M-mode (AMM) image of the LV (bottom), reconstructed from a digitally stored 2D cineloop recording obtained from a right-parasternal short-axis view at the chordal level (top). Notice that the AMM cursor (green line) can be freely positioned on the 2D image, independent of the sector apex, to bisect the IVS, the LV cavity, and the LVPW into two equal parts throughout the cardiac cycle.

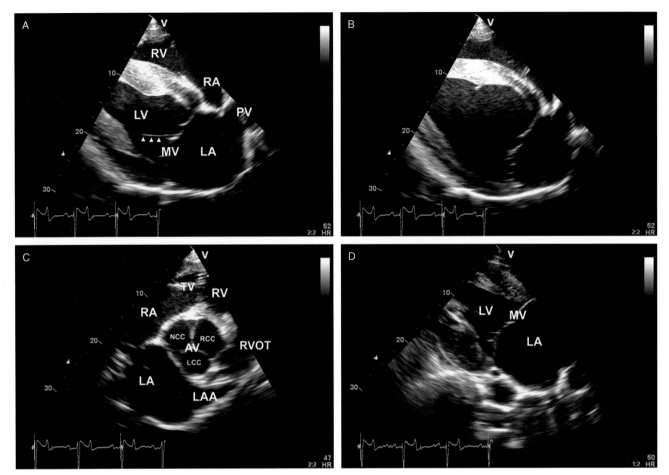

Figure 22.2   Standard echocardiographic views for assessment of left atrial size and function. (A,B) Right-parasternal four-chamber view centered on the left atrium (LA), to image the LA in its entirety throughout the cardiac cycle. At an imaging depth of 30cm, this view is best suited to assess the mitral valve (MV) apparatus, LA dimensions, and LA mechanical function. Only in rare cases (e.g. giant draft breeds, horses with severe cardiomegaly) can the LA not be displayed in its entirety from this window. (A) Image recorded at the end of ventricular systole, one frame prior to opening of the MV, when the LA is at its maximum dimensions. Chordae tendineae are seen in the left ventricular (LV) cavity (arrowheads). (B) Image recorded at the end of diastole, immediately after closure of the MV, when the LA is at its minimum dimensions. Note the obvious change in LA dimensions within a single cardiac cycle (i.e. between A and B), indicating that timing of measurements of LA dimensions is critical. Generally, LA dimensions should be assessed at the end of ventricular systole (A). (C) Right-parasternal short-axis view at the level of the aortic valve. This view is obtained by rotating the transducer 90° clockwise from a right-parasternal left-ventricular outflow tract view (Figure 22.3A). In this view, the aortic valve (AV) with its three cusps is visible in the center of the image. The surrounding structures include right atrium (RA), tricuspid valve, right ventricle (RV), right-ventricular outflow tract (RVOT), LA, and left atrial appendage (LAA). The apparent triangular separation (at the 12 o'clock position) evident between the non-coronary cusp (NCC) and the right coronary cusp (RCC) is a normal finding and does not represent an anomaly. In this view, the end-systolic size of the LA and LAA can be measured and compared to the aortic area. (D) Left-parasternal long-axis view of the LA, MV, and LV. The transducer is positioned in the fifth intercostal space slightly above the olecranon, oriented perpendicular to the chest wall and angled dorsally. This view has traditionally been used for assessment of LA dimensions. However, as opposed to the right-parasternal views (A,B), this view often does not allow imaging of the LA in its entirety due to interference with the ventral lung border. Nonetheless, imaging LA and MV from a left thoracic window provides additional information and should complement the right-parasternal views. LCC: left coronary cusp of the aortic valve; PV: pulmonary vein; TV: tricuspid valve. (Source: Part C – Bonagura, J.D., Reef, V.B., & Schwarzwald, C.C. (2010) [2]. Reproduced with permission of Elsevier.)

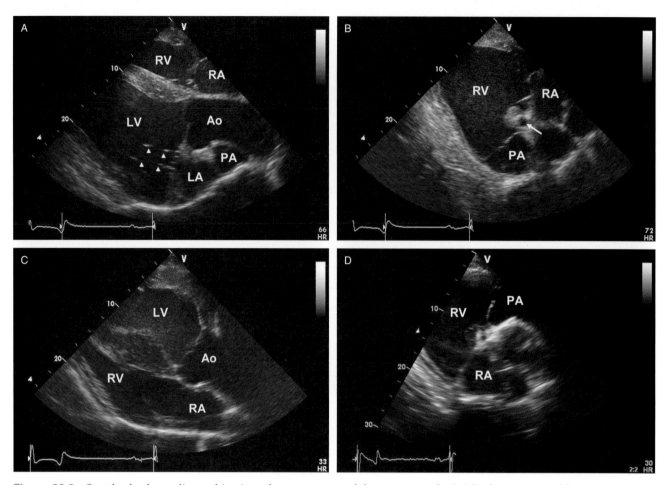

Figure 22.3   Standard echocardiographic views for assessment of the great vessels. (A) Right-parasternal long-axis view of the left ventricular outflow tract (LVOT). Starting from a four-chamber view (Figure 22.1A), the transducer is angled more cranially, tilted dorsally, and rotated to the 2 o'clock position to obtain this view. It is best suited to assess the structures, dimensions, and function of the aortic valve, the sinus of Valsalva, and the ascending aorta (Ao) and the pulmonary artery (PA). The diameter of the PA should be smaller than the diameter of the aorta. (B) Right-parasternal long-axis view of the right ventricular outflow tract (RVOT). Starting from a LVOT view (A), the transducer is angled more cranially to obtain this view; occasionally the transducer will have to be moved one intercostal space cranially. The right atrium (RA), the tricuspid valve, the right ventricle (RV), the RVOT, the pulmonic valve, the pulmonary artery (PA), and a cross-section through the right coronary artery (arrow) can be visualized. (C) Left-parasternal long-axis view of the LVOT. The transducer is positioned in the fifth or fourth intercostal space at a level slightly above the olecranon and angled slightly cranially. (D) Left-parasternal long-axis view of the RVOT. Starting from the LVOT view (C), the transducer is moved one intercostal space cranially to obtain this image. LA: left atrium; LV: left ventricle.

Figure 22.4   Mitral and aortic valve motion. (A) M-mode recording of mitral valve motion obtained from a right-parasternal short-axis view at the level of the mitral valve. The M-mode cursor (dotted line) is placed across the MV leaflets. The motion of the septal mitral leaflet and the time of mitral valve closure (MVC) and opening (MVO) can be identified on the M-mode tracing. The E wave (E) represents early-diastolic opening of the mitral valve during passive inflow of blood from the left atrium into the ventricle. The A wave (A) represents late-diastolic opening of the mitral valve during atrial contraction. The E point-to-septal separation (EPSS) can be increased, seen with aortic regurgitation (regurgitant jet impinging on the valve), LV dilation with left ventricular failure (reduced transmitral flow), or mitral stenosis/tethering (rare defects or acquired from endocarditis). (B) M-mode recording of aortic valve motion obtained from a right-parasternal short-axis view of the aorta. The M-mode cursor (dotted line) is placed across the aortic valve leaflets. Motion of the left-coronary cusp and the time of aortic valve opening (AVO) and aortic valve closure (AVC) can be identified. This view has traditionally been used for assessment of aortic size and left atrial dimensions, but has largely been replaced by two-dimensional methods (Figures 22.2, 22.3). Ao: aorta; LAA: left atrial appendage; RV: right ventricle; TV: tricuspid valve.

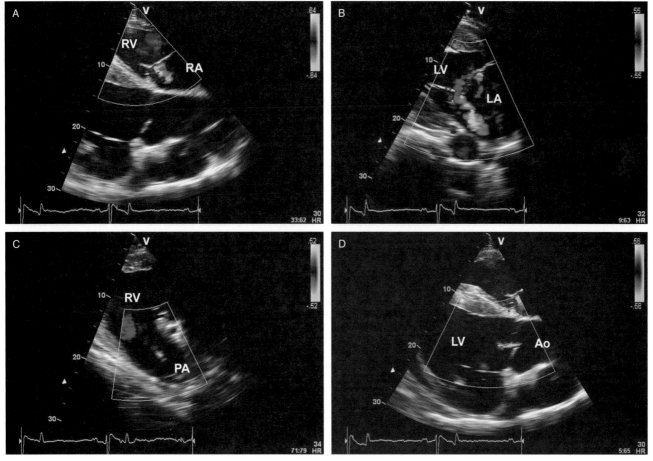

Figure 22.5 Color Doppler findings in apparently healthy horses. Color Doppler recordings obtained from an 8-year-old healthy Hanoverian Warmblood gelding in athletic condition (eventing). Blood flow towards the transducer is coded in red to yellow and flow away from the transducer is coded in shades of blue to cyan. Flow that is turbulent according to the system algorithm is colored in green. Traces of valvular regurgitation are frequently found on echocardiograms of healthy horses with normal exercise capacity, often even in absence of an audible murmur. Many of these small regurgitant jets are evident only in distinct imaging planes and most are not considered clinically relevant. (A) Right-parasternal left ventricular outflow tract view. The region of interest (ROI) is positioned over the tricuspid valve. Trivial tricuspid regurgitation is evident in the right atrium (RA) during systole, color-coded in blue, cyan, and green. (B) Left-parasternal long-axis view with the ROI positioned over the mitral valve. Mild mitral regurgitation is evident in the left atrium (LA) during systole. Two distinct regurgitant jets (color-coded in blue, cyan, and green) are seen: a small jet originating from the parietal leaflet and a larger jet stemming from the septal leaflet. (C) Right-parasternal right ventricular outflow tract (RVOT) view. The ROI is positioned over the pulmonic valve. Trivial, low-velocity pulmonic insufficiency (color-coded in red) is evident in the RVOT during diastole. (D) Right-parasternal left ventricular outflow tract view. The ROI is positioned over the aortic valve. A trace of aortic insufficiency (color-coded in green) can be seen in the left ventricle (LV) at end-diastole, immediately before opening of the aortic valve. Ao: aorta; PA: pulmonary artery; RV: right ventricle.

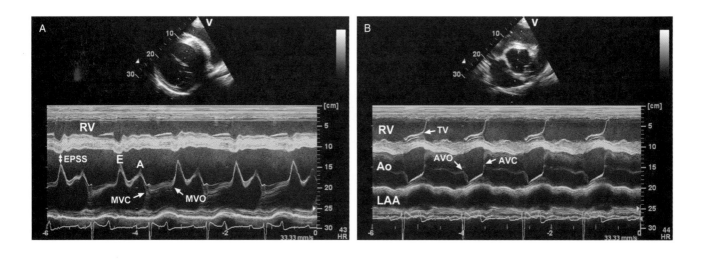

convention, the structures nearest to the transducer are displayed at the top of the screen. The dorsal (in the long-axis views) and cranial (in the short-axis views) structures of the heart are displayed to the right side of the screen.

INDICATIONS AND CLINICAL USE OF ECHOCARDIOGRAPHY IN HORSES

Echocardiography can be used to identify cardiac disorders, assess hemodynamic and structural consequences of disease, and monitor response to treatment and progression of disease (Figures 22.6, 22.7, 22.8, 22.9, 22.10, 22.11, 22.12, 22.13, 22.14, 22.15, 22.16, 22.17, 22.18, 22.19, 22.20, 22.21, 22.22, 22.23, 22.24, 22.25, 22.26, 22.27, 22.28). Echocardiography is indicated in horses with heart murmurs to differentiate physiologic flow murmurs from pathologic murmurs and assess their clinical relevance; to detect underlying cardiac disease in horses with cardiac dysrhythmias; to diagnose or rule out cardiac disease in horses with exercise intolerance, poor performance, collapse, or episodic

weakness; to screen for endocarditis or pericarditis in horses with fever of unknown origin; to diagnose or rule out pericardial disease in horses with muffled heart sounds; to diagnose the cause of persistent tachycardia (e.g. because of severe myocardial disease); to detect pulmonary hypertension in horses with severe respiratory disease; to diagnose suspected congenital cardiac defects in foals; and to determine the cause of heart failure and monitor progression and response to treatment in horses with signs of congestive heart failure.

Assessment of Chamber Dimensions

One of the main goals of echocardiography is detection of cardiac chamber dilation or hypertrophy and grading of the enlargement, if present, as mild, moderate, or severe. Left atrial (LA) and left ventricular (LV) dimensions can be quantified using linear measurements, area measurements, or volumetric estimates that are based on two-dimensional echocardiography (2DE) and M-mode echocardiography (Figures 22.1, 22.2) [3,7,10,11,16,17]. In horses, assessment of LA size has traditionally been limited to subjective evaluation and measurement of the LA diameter from a

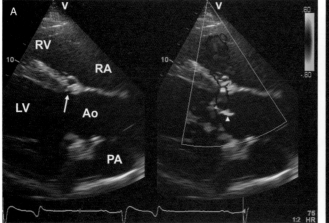 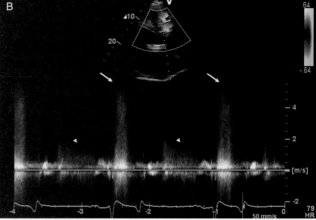

Figure 22.6 Restrictive ventricular septal defect. (A) Right-parasternal long-axis view of the left ventricular outflow tract obtained from a 3-year-old Friesian filly with a restrictive paramembranous ventricular septal defect. The small defect (arrow) can easily be missed on the grayscale image (left). Color flow mapping facilitates identification of the defect and clearly shows trans-septal blood flow (right). Notice the classic color aliasing pattern in which flow changes from dark red, to yellow, to blue, and finally to a green turbulent encoding. A small aortic regurgitant jet is seen as well (arrowhead). The size of the pulmonary artery (PA) relative to the aorta (Ao) appears normal and does not suggest significant pulmonary hypertension. (B) Long-axis echocardiogram and corresponding continuous wave Doppler recording indicating left-to-right shunt flow through the ventricular septal defect. The peak systolic velocity (arrows) is 5.95 m/s, corresponding to a high (normal) left-to-right pressure gradient of 142 mmHg (modified Bernoulli equation: $dp = 4 \times v_{max}^2$). The diastolic flow component (arrowheads) corresponds to aortic regurgitant flow or diastolic shunt flow. LV: left ventricle; RA: right atrium; RV: right ventricle. (Source: Bonagura, J.D., Reef, V.B., & Schwarzwald, C.C. (2010) [2]. Reproduced with permission of Elsevier.)

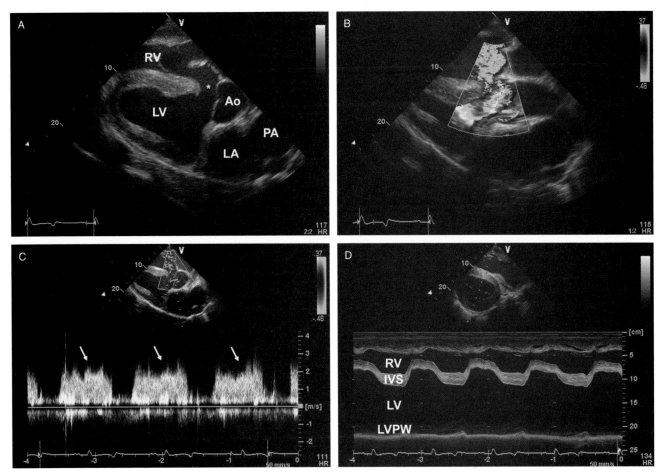

Figure 22.7 Non-restrictive ventricular septal defect. (A) Right-parasternal long-axis view obtained from a 1-year-old Paint filly with a non-restrictive paramembranous ventricular septal defect. Obvious malalignment occurs from the aortic root to the ventricular septum, characterized by over-riding or straddling of the root over the defect. The large defect, with an estimated size of 3.6 cm, is evident immediately below the aortic valve (*). The pulmonary artery (PA) appears enlarged compared to the aorta (Ao), indicating increased transpulmonary flow due to left-to-right shunting or pulmonary hypertension. (B) Color Doppler echocardiogram in a right-parasternal long-axis view indicates systolic flow through the defect. Notice the region of proximal flow convergence in the left ventricular outflow tract, characterized by acceleration of blood flow leading to aliasing (sudden color change from yellow to blue), and the turbulent flow in the right ventricle, color-coded in green. (C) Long-axis echocardiogram and corresponding continuous wave Doppler recording indicating left-to-right shunt flow through the ventricular septal defect (arrows). The peak systolic velocity is 2.6 m/s, corresponding to a (very low) left-to-right pressure gradient of 27 mmHg. Flow is detected during systole and from mid-diastole to end-diastole. The lack of significant flow during early diastole is either due to translational motion of the heart, causing the defect to move out of the cursor line, transient equilibration of early-diastolic ventricular pressures, or cyclical obstruction or diversion of flow by the prolapsing tricuspid valve. (D) Short-axis echocardiogram and corresponding M-mode recording of the left ventricle (LV). The large end-diastolic LV diameter and the hyperkinetic motion of the interventricular septum (IVS) indicate left ventricular volume overload. The fractional shortening of the left ventricle is 39%, indicating that the systolic function of the left ventricle is preserved. LA: left atrium; LVPW: left ventricular peripheral wall; RV: right ventricle. (Source: Parts A, C and D – Bonagura, J.D., Reef, V.B., & Schwarzwald, C.C. (2010) [2]. Reproduced with permission of Elsevier.)

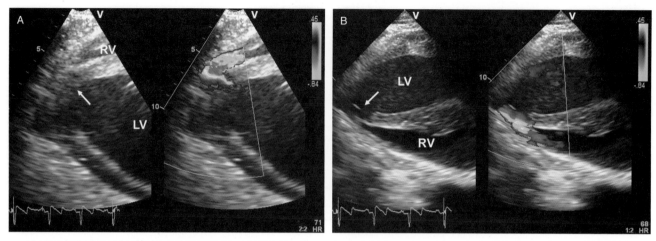

Figure 22.8 Apical muscular ventricular septal defect. Right- (A) and left- (B) parasternal long-axis view of the left (LV) and right ventricle (RV) in a 4-month-old Thoroughbred colt presented with a right-sided grade 3/6 holosystolic apical murmur that had been detected as an incidental finding. The image plane is focused on the apical part of the interventricular septum. In B-mode (A,B: left), a hypoechoic area in the septum (arrows) suggests the presence of a muscular ventricular septal defect. Color Doppler imaging (A,B: right) allowed confirmation of the presence of a defect. Notice the region of proximal flow convergence in the LV (A), characterized by acceleration of blood flow leading to aliasing (sudden color change from yellow to blue). Turbulent flow in the RV is color-coded in green. Post-mortem examination 1 year after the initial examination (for reasons other than the cardiac malformation) revealed severe chronic endocardial fibrosis and complete closure of the ventricular septal defect.

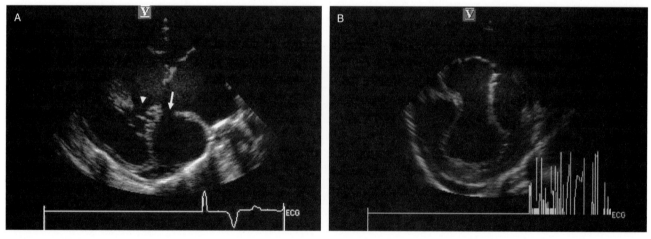

Figure 22.9 Endocardial cushion defect. (A) Right-parasternal four-chamber view obtained from a 4-month-old Morgan colt with a complete endocardial cushion defect. The primum atrial septal defect is evident in the ventral atrial septum (arrow) and an inlet ventricular septal defect component (arrowhead) is observed below the common atrioventricular valve. (B) Right-parasternal short-axis view at the level of the common atrioventricular valve. The ECG electrodes were displaced resulting in the artifact to the right. (Source: Bonagura, J.D., Reef, V.B., & Schwarzwald, C.C. (2010) [2]. Reproduced with permission of Elsevier.)

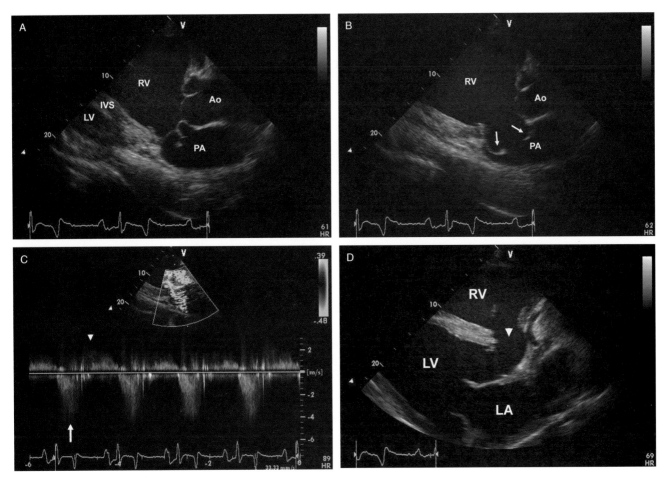

Figure 22.10 Double-outlet right ventricle and endocardial cushion defect. (A) Off-angled right-parasternal long-axis view obtained from a 2-year-old Quarterhorse colt with complex congenital heart disease including double-outlet right ventricle, large atrioventricular septal defect, malformed atrioventricular valves, and valvular pulmonic and aortic stenoses. Both great vessels originate from the right ventricle (RV) and can be displayed side-by-side, typical of double-outlet and/or transposed great vessels. (B) Pulmonary and aortic valvular stenosis related to valvular dysplasia, thickening, and fusion of the leaflets. Doming of the pulmonic valves is visible during systole (arrows). (C) Continuous wave Doppler recording of pulmonic outflow (arrow) and pulmonic regurgitation (arrowhead). The peak systolic outflow velocity is 4.6 m/s (corresponding to a pressure gradient of 85 mmHg), indicating pulmonary valvular stenosis of moderate severity. (D) Right-parasternal four-chamber view. The left ventricle (LV) communicates with the RV across a large atrioventricular septal defect (arrowhead). Ao: aorta; IVS: interventricular septum; LA: left atrium; PA: pulmonary artery. (Source: Bonagura, J.D., Reef, V.B., & Schwarzwald, C.C. (2010) [2]. Reproduced with permission of Elsevier.)

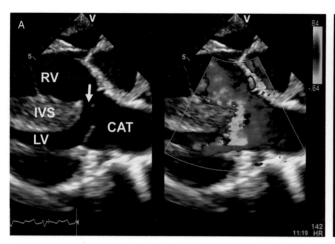
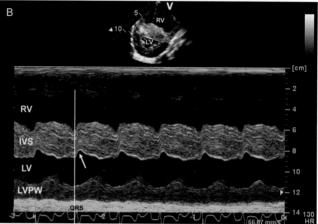

Figure 22.11 Common arterial trunk. (A) B-mode (left) and color Doppler (right) echocardiogram in a right-parasternal long-axis view obtained from a 15-day-old Friesian filly with a common arterial trunk (CAT). Only one great vessel is evident over-riding a ventricular septal defect (arrow) and communicating with both ventricles. (B) M-mode echocardiogram in a right-parasternal short-axis view. The right ventricle (RV) is dilated and hypertrophied, indicating volume and pressure overload. The left ventricle (LV) appears small and its wall is hypertrophied. Notice the flat motion of the interventricular septum (IVS) with early-systolic paradoxical motion (arrow). The vertical line indicates the begin of systole (i.e. the onset of the QRS complex). The LV fractional shortening is low at 26%. LVPW: left ventricular peripheral wall. (Source: Bonagura, J.D., Reef, V.B., & Schwarzwald, C.C. (2010) [2]. Reproduced with permission of Elsevier.)

left-parasternal long-axis view (Figure 22.2D). However, with contemporary echocardiographic systems, right-parasternal long-axis and short-axis views (Figure 22.2A–C) are preferred since they allow visualization of the LA in its entirety and provide sufficient anatomic landmarks for consistent and reliable measurement of LA dimensions.

Objective quantification of the right atrial (RA) and right ventricular (RV) dimensions is difficult, because the geometric shape of the right heart is complex and the internal dimensions of the RA and RV cavities largely depend on transducer placement and imaging plane. Subjective assessment of the right heart chambers in multiple imaging planes is, therefore, important.

Assessment of Systolic Left Ventricular Function

The echocardiographic detection of myocardial failure and deterioration of systolic function has great prognostic implications. Most of the indices used in clinical practice serve to evaluate global systolic LV function. Echocardiographic indices of systolic ventricular function generally do not reflect contractility, but are, to a variable extent, influenced by preload, afterload, heart rate, and rhythm [3,9]. The two-dimensional ejection phase indices are based on measurements of LV dimen-

sions. Left ventricular ejection fraction (EF% = SV/LVEDV × 100; where SV is stroke volume and LVEDV is LV end-diastolic volume) is based on geometrical estimates of LV volumes and has traditionally been the standard index of LV systolic function. The LV fractional shortening (FS% = [LVIDd–LVIDs]/LVIDd × 100; where LVIDd and LVIDs are the LV internal short-axis diameters at end-diastole and at peak systole, respectively), is an approximation of the EF% and is the most commonly used index of LV systolic function in horses. In fact, LV fractional shortening is often the only index used in routine echocardiography because it can be easily calculated from M-mode recordings (Figure 22.1C,D) [3,9,10,18].

Newer echocardiographic methods, including tissue Doppler imaging and 2D speckle tracking (Figure 22.24), allow quantitative assessment of myocardial wall motion velocity, strain (i.e. myocardial deformation), and strain rate (i.e. myocardial deformation rate), and provide additional options for assessment of regional and global ventricular function [4–8,19]. However, further studies are required to investigate their potential clinical utility. To date, whether TDI and 2DST offer substantial advantages over the conventional methods for assessment of systolic ventricular function in horses undergoing routine echocardiographic examination is uncertain.

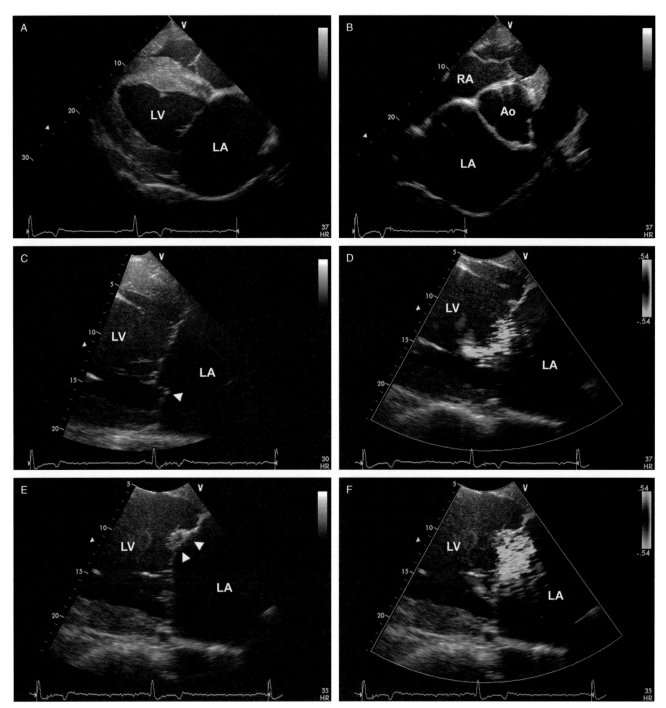

Figure 22.12 Mitral regurgitation. (A) Right-parasternal four-chamber view obtained from a horse with mitral regurgitation. The left atrium (LA) appears markedly enlarged and has a rounded appearance, indicating severe volume overload. (B) Right-parasternal short-axis view at the level of the aorta (Ao) and the left atrium (LA). The LA appears markedly enlarged. (C) Left-parasternal long-axis view. The septal (anterior) mitral valve leaflet is prolapsing into the LA during systole (arrowhead). (D) Color Doppler imaging in the same imaging plane as shown in C indicates turbulent blood flow within the LA (color-coded in green) during systole, consistent with mitral regurgitation. (E) Left-parasternal long-axis view in an imaging plane that is only slightly different from the one shown in C. Nodular thickening of the parietal (posterior) mitral valve leaflet is now visible (arrowheads). (F) Color Doppler imaging in the same plane as shown in E indicates turbulent blood flow within the LA (color-coded in green) during systole. Notice the slightly different appearance of the area of turbulent flow compared to D. Quantification of regurgitation by assessing the area of regurgitant flow within the receiving chamber (i.e. the LA) is problematic, because the Doppler-derived flow signal is largely influenced by imaging plane and direction of flow, gain settings, orifice size and shape, driving pressure, and receiving chamber characteristics. LV: left ventricle; RA: right atrium. (Source: Parts C, D, E and F – Bonagura, J.D., Reef, V.B., & Schwarzwald, C.C. (2010) [2]. Reproduced with permission of Elsevier.)

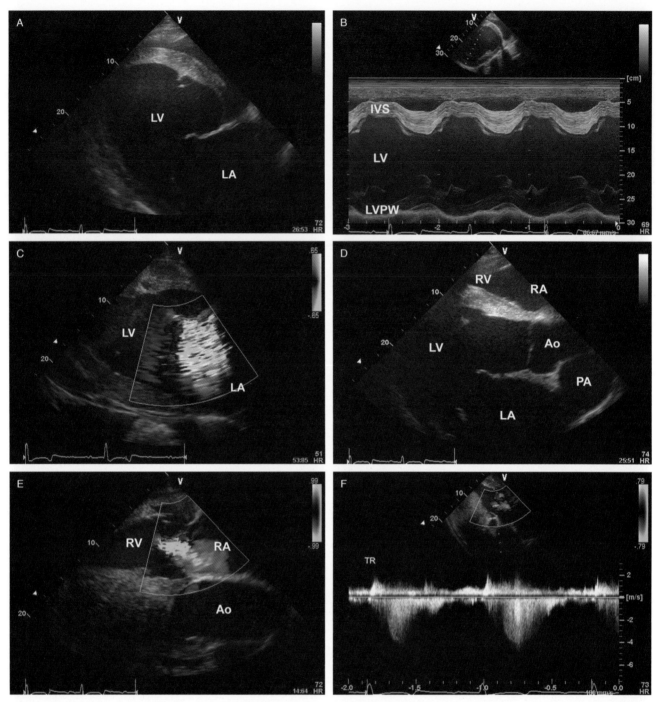

Figure 22.13 Mitral regurgitation and left-sided congestive heart failure. Echocardiogram obtained from a 3-year-old female Standardbred with mitral regurgitation and left-sided congestive heart failure. (A) Right-parasternal long-axis four-chamber view. The left atrium (LA) and the left ventricle (LV) are severely dilated. The right heart appears small. (B) M-mode echocardiogram of the LV in a right-parasternal short-axis view demonstrating LV enlargement and hyperdynamic motion of the interventricular septum (IVS). The LV fractional shortening was 39%. (C) Color Doppler echocardiogram in a left-parasternal long-axis view focused on the mitral valve. A large area of turbulent blood flow (color-coded in yellow and green) is visible during systole in the LA, consistent with mitral regurgitation. (D) Echocardiogram in a right-parasternal long-axis view. The LA and the LV are severely dilated. The pulmonary artery (PA) appears enlarged compared to the aorta (Ao), strongly suggesting pulmonary hypertension secondary to severe mitral regurgitation. (E) Color Doppler echocardiogram in a right-parasternal long-axis view focused on the tricuspid valve. An area of turbulent blood flow (color-coded in green) is visible during systole in the right atrium (RA), consistent with tricuspid regurgitation. (F) Continuous wave Doppler recording of the tricuspid regurgitant jet in a tilted right-parasternal long-axis view. A high-velocity flow pattern is visible during systole. The peak velocity is 4.5 m/s, corresponding to a maximum systolic pressure gradient across the tricuspid valve of 81 mmHg (modified Bernoulli equation: $dp = 4 \times v_{max}^2$). Therefore, the estimated systolic pulmonary artery pressure (assuming a right atrial pressure of 5 mmHg) would be 86 mmHg, indicating pulmonary hypertension secondary to severe mitral regurgitation. Notice that malalignment of the Doppler beam with blood flow may lead to underestimation of peak velocities and pressure gradients. LVPW: left ventricular peripheral wall; RV: right ventricle. (Source: Parts B, D and F – Bonagura, J.D., Reef, V.B., & Schwarzwald, C.C. (2010) [2]. Reproduced with permission of Elsevier.)

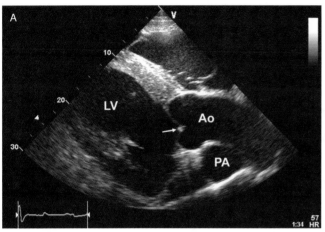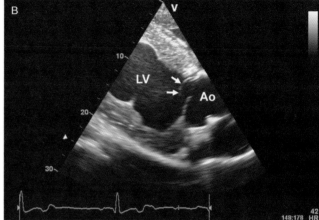

Figure 22.14 Aortic valve lesions. (A) Right-parasternal long-axis view obtained from a 15-year-old Thoroughbred gelding with aortic regurgitation. Nodular thickening of the aortic valve cusps is evident (arrow). (B) Right-parasternal long-axis view obtained from a 12-year-old Arabian gelding with aortic regurgitation. Aortic valve prolapse is evident (arrows). Ao: aorta; LV: left ventricle; PA: pulmonary artery. (Source: Bonagura, J.D., Reef, V.B., & Schwarzwald, C.C. (2010) [2]. Reproduced with permission of Elsevier.)

Assessment of Diastolic Left Ventricular Function

Diastolic ventricular dysfunction may play a role in pericardial and myocardial disease in horses. However, the clinical relevance of diastolic dysfunction in other types of cardiac disease is not clear. Doppler-derived transmitral flow velocities and tissue Doppler analyses of mitral annular or myocardial velocities are commonly used in humans and small animals for assessment of diastolic LV function and filling pressures [3,9]. Transmitral flow velocity profiles can be recorded by PW Doppler, but optimal alignment with blood flow and consistent placement of the sample volume relative to the mitral valve are very difficult in adult horses. Therefore, transmitral flow velocity measurements in horses are relatively unreliable and may not be suitable to detect minor changes in diastolic LV function [16,17,20]. Conversely, TDI indices of LV wall motion are easier to obtain than transmitral flow velocity measurements and can be helpful for assessment of LV diastolic function in horses (Figure 22.24) [5,21].

Assessment of Left Atrial Function

Currently, LA function is rarely considered during routine echocardiography and the clinical relevance of LA dysfunction is not well known in horses. However, LA function is impaired in horses with atrial fibrillation (AF) and may also be altered in horses suffering from mitral regurgitation or other cardiac disease. Per-

sistent LA contractile dysfunction can be detected in horses after conversion from AF to sinus rhythm, likely attributed to AF-induced atrial remodeling [17,22]. LA size and LA mechanical function can easily be assessed in horses by use of 2DE variables, including LA area and LA fractional area changes (Figure 22.2) [16].

Hemodynamic Assessment

The hemodynamic load placed on the heart by cardiac disorders can be estimated by combining echocardiographic information on chamber size, myocardial motion, LV systolic and diastolic function, and intracardiac blood flow. Doppler studies can be used to assess intracardiac pressures and pressure gradients. Normal pressure gradients driving blood flow through heart, valves, and large vessels range from 0.25–1.5 meters per second (m/s). Abnormally high velocities can be found in many cardiac conditions, including ventricular septal defects and valvular regurgitations, in which pressure gradients drive blood across a restrictive orifice (Figures 22.6, 22.7, 22.10, 22.13, 22.15, 22.17, 22.18, 22.19, 22.28). The pressure gradients are either reflections of normal intracardiac pressures or consequences of pathologically increased pressures. Pressure gradients can be estimated using Doppler echocardiography by employing the simplified Bernoulli equation ($dp = 4 \times v_{max}^2$; where dp is the pressure gradient in mmHg and v_{max} is the peak velocity in m/s). The main indications to measure pressure gradients in horses are the diagnosis of pulmonary

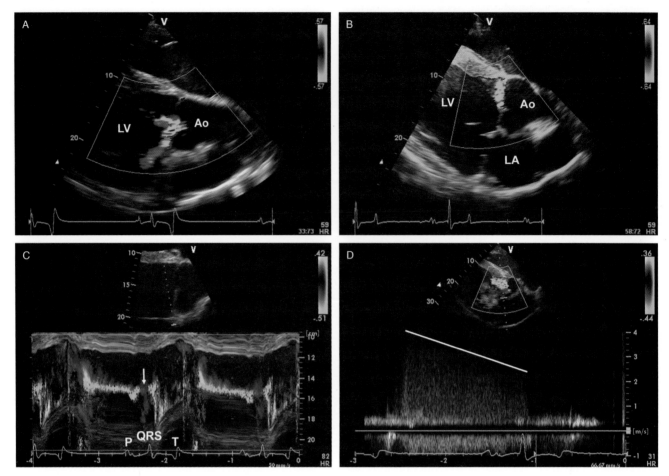

Figure 22.15 Aortic regurgitation. (A) Color Doppler echocardiogram in a right-parasternal long-axis view obtained from a 13-year-old Warmblood mare with aortic regurgitation. The diastolic regurgitant jet is visible as a small area of turbulent flow (color-coded in green) at the coaptation points of the valve leaflets. The image has the appearance of two jets: a central jet and an eccentric jet directed towards the mitral valve. Based on receiving chamber analysis, the severity of the regurgitation would be graded as mild. (B) Color Doppler echocardiogram in a right-parasternal long-axis view obtained from a 15-year-old Warmblood mare with aortic regurgitation. The diastolic regurgitant jet is visible as an area of turbulent flow (color-coded in green) that appears to be directed towards the interventricular septum. Based on receiving chamber analysis, the severity of the regurgitation would be graded as mild. (C) Color M-mode echocardiogram in a right-parasternal long-axis view obtained from a horse with aortic regurgitation. The cursor line is placed immediately below the aortic valve (top). An ECG is recorded simultaneously for timing. This imaging mode is particularly useful for timing of flow events and identifying brief regurgitant signals or normal valve closure noise. In this case, an aortic regurgitant jet is visible as a turbulent flow pattern (color-coded in green), starting at the beginning of diastole (i.e. after the T wave) and ending at the onset of systole (i.e. immediately after the QRS complex). Notice the absence of turbulent flow during the PQ interval (arrow). This can be explained by a change in left ventricular pressure occurring after atrial contraction or a reorientation of the regurgitant jet relative to the cursor owing to translational movement of the heart. (D) Continuous wave Doppler recording of a diastolic aortic regurgitant jet from a right-parasternal long-axis view. The absolute velocities are not accurate in this recording because of lack of adequate alignment with blood flow. However, this recording can be used for timing of flow events (an ECG is recorded simultaneously for timing). Furthermore, the change in jet velocity (which can be expressed as "pressure half-time") reflects the rate of decline in pressure gradient between the aorta and the left ventricle and may be useful to assess the severity of regurgitation as long as ventricular relaxation is normal; a relatively flat or gradual slope of the velocity envelope (white line) indicates mild aortic regurgitation (AR), a steep slope indicates severe AR. Ao: aorta; LA: left atrium; LV: left ventricle; PA: pulmonary artery. (Source: Parts C and D – Bonagura, J.D., Reef, V.B., & Schwarzwald, C.C. (2010) [2]. Reproduced with permission of Elsevier.)

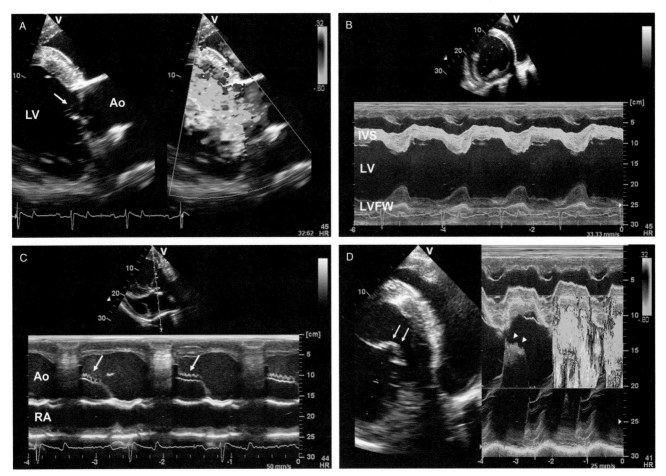

Figure 22.16 Aortic regurgitation. Echocardiogram of a 21-year-old Hanoverian Warmblood gelding with severe aortic regurgitation and left ventricular volume overload. (A) B-mode (left) and color Doppler (right) echocardiogram of the left ventricular outflow tract in a right-parasternal long-axis view. The aortic valve cusps are irregularly thickened and aortic valve prolapse is evident during diastole (arrow). A large regurgitant jet is visible in the left ventricular outflow tract during diastole (green). (B) M-mode echocardiogram of the left ventricle (LV) in a right-parasternal short-axis view demonstrating LV enlargement and hyperdynamic motion of the interventricular septum (IVS). The LV fractional shortening was 46%. (C) M-mode echocardiogram of the aortic valve in a left-parasternal long-axis view. Notice the high-frequency vibrations of the aortic cusp during diastole (arrows) caused by the regurgitant blood flow. (D) Two-dimensional (left), M-mode (middle) and color M-mode (right) echocardiogram of the mitral valve in a right-parasternal short-axis view. Notice the prolapse (arrows) and the high-frequency vibrations (arrowheads) of the septal leaflet of the mitral valve, caused by rapid, turbulent regurgitant flow in the left ventricular outflow tract during diastole (color-coded in green). Ao: aorta; LVFW: left ventricular free wall; RA: right atrium.

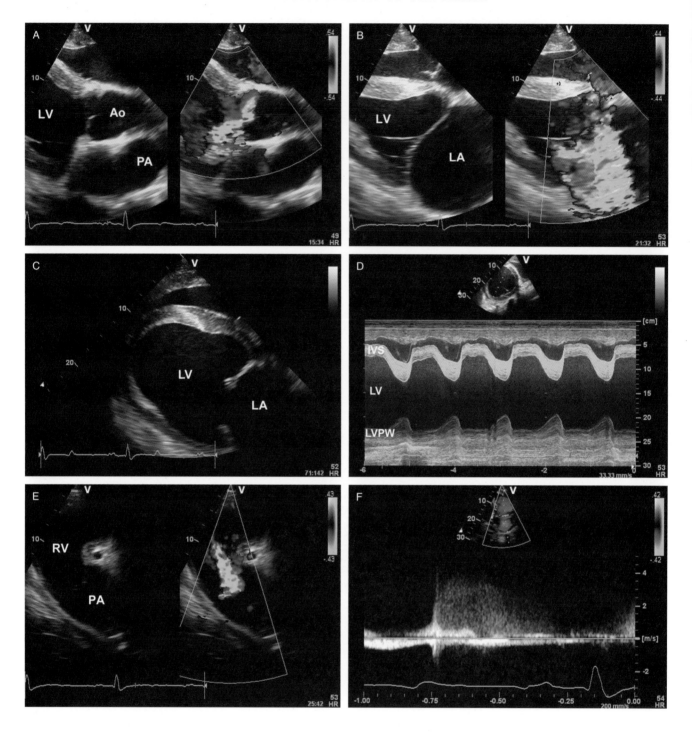

Figure 22.17 Aortic regurgitation, mitral regurgitation, and pulmonary hypertension. Echocardiogram of a 7-year old West-phalian Warmblood mare with severe aortic and mitral regurgitation. (A) Right-parasternal view of the left ventricular outflow tract. A B-mode image (left) and a color flow Doppler image (right) are displayed side by side. The aortic cusps are slightly thickened. An eccentric aortic regurgitant jet (color-coded in green) is seen during diastole, directed towards the septal mitral valve leaflet. Notice the prominent appearance of the pulmonary artery (PA) compared to the aortic root (Ao), suggesting increased pulmonary artery pressures. (B) Right-parasternal four-chamber view, focused on the left atrium (LA) and the mitral valve. A B-mode image (left) and a color flow Doppler image (right) are displayed side by side. A large mitral regurgitant jet (color-coded in green) is seen in the LA during systole. The LA appears rounded and severely enlarged. (C) Right-parasternal four-chamber view, focused on the left ventricle (LV). The LV is enlarged and has a rounded appearance, indicating LV volume overload. (D) Short-axis echocardiogram and corresponding M-mode recording of the LV. The large end-diastolic LV diameter and the hyperkinetic motion of the interventricular septum (IVS) indicate severe LV volume overload. The fractional shorten-ing of the left ventricle is 53%, indicating preserved LV systolic function in the presence of an increase in preload (due to volume overload) and a decrease in afterload (due to mitral regurgitation). (E) Right-parasternal view of the right ventricular outflow tract. A B-mode image (left) and a color flow Doppler image (right) are displayed side by side. Color flow mapping shows a pulmonic regurgitant jet during diastole (color-coded in green). (F) Spectral Doppler recording of the pulmonic regurgitant jet. The maximum diastolic velocity of the regurgitant jet is 3.7 m/s, corresponding to a pressure gradient of 55 mmHg (modified Bernoulli equation: $dp = 4 \times v_{max}^2$). Therefore, the estimated mean pulmonary artery pressure (assuming a right atrial pressure of 5 mmHg) would be 60 mmHg, indicating pulmonary hypertension. LVPW: left ventricular peripheral wall; RV: right ventricle. (Source: Parts D and F – Bonagura, J.D., Reef, V.B., & Schwarzwald, C.C. (2010) [2]. Reproduced with permission of Elsevier.)

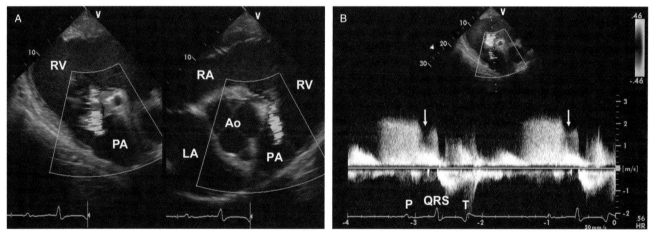

Figure 22.18 Pulmonic insufficiency. (A) Right-parasternal long-axis view of the right ventricular outflow tract (left) and right-parasternal short-axis view at the level of the aortic and pulmonic valve (right). Color Doppler imaging shows diastolic turbulent blood flow within the right ventricular outflow tract (color-coded in green), consistent with pulmonic insufficiency. Pulmonic insufficiency rarely is clinically relevant, but it can be used to estimate mean and diastolic pulmonary artery pres-sures by spectral Doppler. (B) Continuous wave Doppler recording of a pulmonic regurgitation jet in a right-parasternal long-axis view of the right ventricular outflow tract, showing mid- to end-diastolic regurgitant flow. The maximum velocity is approximately 2.35 m/s, corresponding to a transvalvular pressure gradient of 22 mmHg (modified Bernoulli equation: $dp = 4 \times v_{max}^2$). The end-diastolic velocity is approximately 1.75 m/s, corresponding to a transvalvular pressure gradient of 12 mmHg. Therefore, the estimated mean and diastolic pulmonary artery pressures (assuming a right atrial pressure of 5 mmHg) would be 27 and 17 mmHg, which is within normal limits for horses. Notice the sudden decrease in jet velocity during the PQ interval (arrows), which can be explained by a temporary reduction of regurgitant flow caused by a sudden rise in right ventricular pressure occurring after atrial contraction or by transient reorientation of the regurgitant jet relative to the cursor line. Ao: aorta; LA: left atrium; PA: pulmonary artery; RA: right atrium; RV: right ventricle. (Source: Part B – Bonagura, J.D., Reef, V.B., & Schwarzwald, C.C. (2010) [2]. Reproduced with permission of Elsevier.)

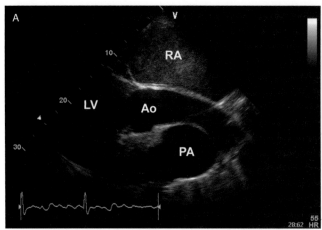
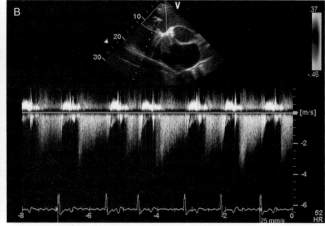

Figure 22.19 Pulmonic insufficiency and pulmonary hypertension. (A) Right-parasternal view of the left ventricular outflow tract obtained from an 11-year-old Paint gelding with severe mitral regurgitation, atrial fibrillation, and left-sided congestive heart failure. Enlargement of the right atrium (RA) and severe pulmonary artery (PA) dilation are evident, consistent with pulmonary hypertension. Notice also the marked spontaneous echo contrast (SEC) in the right atrium. Although some degree of SEC is considered normal in horses, this amount of SEC is unusual. The exact cause of SEC is unknown, but it may be associated with low flow states, systemic inflammation, or abnormal coagulation. (B) Continuous wave Doppler recording of pulmonic insufficiency in a left-parasternal long-axis view of the right ventricular outflow tract, showing diastolic regurgitant flow. The varying peak velocities can be explained by differences in cycle lengths (due to atrial fibrillation), motion of the heart (and the regurgitant jet) relative to the cursor line, and possibly respiratory variations. The highest maximum early-diastolic velocity in this spectral Doppler recording was 4 m/s, corresponding to a transvalvular pressure gradient of 64 mmHg (modified Bernoulli equation: dp = $4 \times v_{max}^2$). Assuming a right atrial pressure of 5 mmHg, the estimated mean pulmonary artery pressure (MPAP) would be at least 69 mmHg, indicating marked pulmonary hypertension. Ao: aorta; LV: left ventricle. (Source: Bonagura, J.D., Reef, V.B., & Schwarzwald, C.C. (2010) [2]. Reproduced with permission of Elsevier.)

hypertension by interrogation of regurgitant flow at the tricuspid valve and the pulmonic valve (Figures 22.10, 22.13, 22.17, 22.18, 22.19) and the assessment of ventricular septal defects by interrogation of shunt flow (Figures 22.6, 22.7). Parallel alignment with blood flow is crucial because excessive angle of interrogation (i.e. >20°) will lead to an underestimation of flow velocities and pressure gradients.

Assessment of Valvular Regurgitation

The Doppler technology of current echocardiographic systems is very sensitive to detect valvular regurgitation and care must be taken not to overinterpret the echo findings, particularly in otherwise healthy animals without abnormal clinical findings and in the absence of heart murmurs. Assessment of valvular regurgitation should be achieved using an integrated qualitative and quantitative approach, combining clinical examination (including auscultation of a typical murmur) and echocardiographic findings. Measurement of cardiac chamber dimensions provides information on the hemodynamic relevance of chronic valvular regurgitation. Abnormal timing and direction of transvalvular flow, as well as flow turbulences, can be detected by 2D color Doppler, color M-mode, and spectral Doppler echocardiography. The regurgitant signal in the "receiving chamber" can be interrogated in multiple imaging planes to identify origin, extent, timing, and duration of the regurgitation. However, color Doppler echocardiography describes blood flow direction and velocity, but not absolute volumetric flow. The Doppler-derived regurgitant signal is largely influenced by gain settings, direction of flow, orifice size and shape, driving pressure, and characteristics of the receiving chamber. Quantification of regurgitation by assessing signal strength of the spectral Doppler regurgitant signal or measuring the area of regurgitation within the receiving chamber is therefore neither very accurate nor reliable.

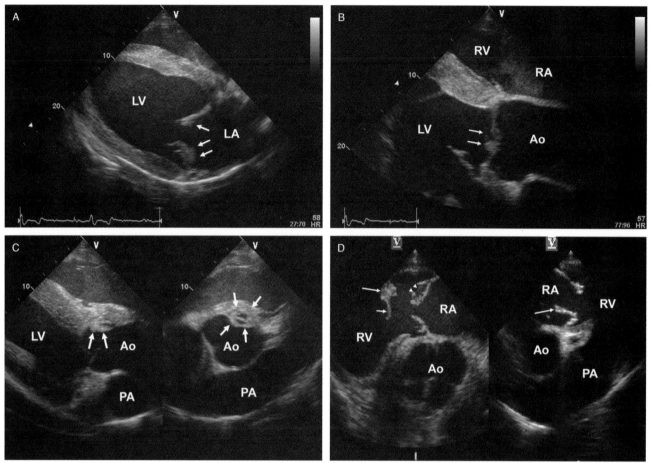

Figure 22.20 Infective endocarditis. (A) Echocardiogram in a right-parasternal four-chamber view. The mitral valve leaflets appear thickened. Echogenic masses are evident, attached to the atrial surface of the mitral valve leaflets (arrows). Focal lesions of endocarditis are typically on the valvular surface facing into the direction of blood flow. (B) Right-parasternal view of the left ventricular outflow tract obtained from a 10-year-old Quarterhorse gelding with bacterial endocarditis. The cusps of the aortic valve appear thickened. Echogenic masses are attached to the free edges of the cusps (arrows). (C) Right-parasternal view of the aortic valve in long-axis (left) and short-axis (right) obtained from a 3-year-old female horse with bacterial endocarditis and aortic root abscess resulting in marked thickening of the aortic wall and periaortic tissues. A vegetative lesion is seen within the sinus of Valsalva (arrows). In short-axis view, the lesion appears as an echogenic, demarcated, loculated mass that is located between the non-coronary and the right-coronary cusp, possibly involving the atrial septum. (D) Echocardiogram obtained from a 6-year-old Quarterhorse mare with severe pleuropneumonia, endocarditis, and tricuspid chordal rupture. In a right-parasternal long-axis view (left), the ruptured chord (short arrow) is visible within the right ventricle (RV). Vegetations are visible at the papillary muscle (long arrow) and at the tricuspid valve leaflet (arrowheads). In short-axis view (right), a flail leaflet (arrow) is visible within the right atrium (RA) during systole. The prominent appearance of the pulmonary artery (PA) compared to the aorta (Ao) is suggestive of pulmonary hypertension. LA: left atrium; LV: left ventricle. (Source: Parts C and D – Bonagura, J.D., Reef, V.B., & Schwarzwald, C.C. (2010) [2]. Reproduced with permission of Elsevier.)

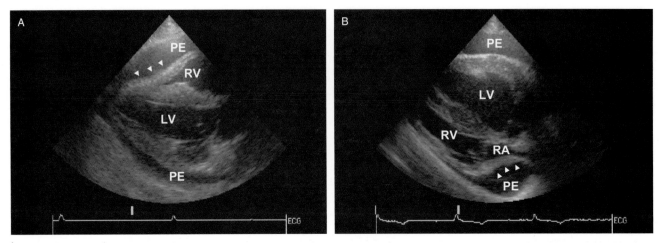

Figure 22.21 Pericardial effusion and cardiac tamponade. (A) Right-parasternal long-axis recording obtained from a horse with pericardial effusion and cardiac tamponade. The heart is surrounded by the anechoic effusion (PE). Right ventricular (RV) collapse is evident (arrowheads). (B) Left-parasternal long-axis recording. Right atrial (RA) collapse becomes obvious in this view (arrowheads), indicating hemodynamically relevant effusion and cardiac tamponade. LV: left ventricle. (Source: Images courtesy of Dr John D Bonagura.)

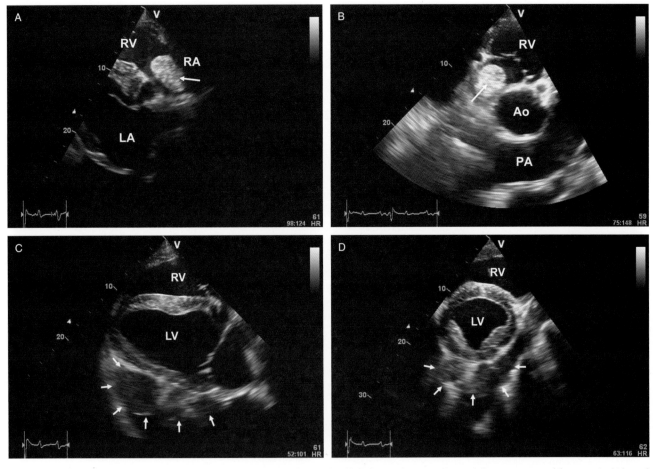

Figure 22.22 Mass lesions in right atrium and pericardium. (A,B) Echocardiogram in a right-parasternal long-axis (A) and short-axis (B) view recorded from a 23-year-old, 380 kg pony gelding with metastasizing adenocarcinoma. A hyperechoic, well demarcated mass (arrow) is visible within the right atrium (RA). In necropsy, this mass was confirmed to be a thrombus containing neoplastic cells, extending from the caudal vena cava to the right atrium. (C,D) Right-parasternal long-axis (C) and short-axis (D) view of the same horse. Multiple hypoechogenic pericardial masses are visible (arrows). Ao: aorta; LA: left atrium; LV: left ventricle; PA: pulmonary artery; RV: right ventricle.

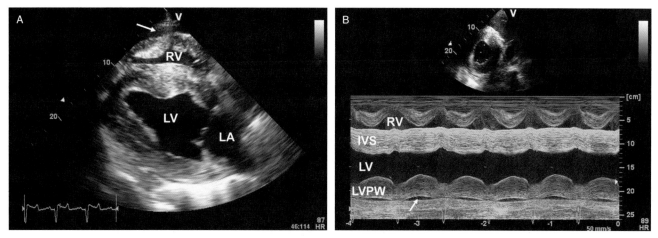

Figure 22.23   Myocarditis. (A) Right-parasternal four-chamber view obtained from a 32-year-old Icelandic Horse gelding with myocarditis of undetermined etiology. The right ventricular (RV) free wall, the interventricular septum, and the left ventricular (LV) peripheral wall are thickened and show heterogeneous echogenicity. Notice the mild pericardial effusion (arrow). (B) Short-axis echocardiogram and corresponding M-mode recording of the LV. The interventricular septum (IVS) and the left ventricular peripheral wall (LVPW) are thickened, whereas the internal dimensions of the LV appear small. The relative wall thickness is 1.03 (normal 0.35–0.6). The motion of the IVS seems flat. The fractional shortening of the left ventricle is 34%. Mild pericardial effusion is evident (arrow). LA: left atrium. (Source: Part B – Bonagura, J.D., Reef, V.B., & Schwarzwald, C.C. (2010) [2]. Reproduced with permission of Elsevier.)

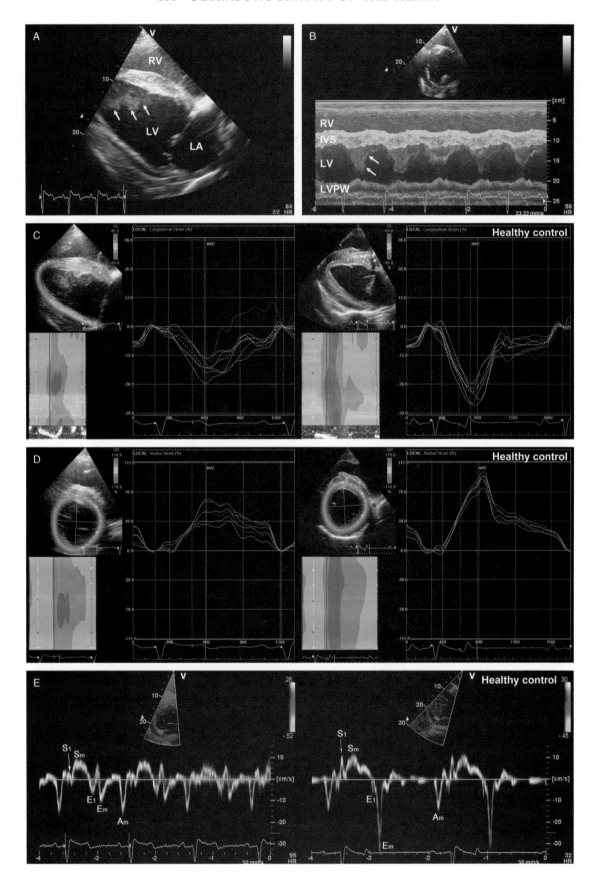

Figure 22.24 Nutritional myocardial damage. Echocardiographic examination in a 22-year-old Arabian mare suffering from nutritional masseter myopathy with concurrent myocardial damage (cardiac troponin I concentration 11.6 ng/mL; normal <0.06 ng/mL). This case study demonstrates the clinical use of novel echocardiographic indices for the assessment of systolic and diastolic LV function in horses with myocardial disease. (A) B-mode recording of the left ventricle in right-parasternal long-axis four-chamber view. Left atrial (LA), left ventricular (LV), and right ventricular (RV) dimensions appear normal. There is marked spontaneous echo contrast in the LV (arrows). This can be found in healthy horses, but may become more distinct with low output states, bradycardia, and possibly systemic inflammation. (B) M-mode recording of the LV in a right-parasternal short-axis view. Notice the flat motion of the interventricular septum (IVS) and the LV peripheral wall (LVPW), suggesting poor LV systolic function (LV fractional shortening 22%; normal 30–45%). Marked spontaneous echo contrast is evident (arrows). (C) Two-dimensional speckle tracking (2DST) analyses of a LV long-axis recording. Trace screens of the 2DST software are shown, displaying the following information: top left, 2D image with the segmented ROI and parametric color-coding at the time of aortic valve closure. Bottom left, M-mode with parametric color-coding. Right, trace display for longitudinal segmental strain (i.e. relative myocardial deformation). The horizontal axis represents the time in ms, the vertical axis represents radial strain in %. The colors of the trace correspond to the colors of the segmented ROI. An ECG is superimposed for timing. The start and the end of the cycle (R waves) are marked on the ECG with yellow dots. Time of aortic valve closure (AVC) is indicated by a green vertical line, dividing the cycle in its systolic and diastolic component. The dotted line indicates the instantaneous average over all segments at the respective time of the cardiac cycle (global strain). Note that peak longitudinal strain in this case (left) is reduced compared to the healthy control (right), indicating depressed LV systolic function. (D) 2DST analyses of a LV short-axis recording. Trace screens of the 2DST software are shown, displaying radial segmental strain (for further explanations see C). Note that peak radial strain (left) in this case is reduced compared to the healthy control (right), indicating depressed LV systolic function. (E) Pulsed wave tissue Doppler (PW TDI) analysis of the LV free wall recorded at the level of the chordae tendineae in a right-parasternal short-axis view. The horizontal scales of the spectral tracings indicate the time in seconds, the vertical scales indicate the wall motion velocity in cm/sec. The E_m/A_m inversion (left) indicates diastolic dysfunction and impaired ventricular relaxation. Notice the normal E_m/A_m ratio in the healthy control (right) for comparison. A_m: peak radial wall motion velocity during late diastole; E_1: peak radial wall motion velocity during isovolumic relaxation; E_m: peak radial wall motion velocity during early diastole; S_1: peak radial wall motion velocity during isovolumic contraction; S_m: peak radial wall motion velocity during ejection.

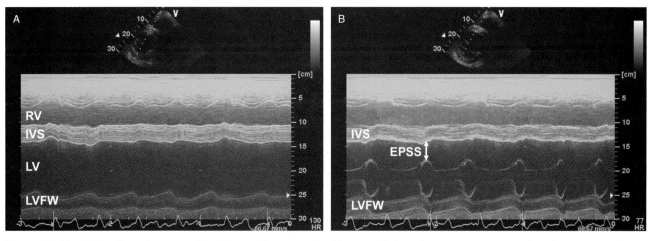

Figure 22.25 Dilated cardiomyopathy. Echocardiogram of a 14-year-old Appaloosa mare presented with congestive heart failure. The findings were compatible with a diagnosis of dilated cardiomyopathy. (A) M-mode echocardiogram in a right-parasternal short-axis view at the level of the chordae tendineae. Notice the hypokinetic motion of the interventricular septum (IVS) and the left ventricular free wall (LVFW), indicating severely depressed left ventricular (LV) systolic function. The LV fractional shortening was 11% (normal 30–45%). (B) M-mode echocardiogram in a right-parasternal short-axis view at the level of the mitral valve. The increased E-point-to-septal separation (EPSS) is consistent with LV dilation and LV failure (resulting in reduced transmitral flow). Other causes for an increased EPSS, such as aortic regurgitation (regurgitant jet impinging on the valve) and mitral stenosis (rare), were ruled out in this case. RV: right ventricle.

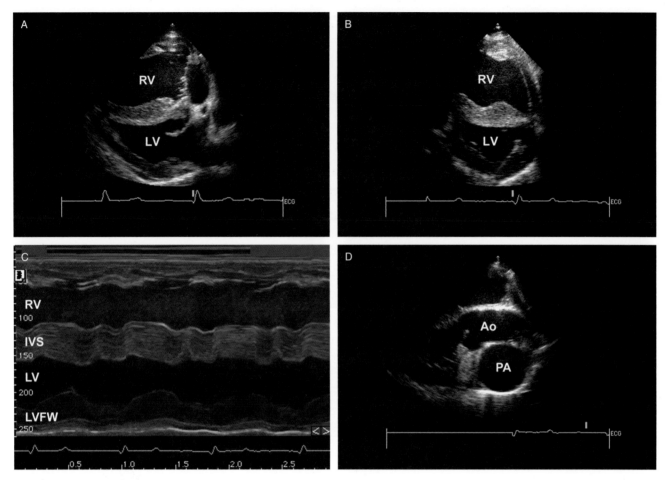

Figure 22.26 Cor pulmonale. Echocardiogram of a 16-year-old American Paint horse gelding with cor pulmonale secondary to severe granulomatous pneumonia. (A,B) Right-parasternal long-axis four-chamber view (A) and right-parasternal short-axis view (B) at end-diastole. Right ventricular (RV) enlargement with bulging of the interventricular septum into the left ventricle (LV) is evident, suggesting chronic RV pressure overload. (C) M-mode echocardiography of the LV in a right-parasternal short-axis view shows enlargement of the RV, small LV, and flattened motion of the interventricular septum (IVS). (D) Right-parasternal long-axis view across the ascending aorta (Ao) and the pulmonary artery (PA). The diameter of the pulmonary artery, seen in short axis, is larger than the aortic diameter, consistent with pulmonary hypertension. This was confirmed by transvenous cardiac catheterization, revealing end-expiratory pulmonary artery pressures of 82/42 mmHg (systolic/diastolic). LVFW: left ventricular free wall.

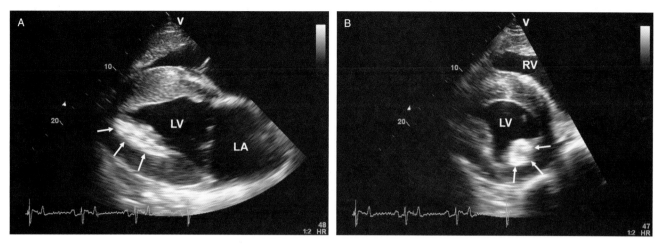

Figure 22.27 Papillary muscle ischemia. Echocardiogram of a 15-year-old Swiss Warmblood gelding with acute transient mitral regurgitation that occurred after physical exhaustion 2 days prior to the examination. Blood cardiac troponin I (cTnI) concentration was 2.15 ng/mL (normal <0.06 ng/mL) on the day of the echocardiographic examination, indicating acute myocardial damage. (A,B) Right-parasternal long-axis four-chamber view (A) and right-parasternal short-axis view at the level of the papillary muscles (B). Notice the distinct hyperechoic area in the region of the parietal papillary muscle of the mitral valve. Differential diagnoses for hyperechoic myocardium include ischemia, infarction, myocarditis, infiltration, amyloidosis, and fibrosis. Based on the history of physical exhaustion and the transient nature of the mitral regurgitation, acute focal ischemia was considered most likely. Blood cTnI concentrations returned to normal within 5 days.

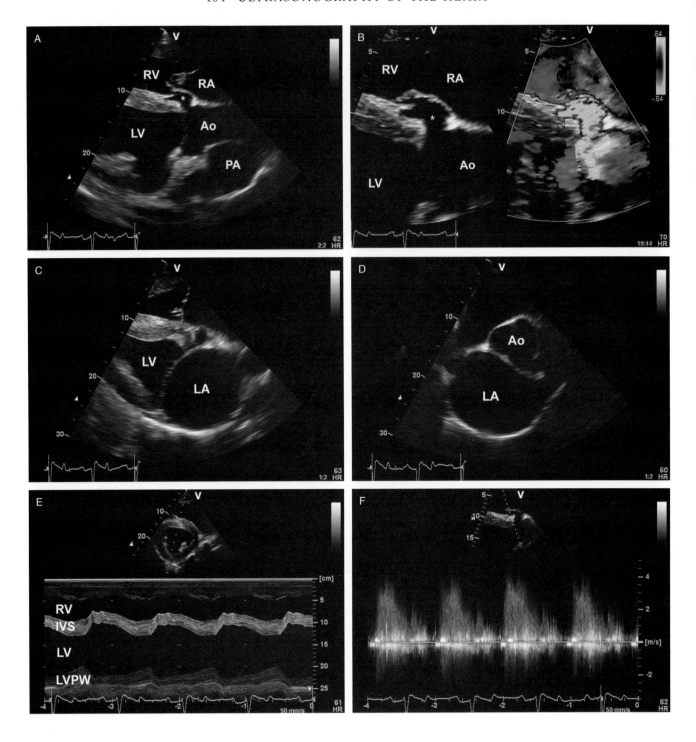

Figure 22.28 Aortic root rupture. (A) Right-parasternal long-axis view of the left ventricular outflow tract obtained from a 21-year-old Paso Fino gelding with a ruptured aortic root. The defect (asterisk) connects the aortic root (Ao) with the right ventricle (RV). The pulmonary artery (PA) appears enlarged relative to the aortic root, indicating increased transpulmonary flow due to left-to-right shunting or pulmonary hypertension. (B) B-mode (left) and color Doppler (right) recording zoomed in on the defect. The defect is located very close to the membranous part of the ventricular septum. However, close inspection of the B-mode recording reveals that the defect is located on the arterial side of the aortic valve, indicating that this defect is an aortic root rupture rather than a ventricular septal defect. Color flow mapping shows left-to-right flow through the defect. Notice the area of proximal flow convergence and concurrent aliasing (sudden color shift from yellow to cyan), visible within the aortic sinus during diastole. (C,D) Right-parasternal four-chamber view (C) and right-parasternal short-axis view (D) of aorta (Ao) and left atrium (LA). The LA is enlarged and has a rounded appearance, indicating left-sided volume overload resulting from left-to-right shunting of blood through the defect. (E) Short-axis echocardiogram and corresponding M-mode recording of the left ventricle (LV). The large end-diastolic LV diameter and the hyperkinetic motion of the interventricular septum (IVS) indicate left ventricular volume overload due to left-to-right shunt. The systolic function of the LV appears adequate, with a fractional shortening of 35%. (F) Continuous wave Doppler (CWD) recording indicating continuous left-to-right shunt flow through the defect, with a predominantly diastolic flow component. The peak velocity is 4.27 m/s, corresponding to a (mid-to-end-diastolic) pressure gradient between Ao and RV of 73 mmHg (modified Bernoulli equation: $dp = 4 \times v_{max}{}^2$). LVPW: left ventricular peripheral wall; RA: right atrium. (Source: Part B – Bonagura, J.D., Reef, V.B., & Schwarzwald, C.C. (2010) [2]. Reproduced with permission of Elsevier.)

REFERENCES

[1] Reef, V.B. (1998) Cardiovascular ultrasonography. In: *Equine Diagnostic Ultrasound*, 1st edn. W.B. Saunders, Philadelphia, 215–272.

[2] Bonagura, J.D., Reef, V.B., & Schwarzwald, C.C. (2010) Cardiovascular diseases. In: *Equine Internal Medicine*, 3rd edn (eds S.M. Reed, W.M. Bayly, & D.C. Sellon). Saunders Elsevier, St. Louis, 372–487.

[3] Boon, J.A. (2011) *Veterinary Echocardiography*. Wiley Blackwell, Oxford.

[4] Sepulveda, M.F., Perkins, J.D., Bowen, I.M., & Marr, C.M. (2005) Demonstration of regional differences in equine ventricular myocardial velocity in normal 2-year-old Thoroughbreds with Doppler tissue imaging. *Equine Veterinary Journal*, 37(3), 222–226.

[5] Schwarzwald, C.C., Bonagura, J.D., & Schober, K.E. (2009) Methods and reliability of tissue Doppler imaging for assessment of left ventricular radial wall motion in horses. *Journal of Veterinary Internal Medicine*, 23(3), 643–652.

[6] Schwarzwald, C.C., Schober, K.E., Berli, A.S.J., & Bonagura, J.D. (2009) Left ventricular radial and circumferential wall motion analysis in horses using strain, strain rate, and displacement by 2D speckle tracking. *Journal of Veterinary Internal Medicine*, 23(4), 890–900.

[7] Schefer, K.D., Bitschnau, C., Weishaupt, M.A., & Schwarzwald, C.C. (2010) Quantitative analysis of stress echocardiograms in healthy horses with 2-dimensional (2D) echocardiography, anatomical M-mode, tissue Doppler imaging, and 2D speckle tracking. *Journal of Veterinary Internal Medicine*, 24(4), 918–931.

[8] Decloedt, A., Verheyen, T., Sys, S., De Clercq, D., & van Loon, G. (2011) Quantification of left ventricular longitudinal strain, strain rate, velocity, and displacement in healthy horses by 2-dimensional speckle tracking. *Journal of Veterinary Internal Medicine*, 25(2), 330–338.

[9] Otto, C.M. (2004) *Textbook of Clinical Echocardiography*. Elsevier Saunders, Philadelphia.

[10] Lang, R.M., Bierig, M., Devereux, R.B., *et al.* (2006) Recommendations for chamber quantification. *European Journal of Echocardiography*, 7(2), 79–108.

[11] Grenacher, P.A. & Schwarzwald, C.C. (2010) Assessment of left ventricular size and function in horses using anatomical M-mode echocardiography. *Journal of Veterinary Cardiology*, 12(2), 111–121.

[12] Patteson, M.W., Gibbs, C., Wotton, P.R., & Cripps, P.J. (1995) Effects of sedation with detomidine hydrochloride on echocardiographic measurements of cardiac dimensions and indices of cardiac function in horses. *Equine Veterinary Journal*, 27(S19), 33–37.

[13] Gehlen, H., Kroker, K., Deegen, E., & Stadler, P. (2004) [Influence of detomidine on cardiac function and hemodynamic in horses with and without heart murmur]. *Schweizer Archiv fur Tierheilkunde*, 146(3), 119–126.

[14] Buhl, R., Ersboll, A.K., Larsen, N.H., Eriksen, L., & Koch, J. (2007) The effects of detomidine, romifidine or acepromazine on echocardiographic measurements and cardiac function in normal horses. *Veterinary Anaesthesia and Analgesia*, 34(1), 1–8.

[15] Menzies-Gow, N.J. (2008) Effects of sedation with acepromazine on echocardiographic measurements in eight healthy thoroughbred horses. *Veterinary Record*, 163(1), 21–25.

[16] Schwarzwald, C.C., Schober, K.E., & Bonagura, J.D. (2007) Methods and reliability of echocardiographic assessment of left atrial size and mechanical function in horses. *American Journal of Veterinary Research*, 68(7), 735–747.

[17] Schwarzwald, C.C., Schober, K.E., & Bonagura, J.D. (2007) Echocardiographic evidence of left atrial mechanical dysfunction after conversion of atrial fibrillation to sinus rhythm in 5 horses. *Journal of Veterinary Internal Medicine*, 21(4), 820–827.

[18] Giguere, S., Bucki, E., Adin, D.B., Valverde, A., Estrada, A.H., & Young, L. (2005) Cardiac output measurement by partial carbon dioxide rebreathing, 2-dimensional echocardiography, and lithium-dilution method in anesthetized neonatal foals. *Journal of Veterinary Internal Medicine*, 19(5), 737–743.

[19] Stoylen A. Strain rate imaging: Cardiac deformation imaging by ultrasound/echocardiography – Tissue Doppler and Speckle tracking. http://folk.ntnu.no/stoylen/strainrate/ (accessed 24 December 2011).

[20] Blissitt, K.J. & Bonagura, J.D. (1995) Pulsed wave Doppler echocardiography in normal horses. *Equine Veterinary Journal*, 27(S19), 38–46.

[21] Schefer, K.D., Hagen, R., Ringer, S.K., & Schwarzwald, C.C. (2011) Laboratory, electrocardiographic, and echocardiographic detection of myocardial damage and dysfunction in an Arabian mare with nutritional masseter myodegeneration. *Journal of Veterinary Internal Medicine*, 25(5), 1171–1180.

[22] De Clercq, D., van Loon, G., Tavernier, R., Duchateau, L., & Deprez, P. (2008) Atrial and ventricular electrical and contractile remodeling and reverse remodeling owing to short-term pacing-induced atrial fibrillation in horses. *Journal of Veterinary Internal Medicine*, 22(6), 1353–1359.

Section 3b: Ultrasonography of the Abdominal Cavity

CHAPTER TWENTY-THREE

Ultrasonography of the Liver, Spleen, Kidney, Bladder, and Peritoneal Cavity

Nathan Slovis

Hagyard Equine Medical Institute, Lexington, KY, USA

Liver

The liver (Figures 23.1, 23.2, 23.3, 23.4, 23.5, 23.6, 23.7, 23.8, 23.9, 23.10) is the largest of the abdominal organs, occupying most of the right quadrant and extending across the midline. The liver can be located in the right cranioventral and mid abdomen between the seventh and fourteenth intercostal spaces (ICS) and dorsally in the fourteenth ICS. It can also be located on the left side cranioventrally between the sixth and ninth ICS. On the right side, the right dorsal colon (RDC) is deep to the liver and the duodenum is located between the RDC and liver in the mid portion of the abdomen. On the left side, the liver will be in contact with the stomach and the spleen. Because the liver lies superficially in the young animal, a 5–7 MHz transducer is optimal, while a 3.5 or even a 2.0 MHz will be necessary in the older, adult horse. Hepatic vessels and bile ducts can be seen diffusely, with the portal vein and caudal vena cava being the largest vessels observed on the right side. The liver is characterized as homogeneously hypoechoic and uniform throughout compared to the spleen.

Spleen

The spleen (Figures 23.11, 23.12, 23.13, 23.14, 23.15, 23.16) is imaged between the seventh ICS and the paralumbar fossa (PLF) on the left side and in the ninth ventral ICS on the right side in contact with the liver. The splenic vein is located on the medial aspect of the spleen, caudal and dorsal to the stomach, in the eleventh to twelfth mid-ICS. The spleen interfaces caudally with the left kidney and is homogeneously echogenic, with few vessels seen. The splenic hilar vessels are usually easily seen while the intrasplenic vessels typically require Doppler for identification.

Kidneys

The left and right kidneys (Figures 23.17, 23.18, 23.19, 23.20, 23.21, 23.22, 23.23, 23.24, 23.25, 23.26, 23.27) differ in ultrasonographic appearance and location. The right kidney is located ventral to the transverse spinous processes between the fourteenth and sixteenth ICS from 2 cm dorsal to the tuber coxae (TC) to 12 cm ventral. The right kidney has a more oval anatomic shape in the longitudinal view than the left kidney. The left kidney can be visualized from the fifteenth ICS to the caudal border of the left PLF and from 2 cm dorsal to 15 cm ventral to the dorsal margin of the TC. From the dorsal plane, the left kidney has a more heart–triangular shape than the right kidney. The renal cortex is hypoechoic compared to the surrounding tissues. However, when compared to the adjacent medulla, it is considered echodense with a slightly mottled appearance. The adjacent medulla is less echogenic than the renal cortex. The renal cortex usually

Atlas of Equine Ultrasonography, First Edition. Edited by Jessica A. Kidd, Kristina G. Lu, and Michele L. Frazer.
© 2014 John Wiley & Sons, Ltd. Published 2014 by John Wiley & Sons, Ltd.
Companion Website: www.wiley.com/go/kidd/equine-ultrasonography

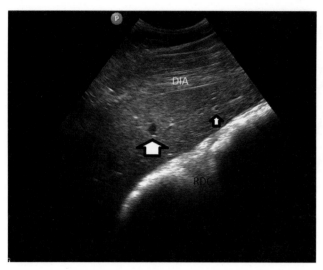

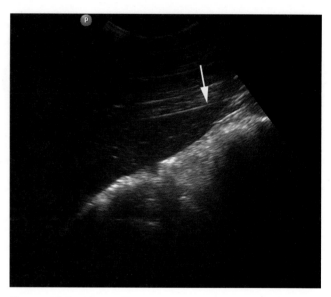

Figure 23.1 Normal liver. This image shows normal liver in a 12-year-old Thoroughbred mare. The hepatic veins (small arrow) image as small, tubular or circular structures with a thin wall. The portal veins (large arrow) usually have a thicker and more echogenic wall than the hepatic veins. The right dorsal colon (RDC) is medial to the right lobe of the liver. The diaphragm (DIA) is superficial to and "covers" the liver. The sonogram was obtained from the right tenth ICS using a curvilinear probe operating at 5.0 MHz at a displayed depth of 18 cm. The left side of this image is dorsal and the right side is ventral.

Figure 23.2 Normal liver. In this image from the mare in Figure 23.1, the liver has normal, tapered edges (arrow). Rounded edges are abnormal and may occur in cases of hepatitis or hepatic lipidosis. The sonogram was obtained from the right tenth ICS, 5–7 cm ventral to the image of Figure 23.1, using a curvilinear probe operating at 5.0 MHz at a displayed depth of 18 cm. The left side of this image is dorsal and the right side is ventral.

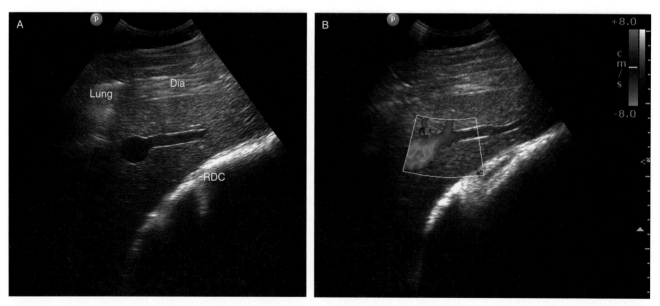

Figure 23.3 Normal liver. (A) In this image from the mare in Figure 23.1, the portal veins are prominent with a thick, echogenic wall. This is a normal anatomic finding of the liver. The ventral tip of the lung can be visualized "covering" the liver on the left side of this image. The diaphragm (Dia) is superficial to the liver. Right dorsal colon (RDC) is visible. The sonogram was obtained from the right eighth ICS using a curvilinear probe operating at 5.0 MHz at a depth of 18 cm. The left side of this image is dorsal and the right side is ventral. (B) Color flow Doppler confirms that the linear structure is the portal vein and not a dilated bile duct.

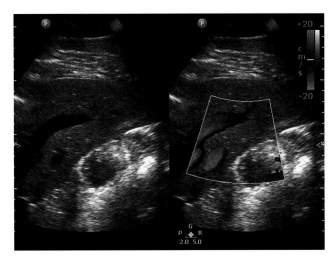

Figure 23.4 Normal portal vein. This image shows the portal vein in a normal, 3-year-old racehorse. The color Doppler was used to confirm that the liner structure was the portal vein and not a dilated bile duct. With color Doppler, direction and velocity of blood flow can be evaluated. Although color may vary with machine, typically, red indicates flow toward the transducer, while blue indicates flow away from the transducer. Brighter hues indicate faster velocity of blood flow, while duller colors indicate slower velocity of blood flow. Turbulent blood flow produces a mixture of colors. This sonogram was obtained from the right abdomen using a curvilinear probe operating at 3.5 MHz at a depth of 18 cm.

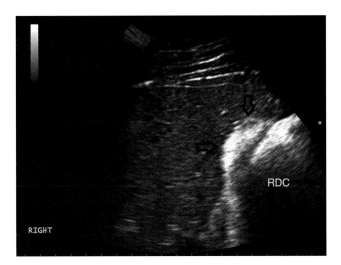

Figure 23.5 Normal liver and duodenum. This image shows the duodenum (arrows) located medial to the right lobe of the liver in a 12-year-old Thoroughbred gelding. The right dorsal colon (RDC) is medial to the duodenum. The duodenum is easily recognized because of its oval and flattened appearance with a hyperechoic center. During peristalsis, the duodenum will have an oval to round-shaped appearance. Note the normal homogeneously hypoechoic sonographic appearance of the liver. The sonogram was obtained from the right fourteenth ICS using a curvilinear probe operating at 3.5 MHz at a displayed depth of 15 cm. The left side of this image is dorsal and the right side is ventral.

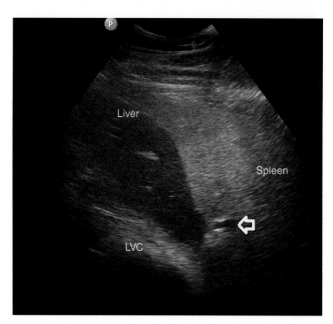

Figure 23.6 Cranioventral abdomen. This image shows the left, cranioventral abdomen obtained from a 12-year-old pregnant Thoroughbred mare. In the normal horse, the spleen is more echogenic and more homogeneous than the liver, which is located medial to the spleen. If the liver is the same echogenicity as the spleen, cholangiohepatitis or hepatitis should be suspected. The hyperechoic, curvilinear structure adjacent to the liver is the left ventral colon (LVC). The splenic vein (small arrow) is visualized in the spleen. The sonogram was obtained from the left, cranioventral abdomen using a curvilinear probe operating at 5.0 MHz at a displayed depth of 17 cm. The left side of this image is dorsal and the right side is ventral.

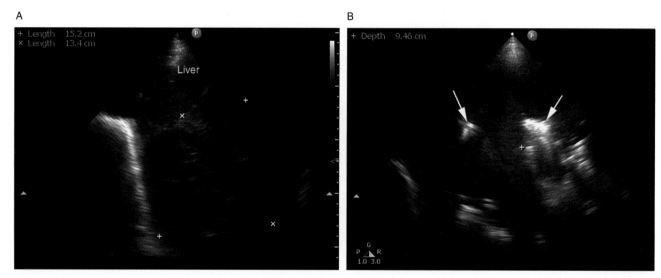

Figure 23.7 Amyloidosis. These images are liver from a 5-year-old Tennessee Walking Horse stallion. The stallion had a history of hyperglobulinemia, anorexia, and intermittent pyrexia for 3 weeks prior to examination. The animal had been treated with sulfadiazine/trimethoprim (30 mg/kg PO q12h) for 3 weeks with minimal improvement. (A) A large mass was imaged adjacent to the liver. In this image, ascertaining if the mass is located medial to the liver or in the liver is difficult. The owners declined a biopsy at the time of the initial examination and the horse was, therefore, discharged with chloramphenicol (50 mg/kg PO q8h) and metronidazole (15 mg/kg PO q8h). The sonogram was obtained from the right ninth ICS using a curvilinear probe operating at 3.0 MHz at a displayed depth of 21 cm. The left side of this image is dorsal and the right side is ventral. (B) The horse was examined again 19 days later for pyrexia and continued anorexia. The sonogram revealed large, hyperechoic structures (arrows) within the liver's parenchyma. Based on histopathology of a biopsy sample, the hyperechoic structures were identified as amyloid deposits and the horse was diagnosed with amyloidosis. The owners opted to euthanize the horse. If the amyloid deposits had been more calcified, an acoustic shadow would have been noted from the near surface of the amyloid deposits. The sonogram was obtained from the right, eleventh ICS using a curvilinear probe operating at 3.0 MHz at a displayed depth of 19 cm. The left side of this image is dorsal and the right side is ventral.

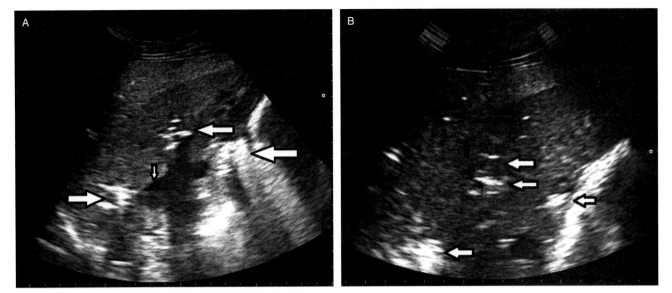

Figure 23.8 Bile duct stricture. This image shows the liver from a 3-month-old Thoroughbred colt diagnosed with a gastric outflow obstruction (stricture) affecting the proximal duodenum. The stricture also incorporated the common bile duct opening. The bile duct stricture resulted in cholestasis and severe suppurative cholangiohepatitis. (A) Note the enlarged bile duct (small arrow) and the abscesses (large arrows) within the liver parenchyma. An acoustic shadow is present medial to the abscess. The foal had a gastrojejunostomy performed and was placed postoperatively on potassium penicillin (22,000 IU/kg IV q6h), metronidazole (15 mg/kg PO q8h), and gentamicin (6 mg/kg IV SID) for 10 days and then changed to chloramphenicol (50 mg/kg PO q6h) along with the metronidazole. The sonogram was obtained from the right eleventh ICS using a curvilinear probe operating at 3.5 MHz at a displayed depth of 17 cm. The left side of this image is dorsal and the right side is ventral. (B) The foal was examined 20 days after discharge from the clinic. His clinical condition had improved and he had been afebrile since treatment. The sonogram of the right lobe of the liver in the twelfth ICS shows a diffuse area of increased echogenicity in the parenchyma of the superficial right lobe representing an area of hepatic cirrhosis. The suppurative hepatitis was responding to the prescribed treatment program based on the horse's improved blood parameters (white blood cell count, sorbitol dehydrogenase (SDH), bile acids, and fibrinogen values in reference range) along with the decreased size of hepatic abscessation (white arrows) from the previous examination. However, the gammaglutamyl transferase (GGT) remained above the reference range secondary to chronic scarring and fibrosis in the liver. The sonogram was obtained from the right twelfth ICS using a curvilinear probe operating at 3.5 MHz at a depth of 13 cm. The left side of this image is dorsal and the right side is ventral.

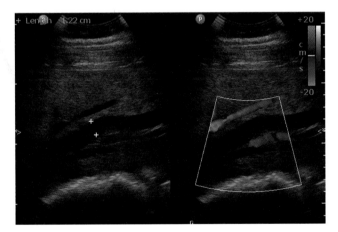

Figure 23.9 Cholangiohepatitis. This image is liver from a mare diagnosed with *Bacteroides fragilis* cholangiohepatitis. On initial examination, the mare had GGT, SDH, and bile acid values above the reference range. Endoscopy of her duodenum revealed a patent bile duct. The mare was treated with potassium penicillin (22,000 IU/kg IV q6h) and metronidazole (15 mg/kg PO q8h) for 2 weeks and then changed to sulfadiazine/trimethoprim (30 mg/kg PO q12h) with metronidazole for another 4 weeks. The mare also received natural vitamin E (10 000 IU PO q24h) and S-adenosyl-l-methionine (20 mg/kg PO q24h). Note the distended bile duct and portal veins indicating portal hypertension. Differentiating a distended hepatic vessel from a bile duct without color flow Doppler may not be possible. The sonogram also shows diffuse, increased echogenicity within the liver. Histopathology of a biopsy sample of the distended bile duct indicated fibrosis around the portal triad. Seven weeks after diagnosis of cholangiohepatitis, the liver values were within the reference range and the bile duct could not be identified ultrasonographically. The diffuse, increased echogenicity was unchanged from initial examination, but the mare had gained weight and delivered a live foal. The sonogram was obtained from the right twelfth ICS using a curvilinear probe operating at 3.5 MHz at a displayed depth of 17 cm. The left side of this image is dorsal and the right side is ventral.

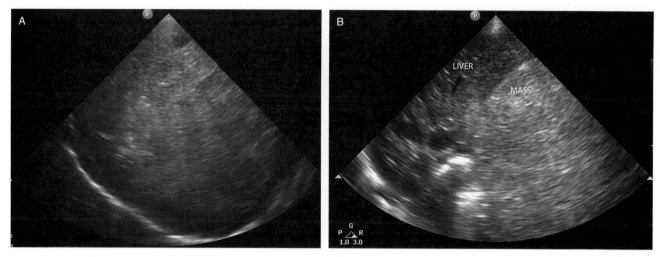

Figure 23.10   Hepatoblastoma. This image shows liver from a 2-week-old premature foal. The foal was referred to the clinic at 2 hours of age for weakness and a pendulous abdomen. Palpation of the abdomen revealed a firm mass in the abdomen. (A) The sonogram revealed a large, 12 cm by 12 cm, heterogeneous, hyperechoic mass within the liver. The mass was a hepatoblastoma involving only the quadrate lobe of the liver. This image was obtained from ventral abdomen using a micro-convex probe operating at 5.0 MHz at a depth of 18 cm. (B) Normal liver has a more homogeneous, hypoechoic architecture compared to the hyperechoic hepatoblastoma (mass) identified in the quadrate lobe. This image was obtained from ventral abdomen, right of midline, with a micro-convex probe operating at 5.0 MHz at a depth of 12 cm.

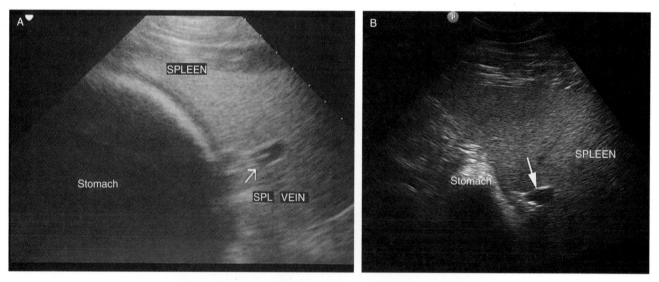

Figure 23.11   Stomach–spleen relationship. (A,B) These images show stomach and spleen from a 3-year-old Thoroughbred filly. The stomach can be easily recognized by its hyperechoic, curvilinear appearance and its location next to the splenic vein (arrow). The spleen is homogeneous and echogenic. The sonogram was obtained at the left ninth ICS using a curvilinear probe operating at 3.5 MHz at a displayed depth of (A) 12 cm and (B) 17 cm. The left side of this image is dorsal and the right side is ventral.

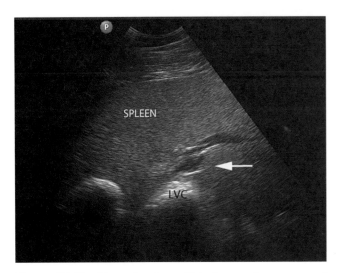

Figure 23.12 Normal spleen. This image shows normal spleen from a 10-year-old pregnant Thoroughbred mare. The spleen is homogeneous and echogenic. Note how the splenic vein (arrow) is easily visualized along the medial aspect of the spleen. Medial to the spleen is the left ventral colon (LVC). This sonogram was obtained from the left twelfth ICS using a curvilinear probe operating at 5 MHz at a displayed depth of 25 cm. The left side of the image is dorsal and the right side is ventral.

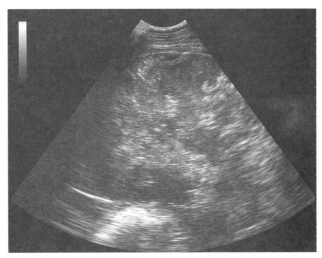

Figure 23.14 Lymphosarcoma. This image is from a yearling Thoroughbred filly with weight loss and intermittent signs of colic. In this image, the spleen has a heterogeneous echogenicity and is swollen with a "round" appearance. The spleen extended across midline 8–10 cm. A biopsy was performed and lymphosarcoma was diagnosed based on histopathology. The sonogram was obtained from the left fourteenth ICS using a curvilinear probe operating at 3.5 MHz at a depth of 27 cm. The left side of this image is dorsal and the right side is ventral.

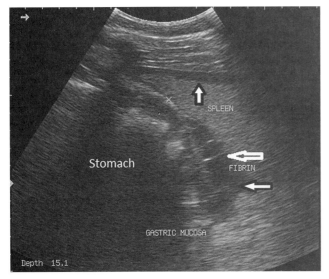

Figure 23.13 Adhesions between spleen and stomach. This image is from a 6-month-old Thoroughbred colt with acute colic signs. The colt, on arrival, had sinus tachycardia (heart rate of 90 beats per minute), injected mucous membranes, and a prolonged capillary refill time. The colt was diagnosed with a perforated gastric ulcer and peritonitis. Fibrin adhesions (white arrow) are seen between the spleen and the stomach. Free fluid (black arrows) is visualized in the abdominal cavity. The normal homogeneous echogenicity of the spleen is maintained. The sonogram was obtained from the left ninth ICS using a curvilinear probe operating at 2.0 MHz at a depth of 15 cm. The left side of this image is dorsal and the right side is ventral.

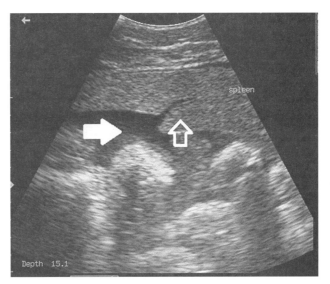

Figure 23.15 Splenic tear. This image is from a Thoroughbred colt. The colt was traumatized on the track when it collided with another horse. The colt presented in hemorrhagic shock and was given 7 liters of whole blood and the hemostatic agent aminocaproic acid (20 mg/kg diluted in liter saline, IV, q6h). The spleen had a tear (hollow arrow) that resulted in hemoabdomen (solid arrow). Note how contracted or thin the spleen is secondary to the large blood loss. The sonogram was obtained just ventral to the paralumbar fossa using a curvilinear probe operating at 2.0 MHz at a displayed depth of 15 cm. The left side of this image is dorsal and the right side is ventral.

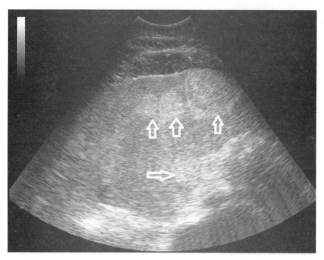

Figure 23.16 Hemangiosarcoma. This image is from a Thoroughbred stallion with weight loss, intermittent colic, and anemia (hematocrit 15%, reference range 34–49%) On arrival, the stallion's mucous membrane color was pale pink with a prolonged capillary refill time. The spleen had a heterogeneous echogenicity with well demarcated masses (white arrows). A biopsy specimen was taken of the spleen and histopathology confirmed hemangiosarcoma. This sonogram was obtained from the left abdomen, caudal to the last rib, with a curvilinear probe operating at 3.5 MHz at a depth of 25 cm.

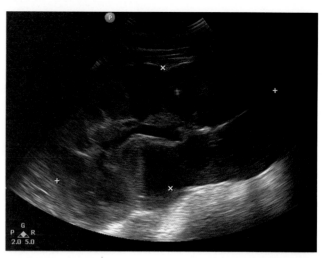

Figure 23.18 Normal right kidney. This image of the right kidney was obtained from a yearling Thoroughbred filly. The kidney was visualized at the sixteenth ICS, just ventral to the tuber coxae. The ureter can be noted adjacent to the renal pelvis. The diameter of the ureter is considered normal. Note the normal heterogeneous echogenicity between the cortex and the medulla. This is a normal size and sonographic appearance for the right kidney. The sonogram was obtained from the right sixteenth ICS with a curvilinear probe operating at 5.0 MHz at a depth of 15 cm. The left side of this image is dorsal and the right side is ventral.

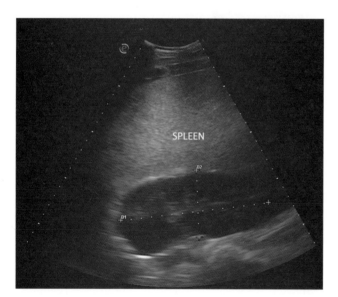

Figure 23.17 Normal left kidney. This image is the left kidney obtained from a 3-year-old Thoroughbred filly. The kidney has a hypoechoic architecture compared to the spleen. Normally, the renal pelvis is echogenic secondary to intrapelvic fat and fibrous tissue. Visualizing the cortex and medulla with adequate detail may be difficult because of the left kidney's depth in the abdomen. Transrectal examination of the left kidney will provide a more detailed view of the organ. The left kidney in an adult horse usually measures 15–16 cm by 10 cm. This sonogram was obtained from the left, lateral abdomen, caudal to the last rib, with a curvilinear probe operating at 3.5 MHz at a depth of 22 cm.

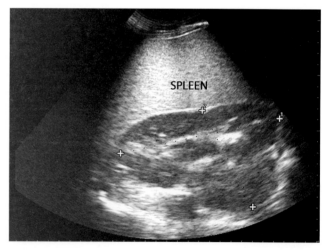

Figure 23.19 Normal left kidney. This image is a normal left kidney in an 8-month-old Thoroughbred colt. Note the heart or triangular shape to the kidney. This view can be difficult at times to obtain in the adult horse due to the left kidney's depth and location. The sonogram was obtained from the left seventeenth ICS using a curvilinear probe operating at 3.5 MHz at a depth of 21 cm. The left side of this image is dorsal and the right side is ventral.

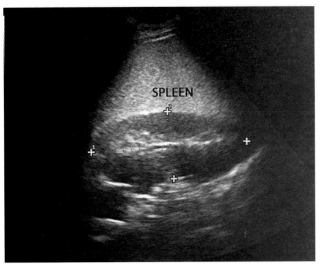

Figure 23.20 Nephritis. This image is from a post-partum, 19-year-old Thoroughbred mare with nephritis. The mare had urinary incontinence immediately after foaling and, 3 weeks later, had intermittent episodes of fever. This image shows an enlarged left kidney measuring 19.23 by 8.09 cm. This image shows similar echogenicity between the cortex and medulla. Therefore, visible delineation is not seen between cortex and medulla. Ascending *Escherichia coli* nephritis was diagnosed based on urine culture and sonographic appearance of the kidney. The mare was treated with sulfadiazine/trimethoprim (30 mg/kg PO q12h) for 2 weeks and the mare recovered from her nephritis. Typically, horses with nephritis have a sonogram appearance of homogeneous echogenicity of the entire kidney with subsequent loss of distinction between the cortex and the medulla. The sonogram was obtained at the paralumbar fossa using a curvilinear probe operating at 3.0 MHz at a depth of 24 cm. The left side of this image is dorsal and the right side is ventral.

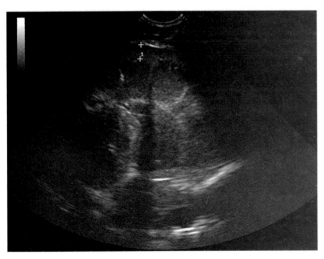

Figure 23.21 Normal right kidney. This image is the right kidney in a yearling, Thoroughbred colt. The cortex (cursors) of this horse's kidney is of normal thickness (<1 cm). Note the normal hyperechogenic appearance of the cortex compared to the hypoechoic echogenicity of the medulla. This sonogram was obtained from the right lateral abdomen, caudal to the last rib with a curvilinear probe operating at 3.5 MHz at a depth of 14 cm.

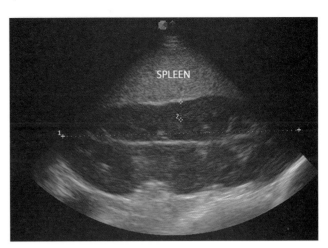

Figure 23.22 Leptospirosis. This image is the left kidney in a 3-month-old Thoroughbred colt with pyrexia and azotemia. The colt was diagnosed with leptospirosis based on positive polymerase chain reaction (PCR) for leptospirosis in a urine sample. The kidney is markedly enlarged (18.7 cm by 13.7 cm) for a 3-month-old foal. The cortical thickness was abnormal at 1.36 cm (normal thickness is <1 cm). The kidney still maintains the normal heterogeneous echogenicity between the cortex and the medulla. The foal was treated with doxycycline (10 mg/kg PO q12h for 14 days) and recovered. The sonogram was obtained at the paralumbar fossa using a curvilinear probe operating at 3.0 MHz at a depth of 16.5 cm. The left side of this image is dorsal and the right side is ventral.

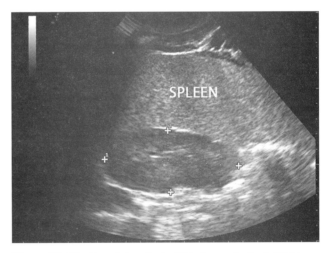

Figure 23.23 Renal dysplasia. This image is the left kidney from a 4-month-old Thoroughbred filly with lethargy and azotemia. This filly had been treated on the farm with intravenous fluids because of azotemia, but the azotemia did not resolve. The left kidney had abnormal sonographic architecture. Note the small size of the kidney along with the homogeneous echogenicity of the kidney. The cortex and the medulla cannot be distinguished from each other and assessing the corticomedullary junction is difficult. The renal pelvis could not be adequately visualized. This filly was diagnosed with bilateral renal dysplasia and was humanely euthanized. The sonogram was obtained ventral to the paralumbar fossa with a curvilinear probe operating at 3.5 MHz at a displayed depth of 15 cm. The left side of this image is dorsal and the right side is ventral.

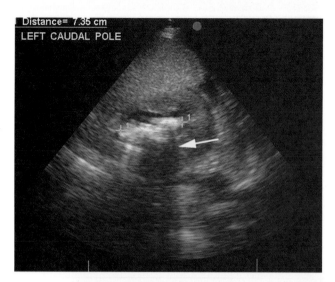

Figure 23.24 Nephrolith. This image is the left kidney in a 10-year-old Thoroughbred mare with a history of intermittent fevers. In this image, the hyperechoic structure casting the acoustic shadow is most likely a nephrolith. The fevers were related to colitis and the nephrolith in the kidney was an incidental finding. Unlike humans, horses can often pass kidney stones with little evidence of pain. The sonogram was obtained ventral to the left paralumbar fossa using a curvilinear probe operating at 2.5 MHz at a depth of 28 cm. The left side of this image is dorsal and the right side is ventral.

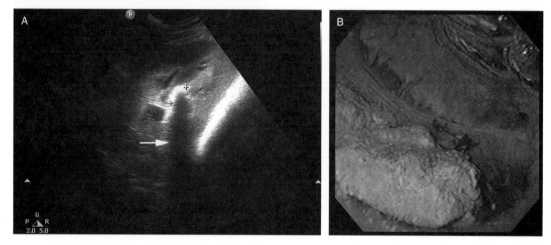

Figure 23.25 Nephrolith. This image is the right kidney in a 12-year-old pregnant Thoroughbred mare with cystitis and nephrolith. (A) This image shows a hyperechoic structure (cursors) that cast an acoustic shadow (arrow) within the renal pelvis. (B) Ureteroscopy revealed a nephrolith and calcium carbonate sediment within the renal pelvis. The mare was treated with 1 oz (28 g) oral of ammonia chloride divided between three feedings and potassium penicillin (20 000 IU IV q6h) for a severe *Streptococcus zooepidemicus* cystitis and nephritis. The sonogram was obtained from the right sixteenth ICS using a curvilinear probe operating at 5.0 MHz at a depth of 21 cm. The left side of this image is dorsal and the right side is ventral.

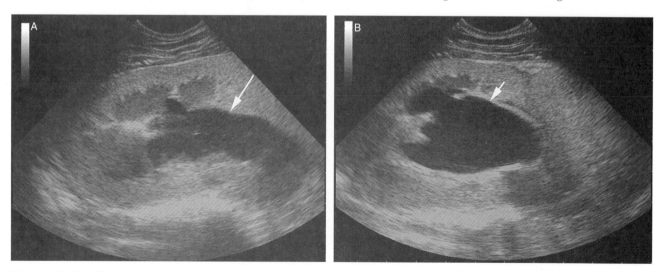

Figure 23.26 Hydroureteronephrosis. (A,B) These images are the right kidney in an aged Thoroughbred mare with hydroureteronephrosis. Endoscopy was used to diagnose stricture of the right ureteral opening at the trigone of the bladder. Only a small amount of urine was observed exiting the strictured ureter into the bladder. This image shows a distended renal pelvis and proximal ureter (arrow) prior to opening the strictured ureter with a splint. The sonogram was characteristic of a hydroureteronephrosis. The sonograms were obtained from the right sixteenth ICS with a curvilinear probe operating at 7.5 MHz at a displayed depth of 8 cm. The left side of these images is dorsal and the right side is ventral.

measures ≤1 cm in thickness. In the cranial and caudal extremities of each kidney, acoustic anisotropy will be observed between the renal cortex and medulla, resulting in the cortex and medulla in these areas appearing more echogenic than in the center of the kidney. The left kidney is generally considered larger than the right kidney, with the length measuring up to 16 cm and the width measuring 10–11 cm in an adult horse. The right kidney usually measures 15 cm in width and 10–11 cm in length in the adult horse.

BLADDER

Bladder (Figures 23.28, 23.29, 23.30, 23.31, 23.32, 23.33, 23.34, 23.35, 23.36, 23.37) can be evaluated transrectally and sometimes transabdominally by scanning the caudal, ventral abdomen in the adult horse. The bladder in the neonate is easily visualized with transabdominal ultrasound. Bladder volume and wall thickness vary with degree of fill.

Uroperitoneum secondary to perforation of the urinary bladder is a common abnormality in the neonate. In the adult horse it is a less common medical diagnosis. Ultrasound imaging of uroperitoneum demonstrates variable volumes of hypoechoic to echogenic peritoneal effusion with free-floating intestinal organs. The bladder walls may be collapsed and folded. Perforations in other areas of the urinary tract other than the bladder may occur. These include rupture of the urachus, ureter, or kidney. Confirmation of uroperitoneum requires analysis of an abdominocentesis sample.

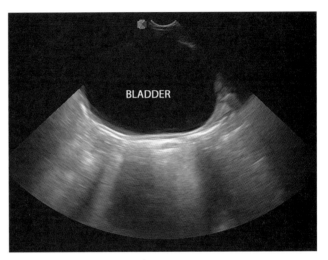

Figure 23.28 This image shows a normal bladder in a neonatal foal. When bladder diameter exceeds 8–9 cm and the walls of the bladder become thin and turgid, the foal may be at risk of rupturing the bladder and catheterization may be warranted. This image was obtained from the caudal aspect of ventral midline with a micro-convex probe operating at 5.0 MHz at a depth of 12 cm.

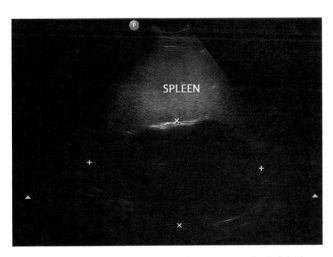

Figure 23.27 Hydronephrosis. This image is the left kidney in an aged pregnant Thoroughbred mare with hydronephrosis. The mare was diagnosed with hydronephrosis secondary to a proximal ureteral stone. The sonogram was obtained from the left paralumbar fossa using a curvilinear probe operating at 5.0 MHz at a depth of 30 cm. The left side of this image is dorsal and the right side is ventral.

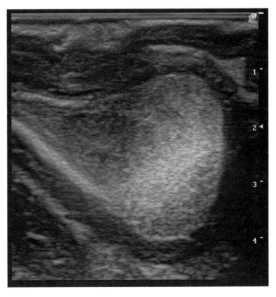

Figure 23.29 This image shows a normal bladder in an adult horse. Note the different echogenicities within the bladder caused by swirling urine. This sonogram was obtained transrectally with a linear probe operating at 7.5 MHz at a depth of 5 cm.

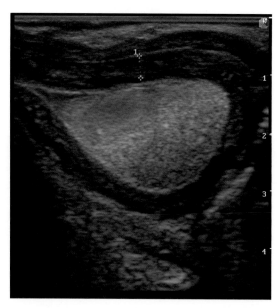

Figure 23.30 Normal bladder in adult. This image is a normal bladder with a small volume of urine in an adult horse. Wall thickness (0.56 cm) is designated by cursors. As the bladder fills with increasing volumes of urine, the bladder walls will stretch and become thin compared to the bladder wall in this image. This sonogram was obtained transrectally with a linear probe operating at 7.5 MHz at a depth of 5 cm.

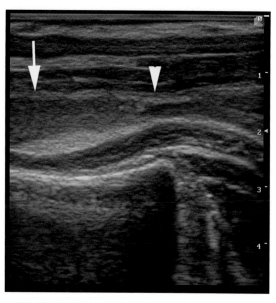

Figure 23.32 Dilated urethra. This image shows the urethra (arrowhead) in an adult horse. Note the area of urethral dilation (arrow). This sonogram was obtained transrectally with a linear probe operating at 7.5 MHz at a depth of 5 cm.

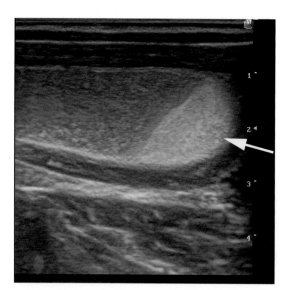

Figure 23.31 Normal bladder with sediment. In this normal bladder, hyperechoic sediment (arrow) is visualized in the bladder. Although some sediment is normal, it can lead to the formation of urinary calculi. This sonogram was obtained transrectally with a linear probe operating at 7.5 MHz at a depth of 5 cm.

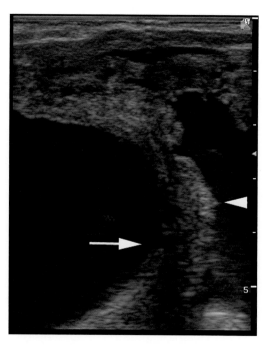

Figure 23.33 Bladder wall defect. This image shows a defect (arrow) in the wall of the bladder. A hyperechoic structure (arrowhead) has formed at the defect and is likely a hematoma. This sonogram was obtained transrectally with a linear probe operating at 7.5 MHz at a depth of 5 cm.

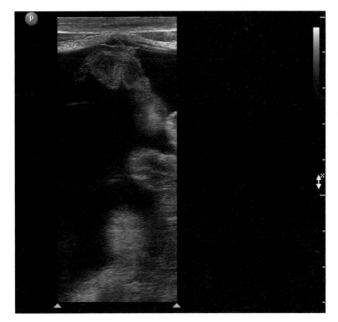

Figure 23.34 Ruptured bladder in foal. This image shows a ruptured bladder in a neonatal foal. Note the collapsed wall of the bladder floating in free peritoneal fluid. This sonogram was obtained from the caudal aspect of the ventral midline with a micro-convex probe operating at 5.0 MHz at a depth of 8 cm.

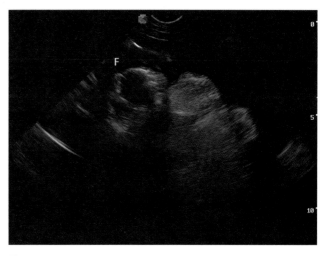

Figure 23.35 Uroperitoneum. This image shows urine (F) in the abdomen of a neonate from ruptured bladder. Note the hypoechoic fluid around the intestine. Uroperitoneum is confirmed by demonstrating a peritoneal fluid creatinine level twice that of the peripheral blood. Although commonly considered a neonatal complication, ruptured bladder can also occur in adults, particularly periparturient mares. This sonogram was obtained from the ventral abdomen with a micro-convex probe operating at 5.0 MHz at a depth of 11 cm.

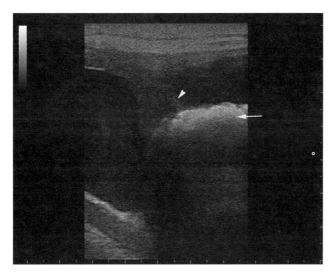

Figure 23.36 Urinary calculi. This image shows a urolith in the bladder of a 20-year-old Arabian stallion presenting for urinary incontinence of 1 month duration. The urolith is delineated by an echogenic surface (arrow) and acoustic shadow ventral to the stone surface. A bladder mucosal adhesion (arrowhead) to the surface of the urolith has occurred. This sonogram was obtained transrectally with a linear probe operating at 5.0 MHz at a depth of 7 cm. (Source: Image courtesy of Dr. Fairfield Bain, University of Queensland Veterinary Medical Centre, Queensland, Australia.)

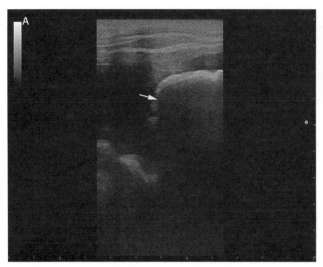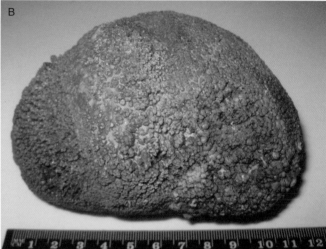

Figure 23.37 Urinary calculi. (A) This image shows another view of the urolith from the horse in Figure 23.36. This sonogram was obtained transrectally with a linear probe operating at 5.0 MHz at a depth of 7 cm. (B) The urolith after surgical removal. (Source: Images courtesy of Dr. Fairfield Bain, University of Queensland Veterinary Medical Centre, Queensland, Australia.)

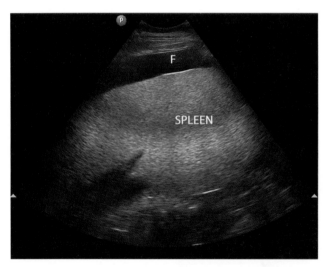

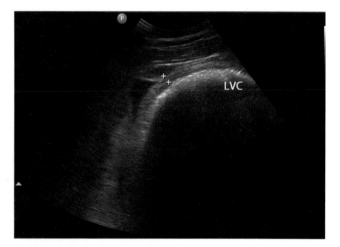

Figure 23.38 Bacterial peritonitis. This image shows peritonitis in a Thoroughbred mare. The free fluid (F) in the abdomen has caused the spleen to move medially, away from the body wall. Bacterial peritonitis was confirmed by cytological analysis of an abdominocentesis sample. This sonogram was obtained from the left fourteenth ICS with a curvilinear probe operating at 5.0 MHz at a depth of 23 cm. The left side of the image is dorsal and the right side is ventral.

Figure 23.39 Intestinal wall in peritonitis case. This image is from the horse with bacterial peritonitis in Figure 23.38. The wall (cursors) of the left ventral colon (LVC) is thickened secondary to the intra-abdominal inflammatory response. This sonogram was obtained from the left ventral abdomen with a curvilinear probe operating at 5.0 MHz at a depth of 15 cm.

Peritoneal Cavity

Ultrasonography is a non-invasive diagnostic tool that can be utilized to evaluate fluid in the peritoneal cavity (Figures 23.38, 23.39, 23.40, 23.41, 23.42, 23.43, 23.44, 23.45, 23.46, 23.47, 23.48, 23.49, 23.50). Normal peritoneal fluid is anechoic and becomes more echogenic with increasing levels of cellularity. Peritonitis is a diffuse inflammatory process in the abdomen, usually of infectious etiology. Ultrasonography helps to quantify the extent of the peritonitis and to characterize the peritoneal fluid. Fibrinous peritonitis can be described as septated because of the loculated appearance of the fluid. The abdomen and associated gastrointestinal and abdominal viscera should be assessed with ultrasound for a cause of peritonitis, including abdominal abscess, tumor, or necrotic bowel.

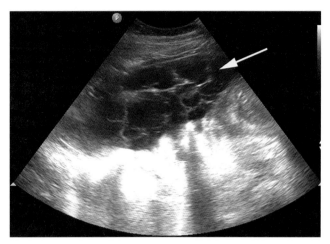

Figure 23.40 Fibrinous peritonitis. This image is from a 10-year-old Thoroughbred mare, 3 days after she had a difficult foaling. The mare was pyrexic (39.2°C, 102.5°F) and colicky. The mare was diagnosed with fibrinous peritonitis, based on her ultrasound findings and after analysis of an abdominocentesis sample. Note the loculated appearance of the fibrin (arrow) characteristic of fibrinous peritonitis. The sonogram was obtained from the right ventral abdomen with a curvilinear probe operating at 5.0 MHz at a depth of 16 cm.

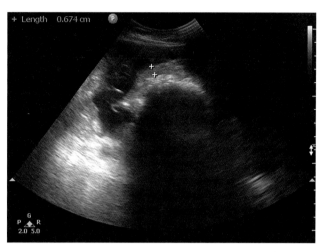

Figure 23.42 Thickened colon wall in fibrinous peritonitis case. This image is from a Warmblood colt presenting for fevers (39.1°C, 102.3°F) and inappetence. The sonogram revealed fibrinous peritonitis with a marked thickened wall (measuring 0.67 cm – cursors) of the left ventral colon. *Actinobacillus* spp was isolated from the abdominal fluid. The sonogram was obtained from the left ventral abdomen with a curvilinear probe operating at 5.0 MHz at a depth of 15 cm.

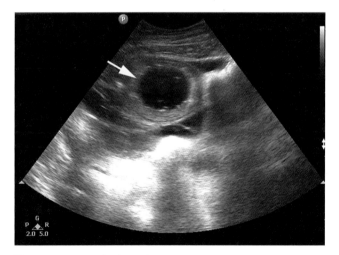

Figure 23.41 Thickened jejunum in peritonitis case. This image shows a loop of jejunum (arrow) with markedly thickened walls in a mare diagnosed with bacterial peritonitis. Note the hypoechoic areas of free peritoneal fluid adjacent to the loop of intestine. Small intestine with thickened walls is commonly diagnosed in cases of severe bacterial peritonitis. Normal wall thickness of small intestine is ≤3 mm. This sonogram was obtained from the right ventral abdomen with a curvilinear probe operating at 5.0 MHz at a depth of 16 cm.

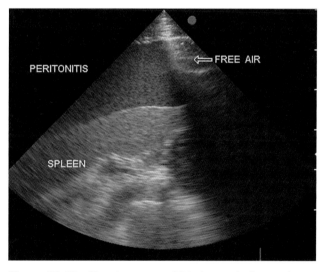

Figure 23.43 Gastric rupture. This image is from a horse diagnosed with gastric rupture. Hyperechoic abdominal fluid and pneumoperitoneum (arrow) are present. This sonogram was obtained from the left thirteenth ICS with a curvilinear probe operating at 3.5 MHz at a depth of 30 cm.

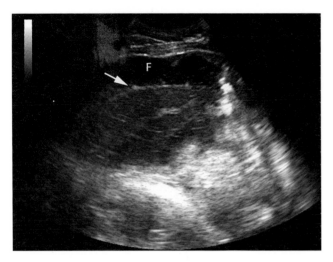

Figure 23.44 Peritoneal fibrin tags. This image is from a 3-month-old Thoroughbred filly presenting for ptyalism and fevers. There are fibrin tags (arrow) on the liver surface and excessive hyperechoic fluid (F) in the abdomen. The sonogram was obtained from the right tenth ICS with a curvilinear probe operating at 3.5 MHz at a depth of 19 cm.

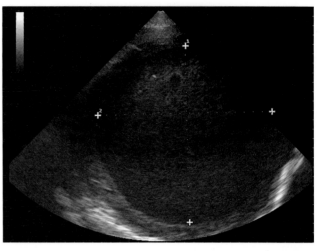

Figure 23.46 Internal abscess. This image is from the filly in Figure 23.45. A large, internal abscess (cursors) is visible in the mesentery of the large colon. *Rhodococcus equi* infection was confirmed at necropsy. This sonogram was obtained from the left ventral abdomen with a curvilinear probe operating at 3.5 MHz at a depth of 25 cm.

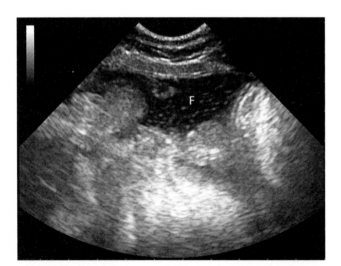

Figure 23.45 Exudative peritonitis. This image shows hyperechoic free fluid (F) in the abdomen. The white blood cell count of the fluid was 84 000 cells/μl. Note the hyperechoic foci in the fluid. This sonogram was obtained from the ventral abdomen with a curvilinear probe operating at 5.0 MHz at a depth of 8 cm.

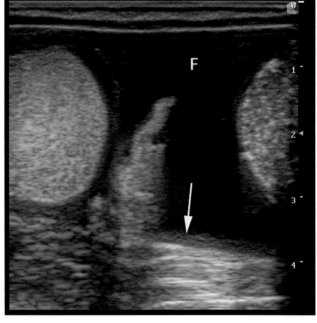

Figure 23.47 Transrectal view of peritonitis. This image shows free fluid (F) in the abdomen of an aged gelding. Note the fibrin tags on the peritoneal surface (arrow). This image was obtained transrectally with a linear probe operating at 5.0 MHz at a depth of 5 cm.

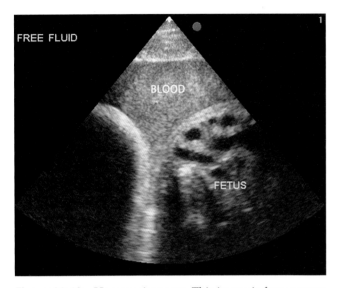

Figure 23.48 Hemoperitoneum. This image is from a mare at 10 months of gestation exhibiting clinical signs of colic. She was diagnosed with periparturient hemorrhage based on ultrasound findings and analysis of an abdominocentesis sample. Hyperechoic, swirling free fluid (blood) is visualized in the abdomen adjacent to the fetus and colon. This sonogram was obtained from the ventral abdomen with a curvilinear probe operating at 22 cm.

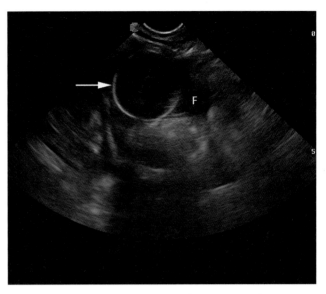

Figure 23.49 Abdominal drain. This image is from a neonatal foal with peritonitis. The thin-walled, circular structure (arrow) is the inflated cuff of an abdominal drain. Note the free peritoneal fluid (F) adjacent to the cuff. This sonogram was obtained from the ventral abdomen with a micro-convex prove operating at 5.0 MHz at a depth of 8 cm.

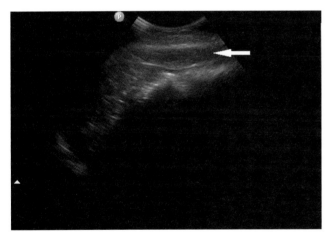

Figure 23.50 Intra-abdominal fat. This image shows intra-abdominal body fat in a gelding. The hyperechoic layer (arrow) is fat and should not be confused with free peritoneal fluid. This image was obtained from the ventral abdomen with a curvilinear probe operating at 3.5 MHz at a depth of 15 cm.

RECOMMENDED READING

Arnold, C.E. & Chaffin, M.K. (2010) Abdominal abscesses in adult horses: 61 cases (1993–2008). *Journal of the American Veterinary Medical Association*, 241(12), 1659–1665.

Budras, K., Sack, W.O., & Röck, S. (2003) *Anatomy of the Horse: An Illustrated Text*, 4th edn. Schlutersche GmbH and Co, Hanover.

Draper, A.C., Bowen, I.M., & Hallowell, G.D. (2012) Reference ranges and reliability of transabdominal ultrasonographic renal dimensions in thoroughbred horses. *Veterinary Radiology & Ultrasound*, 53(3), 336–341.

Ness, S.A.L., Bain, F.T., Zantingh, A.J., *et al.* (2012) Ultrasonographic visualization of colonic mesenteric vasculature as an indicator of large colon right dorsal displacement or 180° volvulus (or both) in horses. *Canadian Veterinary Journal*, 53(4), 378–382.

Reuss, S.M., Chaffin, M.K., Schmitz, D.G., & Norman, T.E. (2011) Sonographic characteristics of intraabdominal abscessation and lymphadenopathy attributable to *Rhodococcus equi* infections in foals. *Veterinary Radiology & Ultrasound*, 52(4), 462–465.

CHAPTER TWENTY-FOUR

ULTRASONOGRAPHY OF THE GASTROINTESTINAL TRACT

Fairfield T. Bain

College of Veterinary Medicine, Washington State University, Pullman, WA, USA

Ultrasonography can be applied to a significant amount of the gastrointestinal tract from the caudal pharynx and esophagus in the neck to the liver, stomach, and large and small intestines within the abdominal cavity. Depending on location and depth required to image the specific structure of interest, probes of multiple frequencies may be utilized. Superficial structures, such as the esophagus, and highest detail of intestinal surfaces may be best imaged using higher-frequency (7.5 MHz or greater) probes. Evaluation of the abdominal cavity as it pertains to the gastrointestinal tract includes evaluation of the liver, stomach, small intestine, and large intestine. The author performs the transabdominal ultrasound examination progressing in a cranial-to-caudal fashion on each side. The exam starts cranially at the third intercostal space, just caudal to the elbow, and progresses in a caudal fashion while scanning dorsal to ventral in each intercostal space from the diaphragm margin ventrad.

Cranially on the left side, the liver is visible adjacent to the spleen. Moving caudally, the stomach is visualized adjacent to the spleen. The stomach is evaluated for contents and size. The normal stomach in the adult horse usually extends over four to five intercostal spaces. Normal small intestine has minimal visible structure. It may be visible with variable motility just ventromedial to the spleen on the left side. The colon is visible ventromedial to the spleen on the left side. On the right side, the large colon is visible in the cranial abdomen. Progressing caudally, the liver is visible ventral to the margin of the lung fields over most of the mid-abdomen. Horses in their mid teens and older may have atrophy of the liver and it may not be readily visualized with ultrasound. The duodenum is visible ventromedial to the liver from the twelfth intercostal

space to just ventral to the right kidney. The right dorsal colon is ventromedial. Ventral–medial to the duodenum is the right dorsal colon. The cecum will be visible in the right paralumbar fossa and extends ventrally along the costal arch and can be distinguished by its lateral vasculature.

On occasion, transrectal ultrasonographic examination may be useful in further characterizing abdominal masses, rectal masses, or intestinal surfaces.

The gastrointestinal anatomy within the abdominal cavity can be dynamic, especially in colic, where abnormal intestinal motility can be involved. Because of this, the author emphasizes the importance of serial sonographic evaluation over time to determine if anatomic changes have occurred, such as position of the colon or amount of gastric or small intestinal distension.

ESOPHAGUS

The esophagus (Figure 24.1) can be imaged from just caudal to the pharynx in the upper neck on the left side along most of its course to the distal neck. It is located just dorsal to the trachea and ventral to the jugular vein and carotid artery. The muscularis appears hypoechoic, whereas the lumen appears echogenic.

STOMACH

The normal stomach (Figures 24.2, 24.3) is imaged adjacent to the spleen on the left side of the abdomen.

Gastric impaction should be considered in animals with a prolonged clinical history of inappetence, mild

Atlas of Equine Ultrasonography, First Edition. Edited by Jessica A. Kidd, Kristina G. Lu, and Michele L. Frazer.
© 2014 John Wiley & Sons, Ltd. Published 2014 by John Wiley & Sons, Ltd.
Companion Website: www.wiley.com/go/kidd/equine-ultrasonography

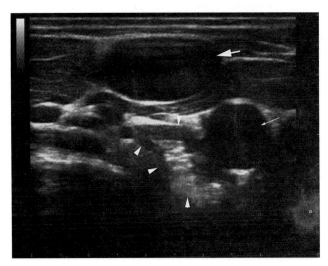

Figure 24.1 Normal esophagus. The normal esophagus is demonstrated by the arrowheads. The trachea is in the bottom left corner of the image. The jugular vein is noted by the large arrow and the carotid artery by the small arrow. This sonogram was obtained from the jugular groove, middle third of the neck, using a linear probe operating at 12 MHz at a depth of 5 cm.

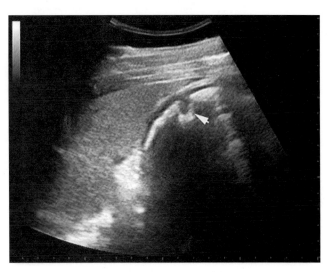

Figure 24.3 Gastric fold. This image shows the normal appearance of stomach adjacent to the spleen in a horse fasted for gastroscopy. A gastric fold (arrowhead) is visible on the surface of the stomach. This sonogram was obtained from the left eleventh ICS using a curvilinear probe operating at 3.5 MHz at a depth of 18 cm.

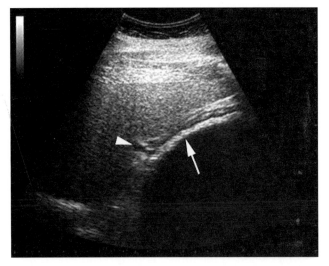

Figure 24.2 Spleen–stomach relationship. This image demonstrates the normal appearance of the stomach adjacent to the spleen. The normal, feed-containing stomach should appear as an echogenic curved line (arrow) against the medial surface of the spleen. The splenic portal vein (arrowhead) is seen along the medial aspect of the spleen. This sonogram was obtained from the left tenth ICS with a curvilinear probe operating at 3.5 MHz at a depth of 18 cm.

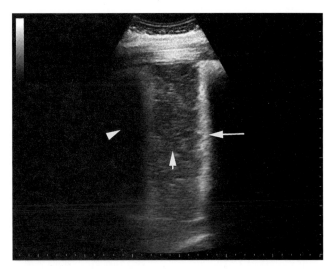

Figure 24.4 Gastric distention. This image demonstrates a fluid-filled, distended stomach (short arrow) in an adult horse. Solid material ventrally (arrowhead) creates an acoustic shadow. A gas–fluid interface (long arrow) is present dorsally. This sonogram was obtained from the left fourteenth ICS with a curvilinear probe operating at 3.5 MHz at a depth of 23 cm.

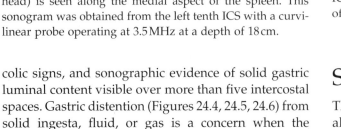

colic signs, and sonographic evidence of solid gastric luminal content visible over more than five intercostal spaces. Gastric distention (Figures 24.4, 24.5, 24.6) from solid ingesta, fluid, or gas is a concern when the stomach extends beyond approximately five rib spaces.

SMALL INTESTINE

The duodenum (Figures 24.7, 24.8) can be imaged along its course on the right side. It is first seen cranially as it appears between the left liver lobe and the

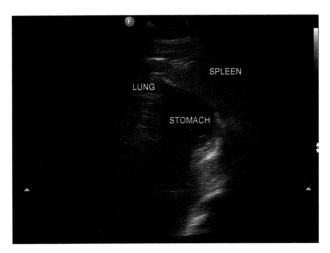

Figure 24.5 Gastric distention. Fluid content is visualized in the stomach. The cranial aspect of the stomach is obscured by the caudodorsal tip of the lung. This sonogram was obtained from the left fourteenth ICS using a curvilinear probe operating a depth of 20 cm. Image is oriented with dorsal to the left side.

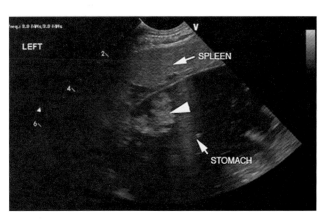

Figure 24.6 Gastric distention with fluid in a neonatal foal. The stomach is markedly distended with a width greater than that of the spleen. Milk clots (arrowhead) are visible within the gastric lumen. This sonogram was obtained from the left twelfth ICS using a curvilinear probe operating at 3.5 MHz at a depth of 6 cm.

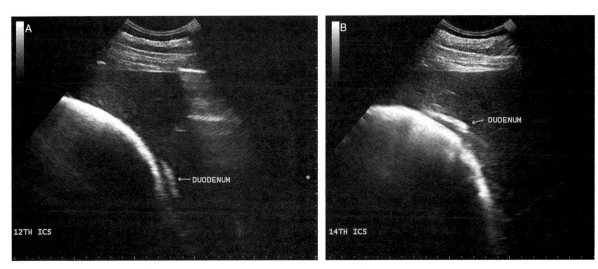

Figure 24.7 Normal duodenum, twelfth and fourteenth ICS. (A,B) These images show normal duodenum. The cranial aspect of the duodenum is visible between the left liver lobe and the right dorsal colon. The echogenic material is luminal content within the duodenum. These sonograms were obtained from the right (A) twelfth and (B) fourteenth ICS using a curvilinear probe operating at 6.6 MHz at a depth of 18 cm.

right dorsal colon, and then progresses caudad to a point ventral to the right kidney.

Duodenal distension (Figure 24.9) can occur with distal small intestinal obstruction, postoperative ileus, or duodenal stricture and obstruction, as well as varying degrees of thickening and distension with enteritis or proximal enteritis syndrome.

Duodenitis (Figure 24.10) and duodenal stricture (Figure 24.11) can produce gastric outflow obstruction in foals. The thickened segment of duodenum can often be imaged along its course on the right side of

the abdomen. Ultrasound can be useful in making the initial diagnosis, as well as monitoring medical therapy and aid in evaluation of postoperative patients that had gastrojejunostomy to relieve the gastric outflow obstruction.

Normal jejunum (Figure 24.12) usually has a nondescript appearance on ultrasound. It is usually visible just ventral and medial to the spleen in the caudal left abdomen around the level of the costal arch.

Small intestinal distension (Figures 24.13, 24.14, 24.15, 24.16, 24.17, 24.18, 24.19, 24.20, 24.21, 24.22,

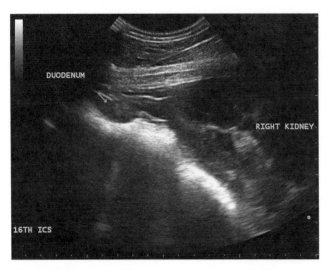

Figure 24.8   Normal duodenum, sixteenth ICS. This image shows normal duodenum ventral to the right kidney and ventromedial to the right dorsal colon. This sonogram was obtained from the right sixteenth ICS with a curvilinear probe operating at 6.6 MHz at a depth of 15 cm.

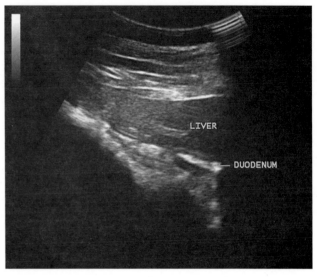

Figure 24.10   Duodenitis. This image demonstrates thick-walled duodenum (arrow) with echogenic luminal material in a 3-year-old Quarterhorse mare that presented with colic and gastric reflux. *Salmonella* spp. was isolated from the gastric fluid suggesting it may have been an etiology for the duodenitis. Normal duodenal wall thickness in an adult horse is ≤3 mm. This sonogram was obtained from the right twelfth ICS with a curvilinear probe operating at 5.0 MHz at a depth of 8 cm.

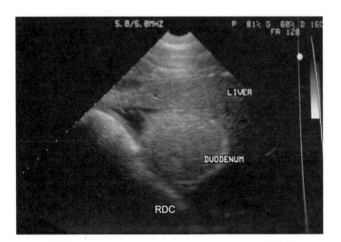

Figure 24.9   Duodenal distension associated with postoperative ileus. The duodenum is imaged between the liver and right dorsal colon (RDC) secondary to postoperative ileus. A small pocket of hypoechoic, free peritoneal fluid is seen adjacent to the duodenum. This sonogram was obtained from the right fourteenth ICS with a curvilinear probe operating at 5.0 MHz at a depth of 15 cm.

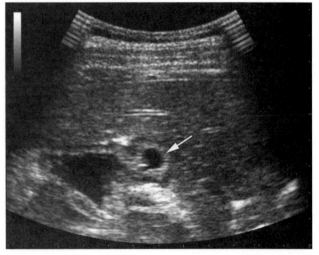

Figure 24.11   Duodenal stricture. This image demonstrates duodenal thickening and stricture producing clinical signs consistent with gastric outflow obstruction in a 6-month-old Hanovarian filly. Duodenal stricture is more common in foals than in adult horses and may be secondary to ulceration of the duodenum and pyloric region. Ulceration can be multifactorial in cause, but may be associated with previous rotavirus infection. This sonogram was obtained from the right fourteenth ICS with a curvilinear probe operating at 6.6 MHz at a depth of 12 cm.

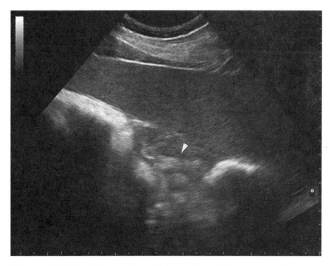

Figure 24.12 Normal small intestine. Normal intestine (arrowhead) is located just medial to the spleen in the caudal left abdomen. It has a nondescript appearance. Wall thickness should not exceed 3 mm. This sonogram was obtained from the caudal left abdomen with a curvilinear probe operating at 6.6 MHz at a depth of 15 cm.

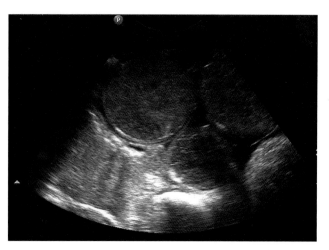

Figure 24.14 Small intestinal volvulus in a yearling. Multiple, fluid-distended, non-motile segments of small intestine are visualized in a yearling presenting for severe abdominal pain of several hours' duration. Eight feet (2.4 m) of non-viable small intestine were resected at surgery. This image was obtained from the ventral abdomen with a curvilinear probe operating at 3.5 MHz at a depth of 15 cm.

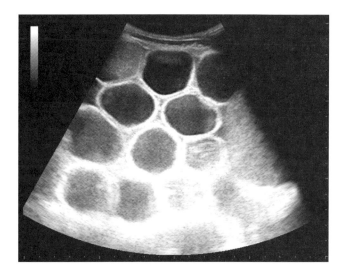

Figure 24.13 Small intestinal volvulus in a foal. Multiple, fluid-distended, non-motile segments of small intestine are imaged in this small intestinal volvulus. This foal presented with acute, severe colic and abdominal distension. This sonogram was obtained from the ventral abdomen with a micro-convex probe operating at 6.6 MHz at a depth of 13 cm.

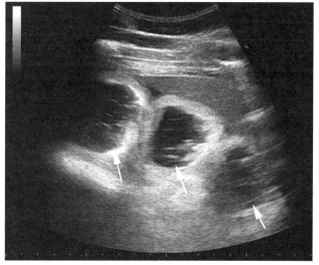

Figure 24.15 Mesenteric defect. Fluid-distended, poorly motile, thick-walled small intestine (arrows) in the left ventral abdomen is imaged in a yearling colt with acute severe colic. The walls of the small intestine measured greater than the normal 3 mm. Serosanguinous peritoneal fluid was observed on abdominocentesis. Multiple segments of thick-walled, red and purple small intestine associated with a mesenteric defect were found at surgery. This sonogram was obtained from the left abdomen with a curvilinear probe operating at 3.5 MHz at a depth of 15 cm.

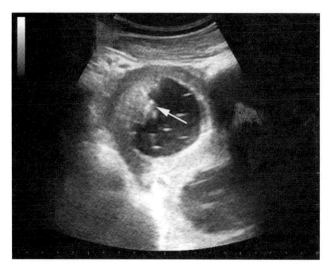

Figure 24.16 Small intestinal strangulation. This image from the patient in Figure 15 shows small intestinal distention from a mesenteric defect. Particulate matter (arrow) has settled to the ventral most aspect of the small intestine. This ventral sedimentation indicates the chronicity of the small intestinal damage. Small intestinal strangulation was confirmed at surgery. This sonogram was obtained from the left abdomen with a curvilinear probe operating at 3.5 MHz at a depth of 15 cm.

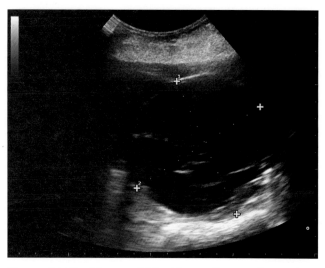

Figure 24.18 Lipoma. This 14-cm, discrete, hypoechoic mass (cursors) was located in the mid-ventral abdomen. Associated sonographic imaging showed dilated, poorly motile small intestine. Post-mortem examination confirmed this mass to be a lipoma strangulating a segment of small intestine. Imaging the lipoma in cases of small intestinal strangulation is rare. The finding of fluid-distended, non-motile and/or thickened small intestine (see Figures 24.19 and 24.20) in an aged animal is the most consistent ultrasound finding with strangulating lipomas. This sonogram was obtained from the ventral abdomen with a curvilinear probe operating at 6.6 MHz at a depth of 14 cm.

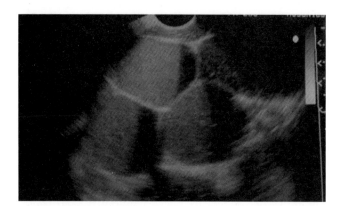

Figure 24.17 Small intestinal volvulus with ventral sedimentation. This image demonstrates fluid distended small intestine with ventral sedimentation of particulate material associated with small intestinal volvulus. Particulate matter has settled ventrally by gravity due to ileus and chronicity of the lesion. Ventral is to the left in this image. This image was obtained from the left abdomen with a curvilinear probe operating at 3.5 MHz at a depth of 15 cm.

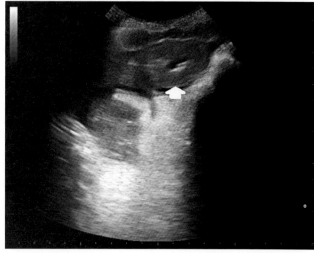

Figure 24.19 Strangulating lipoma. This image demonstrates a thickened segment of small intestine (arrow) consistent with vascular compromise from strangulating lipoma (see Figure 24.18). This sonogram was obtained from ventral abdomen with a curvilinear probe operating at 5.0 MHz at a depth of 15 cm.

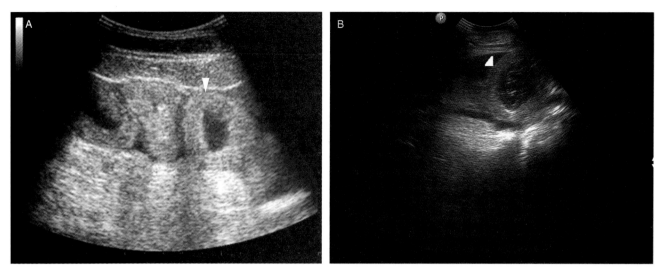

Figure 24.20 Lipoma with strangulated small intestine. (A,B) These images demonstrate strangulated, non-viable small intestine secondary to strangulation around the stalk of a lipoma. Note the thickened and echogenic intestinal walls (arrowheads) consistent with vascular engorgement and stasis and the indistinct serosal surfaces. These images were obtained from ventral abdomen, left of midline with a curvilinear probe operating at (A) 5.0 MHz at a depth of 12 cm and (B) 3.5 MHz at a depth of 20 cm.

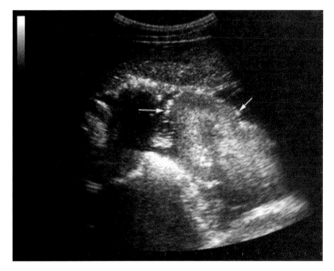

Figure 24.21 Peritonitis with fecal contamination. This image demonstrates peritonitis associated with gastric rupture following small intestinal strangulation around the stalk of a lipoma. Numerous echogenic gas bubbles (arrows) are seen adherent to the intestinal serosa and parietal peritoneal surface. Note the thickened, indistinct intestinal wall of the compromised small intestine. This sonogram was obtained from the ventral abdomen with a curvilinear probe operating at 3.5 MHz at a depth of 15 cm.

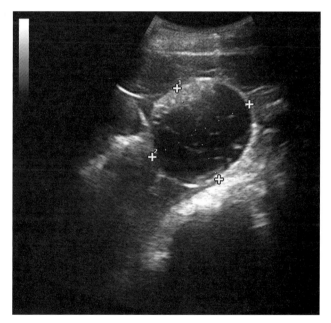

Figure 24.22 Non-strangulating entrapment of small intestine. This image demonstrates marked fluid distension of small intestine (cursors) with poor motility and ventral sedimentation of particulate material in the left ventral abdomen of an adult Quarter Horse. Non-strangulating entrapment of the small intestine associated with large colon impaction was confirmed at surgery. This sonogram was obtained from the left inguinal region with a curvilinear probe operating at 2.5 MHz at a depth of 19 cm.

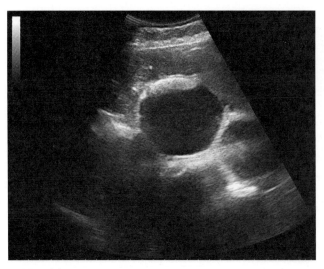

Figure 24.23 Ileal impaction. This image demonstrates poorly motile, fluid-distended small intestine with a small amount of ventral sedimentation of particulate material in the caudal–ventral right abdomen. Ileal impaction was confirmed at surgery. This image was obtained from the ventral abdomen, right of midline, with a curvilinear probe operating at 3.5 MHz at a depth of 21 cm.

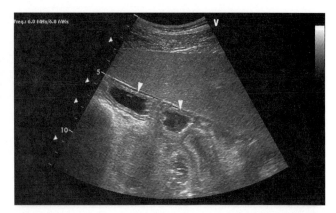

Figure 24.24 Enteritis in an adult horse. This image demonstrates thickened small intestine (arrowheads) associated with enteritis in an adult horse. Multiple echogenic foci within the small intestinal wall are consistent with inflammation. This sonogram was obtained from the left abdomen with a curvilinear probe operating at 6.0 MHz at a depth of 15 cm.

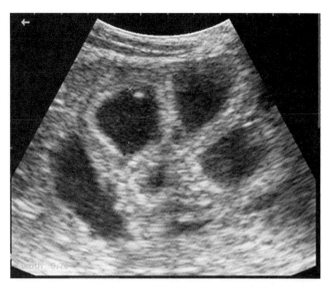

Figure 24.25 Enteritis in a foal. The small intestine has moderate fluid distention and varying degrees of motility. The walls are indistinct and echogenic consistent with inflammatory changes associated with enteritis. This sonogram was obtained from the ventral abdomen with a micro-convex probe operating at 5.0 MHz at a depth of 10 cm.

24.23) can indicate strangulating or non-strangulating obstruction, enteritis, or altered motility such as occurs with postoperative ileus. Clinical history, severity of clinical signs, and occasionally other diagnostic aids, such as abdominocentesis, are required to differentiate between these types of lesions prior to confirmation by exploratory surgery.

The observation of markedly distended, poorly motile segments of small intestine with ventral sedimentation of particulate material (Figure 24.16, 24.17, 24.22, 24.23) is most often suggestive of a strangulating lesion of the small intestine such as small intestinal volvulus, entrapment in a mesenteric tear, or epiploic foramen entrapment. However, this pattern of ultrasonographic change in the small intestine can also be observed with non-strangulating, obstructive lesions such as ileal impactions and non-strangulating entrapment of the small intestine.

Ultrasound imaging can be useful in identifying enteritis (Figure 24.24, 24.25, 24.26) as confirmation of clinical signs (colic, fever) and supportive laboratory data (leucopenia with or without hypoproteinemia). In both foals and adult horses, ultrasound may help identify enteritis by imaging thickened, variably echogenic and variably motile walls of the small intestine that often have some luminal fluid present.

Lawsonia intracellularis infection in weanling to yearling aged animals typically causes thick-walled, edematous small intestine consistent with proliferative enteritis (Figure 24.27). Edematous thickening of the large intestine may also be present as a result of marked hypoalbuminemia.

Jejunojejunal intussusception (Figure 24.28) images as multiple layers of intestine creating a "bull's eye" appearance.

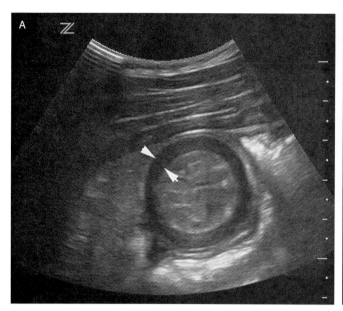
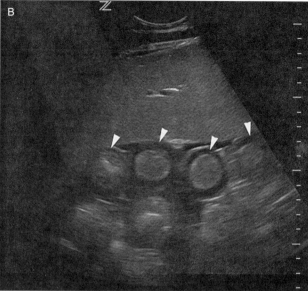

Figure 24.26 Small intestinal muscular hypertrophy. (A) This image demonstrates small intestinal muscular hypertrophy in a 7-year-old Thoroughbred stallion with clinical signs of recurrent colic secondary to non-strangulating obstruction of the small intestine. The arrows indicate the thickened, hypoechoic tunica muscularis layer of the small intestinal wall. (B) This image is another view of the same segment of small intestine showing a thick, hypoechoic layer representing hypertrophy of the tunica muscularis of the small intestine. These sonograms were obtained from left abdomen with a curvilinear probe operating at 3.5 MHz at a depth of 17 cm. (Source: Images courtesy of Dr. Sally Ness, Cornell University, Ithaca, NY, USA.)

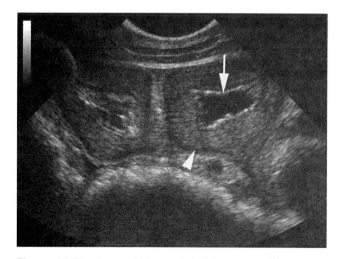

Figure 24.27 *Lawsonia intracellularis* infection. This image demonstrates marked thickening of the small intestinal wall in an 8-month-old Hanovarian colt with peripheral edema, hypoproteinemia, and hypoalbuminemia. The small intestinal changes (thickening of walls) were from proliferative enteropathy secondary to *Lawsonia intracellularis* infection. The arrowhead indicates the serosa and the arrow indicates the mucosal surface of the small intestinal wall. This sonogram was obtained from the ventral abdomen with a microconvex probe operating at 8.0 MHz at a depth of 12 cm.

LARGE INTESTINE

The large colon and cecum normally occupy much of the ventral aspect of the abdominal cavity and are identified sonographically by their location and surface appearance. The right dorsal colon (Figure 24.29) is usually identified by its position just ventral and medial to the right liver lobe. The ventral colon (Figure 24.30) is ventral-most in the abdomen and can sometimes be identified by the sacculations along its surface.

Gas produces a series of horizontal parallel reverberations on ultrasound (Figure 24.31). Gas-distended colon will produce this appearance and can be found with displacements and other obstruction of the large intestine such as impaction or enterolith.

Nephrosplenic entrapment (Figure 24.32) can be demonstrated ultrasonographically by the presence of colon within the nephrosplenic space as seen through the upper left abdominal wall and paralumbar fossa. The colon should obscure visualization of the left kidney and will occasionally displace the spleen away from the body wall.

Right dorsal displacement of the colon (Figure 24.33) can be implied by finding the medial colonic vasculature against the body wall on the right side of the abdomen. This is usually identified over several intercostal spaces, near the ventral aspect of the ribs,

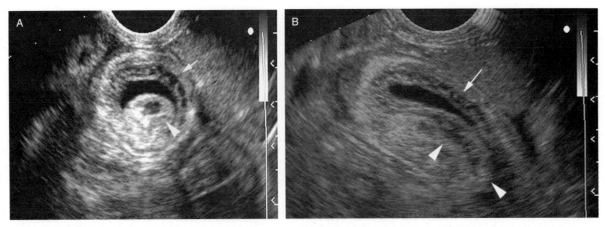

Figure 24.28 Jejunojejunal intussusception. These images demonstrate (A) cross-sectional and (B) longitudinal views of a jejunojejunal intussusception. A loop of jejunum telescoped into another loop of jejunum to create the classic "bull's eye" appearance. Note the layers consisting of the outer intussusception (arrows) and inner intussusception (arrowheads) portions. The lesion can be transient and serial ultrasonographic examination may be needed to identify the lesion. These sonograms were obtained from the ventral abdomen with a micro-convex probe operating at 5.0 MHz at a depth of 6 cm.

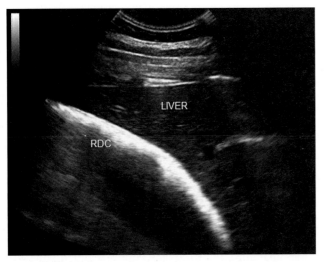

Figure 24.29 Normal right dorsal colon. The curved, echogenic surface of the luminal material of the right dorsal colon (RDC) is imaged from the right side and is located ventral and medial to the right liver lobe. Ventral is to the left in this image. This sonogram was obtained from the right ventral abdomen with a curvilinear probe operating at 6.6 MHz at a depth of 15 cm.

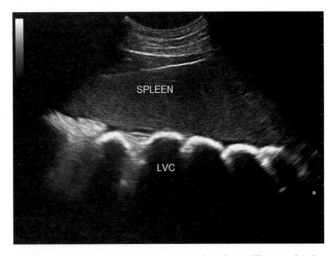

Figure 24.30 Normal left ventral colon. The multiple, short, curved echogenic structures represent the sacculations of the left ventral colon (LVC) as seen on the left side just ventral and medial to the ventral aspect of the spleen. This sonogram was obtained from the left ventral abdomen with a curvilinear probe operating at 6.6 MHz at a depth of 17 cm.

although with time, medical treatment, and mobility of the colon, the location of the vessels can change.

Right dorsal colitis (Figures 24.34, 24.35) is a unique, focal, ulcerative change in the right dorsal colon associated with a history of excessive or prolonged administration of non-steroidal anti-inflammatory medications. Ultrasound imaging can demonstrate edema and thickening of the right dorsal colon along its course on the right side of the abdomen. Serial

evaluation may be useful in following the clinical course and response to medical management.

Colitis (Figures 24.36, 24.37, 24.38) is usually differentiated clinically from other causes of colic by the lesser degree of pain and presence of fever, diarrhea, and leucopenia. In some instances, the patient will present prior to the onset of diarrhea, and ultrasound examination will be useful in providing information to support the diagnosis of colitis by demonstration of a thick, edematous colon wall.

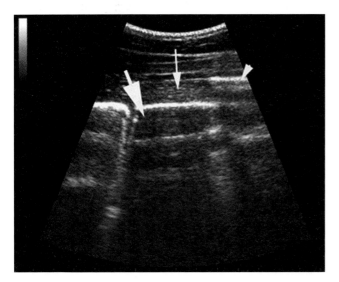

Figure 24.31 Colonic tympany. Colonic tympany images as horizontal reverberations from the colon wall. Causes for gas-distended colon include large intestinal displacement, impactions, or enteroliths. Gas-distended colon (thick arrow), the diaphragm (thin arrow), and the air-filled lung (arrowhead) are visible. This sonogram was obtained from left ventral abdomen with a curvilinear probe operating at 5.0 MHz at a depth of 12 cm.

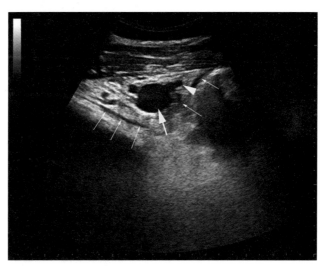

Figure 24.33 Right dorsal displacement of the colon. Right dorsal displacement of the colon may result in engorgement of the colonic vessels. Distended colonic vein (arrow) and artery (arrowhead) and medial mesocolon (long thin arrows) are imaged adjacent to the right body wall just ventral to the twelfth intercostal space. This sonogram was obtained from the right ventral abdomen with a curvilinear probe operating at 3.5 MHz at a depth of 17 cm.

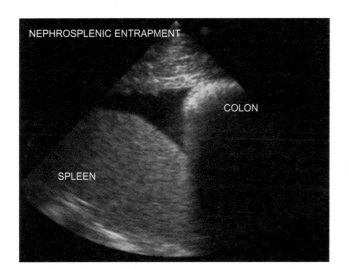

Figure 24.32 Nephrosplenic entrapment. Nephrosplenic entrapment, or left dorsal displacement of the colon, images as colon in the nephrosplenic space. The colon obscures the ultrasound view of the left kidney and may force the spleen medial off the body wall. Pockets of free peritoneal fluid may be present around the spleen and colon. This sonogram was obtained from the left lateral abdomen with a curvilinear probe operating at 3.5 MHz at a depth of 18 cm.

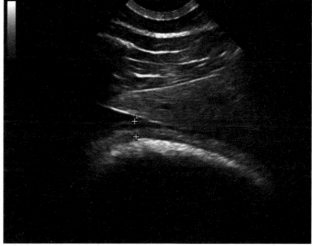

Figure 24.34 Right dorsal colitis. This image demonstrates right dorsal colitis secondary to administration of non-steroidal anti-inflammatory drugs (NSAIDs). Note the thickened wall of the right dorsal colon. This case was from a 2-year-old colt with history of NSAID use following throat surgery. The colt was febrile, hypoproteinemic, and hypoalbuminemic. This sonogram was obtained from the right abdomen with a curvilinear probe operating at 6.6 MHz at a depth of 21 cm.

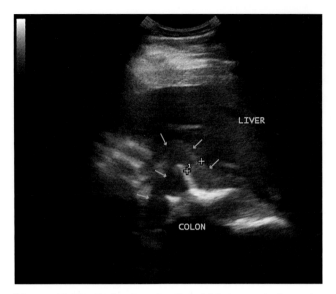

Figure 24.35   Right dorsal colitis. This image is from the patient in Figure 24.34 1 month after initial presentation. The colon wall is thickened and echogenic (cursors). A thin, hypoechoic layer below the serosa is suggestive of edema. This is compatible with mucosal fibrosis of a healing mucosal ulceration of the right dorsal colon. This sonogram was obtained from the right abdomen with a curvilinear probe operating at 6.6 MHz at a depth of 21 cm.

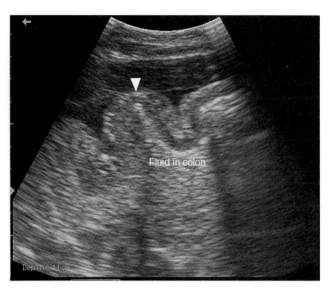

Figure 24.37   Colitis from salmonellosis. This image demonstrates thickened and edematous colon in a horse diagnosed with salmonellosis. Note the visible fluid content in the lumen of the colon. This image was obtained from the left ventral abdomen with a curvilinear probe operating at 2.0 MHz at a depth of 12 cm. (Source: Image courtesy of Dr. Nathan Slovis, Hagyard Equine Medical Institute, Lexington, KY, USA.)

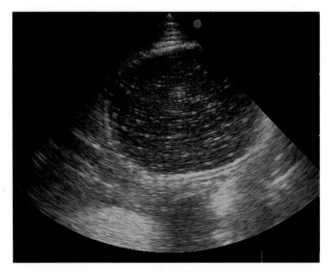

Figure 24.36   Colonic fluid. This image demonstrates increased fluid content in the lumen of the large colon. This image was obtained from the ventral abdomen with a curvilinear probe operating at 2.0 MHz at a depth of 20 cm. (Source: Image courtesy of Dr. Nathan Slovis, Hagyard Equine Medical Institute, Lexington, KY, USA.)

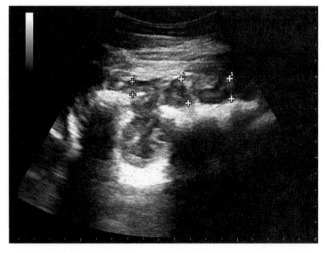

Figure 24.38   Colitis in adult. This image demonstrates a thickened and edematous colon wall from a horse with colitis. The corrugated appearance is sometimes seen with inflammatory processes. This image was obtained from the left abdomen with a curvilinear probe operating at depth of 14 cm.

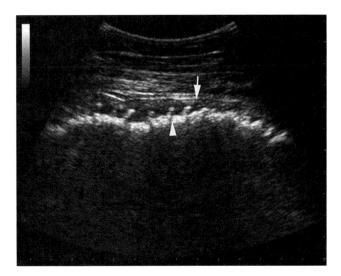

Figure 24.39 Colon torsion. Colon torsion may result in vascular compromise to the colon resulting in wall edema. This image is from a mare with colon torsion prior to surgical correction. The colon wall (arrow) is thickened and edematous. Luminal content (arrowhead) is visualized adjacent to the colon wall. This sonogram was obtained from the ventral abdomen with a curvilinear probe operating at 3.5 MHz at a depth of 11 cm.

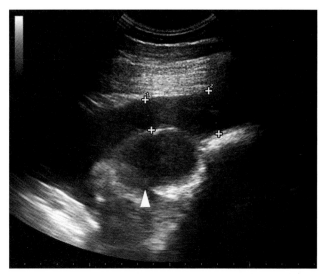

Figure 24.40 Reperfusion injury after correction of colon torsion. This image is from a 12-year-old Thoroughbred mare 12 hours after surgical correction of a colon torsion. The right dorsal colon is imaged through the tenth ICS. Thickening of the colon wall from edema (cursors) is suggestive of significant reperfusion injury. A focally, extensive, hypoechoic area (arrowhead) within the submucosa is suggestive of a submucosal hematoma. Hematoma formation within the colon wall may indicate a coagulopathy associated with large and small vessel injury secondary to the colon torsion. The mare's clinical status deteriorated and she was euthanized 6 hours after this ultrasound examination. This sonogram was obtained from the ventral abdomen with a curvilinear probe operating at 6.6 MHz at a depth of 15 cm.

Torsion or volvulus of the colon (Figures 24.39, 24.40) most often is diagnosed in a post-partum mare with acute onset of severe abdominal pain with abdominal distension and palpation of a gas-distended large intestine on rectal examination. Ultrasound can provide information as to wall thickness and potential for vascular compromise.

The cecum (Figure 24.41) can be imaged from its base in the upper right paralumbar fossa, along the costal arch, down to its apex near the ventral abdomen. The lateral vessels of the cecum can usually be seen on ultrasonography.

Cecal impaction (Figure 24.42) is most often diagnosed by rectal palpation of a firm mass within the cecal base. Ultrasonography can determine the extent of cecal distension and character of the cecal wall.

Cecocolic intussusception (Figure 24.43) can be observed on ultrasonography where the trilayer appearance of thickened, edematous, intussuscepted cecal wall is seen within the lumen of the right ventral colon. The trilayer is composed of the outermost mucosa with the central echogenic layer of muscularis and innermost layer of serosa. The intussusception can be demonstrated more easily when it is surrounded by liquid luminal content within the right ventral colon. Cecal inversion (Figure 24.44) also appears as a trilayer appearance consisting of cecal wall and the inverted cecal apex.

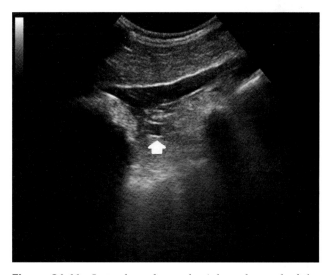

Figure 24.41 Lateral cecal vessels. A lateral vessel of the cecum (arrow) is visible just caudal to the costal arch on the right side of the abdomen. This sonogram was obtained from the right abdomen with a curvilinear probe operating at 6.6 MHz at a depth of 14 cm.

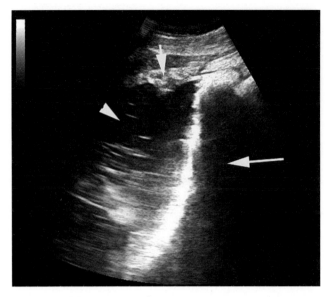

Figure 24.42 Cecal impaction. Cecal impaction is usually diagnosed by rectal palpation, but may be visible ultrasonographically. The solid, intraluminal mass (long arrow) in the cecal base is visible adjacent to the fluid-filled cecal lumen (arrowhead) ventrally. The lateral cecal wall (short arrow) is visible. This sonogram was obtained from the right lateral abdomen with a curvilinear probe operating at 2.5 MHz at a depth of 23 cm.

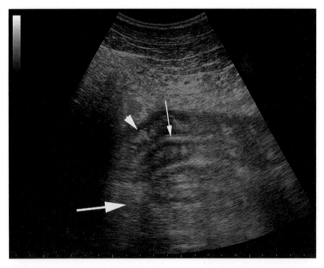

Figure 24.43 Cecocolic intussusception. The cecum is intussuscepted into the lumen of the right ventral colon (long thick arrow). The cecal mucosal surface (arrowhead) and serosal surface (long thin arrow) are visible. Cranial is to the left in this image. This sonogram was obtained from right ventral abdomen with a curvilinear probe operating at 5.0 MHz at a depth of 17 cm.

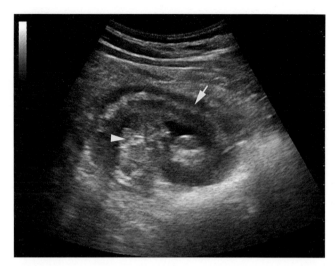

Figure 24.44 Cecal inversion. Cecal inversion images as edematous trilayer appearance of cecal wall (arrow) with inverted cecal apex (arrowhead). This lesion was present in the midventral abdomen of a weanling Quarterhorse foal with clinical signs of intermittent colic over 2 days. Cecal inversion was confirmed at surgery. This image was obtained from ventral abdomen with a curvilinear probe operating at 6.6 MHz at a depth of 13 cm.

Ultrasound changes seen with typhlitis (Figure 24.45) include thickening of the cecal base wall.

Rectum

Transrectal ultrasound may be used to image abnormalities including abscesses (Figure 24.46) in the rectum wall.

Neonatal Ultrasonography

Ultrasonography of the neonatal gastrointestinal tract is similar in technique to that of the adult, although occasional age-related differences, such as typical fluid content of the normal neonatal stomach, occur. Some unique pathologic alterations can be identified with ultrasonography of the neonatal abdomen.

Meconium impaction (Figure 24.47) represents a neonatal form of colonic obstruction. The solid meconium masses can often be demonstrated within the large and small colon on ultrasound examination. Secondary evidence of colonic obstruction with meconium can include colonic tympany. In the absence of fecal passage of meconium in a foal with sonographic

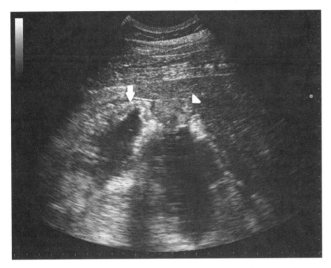

Figure 24.45   Typhlitis. The thickened wall of the cecal base (arrow) is consistent with typhlitis. The duodenum (arrowhead) is visible dorsally. This sonogram was obtained from the right lateral abdomen with a curvilinear probe operating at 6.6 MHz at a depth of 19 cm.

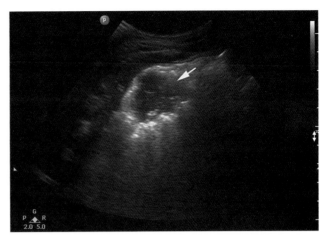

Figure 24.47   Meconium impaction. Meconium impaction is obstruction of the large intestine with meconium in neonatal foals. Solid meconium mass (arrow) images as echolucent material within the large colon. This sonogram was obtained from the right ventral abdomen with a micro-convex probe operating at 6.6 MHz at a depth of 9 cm.

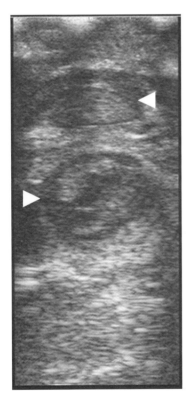

Figure 24.46   Perirectal abscess. This image shows two abscesses (arrowheads) in the dorsal wall of the rectum. This sonogram was obtained transrectally with a linear probe operating at 5.0 MHz at a depth of 8 cm. (Source: Image courtesy of Dr. Nathan Slovis, Hagyard Equine Institute, Lexington, KY, USA.)

evidence of colon tympany, the differential diagnosis of atresia coli should be considered.

RECOMMENDED READING

Bithell, S., Habershon-Butcher, J.L., Bowen, I.M., & Hallowell, G.D. (2010) Repeatability and reproducibility of transabdominal ultrasonographic intestinal wall thickness measurements in Thoroughbred horses. *Veterinary Radiology & Ultrasound*, 51(6), 647–651.

Busoni, V., De Busscher, V., Lopez, D., Verwilghen, D., & Cassart, D. (2011) Evaluation of a protocol for fast localised abdominal sonography of horses (FLASH) admitted for colic. *Veterinary Journal*, 188(1), 77–82. doi: 10.1016/j.tvjl.2010.02.017. Epub 2010 Mar 26.

Epstein, K., Short, D., Parente, E., *et al.* (2008) Gastrointestinal ultrasonography in normal adult ponies. *Veterinary Radiology & Ultrasound*, 49(3), 282–286.

Epstein, K., Short, D., Parente, E., *et al.* (2008) Serial gastrointestinal ultrasonography following exploratory celiotomy in normal adult ponies. *Veterinary Radiology & Ultrasound*, 49(6), 584–588.

Gomaa, N., Uhlig, A., & Schusser, G.F. (2011) Effect of Buscopan compositum on the motility of the duodenum, cecum and left ventral colon in healthy conscious horses. *Berliner und Münchener tierärztliche Wochenschrift*, 124(3–4), 168–174.

Hendrickson, E.H., Malone, E.D., & Sage, A.M. (2007) Identification of normal parameters for ultrasonographic examination of the equine large colon and cecum. *Canadian Veterinary Journal*, 48(3), 289–291.

Kihurani, D.O., Carstens, A., Saulez, M.N., & Donnellan, C.M. (2009) Transcutaneous ultrasonographic evaluation of the air-filled equine stomach and duodenum following gastroscopy. *Veterinary Radiology & Ultrasound*, 51(4), 429–435.

Lores, M., Stryhn, H., McDuffee, L., Rose, P., & Muirhead, T. (2007) Transcutaneous ultrasonographic evaluation of gastric distension with fluid in horses. *America Journal of Veterinary Research*, 68(2), 153–157.

Mitchell, C.F., Malone, E.D., Sage, A.M., & Nilsich, K. (2005) Evaluation of gastrointestinal activity patterns in healthy horses using B mode and Doppler ultrasonography. *Canadian Veterinary Journal*, 46(2), 134–140.

Norman, T., Chaffin, K., & Schmitz, D. (2010) Effects of fasting and intraluminal contrast enhancement on ultrasonographic appearance of the equine small intestine. *Veterinary Radiology & Ultrasound*, 51(6), 642–646.

Section 3c: Ultrasonography of Small Structures

CHAPTER TWENTY-FIVE

ULTRASONOGRAPHY OF THE EYE AND ORBIT

Caryn E. Plummer[1] and David J. Reese[2]

[1]University of Florida, Gainesville, FL, USA
[2]College of Veterinary Medicine, Murdoch University, Murdoch, WA, Australia

Ultrasonography as an examination and diagnostic tool in human and veterinary ophthalmology has been in use since the 1960s [1,2,3]. With development of portable ultrasound units, ultrasonography has grown significantly in many aspects of equine practice [2]. Strikingly, despite ease of use and availability, ultrasonography has not routinely been employed for examination of the eye and orbital structures in horses. As a non-invasive imaging technique that can be performed in the standing horse, ultrasound can provide invaluable qualitative and quantitative information about intraocular and orbital structures [4,5,6,7,8,9]. Ocular ultrasonography is indicated in cases of corneal edema, cataracts, or intraocular hemorrhage, because the normally clear ocular media has become opaque and visualization of the interior structures of the globe is restricted. It is indicated in ocular trauma and when eyelid swelling prevents access to the globe. Ultrasonography may also provide biometric data, such as absolute and relative size and positions of ocular and orbital structures [8,9,10,11]. Measurement of the fetal eye size has even been used as a tool for predicting parturition in horses [12]. Ultrasound measurements of preoperative axial globe length is an important criterion for the calculation of diopter strength of artificial lens implants when performing lens replacement surgery [13,14,15].

Technological advancements have introduced various methods of ultrasonography to the field of ophthalmology. The original form, known as amplitude modulation (A-mode), displays echoes received by the transducer in one dimension and relative to time as vertical amplitudes from a baseline [3,5]. The height of each spike represents the intensity of the echo and the spacing of the spikes represents the spatial distribution of the structures being examined. This technique is the method of choice for *in vivo* measurements of intraocular distances such as depth of anterior and vitreal chambers, lens thickness, and axial globe length. Vector A-scan can be combined with brightness mode (B-mode) ultrasound to provide information on both the topography of a lesion (B-mode) and objective information on the lesion size and character (A-mode) [4]. The most commonly employed method of ultrasonography in clinical ophthalmology, however, is B-mode using a 10 MHz transducer with a 3–4 cm focal range and a small scan head [4,5]. Lower-frequency probes, such as 5 MHz and 7.5 MHz, may also provide adequate images and will image deeper tissues for examination of retrobulbar lesions. Color Doppler technique is used to visualize blood vessels and their flow characteristics within the eye and orbit. Normal reference values for blood velocity and vascular resistance patterns have not yet been determined in the equine eye, so comparing these parameters between seemingly normal and diseased eyes is not possible. This tool is helpful, however, in determining if a structure, such as an intraocular or orbital mass lesion, is vascular or avascular.

The latest form of ultrasonography to be employed for diagnostic purposes in the veterinary patient is high-frequency ultrasound biomicroscopy [16,17]. This method is similar to traditional B-mode ultrasonography but uses frequencies between 50 and 100 MHz. With this technique, tissue resolution is dramatically improved, permitting visualization and discrimination of structures as small as 50 μm, nearly on par with microscopic resolution [16,17]. However, tissue penetration is limited to depths of only 4–5 mm and the horse must be heavily sedated or placed under general anesthesia to avoid any movement and potential artifact. In the horse, this typically permits examination of the cornea, sclera, iridocorneal angle, and part of the anterior chamber. The clinical value of

Atlas of Equine Ultrasonography, First Edition. Edited by Jessica A. Kidd, Kristina G. Lu, and Michele L. Frazer.
© 2014 John Wiley & Sons, Ltd. Published 2014 by John Wiley & Sons, Ltd.
Companion Website: www.wiley.com/go/kidd/equine-ultrasonography

the technique in the horse eye is in determining depth and extent of lesions (e.g. corneolimbal squamous cell carcinoma) in the cornea and rostral sclera, especially prior to surgical intervention [4,16,17]. Transducers with frequencies between 25 and 50 MHz are available and allow examination of the anterior chamber. As with traditional B-mode transducers, these lower-operating-frequency transducers have a lower resolution compared to the higher-frequency transducers. However, these transducers are less prone to artifacts and may be used in standing, sedated animals.

ULTRASONOGRAPHIC TECHNIQUE IN THE NORMAL EYE

Ocular and orbital ultrasonography is usually easily performed in the standing horse following sedation, an auriculopalpebral nerve block, and the application of topical anesthetic (e.g. proparacaine, tetracaine) to the ocular surface. The examination can be performed by placing the transducer directly on the cornea or by scanning through the closed eyelids [1,2,3,4,5,6,7]. The best possible image of the globe and orbit is achieved by placing the transducer directly on the cornea with coupling gel as a standoff medium. Scanning through closed eyelids or with a standoff device may produce sound attenuation and, therefore, may require an increase in gain setting. However, it facilitates examination of the anterior segment and is recommended in cases of corneal injury, ocular trauma, or following intraocular surgery to avoid further damage to the cornea. Standard ultrasound coupling gels should be avoided during examination of the eye and orbital structures since they can cause ocular surface irritation. Sterile methocellulose gel, such as K-Y jelly, is preferred and should be irrigated from the eye upon completion of the examination.

The eye is routinely examined in both vertical and horizontal planes through the visual axis by initially using the lens as a landmark for orientation. Once the examiner is oriented, the transducer is carefully and slowly directed off of the central axis, either rostrolateral or dorsoventral. The meridian between 12 o'clock and 6 o'clock is examined in the vertical axis, while the meridian between 9 o'clock and 3 o'clock is examined in the horizontal axis. In each plane, the transducer should be slightly tilted both dorsally and ventrally to examine the most peripheral portions of the spherical globe. Oblique positioning can sometimes add useful additional information. When orbital lesions are a concern, the transducer can also be positioned dorsal to the zygomatic arch and over the supraorbital fossa [4]. If the fellow eye in a patient is normal, it can serve as control for comparison purposes.

As with other structures of the body, ultrasonographic images of the eye are described as anechoic, hypoechoic, or hyperechoic (Figure 25.1). Four main

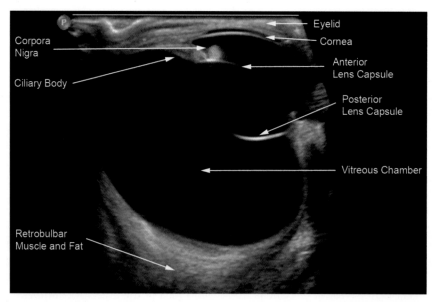

Figure 25.1 Normal anatomic structures in the eye. This image shows normal anatomic structures labeled in a normal equine eye. The anterior cornea, anterior lens capsule, posterior lens capsule, ciliary body, and extraocular muscles are hyperechoic structures. The corpora nigra is a well defined, hyperechoic structure located at the pupillary margin and extending into the anterior chamber. The anterior, posterior, and vitreal chambers should be anechoic in the normal eye.

ocular acoustic echoes are generated within the normal eye. These hyperechoic structures are the anterior cornea, anterior lens capsule, posterior lens capsule, and retina/choroid/sclera (as a single entity since these structures cannot normally be differentiated from one another with standard ultrasonography) [1,2,3,4,5,6,9]. Additionally, more hypoechoic, echogenicities can be generated by the iris, corpora nigra, ciliary body, optic nerve, orbital fat, and extraocular muscles [1,2,3,4,5,6,9]. The corpora nigrum typically appears as a well defined hyperechoic structure protruding into the anterior chamber at the pupillary margin. The anterior, posterior, and vitreal chambers, as well as the lens cortex and nucleus, are normally anechoic. The optic nerve head is typically hyperechoic, while the remainder of the nerve as it courses posterior is a relatively hypoechoic structure [1,2,3,4,5,6,9]. The orbital muscle cone, as it extends posterior from the equator to converge at the orbital apex, is a hyperechoic structure surrounding the optic nerve [1,2,3,4,5,6,9].

ULTRASONOGRAPHIC CHANGES IN THE ABNORMAL EYE

See Figures 25.2, 25.3, 25.4, 25.5, 25.6, 25.7, 25.8, 25.9, 25.10, 25.11, 25.12, 25.13, 25.14, 25.15, 25.16, 25.17, 25.18.

Anterior Segment

The anterior segment consists of the ocular structures anterior to and including the crystalline lens. Detailed examination of the cornea, particularly the layers, is not possible without a high-frequency transducer and a standoff device, but overall corneal integrity can be

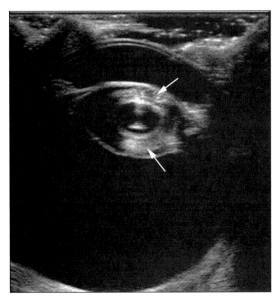

Figure 25.3 Cataract. The hyperechoic material (arrows) in the region of the lens cortex is a cataract. In the normal eye, only the anterior and posterior lens capsule should generate hyperechoic margins.

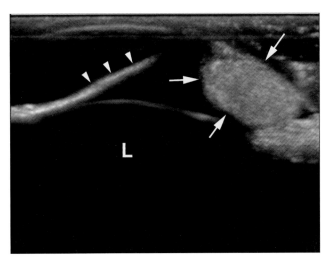

Figure 25.2 Anterior uveal mass lesion. A homogeneous neoplastic mass (arrows) arises from the base of the iris and protrudes into the anterior chamber and contacts the endothelial surface of the cornea. Arrowheads delineate the continuation of the peripheral iris leaflet. L: crystalline lens.

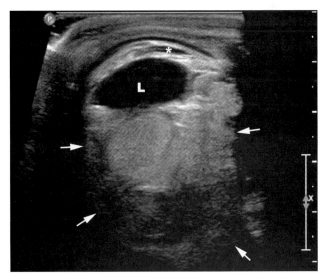

Figure 25.4 Ocular trauma. This image shows the crystalline lens (L) anteriorly luxated after trauma to the eye. The anterior chamber (*) is shallow. Hemorrhage has occurred in the vitreal chamber (arrows).

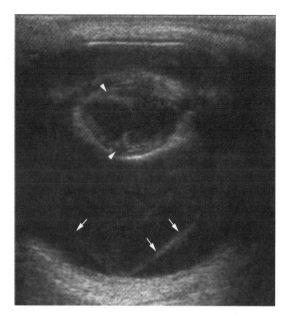

Figure 25.5 Cataract and retinal detachment. The anterior and posterior lens cortices have cataractous changes (arrowheads). Retinal elevation (arrows) is seen indicating retinal detachment. Note that the retina remains attached at the level of the optic nerve head.

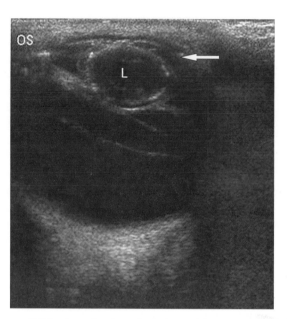

Figure 25.7 Anterior lens luxation with anterior uveitis and vitreal debris. This image is from an adult horse with chronic anterior uveitis. Note the shallow anterior chamber (arrow) and the position of the lens (L) within the anterior chamber in front of the iris leaflets. Thin, hyperechoic strands behind the iris represent vitreal debris, likely fibrin and vitreal degeneration.

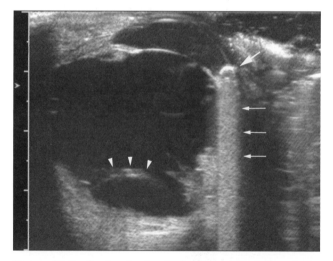

Figure 25.6 Ocular foreign body. A metallic foreign body (large arrow) is located in the ventral anterior chamber. Note the comet tail artifact (arrows) from the foreign body. A partial retinal detachment (arrowheads) is also present.

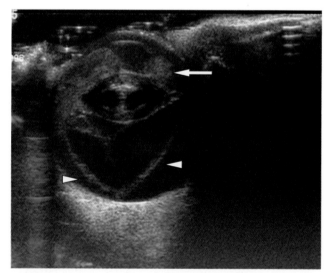

Figure 25.8 Cataract with retinal detachment, fibrin, and hyphema in the anterior chamber. This image is from an adult horse following blunt trauma to the globe. The anterior chamber (arrow) is obscured with hyperechoic material which is consistent with hyphema. The increased echogenicity of the lenticular fibers represents cataract. The thin, hyperechoic lines in the vitreal chamber (arrowheads) represent a complete retinal detachment. Note the attachments that remain at the level of the optic disc and near the ora ciliaris retinae near the equator, which provide the classic "seagull" sign indicative of retinal detachment.

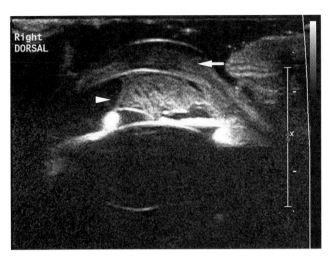

Figure 25.9 Corneal stromal abscess with fibrin and hypopyon in the anterior chamber. This image is from an adult horse with profound increase in corneal thickness (arrow). The increased echogenicity within the cornea is the result of a corneal stromal abscess and corresponding edema. This condition is typically accompanied by significant anterior uveitis, which is evidenced here by miosis (small pupil, note the location of the corpora nigrum and the dependent iris leaflet nearer to the central axis of the eye than usual) and fibrin within the anterior chamber (arrowhead).

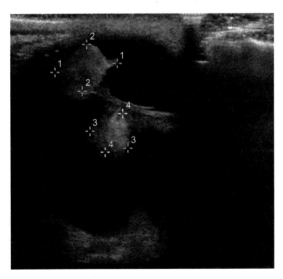

Figure 25.10 Iris and ciliary body. This image is from an adult horse presenting for evaluation of an iris mass. This is an image of a peripheral section of the eye. Two mass lesions are appreciated: one (1–2) is associated with the iris and is protruding into the anterior chamber and the other mass (3–4) is located within the posterior chamber and is associated with the ciliary body. Both lesions were contiguous in other sections and were diagnosed as melanoma from histopathology.

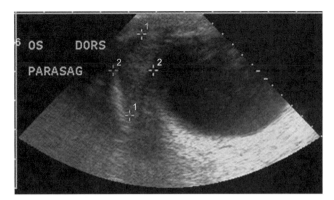

Figure 25.11 Lacrimal gland abscess. This image is from an adult horse presenting with swelling underneath the upper eyelid. This image was acquired by placing the transducer above the eyelid and imaging from the dorsal plane. Note the mixed echogenic mass lesion dorsal to the globe. This was an abscess within the orbital lacrimal gland.

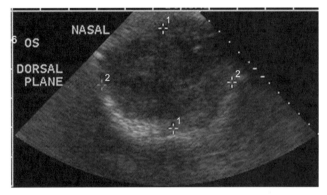

Figure 25.12 Lacrimal gland abscess. This image is an abscess within the dorsal orbital lacrimal gland. Note the distinctly hyperechoic gland capsule and the mixed echogenic center.

assessed with traditional transducers. This is especially true in ocular trauma, when the contour of the cornea may be altered. Ocular trauma, both penetrating and blunt, can result in significant intraocular changes. The anterior chamber may be shallow and contain fibrin, hypopyon, or hyphema, which often results in an increase in echogenicity associated with the aqueous humor. Lenticular changes may occur, such as cataracts, lens capsule ruptures, partial or complete lens luxations, or expulsions of the lens through a corneal or scleral rent [4,6].

In inflammatory conditions, regardless of etiology, infiltrates may be present that are appreciable with ultrasound. Fibrin typically appears as well defined, hyperechoic, disconnected strands throughout the

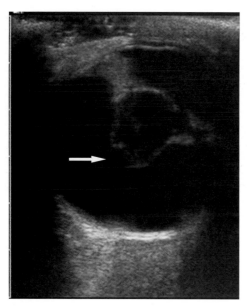

Figure 25.13 Posterior lens capsule rupture. This image is from an adult horse presenting for acute worsening of anterior uveitis. A cataract was noted in the lens and the integrity of the posterior lens capsule was compromised, consistent with a capsular rupture (arrow), resulting in exposure of intralenticular antigen and phacoclastic uveitis.

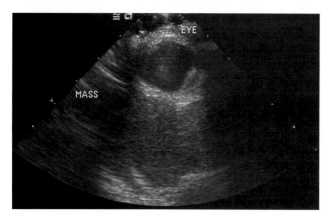

Figure 25.14 Retrobulbar mass. This image is from an adult horse presenting for exophthalmos and exposure keratitis. A hyperechoic mass lesion is present posterior to the globe. The contour of the posterior globe is abnormal, suggesting that the mass lesion is deforming the globe. Histopathology of a biopsy sample confirmed a diagnosis of squamous cell carcinoma.

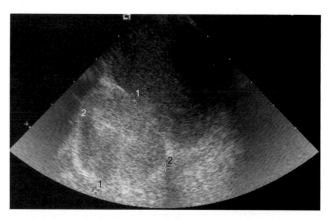

Figure 25.15 Retrobulbar abscess. This image is from an adult horse presenting for exophthalmos. A hyperechoic mass (1–2) is present posterior to the globe that is deforming the posterior contour of the globe.

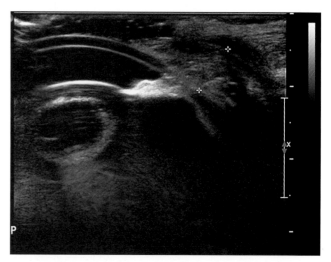

Figure 25.16 Lymphoma with severe chemosis and normal globe. This image is from an adult horse presenting for severe chemosis. The asterisks mark the borders of the globe and the eyelid which should be in contact in the normal state. The intervening space is filled with severely thickened and edematous conjunctiva. Histopathology of a biopsy sample from the conjunctiva confirmed a diagnosis of lymphoma. The circular or ring opacity within the lens delineates the lens cortex from its nucleus and is a marker of nuclear sclerosis.

anterior chamber [4,6]. Hypopyon results in homogeneous, hyperechoic material in the ventral aspect of the chamber [4,6]. Hyphema is usually hyperechoic and may be located ventrally if it is beginning to settle. If it has not settled or if intraocular hemorrhage continues, hyphema appears as echogenic aqueous humor throughout the anterior chamber. The iris and ciliary body may appear thickened or have deviations from the normal echogenicity when inflamed.

Anterior segment mass lesions may be inflammatory, neoplastic, or cystic in origin [4,5,6,18]. In the horse, they typically arise from, or are associated with, the anterior uvea and protrude into the anterior chamber. Pigmented lesions that cannot be transilluminated on clinical examination may be either melano-

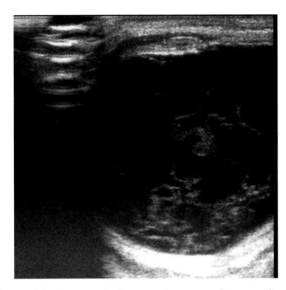

Figure 25.17 Vitreal degeneration secondary to chronic uveitis. Chronic inflammation in this horse with equine recurrent uveitis resulted in severe vitreal degeneration. Note the wispy, flowing, linear opacities the vitreal chamber. These are often observed to float about during ultrasonographic examination if the patient moves the globe.

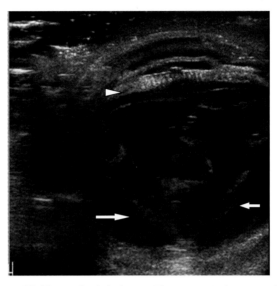

Figure 25.18 Endophthalmitis. This image is from an adult horse following a penetrating wound to the globe. Note the complete retinal detachment (arrows) and profound thickening of uveal tissue (arrowhead). A vitreal aspirate revealed the presence of a *Streptococcus* spp. within the globe.

mas or cysts. Cysts of the corpora nigra are relatively common in the horse and have a hyperechoic wall with an anechoic (fluid-filled) center. Neoplastic lesions, such as intraocular melanomas, are usually hyperechoic and homogeneous. Space-occupying intraocular lesions will occasionally displace normal intraocular structures such as the lens or iris leaflets.

Normally, the lens appears as two distinct hyperechogenicities: a slightly convex echo at the anterior capsule and a slightly concave echo at the posterior capsule. The center of the lens is anechoic and lens equators are not visible [4,6]. When a cataract is present, the internal reflectivity of the lens increases and internal echoes are visible. Also, the periphery (equator) of the lens will be more easily visualized. The stage and location of the cataract will determine the ultrasonographic appearance, but, typically, the more mature the cataract, the stronger and brighter the internal echoes. Lens capsule ruptures can be difficult to confirm, but they often appear as irregularities along the normally smooth capsular margin, often with hyperechoic material either extruding from the lens or attaching to the surface. Lens size can be appreciated as well. Hypermature, resorbing cataracts or microphakic lenses will be decreased in size as measured from anterior to posterior along the central axis. Lens luxations or subluxations will present with alterations in the relative depth of the anterior and vitreal chambers [1,2,3,4,5,6,7,19].

Posterior Segment

The posterior segment includes the vitreal chamber, the posterior wall of the globe, and the anterior-most section of the optic nerve. Ultrasonographic evaluation of the posterior segment is most commonly employed in trauma or if a cataract is present and precludes clinical examination of the fundus [1,2,3,4,5,6,7,13,19,20]. Ocular trauma can result in vitreal hemorrhage, retinal detachments and tears, choroidal detachments, and sclera ruptures that may be visualized ultrasonographically [4,5,6,19,20]. This information is crucial to clinical decision making and estimations of prognosis. Preoperative ultrasonography is a critical step in determining if the retina is in correct anatomic position prior to cataract removal and to determine if surgery is indicated [13,19].

Abnormalities of the vitreous appear as echogenicities within the normally anechoic space. Vitreal degeneration, either post-inflammatory or age-related, will appear as either linear hyperechoic structures or multiple hyperechoic foci in the central vitreal cavity [4,5,6,19]. Increase the far-field gain setting during scanning of the vitreous to help detect subtle lesions that might otherwise go unnoticed [4]. Vitreal hemorrhage appears as discrete to diffuse medium echogenicities that may appear to float, particularly if acute. Vitreous inflammation, either fibrinous or cellular, appears as disconnected and irregular, multifocal, hyperechoic material.

The discrete retinal echo is normally indistinguishable from the choroidal and scleral echoes unless pathology is present. A retinal detachment appears as a continuous, thin, linear, hyperechoic structure protruding into the vitreal chamber. Most commonly, the retina remains attached at the optic nerve and ora ciliaris retinae, resulting in a gull-wing appearance; however, partial detachments or disinsertions can be present and will not present the classic "sea-gull" sign [1,2,3,4,5,6,7,19,20]. Early detachments will often undulate in real-time, but more chronic detachments will fibrose and become fixed. Examination of the subretinal space should be performed. An anechoic space suggests fluid such as a transudate; while a hyperechoic appearance may indicate neoplasia, inflammatory infiltrate, or subretinal hemorrhage.

If the posterior globe has been ruptured, the normal bright echo of the retinal/choroidal/scleral unit will be disrupted. Irregular shaped hyperechoic material in the vitreal chamber and a homogeneous structure in the orbit posterior to the globe suggestive of hemorrhage are typically visualized with rupture. The optic nerve may not be visualized or may be displaced.

Orbit

Exophthalmos and trauma are the most common indications for orbital ultrasonography. The size, character, and location of lesions within the orbit can be determined. Orbital masses (neoplasia, hemorrhage, cellulitis, or abscessation) may be characterized as solid or cystic; further characterization usually requires additional diagnostics [1,2,3,4,5,6,7]. Ultrasound-guided aspiration and biopsy are useful tools for diagnosis and therapeutic planning. Ultrasonography after traumatic insults is useful to evaluate the retrobulbar space for displaced orbital fractures, hemorrhage, compression or entrapment of the optic nerve, and loss of integrity of the posterior wall of the globe [1,2,3,4,5,6,7,19]. Although ultrasonography is a useful first step, more advanced imaging techniques, such as computed tomography or magnetic resonance imaging, may be necessary to determine the extent of an orbital disease process, especially if neoplasia is present [5].

Most orbital abnormalities will generally have a more homogeneous appearance than the normal, varied orbital tissue. If they are large enough to produce clinical signs, they should be easily detected with ultrasound [4,5,6]. The echogenicity of the lesion will depend upon its cause and severity. Inflammatory conditions often exhibit hypoechoic regions, especially if pockets of exudates appear, while neoplastic conditions are typically characterized by more hyperechoic lesions [5].

Another condition that may be diagnosed with orbital ultrasonography is dacryoadenitis. Patients present with severe eyelid swelling and ultrasonography will reveal an enlarged structure protruding from under the dorsal orbital rim. The inflamed lacrimal gland will have a mottled, slightly heterogeneous appearance [21]. The non-inflamed gland is difficult to visualize due to its location under the dorsal orbital rim.

ARTIFACTS

Acoustic artifacts may confound examination of the eye and orbital structures. Reverberation artifacts are especially common and may occur from air trapped between the transducer and the eye (especially with transpalpebral examinations) or from a particularly reflective structure, such as the lens capsule, an artificial lens implant, the sclera, or an orbital bone [19]. The most common reverberation artifact occurs from the lens capsule and appears as evenly spaced repeating hyperechoic lines in the mid to posterior axial vitreous and can be confused with hemorrhage, inflammation, or degeneration [4,5,6]. Another artifact that may confuse the examiner is Baum's bumps, also known as a speed propagation artifact [6]. These are artifacts that appear as retinal elevations and may masquerade as retinal lesions. They occur because the sound from the transducer travels more quickly through the peripheral lens than the center, so the posterior wall appears closer to the probe, resulting in discrete bumps. Imaging the region in a different axis may help differentiate a true lesion from an artifact. Shadowing artifacts may occur with dense cataracts or intraocular foreign bodies. Artifacts can be distinguished from true lesions by their tendencies to remain equidistant from an anterior structure, to decrease in strength, and to move with movement of the transducer.

REFERENCES

[1] Rubin, L.F. & Koch, S.A. (1968) Ocular diagnostic ultrasonography. *Journal of the American Veterinary Medical Association*, 153(12), 1706–1716.

[2] Rantanen, N.W. & Ewing, R.L. (1981) Principles of ultrasound application in animals. *Veterinary Radiology*, 22, 196–203.

[3] Ossoinig, K.C. (1979) Standardized echography: basic principles, clinical applications, and results. *International Ophthalmology Clinics*, 19, 127–210.

[4] Gilger, B.C. & Stoppini, R. (2011) Equine ocular examination: routine and advanced diagnostic techniques. In: *Equine Ophthalmology*, 2nd edn. (ed. B.C. Gilger). Elsevier, Maryland Heights, 1–51.

[5] Dietrich, U.M. (2007) Ophthalmic examination and diagnostics: diagnostic ultrasonography. In: *Veterinary Ophthalmology*, 4th edn. (ed. K.N. Gelatt). Blackwell Publishing, Ames, 507–519.

[6] Williams, J. & Wilkie, D. (1996) Ultrasonography of the eye. *Compendium of Continuing Education for the Practicing Veterinarian*, 8, 667–677.

[7] Eisenberg, H.M. (1985) Ultrasonography of the eye and orbit. *Veterinary Clinics of North America: Small Animal Practice*,15(6), 1263–1274.

[8] Rogers, M. & Cartee, R. (1986) Evaluation of the extirpated equine eye using B-mode ultrasonography. *Veterinary Radiology*, 27, 24–29.

[9] Byrne, S.F. & Green, R.L. (2002) *Ultrasound of the Eye and Orbit*, 2nd edn. Mosby, St. Louis.

[10] Grinninger, P., Skalicky, M., & Nell, B. (2010) Evaluation of healthy equine eyes by use of retinoscopy, keratometry, and ultrasonographic biometry. *American Journal of Veterinary Research*, 71(6), 677–681.

[11] Plummer C.E., Ramsey D.T., Hauptman J.G. (2003) Assessment of corneal thickness, intraocular pressure, optical corneal diameter, and axial globe dimensions in Miniature Horses. *American Journal of Veterinary Research*, 64(6), 661–665.

[12] Turner, R.M., McDonnell, S.M., Feit, E.M., Grogan, E.H., & Foglia, R. (2006) Real-time ultrasound measure of the fetal eye (vitreous body) for prediction of parturition date in small ponies. *Theriogenology*, 66(2), 331–337.

[13] McMullen, R.J. Jr & Utter, M.E. (2010) Current developments in equine cataract surgery. *Equine Veterinary Journal*, suppl 37, 38–45.

[14] McMullen, R.J. Jr & Gilger, B.C. (2006) Keratometry, biometry and prediction of intraocular lens power in the equine eye. *Veterinary Ophthalmology*, 9(5), 357–360.

[15] McMullen, R.J., Davidson, M.G., Campbell, N.B., Salmon, J.H., & Gilger, B.C. (2010) Evaluation of 30- and 25-diopter intraocular lens implants in equine eyes after surgical extraction of the lens. *American Journal of Veterinary Research*, 71(7), 809–816.

[16] Bentley, E., Miller, P.E., & Diehl, K.A. (2003) Use of high-resolution ultrasound as a diagnostic tool in veterinary ophthalmology. *Journal of the American Veterinary Medical Association*, 223(11), 1617–1622.

[17] Dietrich, U. & Moore, P.A. (2002) Clinical application of ultrasound biomicroscopy in veterinary ophthalmology (abstract). *Veterinary Ophthalmology*, 5, 292.

[18] Miller, W.W. & Cartee, R.E. (1985) B-scan ultrasonography for the detection of space-occupying ocular masses. *Journal of the American Veterinary Medical Association*, 187(1), 66–68.

[19] Scotty, N.C., Cutler, T.J., Brooks, D.E., & Ferrell, E. (2004) Diagnostic ultrasonography of equine lens and posterior segment abnormalities. *Veterinary Ophthalmology*, 7(2), 127–139.

[20] Strobel, B.W., Wilkie, D.A., & Gilger, B.C. (2007) Retinal detachment in horses: 40 cases (1998–2005). *Veterinary Ophthalmology*, 10(6), 380–385.

[21] Reimer, J.M. & Latimer, C.S. (2011) Ultrasound findings in horses with severe eyelid swelling, and recognition of acute dacryoadenitis: 10 cases (2004–2010). *Veterinary Ophthalmology*, 14(2), 86–92.

CHAPTER TWENTY-SIX

ULTRASONOGRAPHY OF THE SOFT TISSUE STRUCTURES OF THE NECK

Massimo Magri

Clinica Veterinaria Spirano, Spirano (BG), Italy

PREPARATION AND SCANNING TECHNIQUE

Optimal equipment for ultrasonography of structures of the neck should include a high frequency, 10–12 MHz linear probe and a 6.6 MHz micro-convex probe. These two probes allow visualization with maximal definition of both superficial and deep structures. However, many structures of the neck can be visualized using only a 5–7.5 MHz linear probe typically used for equine obstetrics. Best images are obtained by clipping the hair with a surgical clipper blade and applying coupling gel; however, alcohol will also serve as an adequate contact medium. Ideally, place an examination glove or similar over the probe because continued exposure to coupling gel, particularly alcohol, can cause degradation of the probe and potentially affect image quality and life span of the probe (Figure 26.1).

Orientation of the probe must be kept constant over time to obtain comparable images. When scanning in the longitudinal axis (Figure 26.2A), orientate the probe so that distal structures are on the left side of the screen and proximal structures are on the right (Figure 26.2B). When scanning in the cross (short) axis (Figure 26.2C), orientate the probe so that ventral structures are on the left side of the screen and dorsal structures are on the right (Figure 26.2D).

Structures visualized when scanning the neck include major blood vessels (jugular veins and carotid arteries), parotid salivary glands, guttural pouches, thyroid glands, lymph nodes, esophagus, trachea, and

muscle (Figure 26.3). All structures are bilateral, except for the esophagus, trachea, sternohyoideus muscle, and sternothyroideus muscle, so suspect images can be compared to the opposite side assuming a lesion or abnormality is unilateral.

JUGULAR VEIN

The jugular vein (Figures 26.4, 26.5, 26.6, 26.7, 26.8, 26.9, 26.10, 26.11) is visible in the jugular groove, from the mandibular branch to the thoracic inlet. Normally, it is thin walled and easily compressible with the ultrasound probe. The blood inside the jugular vein has a hyperechoic, swirling appearance when compared to blood in the adjacent carotid artery. The distal part of the vein should be compressed to dilate the proximal portion of the vessel being scanned to aid in correctly visualizing all the structures, including the valves of the vein. Valves are normal structures that can easily be confused with a small thrombus. Valves appear as thin structures adjacent to the walls of the vessel and move in synchrony with blood flow.

Ultrasound of the jugular vein can confirm correct placement of an intravenous catheter in the vessel lumen and may aid in detecting early signs of thrombus formation associated with the catheter, although thrombi may also form in the jugular vein in the absence of an intravenous catheter or any other known trauma to the vessel. Thrombi appear as hyperechoic structures in the vessel lumen or attached to the vessel

Atlas of Equine Ultrasonography, First Edition. Edited by Jessica A. Kidd, Kristina G. Lu, and Michele L. Frazer.
© 2014 John Wiley & Sons, Ltd. Published 2014 by John Wiley & Sons, Ltd.
Companion Website: www.wiley.com/go/kidd/equine-ultrasonography

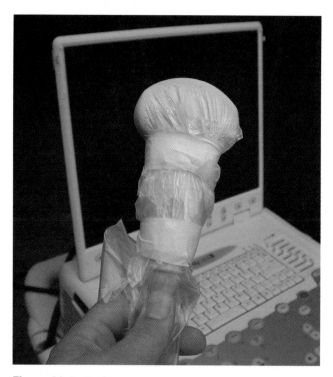

Figure 26.1 Probe protection. Protect the probe from coupling gel or alcohol with an examination glove or similar covering.

wall. Margins may be smooth and well demarcated or pedunculated in appearance. If an intravenous catheter is in the vein, a fibrin envelope or sleeve may be visualized around the catheter before a thrombus forms [1]. Initially, blood flow is maintained, but the thrombus may increase in size to cause inflammation of the vessel (thrombophlebitis) and, potentially, complete occlusion of the vessel. Other changes associated with thrombophlebitis include perivasculitis of the surrounding soft tissue and thickening of the vessel wall [1].

CAROTID ARTERY

The carotid artery (Figures 26.4, 26.5, 26.6, 26.8) is visible in the jugular groove medial to the jugular vein and lateral to the trachea. The wall is thicker than that of the jugular vein and the vessel is not compressible. The blood is hypoechoic compared to blood in the jugular vein. In the proximal neck, the carotid artery is separated from the jugular vein by the omohyoideus muscle, but in the middle and distal neck, the muscle thins and the carotid artery and jugular vein are in close proximity to each other.

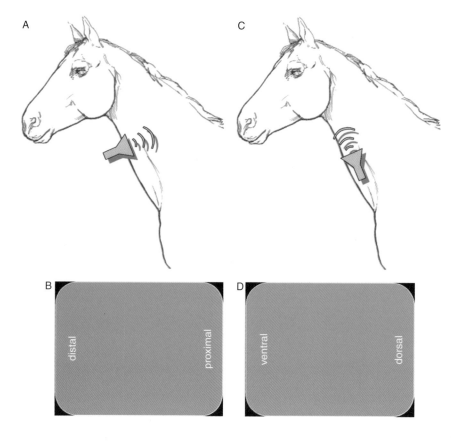

Figure 26.2 Probe orientation. (A) This image shows orientation of probe for obtaining longitudinal view. (B) Position the probe so the distal aspect of the neck is on the left side of the screen and the proximal aspect is on the right. (C) This image shows orientation of probe for cross-sectional view. (D) Position the probe so the ventral aspect of the neck is on the left side of the screen and the dorsal is on the right.

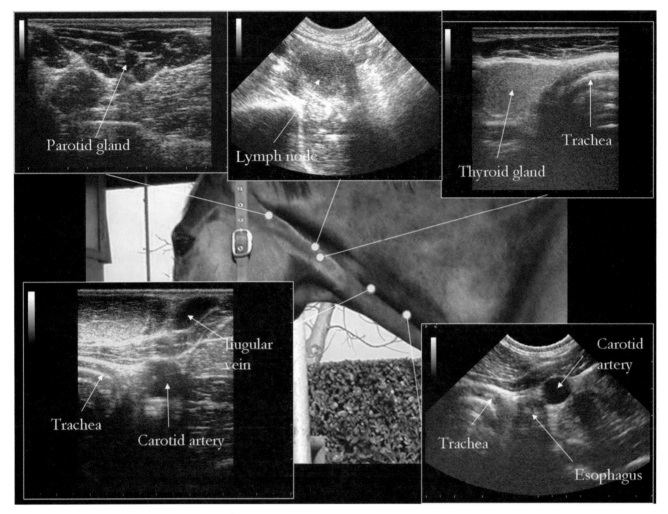

Figure 26.3 The main ultrasound sites and associated structures in the neck. This picture illustrates areas on the neck to obtain images of the parotid gland, lymph nodes, thyroid gland, trachea, carotid artery, jugular vein, and esophagus.

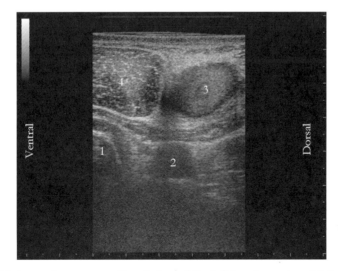

Figure 26.4 Jugular vein. This image is a cross-sectional view of the left jugular region obtained from a normal adult horse. The jugular vein (3) has been occluded in the distal cervical region. Therefore, the jugular vein remains distended when pressure is applied from the ultrasound probe. The blood inside the vein has a hyperechoic, swirling appearance. The carotid artery (2) is deeper than the jugular vein and the blood has a hypoechoic appearance. The trachea (1) is on the median axis. This sonogram was obtained with a wide-bandwidth 10.0 MHz linear array transducer, operating at 12.0 MHz, at a display depth of 6 cm.

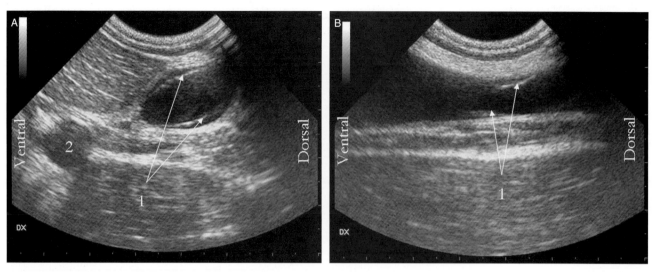

Figure 26.5 Jugular vein. These images are (A) cross-sectional and (B) longitudinal views of the left jugular region from a normal adult horse. Valves (1) are visualized adjacent to the vessel wall. The carotid artery (2) is deep to the jugular vein. This sonogram was obtained with a wide-bandwidth 6.6 MHz micro-convex linear array transducer, operating at 8.0 MHz, at a display depth of 5 cm.

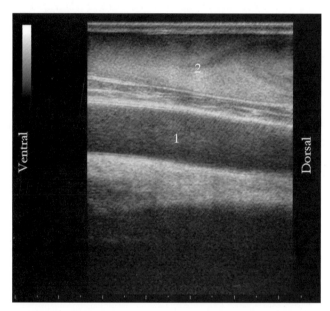

Figure 26.6 Jugular vein. This image is a longitudinal view of the left jugular region obtained from a normal adult horse. The carotid artery (1) is deep to the jugular vein (2). The jugular vein has a thin wall, while the carotid artery has a thick wall. Blood in the carotid artery is hypoechoic, while blood in the jugular vein is hyperechoic and swirling. This sonogram was obtained with a wide-bandwidth 10.0 MHz linear array transducer, operating at 12.0 MHz, at a display depth of 5 cm.

GUTTURAL POUCHES

The guttural pouches are ventral diverticula of the eustachian tube and extend from the nasopharynx to the middle ear. They contain air and have a capacity of 300–500 ml in adults. These structures are usually not detectable by ultrasound examination except in the diseased state.

Guttural pouch tympany (Figure 26.12) occurs in young animals, usually less than 1 year of age, when the plica salpingopharyngea, the flap of tissue covering the pharyngeal opening, fails to let air escape the

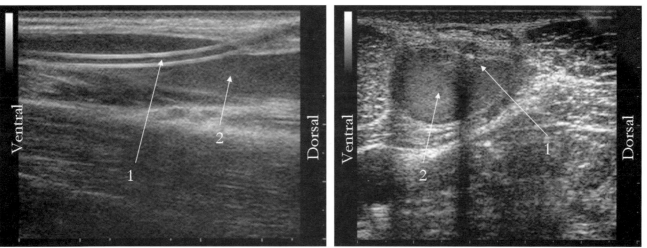

Figure 26.7 Jugular vein. These images are (A) longitudinal and (B) cross-sectional views of the left jugular region from an adult horse with an intravenous catheter. The intravenous catheter (1) is visualized in the lumen of the jugular vein (2). This sonogram was obtained with a wide-bandwidth 10.0 MHz linear array transducer, operating at 12.0 MHz, at a display depth of 5 cm.

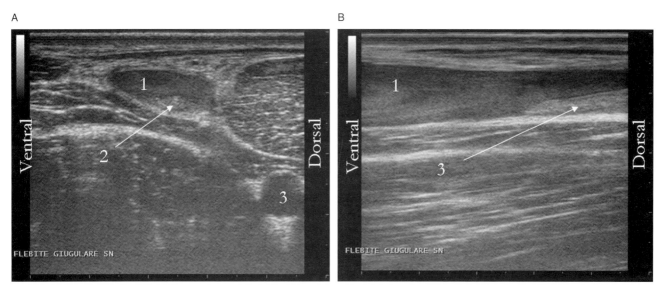

Figure 26.8 Jugular vein. These images are (A) cross-sectional and (B) longitudinal views of the left jugular vein from an adult horse with an intravenous catheter. A hyperechoic clot (2) with well defined margins is visible inside the jugular vein (1). The carotid artery (3) is visualized deep to the jugular vein. These sonograms were obtained with a wide-bandwidth 10.0 MHz linear array transducer, operating at 12.0 MHz, at a display depth of 4 cm.

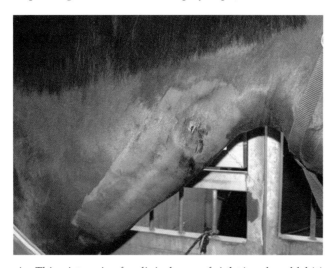

Figure 26.9 Jugular vein. This picture is of a clinical case of right jugular phlebitis with a draining track.

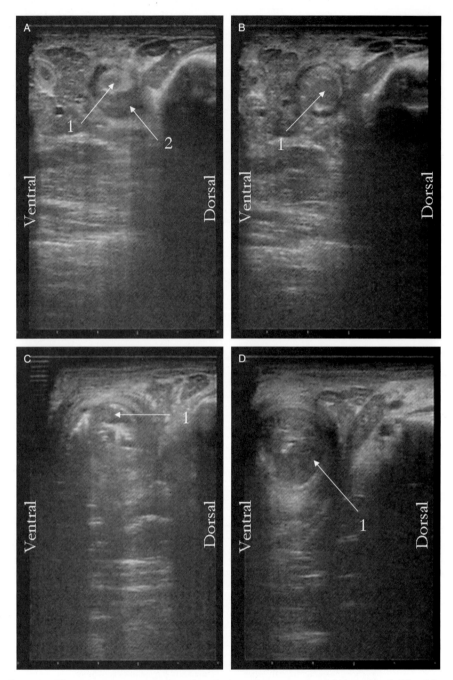

Figure 26.10 Jugular vein. These images are cross-sectional views from proximal (A) to distal (D) of the right jugular region obtained from the clinical case in Figure 26.9. A well demarcated, hyperechoic clot (1) is visible inside the jugular vein (2).

guttural pouch. With the flap functioning as a one-way valve, the pouch fills with air. Some cases are mild, while others progress to respiratory distress from occlusion of the pharyngeal area from the distended guttural pouch [2].

Guttural pouches may contain exudate or chondroids (inspissated pus) with guttural pouch empyema (Figures 26.13, 26.14). Empyema may occur secondary to any respiratory disease, but infection with *Strepto-coccus equi* is a common finding. The pouches may contain blood if trauma occurs to any structure associated with the guttural pouch. A common finding in guttural pouch trauma and hemorrhage is fracture of the stylohyoid bone. Another cause of blood in the pouch is guttural pouch mycosis. A fungal plaque forms in the pouch and causes erosion of a blood vessel, usually the internal carotid artery, resulting in hemorrhage into the guttural pouch.

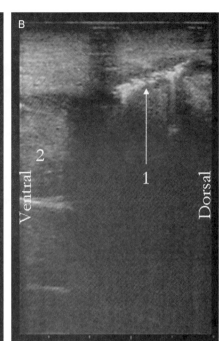

Figure 26.11 Jugular vein. These images are longitudinal views from proximal (A) to distal (B) of the right jugular region obtained from the clinical case in Figure 26.9. A draining track (1) is visible coming from the jugular vein (2). These sonograms were obtained with a wide-bandwidth 10.0 MHz linear array transducer, operating at 12.0 MHz, at a display depth of 4 cm.

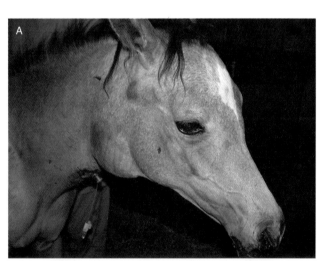

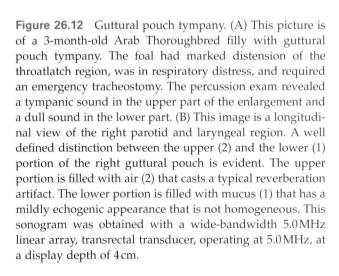

Figure 26.12 Guttural pouch tympany. (A) This picture is of a 3-month-old Arab Thoroughbred filly with guttural pouch tympany. The foal had marked distension of the throatlatch region, was in respiratory distress, and required an emergency tracheostomy. The percussion exam revealed a tympanic sound in the upper part of the enlargement and a dull sound in the lower part. (B) This image is a longitudinal view of the right parotid and laryngeal region. A well defined distinction between the upper (2) and the lower (1) portion of the right guttural pouch is evident. The upper portion is filled with air (2) that casts a typical reverberation artifact. The lower portion is filled with mucus (1) that has a mildly echogenic appearance that is not homogeneous. This sonogram was obtained with a wide-bandwidth 5.0 MHz linear array, transrectal transducer, operating at 5.0 MHz, at a display depth of 4 cm.

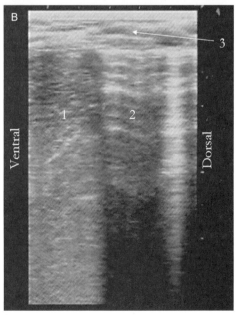

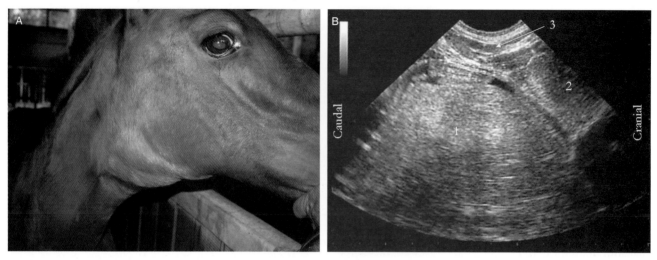

Figure 26.13   Guttural pouch empyema. (A) This picture is of a 5-month-old Spanish colt with guttural pouch empyema with an abscess inside the pouch. The foal had marked distension of the throatlatch region and clinical signs of respiratory distress. The mass was firm, not painful, and not adhered to the skin. (B) This image is a cross-sectional view of the right, lateral, laryngeal region. A well demarcated hyperechoic mass (1) is visible deep to the parotid salivary gland (3) and in contact with an enlarged, but architecturally normal, lymph node (2). This mass is inside the guttural pouch which has a visible wall and peripheral layer of hypoechogenic material. This sonogram was obtained with a wide-bandwidth 6.6 MHz micro-convex linear array transducer, operating at 6.6 MHz, at a display depth of 9 cm.

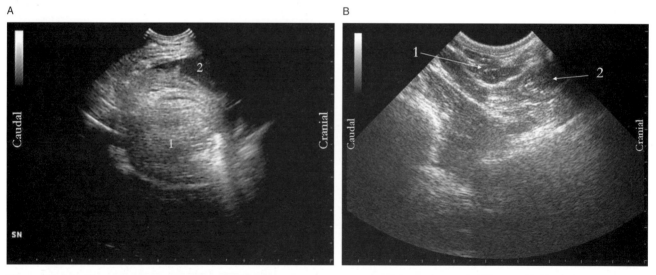

Figure 26.14   Guttural pouch empyema. (A) This image is a cross-sectional view of the right lateral laryngeal region obtained from the case in Figure 26.13 after insertion of a foley catheter and copious lavages of the guttural pouch with a diluted acetylcysteine solution. The echogenic mass (1) is still clearly visible and well defined, but the outer layers are slowly dissolving in the lavage fluid (2). This sonogram was obtained with a wide-bandwidth 6.6 MHz micro-convex linear array transducer, operating at 6.6 MHz, at a display depth of 7 cm. (B) This image is a cross-sectional view of the right lateral laryngeal region obtained from the case in Figure 26.13 after clinical resolution of guttural pouch empyema. The echogenic mass has completely disappeared and the normal structures of the region, the parotid salivary gland (1) and the lymph node (2), are visible. This sonogram was obtained with a wide-bandwidth 6.6 MHz micro-convex linear array transducer, operating at 6.6 MHz, at a display depth of 14 cm.

PAROTID SALIVARY GLANDS

The parotid salivary gland (Figures 26.15, 26.16, 26.17, 26.18) is a well demarcated, bilateral, multilobulated structure located in the proximal cervical region, below the ear, immediately underneath the skin. The gland extends from the vertical ramus of the mandible and wing of the atlas cranially to the linguofacial vein distally. Medially, it is adjacent to the guttural pouches and retropharyngeal lymph nodes. The gland has a hyperechoic capsule and septae and a hypoechoic to anechoic parenchyma. It is approximately 2 cm thick and 20 cm long. The salivary duct (Stenone's duct) is normally not visible with ultrasonography. Abnormalities of the parotid salivary gland are rare, but obstruction of the duct may cause dilation of the salivary duct.

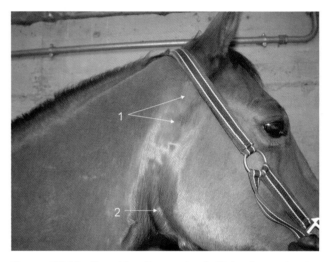

Figure 26.15 Parotid salivary gland. This image is a cross-sectional view of the left parotid salivary gland obtained from a normal adult horse. Hypoechoic, multilobulated, structures of the glandular parenchyma (1) are surrounded by hyperechoic capsule and septae. This sonogram was obtained with a wide-bandwidth 10.0 MHz linear array transducer, operating at 12.0 MHz, at a display depth of 5 cm.

Figure 26.16 Parotid salivary gland. This picture is of a 9-year-old Criollo gelding with a marked atrophy of the right parotid salivary gland (1) and a prominent ectatic duct (2).

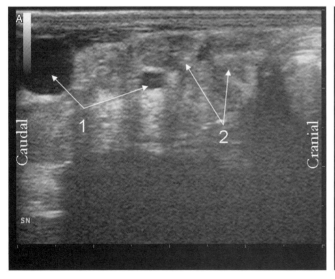
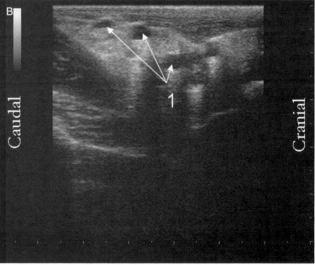

Figure 26.17 Parotid salivary gland. (A,B) These sonograms are of the right proximal cervical region obtained from the case in Figure 26.16. The glandular parenchyma (2) is visible only in a very small area. The remaining area of the parotid region is characterized by the presence of the ectatic duct (1) and fibrous tissue that is not homogeneous. A marked acoustic enhancement artifact is present in the far wall of the dilated ducts, confirming that these structures are fluid filled. These sonograms were obtained with a wide-bandwidth 10.0 MHz linear array transducer, operating at 12.0 MHz, at a display depth of 5 cm.

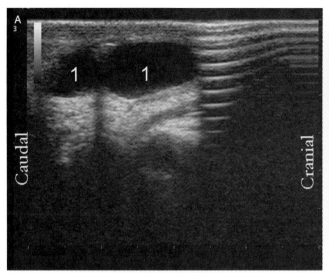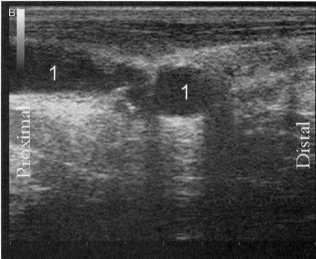

Figure 26.18 Parotid salivary gland. These images are (A) cross-sectional and (B) longitudinal views of the right mandibular edge obtained from the case in Figure 26.16. The parotid salivary duct (1) is distended and anechoic. The duct has a tortuous course and a thickened wall. These sonograms were obtained with a wide-bandwidth 10.0 MHz linear array transducer, operating at 12.0 MHz, at a display depth of 5 cm.

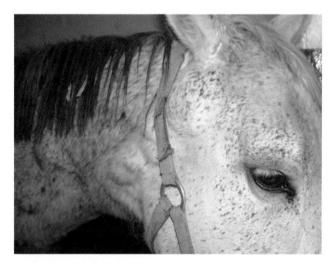

Figure 26.19 Melanoma. This picture is of a 20-year-old grey horse diagnosed with melanoma. The swelling in the proximal cervical region was irregular, firm, nodular, and not painful.

Also, neoplasia, particularly melanomas (Figures 26.19, 26.20), may infiltrate this gland.

THYROID GLAND

The thyroid gland (Figure 26.21) is bilateral with a narrow isthmus connecting the two lobes. It is located in the proximal cervical region, caudal to the larynx, at the level of the second to fourth tracheal rings, just below the skin surface. It is approximately 2 cm thick, 2 cm wide, and 5 cm long. Ultrasonographically, it appears as an oval, homogeneous, echogenic structure. Although abnormalities are rare, enlargement can occur with hyperthyroidism, hypothyroidism, euthyroidism, abscesses, hematomas, tumors, or as an incidental finding.

LYMPH NODES

Lymph nodes (Figure 26.22) are well demarcated structures with a hyperechoic capsule and a hypoechoic, homogeneous parenchyma. Major lymph nodes of the neck include the parotid lymph node, located under the cranial aspect of the parotid salivary gland, the retropharyngeal lymph nodes, located around the pharyngeal area and between the larynx and wing of the atlas, superficial cervical lymph nodes, located cranial to the shoulder under the superficial neck muscles, and deep lymph nodes, located along the trachea [3].

Lymph nodes may enlarge secondary to lymphadenitis or infection (Figures 26.23, 26.24, 26.25). When abscesses form in lymph nodes, the parenchyma loses its homogeneous appearance and typically appears hypoechoic to anechoic. Necrotic material and cellular debris may appear as hyperechoic areas in the abscessed lymph node. Draining tracts may be visualized ultrasonographically, coursing from the abscessed

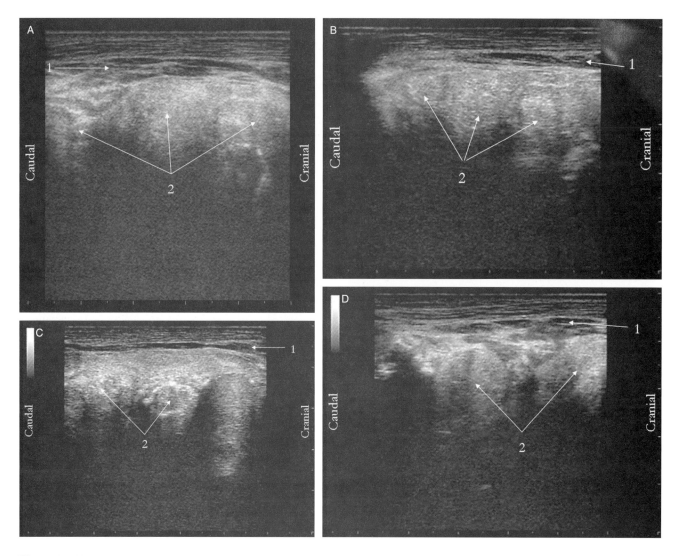

Figure 26.20 Melanoma. This series of sonograms (A,B,C,D) is of the right proximal cervical region obtained from the case in Figure 26.19. The glandular parenchyma (1) is reduced to a thin layer; beneath it various hyperechoic masses (2) characterized by a variable echogenicity are present. These sonograms were obtained with a wide-bandwidth 10.0 MHz linear array transducer, operating at 12.0 MHz, at a display depth of 5 cm.

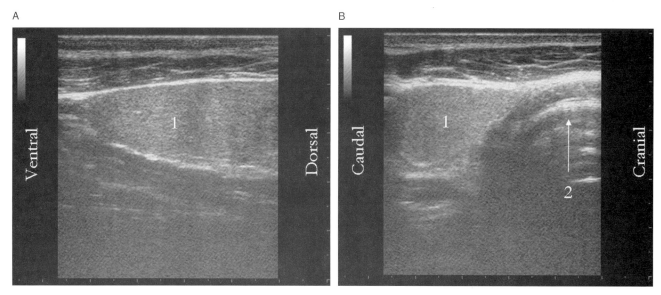

Figure 26.21 Thyroid gland. These images are (A) longitudinal and (B) cross-sectional views of the left thyroid gland obtained from a normal adult horse. The glandular parenchyma (1) has a homogeneous echogenic appearance with a well defined capsule. It is approximately 2 cm thick and 5 cm long. It has a round elongated aspect and a thinner part adjacent to the trachea (2). This sonogram was obtained with a wide-bandwidth 10.0 MHz linear array transducer, operating at 12.0 MHz, at a display depth of 5 cm.

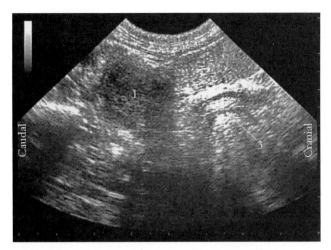

Figure 26.22   Normal lymph node. This image is a cross-sectional view of the left lateral laryngeal region of a normal adult horse. A lymph node (1) is visible with its characteristic hypoechoic, homogeneous appearance. It is near the thyroid gland (2) and lateral to the trachea (3). This sonogram was obtained with a wide-bandwidth 6.6 MHz micro-convex linear array transducer, operating at 6.6 MHz, at a display depth of 6 cm.

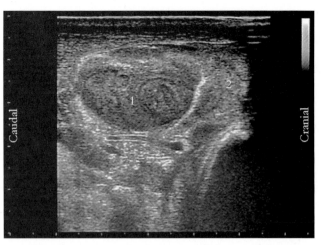

Figure 26.23   Laryngeal lymph node abscess. This image is a cross-sectional view of the left lateral laryngeal region of a 6-month-old filly. An abscess (1) is visible where a lymph node is normally located near the thyroid gland (2). The abscess has a well defined, hyperechoic capsule with hypoechoic contents and a swirling appearance. This sonogram was obtained with a wide-bandwidth 10.0 MHz linear array transducer, operating at 12.0 MHz, at a display depth of 5 cm.

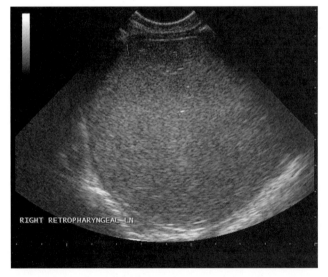

Figure 26.24   Retropharyngeal lymph node abscess. This image is a cross-sectional view of the right retropharyngeal region of a weanling. An abscess is visible where a lymph node is normally located in the retropharyngeal area. The horse was diagnosed with *Streptococcus equi* (strangles) based on culture results of a fine-needle aspirate from the abscess. This sonogram was obtained with a micro-convex transducer, operating at 6.6 MHz, at a display depth of 8 cm. (Source: Image courtesy of Dr. Michael Beyer, Equine Health Care PSC, Versailles, KY, USA.)

lymph node to other internal structures or to the exterior. Neoplastic infiltrates to lymph nodes image as areas of increased echogenicity or complete loss of normal lymph node architecture.

Esophagus

The esophagus (Figures 26.26, 26.27, 26.28) is a tubular structure with a 3–4 mm thick wall formed by an outer, hyperechoic, serosal layer and an inner, hypoechoic muscular layer. The lumen is irregular and hyperechoic due to the mucosal folds covered by mucus containing gas. In the cranial third of the neck, the esophagus is located on the median line, deep to the trachea. In the middle and caudal thirds of the neck, it is usually located left of the trachea. However, some normal horses will have an esophagus located to the right of the trachea. The esophagus is normally collapsed except during swallowing.

Esophageal obstruction (Figures 26.29, 26.30), commonly referred to as choke, is a leading cause of esophageal pathology. Feed material is the most common cause of obstruction and appears as an echogenic mass in the lumen of the esophagus. Initially, obstruction results in esophageal dilation, but prolonged or repeat episodes may lead to esophageal

A

B

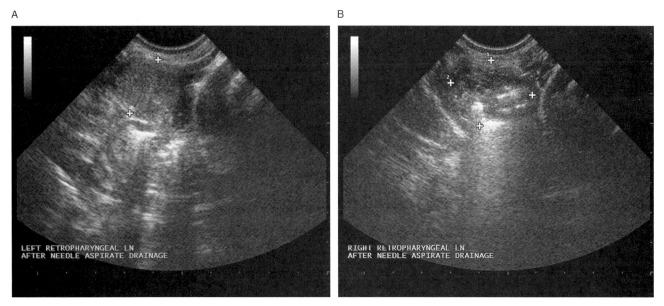

Figure 26.25   Retropharygneal lymph node abscess after aspirate. These images are cross-sectional views of the retropharyngeal region of the weanling in Figure 26.24. These images show the left (A) and right (B) retropharyngeal lymph nodes after a fine-needle aspirate and drainage of exudate. These sonograms were obtained with a micro-convex transducer, operating at 6.6 MHz, at a display depth of 8 cm. (Source: Images courtesy of Dr. Michael Beyer, Equine Health Care PSC, Versailles, KY, USA.)

A

B

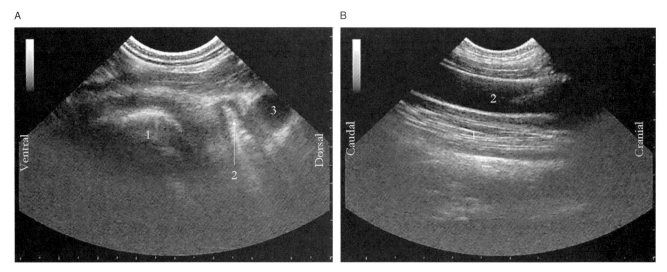

Figure 26.26   Normal esophagus. These images are (A) cross-sectional and (B) longitudinal views of the left jugular region from a normal adult horse. The esophagus (2) is visible between the carotid artery (3) and the trachea (1). The esophageal mucosal folds appear as alternating hyperechoic and hypoechoic lines. The esophageal wall has a hypoechoic appearance. These sonograms were obtained with a wide-bandwidth 6.6 MHz micro-convex linear array transducer, operating at 6.6 MHz, at a display depth of (A) 6 and (B) 8 cm.

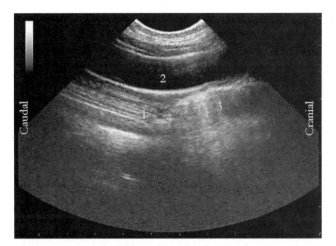

Figure 26.27 Normal esophagus with food bolus. This image is a longitudinal view of the left jugular region of a normal adult horse. The normal esophagus (1) with a food bolus (3) is visible deep to the carotid artery (2). This sonogram was obtained with a wide-bandwidth 6.6 MHz microconvex linear array transducer, operating at 6.6 MHz, at a display depth of 8 cm.

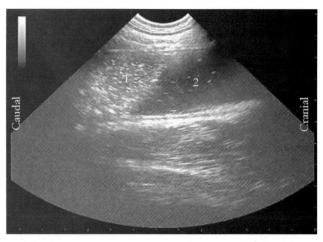

Figure 26.29 Esophageal choke. This image is a longitudinal view of the left distal jugular region of a Spanish adult horse with esophageal choke. The cranial part of the esophagus is filled with fluid (2), while the more caudal part has solid content (1). This sonogram was obtained with a wide-bandwidth 6.6 MHz micro-convex linear array transducer, operating at 6.6 MHz, at a display depth of 10 cm.

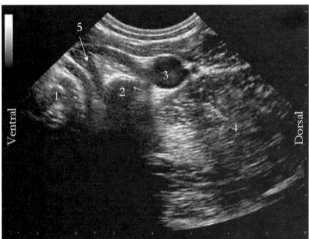

Figure 26.28 Esophagus with nasogastric tube. This image is a cross-sectional view of the left jugular region of a normal adult horse with a nasogastric tube in the esophagus. The esophagus (5) is visible between the carotid artery (3) and the trachea (1) near the scalenus muscle (4). The nasogastric tube (2) is well identified inside the esophageal lumen, confirming its correct positioning. This sonogram was obtained with a wide-bandwidth 6.6 MHz micro-convex linear array transducer, operating at 6.6 MHz, at a display depth of 6 cm.

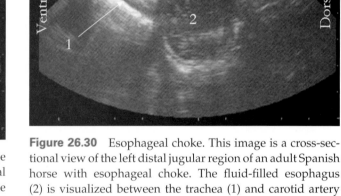

Figure 26.30 Esophageal choke. This image is a cross-sectional view of the left distal jugular region of an adult Spanish horse with esophageal choke. The fluid-filled esophagus (2) is visualized between the trachea (1) and carotid artery (3). This sonogram was obtained with a wide-bandwidth 6.6 MHz micro-convex linear array transducer, operating at 6.6 MHz, at a display depth of 8 cm.

stricture, diverticula, or rupture. External trauma, such as a kick, or use of a nasogastric tube may also result in esophageal pathology. Megaesophagus (Figures 26.31, 26.32), or profound dilation of the esophagus, may occur from a congenital defect or secondary to obstruction or other esophageal trauma.

Esophageal fistulas (Figure 26.33) may develop secondary to trauma or as a result of passage of a nasogastric tube.

TRACHEA

The trachea (Figure 26.34) is a tubular structure composed of tracheal rings, that image as hypoechoic

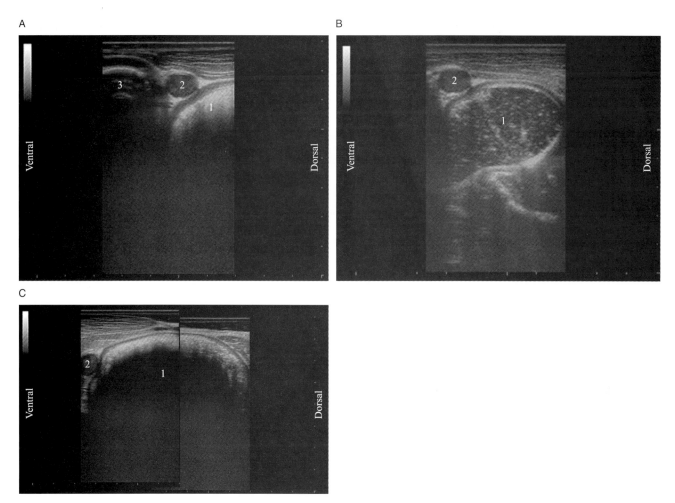

Figure 26.31 Megaesophagus. These images are cross-sectional views of the left distal jugular region of a 13-year-old Welsh pony with megaesophagus. (A) The esophagus (1) is distended and has a thickened wall with hyperechoic material in the lumen. The location between the carotid artery (2) and the trachea (3) is abnormal. (B) The esophagus (1) is filled with fluid and visualized near the carotid artery (2). (C) At the base of the neck, the esophagus (1) is dilated to almost 8 cm in diameter. Two image planes were required to visualize the extent of the megaesophagus. The carotid artery (2) is adjacent to the megaesophagus. These sonograms were obtained with a wide-bandwidth 10.0 MHz linear array transducer, operating at 12.0 MHz, at a display depth of 8 cm.

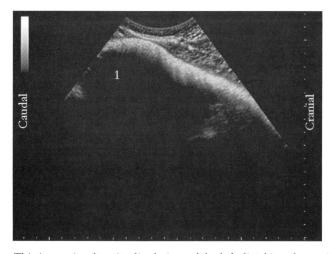

Figure 26.32 Megaesophagus. This image is a longitudinal view of the left distal jugular region of a 13-year-old Welsh pony with megaesophagus. In this part of the esophagus (1), a 2 cm layer of hyperechoic material is present. This sonogram was obtained with a wide-bandwidth 3.5 MHz convex linear array transducer, operating at 3.5 MHz, at a display depth of 15 cm.

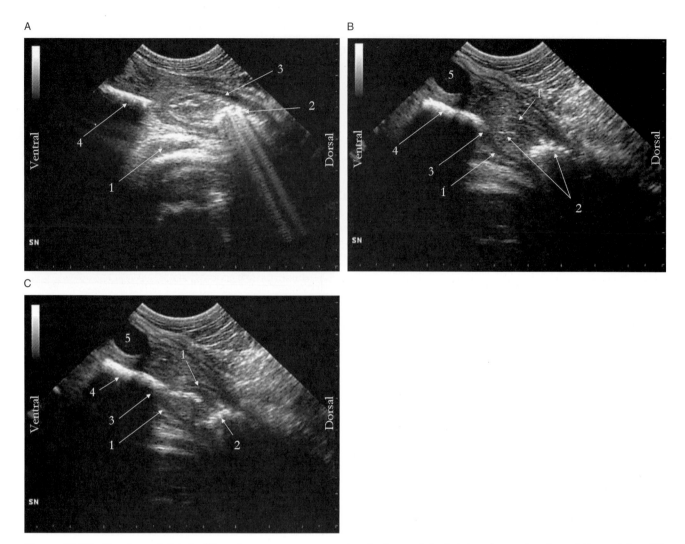

Figure 26.33 Esophageal fistula. These images are cross-sectional views of the left jugular region from (A) cranial to (C) caudal of a 9-year-old Standardbred mare with an esophageal fistula and diffuse cellulitis at the base of the neck. (A) The hypoechoic esophageal wall (3) surrounds hyperechoic material in the esophageal lumen. The trachea (1) is deep to the esophagus. Hyperechoic material (4) is present outside the esophageal lumen. An acoustic shadow artifact (2) is present. (B) The esophageal wall (1) is visible with hyperechoic material inside the esophageal lumen (2). Hyperechoic material is present outside the esophageal lumen (4) secondary to an esophageal fistula (3). The jugular vein (5) is visible. (C) Esophageal wall (1), hyperechoic material inside the esophageal lumen (2), point of rupture of the esophageal wall (3), hyperechoic material crossing the esophageal wall (4). The jugular vein (5) is visible. These sonograms were obtained with a wide-bandwidth 6.6 MHz micro-convex linear array transducer, operating at 6.6 MHz, at a display depth of 7 cm.

areas, and tough membranes, that image as hyperechoic areas. The inner surface is hyperechoic because of mucus containing gas microbubbles. The trachea is located along the median, ventral ridge of the neck. Trauma may result in tracheal rupture and subcutaneous emphysema. Abscesses may form around the trachea from trauma or at transtracheal wash sites.

MUSCLES

Muscle (Figure 26.35) has hypoechoic fibers and hyperechoic fascia. The ultrasonographic appearance of each muscle varies depending on the quantity of connective tissue and fat present inside it. The omohyoideus muscle forms the medial border of the jugular groove;

A

B

C

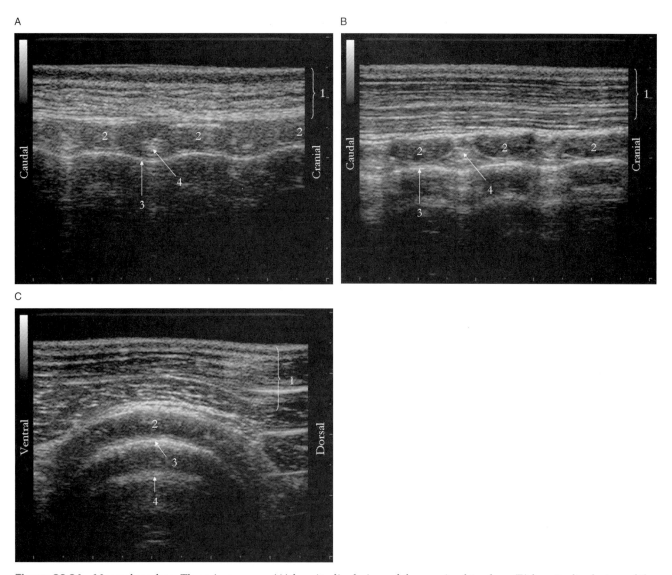

Figure 26.34   Normal trachea. These images are (A) longitudinal view of the proximal trachea, (B) longitudinal view of the middle trachea, and (C) cross-sectional view of the middle trachea in a normal adult horse. Cutis, subcutis and muscles (1) are superficial to the trachea. Tracheal rings (2) are hyperechoic in the proximal part and hypoechoic in the middle and distal parts of the trachea. The mucosal surface of the trachea (3) is hyperechoic and casts a reverberation artifact due to the presence of air in the mucus. The membranes between the tracheal rings (4) are hyperechoic. These sonograms were obtained with a wide-bandwidth 10.0 MHz linear array transducer, operating at 12.0 MHz, at a display depth of 4 cm.

it originates at the subscapular fascia and inserts on the basihyoid bone. The sternohyoideus and sternothyroideus muscles, often called the strap muscles, course along the ventral surface of the trachea. Both muscles originate at the sternum, but the sternohyoid inserts on the basihyoid bone, while the sternothyroideus inserts on the thyroid cartilage of the larynx. The sternocephalicus muscle forms the ventral border of the jugular groove and extends from the sternum to the head. The brachiocephalic muscle forms the dorsal border of the jugular groove; it originates on the head

of the humerus and inserts at the poll. Other superficial muscles of the neck include the splenius, cervical rhomboid, and cervical ventral serratus [4].

Swellings in muscle should be scanned to assess the nature, depth, and topographic relationship with normal structures of the neck, particularly blood vessels. The ultrasound appearance of muscle swelling is highly variable depending on cause. Diffuse infection, abscesses (Figures 26.36, 26.37), and neoplasia (Figure 26.38) are differentials for swelling in or adjacent to muscles of the neck.

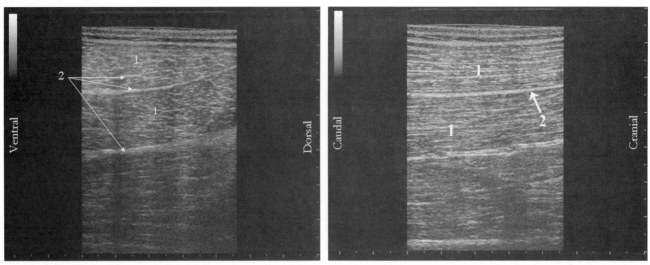

Figure 26.35 Neck muscles. These images are (A) cross-sectional and (B) longitudinal views of the lateral neck in a normal adult horse. The muscle fibers (1) have a hypoechoic, heterogeneous appearance, while the fascia (2) is hyperechoic. These sonograms were obtained with a wide-bandwidth 10.0 MHz linear array transducer, operating at 12.0 MHz, at a display depth of 7 cm.

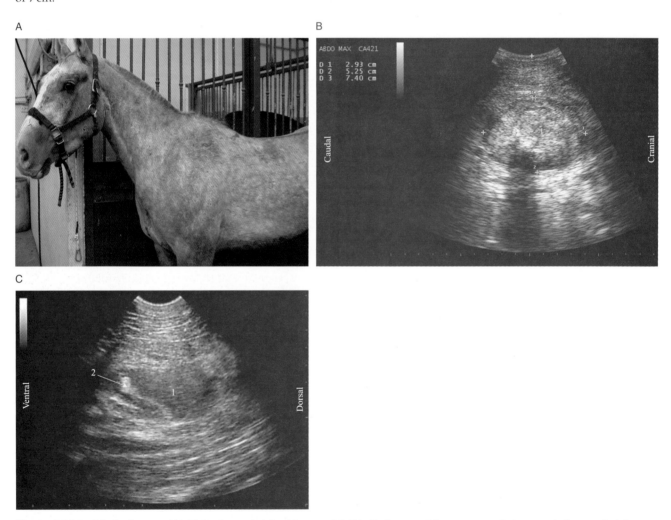

Figure 26.36 Neck abscess. (A) This picture is of a 13-year-old Criollo horse with a suspected abscess. A firm, painful mass and a fistula with mucopurulent exudate is present at the base of the neck to the left of the trachea. (B) This image is a longitudinal view of the base of the neck. A well defined mass (1) is visible 2.52 cm deep. This mass has a homogeneous, hypoechoic structure with a thick and well demarcated hyperechoic capsule. (C) This image is a cross-sectional view of the base of the neck. The same hypoechoic mass (1) is visible with a hyperechoic structure identified as a necrotic fragment (2). These sonograms were obtained with a wide-bandwidth 3.5 MHz convex linear array transducer, operating at 5.0 MHz, at a display depth of 12 cm.

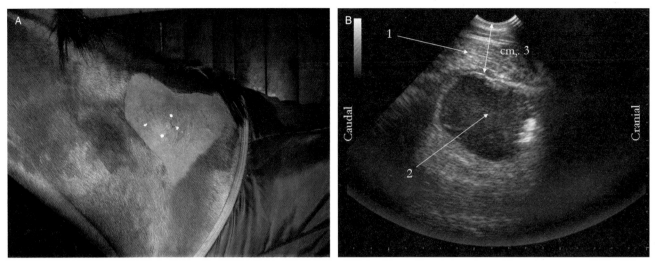

Figure 26.37 Neck abscess. (A) This picture is of a 9-year-old Hanover horse with a suspected abscess. A firm, painful mass is present on the lateral side of the neck. (B) This image is a longitudinal view of the lateral side of the neck. A hypoechoic mass (2) is visible, 3 cm deep, with a well defined hyperechoic capsule. The superficial muscle layer (1) is visible. This sonogram was obtained with a wide-bandwidth 3.5 MHz convex linear array transducer, operating at 5.0 MHz, at a display depth of 13 cm.

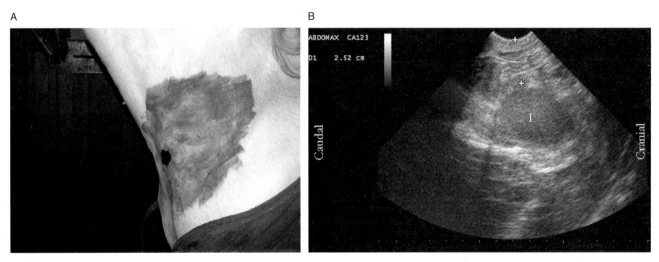

Figure 26.38 Melanoma. (A) This picture is of a 10-year-old Spanish horse with suspect melanoma. A firm, slightly painful mass and a fistula with black exudate is present at the base of the neck to the left of the trachea. (B) This image is a longitudinal view of the base of the neck. A well defined mass (1) is visible 2.93 cm deep, measuring 5.25 cm by 7.40 cm. The mass does not have a homogeneous echogenic appearance. This sonogram was obtained with a wide-bandwidth 3.5 MHz convex linear array transducer, operating at 3.5 MHz, at a display depth of 15 cm.

REFERENCES

[1] Gardner, S.Y., Reef, M.B., & Spencer, P.A. (1991) Ultrasonographic evaluation of 46 horses with jugular vein thrombophlebitis: 1985–1988. *Journal of the American Veterinary Medical Association*, 199, 370–373.

[2] Wheat, J.D. (1962) Tympanites of the guttural pouch of the horse. *Journal of the American Veterinary Medical Association*, 140, 453–454.

[3] Pasquini, P., Spurgeon, T., & Pasquini, S. (2003) General. In: *Anatomy of Domestic Animals*, 10th edn. Sudz, Pilot Point, 439–440.

[4] Pasquini, P., Spurgeon, T., & Pasquini, S. (2003) Muscle. In: *Anatomy of Domestic Animals*, 10th edn. Sudz, Pilot Point, 210–211.

CHAPTER TWENTY-SEVEN

ULTRASONOGRAPHY OF VASCULAR STRUCTURES

Fairfield T. Bain

College of Veterinary Medicine, Washington State University, Pullman, WA, USA

JUGULAR VEIN

Ultrasound imaging of the vascular system most often includes evaluation of the jugular vein (Figures 27.1, 27.2, 27.3, 27.4, 27.5, 27.6, 27.7, 27.8, 27.9, 27.10). It is most often performed when thrombophlebitis is suspected, especially in sick horses with intravenous catheters in place. The jugular vein can be imaged from its entry into the thoracic inlet distally on the neck and throughout its course in the neck to its bifurcation into the internal and external jugular vein branches just caudal to the ramus of the mandible. As with most structures, the jugular vein should be imaged in two planes: longitudinal and transverse. The vein is best imaged when distended, which can be accomplished by occlusion of the vein distally near the thoracic inlet with the thumb of the opposite hand from the hand performing the sonography. The ultrasound probe can then be placed over the vein and the course of the vein traced with the probe. The author likes to scan from distal to proximal on the vein and then focus on the particular region of concern (e.g. site of intravenous catheter insertion or palpable thickening of the vein or perivenous tissues).

DISTAL LIMB VASCULATURE

In addition to ultrasound of the jugular vein, imaging of the vascular system can include examination of distal limb vasculature (Figures 27.11, 27.12). This is most often performed when a horse has persistent swelling in a limb or has a pattern of tortuous, distended cutaneous vessel.

LATERAL THORACIC VEIN

The lateral thoracic vein (Figure 27.13) can be imaged along the lateral aspect of the thorax just caudal to the point of the elbow. This vessel may be imaged to assist in intravenous catheter placement when the jugular vein cannot be used for intravenous catheter access.

ILIAC ARTERIES AND AORTA

Transrectal ultrasound evaluation of the iliac arteries (Figures 27.14, 27.15) is performed to diagnose possible thrombosis. Historically, thrombosis of these arteries has been associated with *Strongylus vulgaris* infection. However, other causes include trauma, foaling complication, or the presence of a hypercoagulable state from another disease process. Thrombosis of an iliac artery should be considered in horses with undiagnosed hind limb lameness or a hind limb that is cooler than body temperature. The distal aorta (Figure 27.16) may also be imaged transrectally.

Atlas of Equine Ultrasonography, First Edition. Edited by Jessica A. Kidd, Kristina G. Lu, and Michele L. Frazer.
© 2014 John Wiley & Sons, Ltd. Published 2014 by John Wiley & Sons, Ltd.
Companion Website: www.wiley.com/go/kidd/equine-ultrasonography

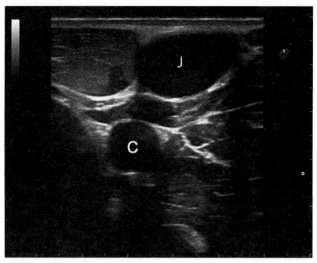

Figure 27.1 Normal jugular vein. The normal jugular vein and its relation to the underlying carotid artery and esophagus vary along its course in the neck. This image shows the close approximation of the jugular vein (J) and carotid artery (C) in the distal third of the neck. The jugular vein is distended with some increasing echogenicity of the blood from stasis. The walls of this normal vein are thin and crisply echogenic. The normal musculature of the neck can be seen surrounding the vein and artery. This sonogram was obtained from the jugular groove with a linear probe operating at 7.5 MHz at a depth of 5 cm.

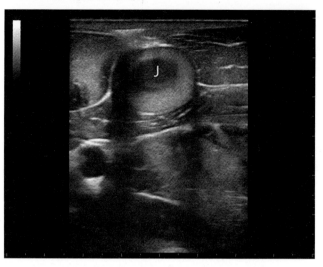

Figure 27.2 Occluded jugular vein. This image shows the jugular vein (J) occluded distally. Occlusion of the jugular vein will obstruct normal blood flow and swirling echogenicity of the normal blood will be observed during the first several seconds after occlusion. This sonogram was obtained from the jugular groove with a linear probe operating at 7.5 MHz at a depth of 5 cm.

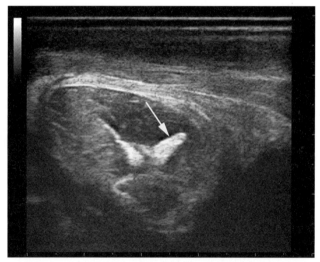

Figure 27.3 Myositis near jugular vein. The main indication for imaging the jugular vein is concern for possible thrombosis. Clinical evaluation of the vein would include palpation of the vein along its course, both before and after distal occlusion. Some patients may have significant perivenous swelling or swelling along the jugular groove of the neck, and ultrasonography can be useful to differentiate perivenous inflammation from actual jugular thrombosis or thrombophlebitis. This sonogram shows a central region of echogenicity (arrow) within the cervical muscles consistent with inflammation from intramuscular injection from attempted venous injection in a fractious horse. In this patient, the swelling in the neck was from the focal myositis rather than the jugular vein. This sonogram was obtained from the jugular groove with a linear probe operating at 7.5 MHz at a depth of 4 cm.

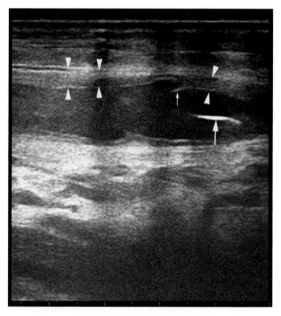

Figure 27.4 Intravenous catheter. Swelling, firmness, or thickening of the jugular vein associated with the presence of an intravenous catheter is one of the more common indications for ultrasound evaluation of the jugular vein. This patient with an intravenous catheter in place (arrow) has sonographic evidence of early phlebitis with thickening of the jugular vein wall (arrowheads). A venous valve (small arrow) is also seen in this image. This sonogram was obtained from the jugular groove with a linear probe operating at 7.5 MHz at a depth of 5 cm.

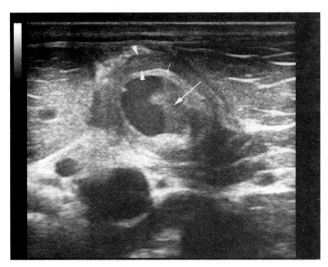

Figure 27.5 Jugular thrombosis. Jugular thrombosis often starts at the site of a traumatic venipuncture in an animal with a prothrombotic state or at the site of entry into the vein of an intravenous catheter. This image shows an asymmetric jugular venous thrombus (long arrow) in a transverse image of the jugular vein. The vein has thickening of the tunica media (arrowheads) and also thickening of the intimal layer (short arrow). These findings indicate jugular phlebitis with developing luminal thrombus formation. This sonogram was obtained from the jugular groove with a linear probe operating at 7.5 MHz at a depth of 4 cm.

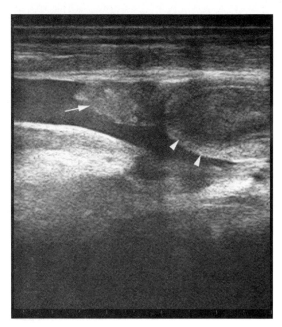

Figure 27.6 Intraluminal thrombus. This image is a longitudinal view of a jugular vein with an intraluminal thrombus. The smooth margins of the older component of the thrombus are seen (arrowheads) along with a more recent, actively proliferating clot (arrow) on the distal edge of the thrombus. The proximal aspect (cranial on the horse) of the vein is to the right. This sonogram was obtained from the jugular groove with a linear probe operating at 7.5 MHz at a depth of 5 cm.

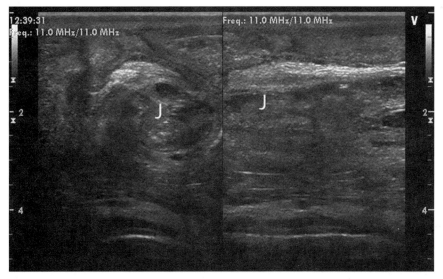

Figure 27.7 Thrombophlebitis of jugular vein. Jugular thrombophlebitis may progress from a partially occlusive thrombus to complete occlusion of the vein. Ultrasound imaging is helpful in differentiating the process of thrombosis from septic thrombophlebitis. This patient had complete occlusion of the jugular vein (J) with an irregular, laminar pattern of thrombosis. The vein has multiple, small echogenic foci that give some concern for possible sepsis. Transverse (left) and longitudinal (right) views are included. This sonogram was obtained from the jugular groove with a linear probe operating at 7.5 MHz at a depth of 5 cm.

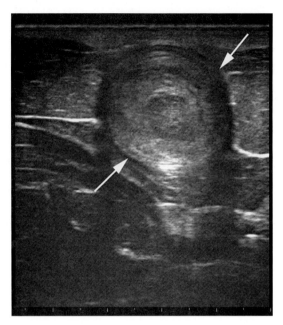

Figure 27.8 Chronic jugular vein thrombosis. This image is a transverse view of a chronic, organized jugular vein thrombosis (arrows indicate outer border of jugular vein) with complete occlusion of the lumen. The thrombus has a laminar pattern. This sonogram was obtained from the jugular groove with a linear probe operating at 7.5 MHz at a depth of 5 cm.

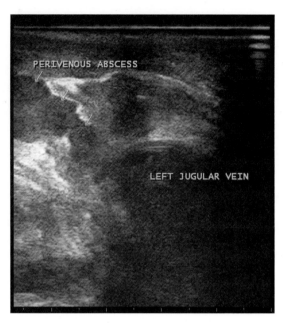

Figure 27.9 Thrombophlebitis from intravenous catheter. Some cases of jugular thrombophlebitis will occur as extensions from a perivenous, subcutaneous infection along the tract created by an intravenous catheter. This patient had a perivenous abscess present along the catheter tract in addition to thrombosis of the jugular vein. This sonogram was obtained from the jugular groove with a linear probe operating at 7.5 MHz at a depth of 5 m.

A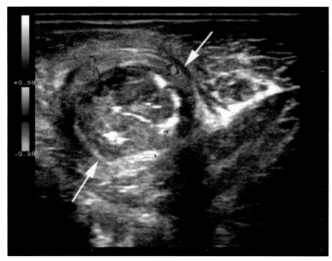

B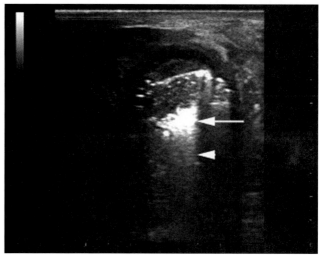

C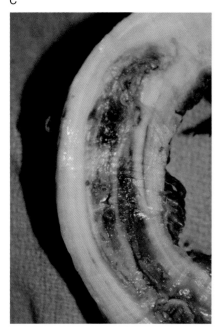

Figure 27.10 Jugular thrombophlebitis from anaerobic infection. This patient had a progressive, septic jugular thrombophlebitis with an anaerobic infection following a dental procedure involving an infected tooth root. The vein had rapid occlusion with a thrombus containing multiple echogenic foci and regions of obvious intraluminal gas. Post-mortem evaluation revealed the mixed laminated pattern with regions of suppurative exudate. (A) This image shows septic jugular thrombophlebitis (arrows mark outer border of jugular vein) with echogenic regions consistent with suppurative exudate. Color flow Doppler indicates absence of luminal blood flow. (B) This image shows echogenic shadowing (arrowhead) consistent with suppurative exudate containing gas (arrow). This was associated with a septic anaerobic infection of the jugular thrombophlebitis. These sonograms were obtained from the jugular groove with a linear probe operating at 7.5 MHz at a depth of 4 cm. (C) This image is a post-mortem longitudinal section of the septic anaerobic jugular thrombophlebitis demonstrating the mixed laminated appearance of the luminal thrombosis with intervening regions of suppurative exudate.

A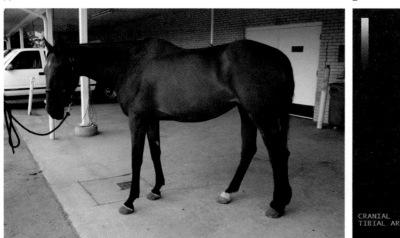

B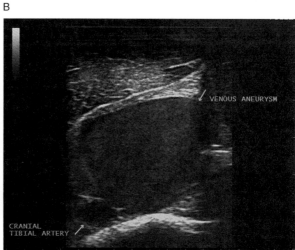

Figure 27.11 Arteriovenous fistula. (A) This image is of a horse with a 3-month history of hind limb swelling following trauma to the dorsum of the hock. The left hind leg had a pattern of distended veins in the skin on the gaskin along the proximal margin of the swelling. (B) Ultrasound image (transverse view) of the tortuous skin vessels in the hind limb shows a dilated region (aneurysm) within the vein adjacent to the underlying cranial tibial artery suggesting the presence of an arteriovenous fistula creating turbulent blood flow. This sonogram was obtained from the craniolateral aspect of the hind limb, near the hock, with a linear probe operating at 7.5 MHz at a depth of 6 cm.

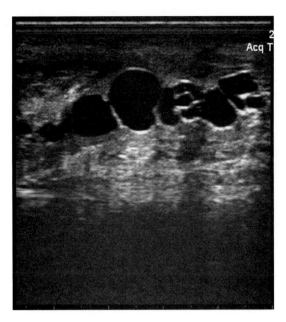

Figure 27.12 Chronic lymphangitis. This longitudinal ultrasound image of the swollen distal limb in Figure 27.11 shows multiple, tortuous, dilated lymphatic vessels within the subcutaneous tissues consistent with lymphatic obstruction. This is a common finding with clinical cases of chronic lymphangitis. This sonogram was obtained from the craniolateral aspect of the hind limb, near the hock, with a linear probe operating at 7.5 MHz at a depth of 6 cm.

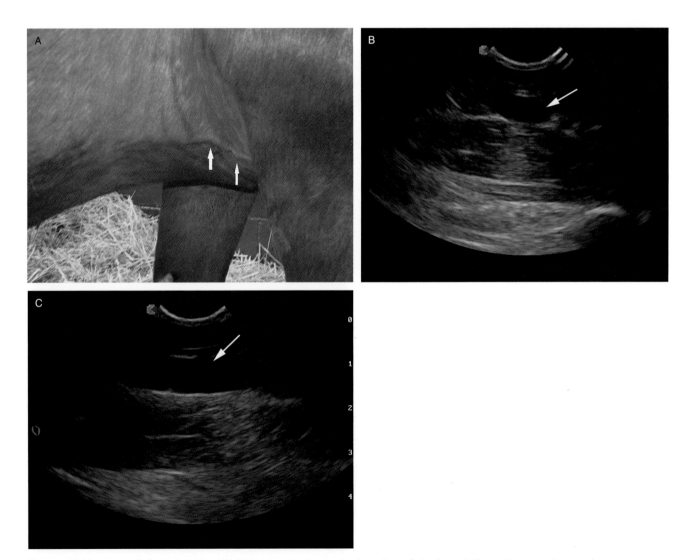

Figure 27.13 Lateral thoracic vein. (A) This picture shows the location of the lateral thoracic artery (arrows) in a pregnant broodmare. (B) Cross-sectional and (C) longitudinal views of the lateral thoracic vein (arrow). The vein courses superficially along the ventrolateral aspect of the thoracic cavity caudal to the elbow. This vessel can be used for intravenous catheter placement when the jugular vein can not be used. This sonogram was obtained from the lateral chest wall, caudal to the seventh ICS, with a linear probe operating at 5.0 MHz at a depth of 5 cm.

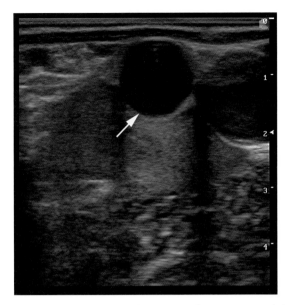

Figure 27.14   Iliac artery. This image shows a normal iliac artery (arrow) in a gelding. This sonogram was obtained transrectally using a linear probe operating at 5.0 MHz at a depth of 5 cm.

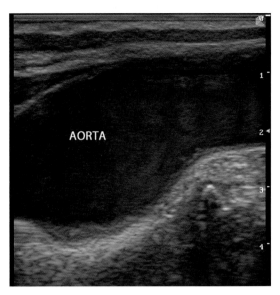

Figure 27.16   Aorta. This image was obtained transrectally using a linear probe operating at 5.0 MHz at a depth of 5 cm.

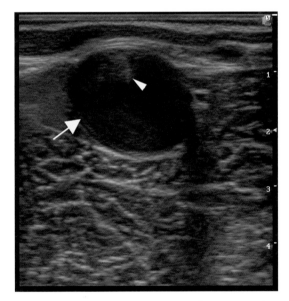

Figure 27.15   Plaque in iliac artery. This image shows a hyperechoic structure (arrowhead) in an iliac artery (arrow). This small plaque was an incidental finding in an aged gelding. Clinical signs from thrombosed iliac artery do not usually occur until the vessel lumen is almost completely occluded. Most thrombosed iliac arteries are chronic before they are diagnosed. This image was obtained transrectally using a linear probe operating at 5.0 MHz at a depth of 5 cm.

RECOMMENDED READING

Duggan, V.E., Holbroo, T.C., Dechant, J.E., *et al.* (2004) Diagnosis of aorto-iliac thrombosis in a quarter horse foal using Doppler ultrasound and nuclear scintigraphy. *Journal of Veterinary Internal Medicine*, 18(5), 753–756.

Geraghty, T.E., Love, S., Taylor, D.J. *et al.* (2009) Assessment of subclinical venous catheter-related diseases in horses and associated risk factors. *Veterinary Record*, 164(8), 227–231.

Hilton, H., Aleman, M., Textor, J., *et al.* (2008) Ultrasound-guided balloon thrombectomy for treatment of aorto-iliac-femoral thrombosis in a horse. *Journal of Veterinary Internal Medicine*, 22(3), 679–683.

Vaughan, B., Whitcomb, M.B., Puchalski, S.M., *et al.* (2010) Imaging diagnosis – arterial and venous thromboses of the proximal limb in two thoroughbred racehorses. *Veterinary Radiology & Ultrasound*, 51(3), 305–310.

CHAPTER TWENTY-EIGHT

Ultrasonography of Umbilical Structures

Massimo Magri

Clinica Veterinaria Spirano, Spirano (BG), Italy

Preparation and Scanning Technique

Optimal equipment to scan the umbilical remnant in the foal is a high-frequency, 10–12 MHz linear probe, although a cursory examination can be performed with a transrectal, 5–7.5 MHz linear probe. Ideally, clip the hair with a #40 surgical clipper blade from the xiphoid caudal to the inguinal region and apply coupling gel. However, wetting the area with alcohol is often sufficient. The probe should be covered with an examination glove or similar to prevent damage to the probe from alcohol (Figure 28.1).

Although most foals tolerate this procedure without sedation, it may be required in some foals to minimize stress of the procedure. In the author's experience, the best way to perform this examination is to stand beside the foal, with an assistant restraining the foal at the shoulder, next to the mare. One hand holds the probe while the other stretches the skin. The umbilical remnant can also be scanned with the foal in lateral recumbency. The ultrasonographer is behind the foal's back with head and legs restrained by an assistant.

Orientation of the probe must be kept constant over time to obtain comparable images. In the longitudinal axis view, orientate the probe so the caudal abdomen is on the left side of the screen, and the proximal abdomen is on the right. In the transverse (short) axis view, orientate the probe so the right abdomen is on the left side of the screen and the left abdomen is on the right (Figure 28.2).

Structures imaged when scanning the umbilical area include the external umbilical remnant, umbilical vein, umbilical arteries, urachus, and umbilical hernia if present. The umbilical remnant is located along the ventral midline of the abdomen (Figure 28.3), a few centimeters from the surface. To locate and recognize the different structures, the easiest way is to start with the cross-sectional view of the external umbilical remnant and move cranially to the xiphoid cartilage. Then, start at the external umbilical remnant again and move caudally to the pelvic rim. In the male, the presence of the penis makes scanning the most caudal part difficult. If an abnormal structure is suspected, a longitudinal scan should be performed. This scan plane is more difficult to visualize due to the tubular structure of the umbilical structures.

External Umbilical Remnant

The external umbilical remnant contains the umbilical vein, the two umbilical arteries, and the urachus (Figure 28.4). These structures normally atrophy within a few days after birth and detach from the skin.

Infection is the main pathology of the external umbilical remnant. Clinically this pathology is characterized by a local swelling and a draining tract (Figure 28.5a). Sonographically, it is characterized by an enlarged external umbilical remnant filled with hypoechoic to echoic fluid (Figure 28.5b).

Umbilical Vein

The umbilical vein runs cranially from the umbilicus to the xiphoid cartilage, along the midline, very close to the skin surface (Figure 28.6a). When it reaches the xiphoid cartilage, it courses deep to reach the liver

Atlas of Equine Ultrasonography, First Edition. Edited by Jessica A. Kidd, Kristina G. Lu, and Michele L. Frazer.
© 2014 John Wiley & Sons, Ltd. Published 2014 by John Wiley & Sons, Ltd.
Companion Website: www.wiley.com/go/kidd/equine-ultrasonography

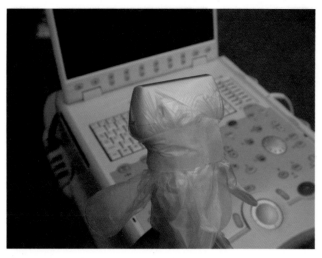

Figure 28.1   Probe protection. Protect the probe from coupling gel or alcohol with an examination glove or similar covering.

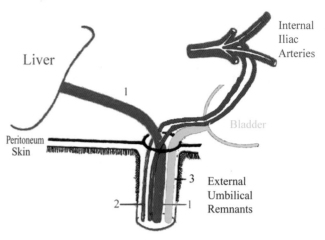

Figure 28.3   Umbilical remnants. This diagram illustrates the umbilical remnants including umbilical vein (1), umbilical arteries (2), and urachus (3).

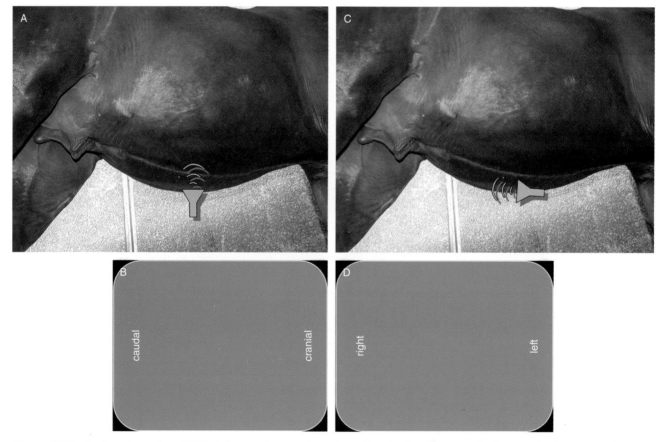

Figure 28.2   Probe orientation. (A) This image shows orientation of probe for obtaining the longitudinal view. (B) Position the probe so the caudal aspect of the umbilical structures are on the left side of the screen and the cranial aspect is on the right. (C) This image shows orientation of probe for the cross-sectional view. (D) Position the probe so the right aspect of the umbilical structures is on the left side of the screen and the left is on the right.

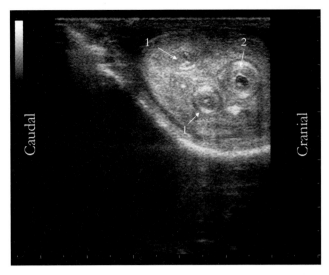

Figure 28.4 Longitudinal view of external umbilical remnant obtained from a normal 3-day-old foal. The two umbilical arteries (1) and umbilical vein (2) are identified. The vein has a thicker wall than the arteries and has a hypoechoic center. The urachus is in the space between the two arteries, but it is not possible to distinguish it from the surrounding tissues. This sonogram was obtained with a wide-bandwidth 10.0 MHz linear array transducer, operating at 12 MHz, at a display depth of 5 cm.

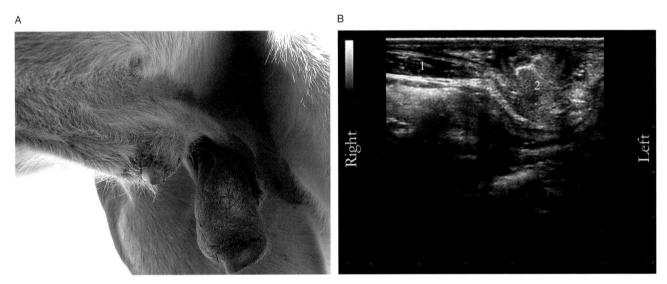

Figure 28.5 Infected external umbilical remnant. (A) This picture of a foal shows an infected external umbilical remnant. (B) This image shows the cross-sectional view of the external umbilical remnant. Echogenic material (2) is present inside the external umbilical remnant outside the abdominal wall (1). The umbilical vein and arteries are not identifiable. This sonogram was obtained with a wide-bandwidth 10.0 MHz linear array transducer, operating at 12.0 MHz, at a display depth of 5 cm.

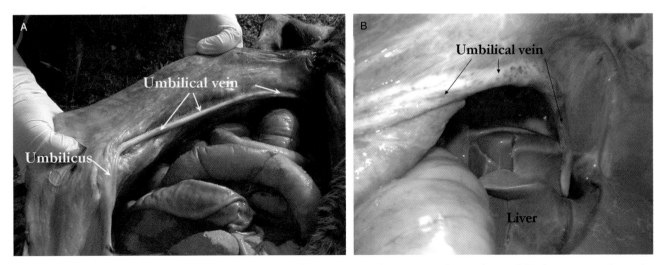

Figure 28.6 Umbilical structures. (A) This picture of an anatomical specimen shows the umbilical structures from the umbilicus cranially. (B) This picture of a post-mortem specimen shows the umbilical vein deepening to the liver.

(Figure 28.6b). In the fetus, the umbilical vein transports blood from the placenta to the fetal liver. The umbilical vein is connected to the abdominal wall by a reflection of the peritoneum (Figure 28.7). It atrophies after birth and becomes the round ligament of the liver, part of the falciform ligament.

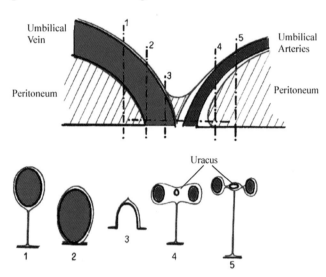

Figure 28.7 Umbilical remnants. The diagram of the umbilical remnants shows the relationship between the umbilical structures and the peritoneum.

The umbilical vein is an oval or elliptical structure with a thin echogenic wall and a hypoechoic center. Its diameter is 10 mm (or less) near the umbilicus (Figure 28.8a), but diameter decreases moving cranially (Figure 28.8b). It is located directly over the linea alba and this is used as the landmark to identify the vein. The vein can move laterally only a few centimeters from this landmark due to the peritoneal reflection. However, this slight lateral movement may occur when the scan is performed in lateral recumbency.

Infection is the main pathology of the umbilical vein, although it is less common than infection of the umbilical arteries and the urachus. The infected umbilical vein is enlarged (more than 10 mm), with hypoechoic to echoic material within it (Figures 28.9, 28.10).

UMBILICAL ARTERIES

The umbilical arteries (Figures 28.11, 28.12, 28.13) run caudally from the umbilicus toward the bladder. The urachus is located between the two arteries. When the umbilical arteries reach the bladder, they move away from each other, running close to the lateral aspect of the bladder. In the fetus, the arteries transport blood

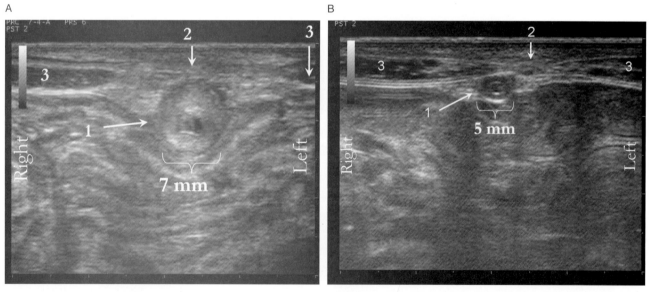

Figure 28.8 Umbilical vein. (A) This image is a cross-sectional view of the umbilical vein, near the umbilicus, in a normal, 4-day-old foal in the standing position. The umbilical vein (1) is well defined, with a 2–3 mm echoic wall and a hypoechoic center. It is close to the linea alba (2), located between the abdominal wall muscles (3). The linea alba is used as a landmark to identify the umbilical vein. This sonogram was obtained with a wide-bandwidth 10.0 MHz linear array transducer, operating at 12.0 MHz, at a display depth of 3 cm. (B) This image is a cross-sectional view of the umbilical vein, near the xyphoid, in a normal, 4-day-old foal in right lateral recumbency. The umbilical vein (1) is well defined with a 2 mm hypoechoic wall, an echoic inner and outer rim, and a hypoechoic center. The diameter is smaller at the xyphoid than at the umbilicus. It is located to the right side of the linea alba (2) due to the recumbent position. The abdominal wall muscles (3) are easily identified on both sides of the linea alba. This sonogram was obtained with a wide-bandwidth 10.0 MHz linear array transducer, operating at 12.0 MHz, at a display depth of 3 cm.

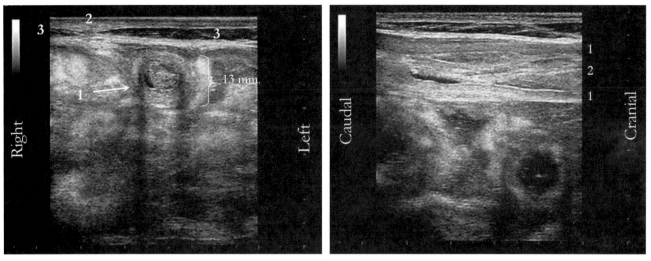

Figure 28.9 Umbilical pathology in 7-day-old foal. (A) This image is a cross-sectional view of the umbilical vein with foal in left lateral recumbency. The umbilical vein (1) appears thickened, with an echoic wall and an echoic center and is surrounded by a thin layer of hypoechoic fluid. The diameter is larger than normal at 13 mm. It is located to the left side of the linea alba (2) due to the recumbent position. The abdominal wall muscles (3) are easily identified at both sides of the linea alba. This sonogram was obtained with a wide-bandwidth 10.0 MHz linear array transducer, operating at 12.0 MHz, at a display depth of 5 cm. (B) This image is a longitudinal view of the umbilical vein with the foal in left lateral recumbency. The umbilical vein appears thickened with an echoic wall (1) and luminal content (2) of various echogenicities. This sonogram was obtained with a wide-bandwidth 10.0 MHz linear array transducer, operating at 12.0 MHz, at a display depth of 5 cm.

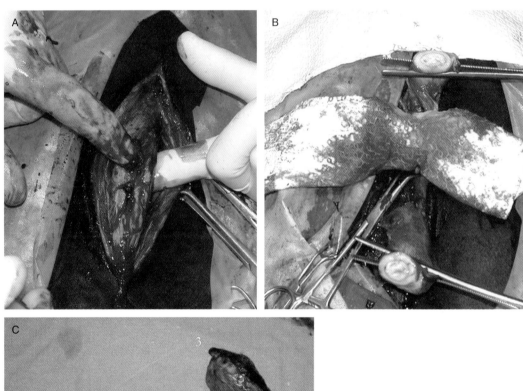

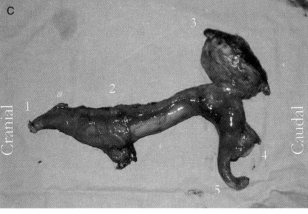

Figure 28.10 Intraoperative findings infected umbilicus. These images are from the case in Figure 28.9. (A) The umbilical vein is thickened. (B) Purulent material is present inside the thickened umbilical vein. (C) This picture is an anatomical specimen identifying the normal umbilical vein (1), thickened and infected umbilical vein (2), umbilicus (3), urachus (4), and umbilical artery (5).

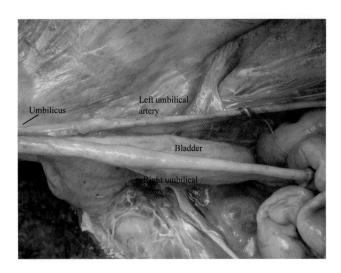

Figure 28.11 Umbilical structures. This picture of an anatomical specimen shows the umbilical structures from the umbilicus caudally.

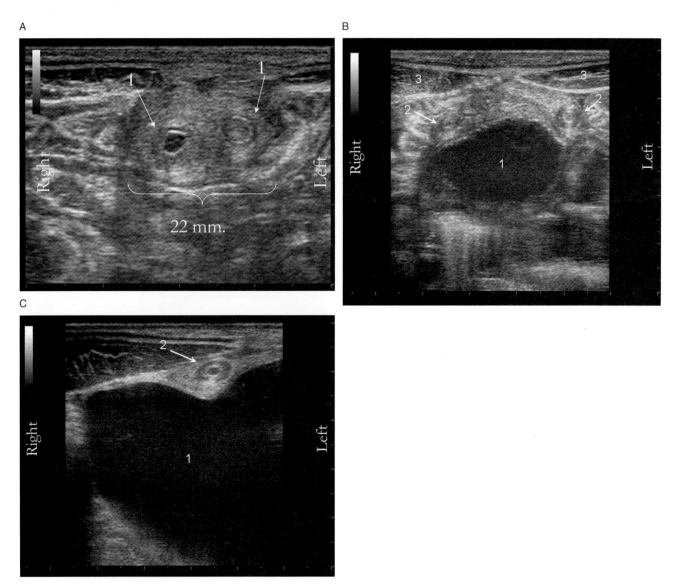

Figure 28.12 Cross-sectional views of umbilical arteries in a normal, 4-day-old foal in standing position. (A) Near the umbilicus, the umbilical arteries (1) have a 2–3 mm echoic wall and a hypoechoic (right artery) to echoic (left artery) center. The urachus is not identifiable in this sonogram. The total measure of the umbilical arteries–urachus complex is normally less than 25 mm. This sonogram was obtained with a wide-bandwidth 10.0 MHz linear array transducer, operating at 12.0 MHz, at a display depth of 3 cm. (B) At the level of the bladder (1), the umbilical arteries (2) normally have a diameter less than 12 mm. Abdominal wall muscles (3) are seen on both sides of bladder. This sonogram was obtained with a wide-bandwidth 10.0 MHz linear array transducer, operating at 12.0 MHz, at a display depth of 5 cm. (C) The umbilical artery (2) is visible along the bladder (1). The diameter of the umbilical arteries does not change from the umbilicus to the bladder. This sonogram was obtained with a wide-bandwidth 10.0 MHz linear array transducer, operating at 12.0 MHz, at a display depth of 5 cm.

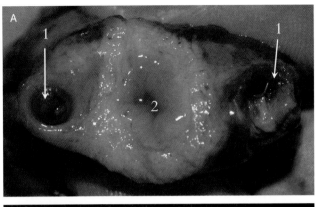

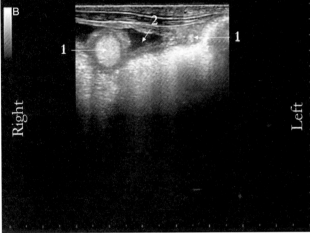

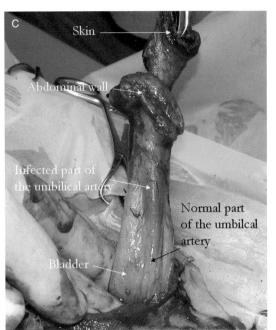

Figure 28.13 Umbilical arteries. (A) This picture of an anatomical specimen shows the umbilical arteries (1) and the transition point between the urachus and the bladder (2). (B) This image is a cross-sectional view of the umbilical arteries (1), along the bladder (2), obtained from a 9-day-old foal with suspected umbilical pathology. The right umbilical artery is enlarged, with a hypoechoic wall and echogenic material inside. This sonogram was obtained with a wide-bandwidth 10.0 MHz linear array transducer, operating at 12.0 MHz, at a display depth of 5 cm. (C) This image is intraoperative findings of an infection of the left umbilical artery.

from the internal iliac arteries to the placenta. They atrophy after birth and become the round ligaments of the bladder.

The diameter of the two arteries and urachus near the umbilical stump should be 24 mm or less. They can be visualized ultrasonographically for almost the entire length of the bladder.

Infection of the umbilical arteries and of the urachus is the most common pathology of the internal umbilical remnant. An infected umbilical artery becomes enlarged, with a thickened wall and hypoechogenic to echogenic material inside the lumen.

URACHUS

The urachus (Figure 28.14) is located between the umbilical arteries. In the fetus, the urachus transports urine from the fetal bladder to the allantoic cavity. It closes and atrophies along its entire length after birth and becomes the median ligament of the bladder. The urachus is only a potential space and normally does not contain fluid, so it is not a distinct structure ultrasonographically.

Patent urachus is a frequent pathology of the neonate. The urachus may not atrophy correctly and, thus, maintains a degree of patency. Also, it may begin to atrophy but become patent after a few days as a consequence of other pathology. The urine normally drains continuously in small quantities, so identifying this structure ultrasonographically may not be possible. Therefore, a patent urachus may appear sonographically normal. When infected, the urachus enlarges causing an increase in diameter of the umbilical arteries–urachus complex. The infected urachus typically has a thin wall with hypoechoic to hyperechoic material in the lumen (Figure 28.15).

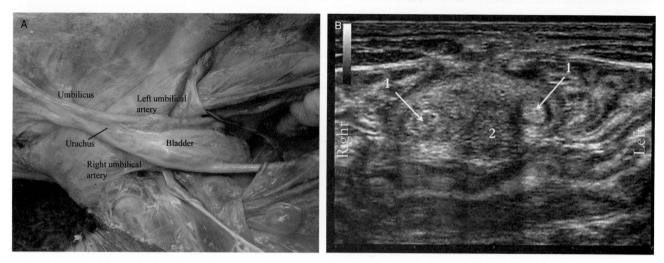

Figure 28.14 Umbilical structures. (A) This picture of an anatomical specimen shows the umbilical structures from the umbilicus caudally. (B) This image is a cross-sectional view of internal umbilical remnant, caudal to the umbilicus, obtained from a normal, 4-day-old foal in the standing position. The urachus (2) is a poorly defined structure between the umbilical arteries (1). This sonogram was obtained with a wide-bandwidth 10.0 MHz linear array transducer, operating at 12.0 MHz, at a display depth of 3 cm.

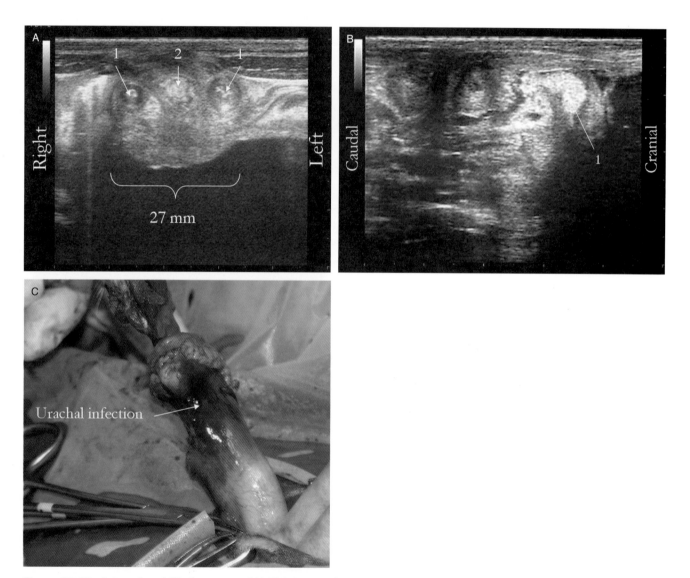

Figure 28.15 Internal umbilical remnant. (A) This image shows a cross-sectional view of the internal umbilical remnant, caudal to the umbilicus, obtained from a 7-day-old foal with suspected umbilical pathology. The infected urachus (2) is a well defined echoic structure between the umbilical arteries (1). The diameter of the umbilical arteries–urachus complex is 27 mm. (B) This image is a longitudinal view of the infected urachus from the same foal. The infected urachus (1) is a well defined, not linear, echoic structure. These sonograms were obtained with a wide-bandwidth 10.0 MHz linear array transducer, operating at 12.0 MHz, at a display depth of 4 cm. (C) Intraoperative findings of an urachal infection.

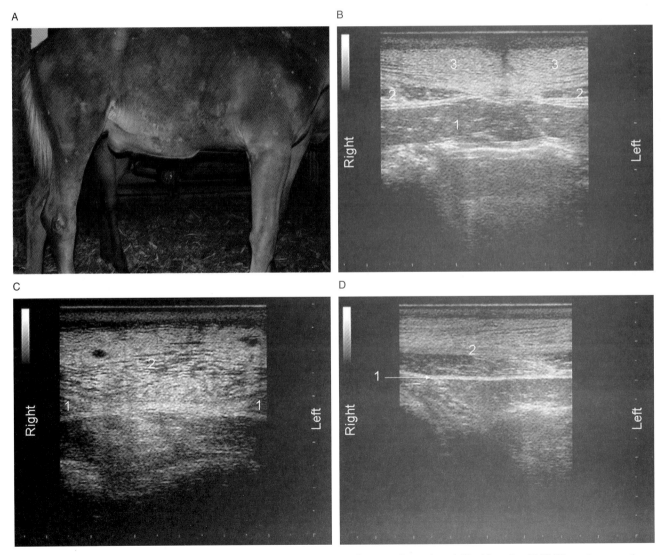

Figure 28.16 Umbilical hernia. (A) This picture is an umbilical hernia in a foal. (B) This image shows a cross-sectional view of an umbilical hernia. Anechoic peritoneal fluid surrounds the umbilical arteries (1), umbilical vein (2), and a loop of small intestine (3). This sonogram was obtained with a wide-bandwidth 6.6 MHz micro-convex linear array transducer, operating at 8.0 MHz, at a display depth of 6 cm.

Figure 28.17 Complicated umbilical hernia. (A) This picture is of a complicated umbilical hernia. (B,C) These images show a cross-sectional view of the abdominal wall. Subcutaneous edema (3) is visualized outside the abdominal muscular wall (2) and retroperitoneal fat (1) is visualized inside the abdomen. These sonograms were obtained with a wide-bandwidth 10.0 MHz linear array transducer, operating at 12.0 MHz, at a display depth of 5 cm. (D) This image is a longitudinal view of the abdominal wall near the umbilicus. A thick layer of subcutaneous edema (2) is outside the abdominal wall (1). This sonogram was obtained with a wide-bandwidth 10.0 MHz linear array transducer, operating at 12.0 MHz, at a display depth of 6 cm.

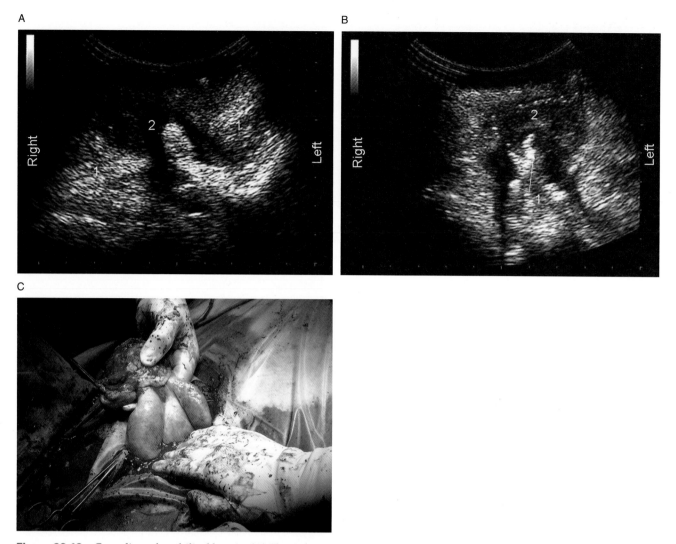

Figure 28.18 Complicated umbilical hernia. (A) This image shows a cross-sectional view of the complicated umbilical hernia from Figure 28.17. A structure with hypoechoic external layer (2) and an echoic internal layer is visualized in the abdominal wall defect (1). This sonogram was obtained with a wide-bandwidth 3.5 MHz convex linear array transducer, operating at 5.0 MHz, at a display depth of 8 cm. (B) Cross-sectional view of complicated umbilical hernia. The structure (2) inside the hernia has a well defined echoic structure (1) that is suggestive of intestine in the hernia sac. This sonogram was obtained with a wide-bandwidth 3.5 MHz convex linear array transducer, operating at 5.0 MHz, at a display depth of 8 cm. (C) Intra-operative findings of the previous case. Part of the cecum is adhered to the hernia sac.

Infection of the urachus can result in leakage of urine into the abdomen resulting in uroperitoneum. Urine may also leak from the urachus into the subcutaneous tissue of the body wall resulting in body wall edema.

UMBILICAL HERNIA

The most frequent umbilical hernia (Figure 28.16, 28.17, 28.18) in the foal is small (2–3 cm), manually reducible, and not painful. It usually contains peritoneal fluid, the umbilical remnant, and sometimes omentum or small intestine (Figure 28.16B). Rarely a part of the large colon or cecum can be involved. A complicated hernia has a varied clinical appearance, but it is usually characterized by swelling of the ventral part of the abdomen, is painful, and is not manually reducible. A draining tract can be present. A complete ultrasound examination is very important to evaluate the presence of infection and of intestinal portions.

RECOMMENDED READING

Franklin, R.P. & Ferrell, E.A. (2002) How to perform umbilical sonograms in the neonate. In: *Proceedings of the 48th American Association of Equine Practitioners Annual Convention*.

Lavan, R.P., Crayer, T., & Madigan, J.E. (1977) Practical method of umbilical ultrasonographic examination of one-week old foals: the procedure and the interpretation of age-correlated size ranges of umbilical structures. *Journal of Equine Veterinary Science*, 17, 96.

Pokar, J. (2004) Diseases of umbilical structures and urinary bladder in foals: ultrasound as a valuable aid for diagnosis and therapy. *Praktische Tierarzt*, 85, 646–653.

Reef, V.B. & Collatos, C.A. (1998) Ultrasonography of the umbilical structures in clinically normal foals. *American Journal of Veterinary Research*, 49, 2143–2146.

Reef, V.B. (1998) Pediatric abdominal ultrasonography. In: *Equine Diagnostic Ultrasound* (ed. V.B. Reef). Saunders, Philadelphia, 364–403.

Reimer, J.M. (1993) Ultrasonography of umbilical remnant infections in foals. In: *Proceedings of the 39th American Association of Equine Practitioners Annual Convention*, 247.

Reimer, J.M. The gastrointestinal tract: the foal. In: *Atlas of Equine Ultrasonography* (ed. J.M. Reimer). Mosby, St.Louis, 200–211.

Reimer, J.M. & Bernand, W.V. Abdominal sonography of the foal. In: *Equine Diagnostic Ultrasound* (eds W.N. Rantanen & A.O. Kinnon), 1st edn. Wiley, Philadelphia.

Walston, R.N. (2006) Case 12-1 Umbilical infection/patent urachus. In: *Equine Neonatal Medicine – A Case Based Approach* (ed. M.R. Paradis), 1st edn. Elsevier Saunders, Philadelphia, 233–238.

INDEX

Atlas of Equine Ultrasonography, First Edition. Edited by Jessica A. Kidd, Kristina G. Lu, and Michele L. Frazer.
© 2014 John Wiley & Sons, Ltd. Published 2014 by John Wiley & Sons, Ltd.
Companion Website: www.wiley.com/go/kidd/equine-ultrasonography